ESSENTIALS OF HUMAN EMBRYOLOGY

ESSENTIALS OF HUMAN EMBRYOLOGY

William J. Larsen, Ph.D.

Professor, Department of Cell Biology, Neurobiology and Anatomy
Faculty Member, Developmental Biology Graduate Program
University of Cincinnati College of Medicine
Research Faculty, Perinatal Research Institute
Children's Hospital and University of Cincinnati College of Medicine
Cincinnati, Ohio

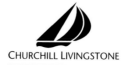

CHURCHILL LIVINGSTONE

New York, Edinburgh, London, Madrid, Melbourne, San Francisco, Tokyo

Library of Congress Cataloging-in-Publication Data

Larsen, William J. (William James)
    Essentials of human embryology / William J. Larsen.
       p.   cm.
    Based on the first edition of Human embryology, published in 1993.
    Includes bibliographical references and index.
    ISBN 0-443-07514-X (alk. paper)
     1. Embryology, Human.   I. Larsen, William J. (William James).
    Human embryology. II. Title.
     [DNLM: 1. Embryology.   QS 604 L334e 1998]
    QM601.L369   1998
    612.6′4—dc21
    DNLM/DLC
    for Library of Congress   97-17953
                                       CIP

Distributed in the United Kingdom by Churchill Livingstone, Robert Stevenson House, 1–3 Baxter's Place, Leith Walk, Edinburgh EH1 3AF, and by associated companies, branches, and representatives throughout the world.

Medical knowledge is constantly changing. As new information becomes available, changes in treatment, procedures, equipment and the use of drugs become necessary. The editors/authors/contributors and the publishers have, as far as it is possible, taken care to ensure that the information given in this text is accurate and up to date. However, readers are strongly advised to confirm that the information, especially with regard to drug usage, complies with the latest legislation and standards of practice.

The Publishers have made every effort to trace the copyright holders for borrowed material. If they have inadvertently overlooked any, they will be pleased to make the necessary arrangements at the first opportunity.

Acquisitions Editor: *Marc Strauss*
Production Editor: *Dave Terry*
Production Supervisor: *Sharon Tuder*
Desktop Coordinator: *Barbara Ulbrich*
Cover Design: *Jeannette Jacobs*
Illustrators: *Margie Caldwell-Gill;* with *Marcia Hartsock, Kathleen I. Jung, Kevin A. Somerville, Rebekah Dodson,* and *Beth Ann Willert*

Printed in Singapore

First published in 1998   7 6 5 4 3 2 1

To my innumerable skeptical students
and to my spirited and forgiving family:
Judy, Britt, and Eric

Preface

This concise textbook of human embryology is written in response to the needs of institutions that have streamlined their instruction in human embryology and should be useful for a variety of teaching programs in the allied health sciences.

The major part of this text is devoted to the basic descriptive human embryology upon which more and more clinical practice is based. These sections are profusely illustrated with modern three-dimensional drawings and scanning electron micrographs especially designed to show the continuity of pertinent developmental processes. The drawings are also used as the basis for animations of developmental mechanisms on a web site designed to support this textbook and the second edition of *Human Embryology* (Churchill Livingstone, 1997). The address of the web site is http://www.med.uc.edu/embryology. Other features of the web site include a self-testing program based on single-best-answer questions and updates of new developments in human developmental biology and clinical practice. In addition, a glossary of common concepts and terms is provided in this more concise introduction to the study of human embryology.

Essentials of Human Embryology is based on the first edition of *Human Embryology,* published in 1993 as one of the first textbooks of human embryology that recognized the ascending importance of human genetics and molecular biology in the clinical practice of pediatrics and neonatology. Indeed, it would have been difficult to incorporate much of this information into the embryology curriculum prior to this date since the molecular and genetic bases of human development and congenital disease were just emerging during this period. An explosion of information since this time, however, has demonstrated the importance of this new information to clinical practice. Indeed, in response, the National Board of Medical Examiners has established a task force in "Development and Human Genetics" to incorporate this emerging knowledge into Step-1 examinations in coming years. Further evidence of the applicability of this new information is the development of numerous new genetic counseling programs throughout the United States and the ascending stature of human genetics programs in the clinical research setting. For these reasons, the first thirteen chapters of *Essentials of Human Embryology* include Applications to Clinical Practice sections that introduce the student to these new developments. While an attempt has been made to restrict these sections to subjects of clear clinical relevance, there is little doubt that these sections will expand in the near future as new molecular and genetic information give rise to new diagnoses and therapies.

It should be noted that the organization of *Essentials of Human Embryology* closely follows the organization of the second edition of *Human Embryology.* This more thorough textbook (along with the web site) offers both students and instructors opportunities to dig more deeply into the emerging molecular and genetic information and to keep abreast of new developments.

I owe a debt of sincere gratitude to the many colleagues who graciously contributed figures or who read and critiqued parts of this book. They include George Daston, David Repaske, William J. Scott, Sheila Bell, Cliff Tabin, Andrew McMahon, Larry Sherman, Steve Potter, Dorothy Supp, Jay Hoying, Robert Gendron, Peter Stambrook, Gail Benson, Tom Doetschman, Stephen D. Smith, Richard Maas, R. A. Conlon, Mario Cappechi, Susan Wert, Kathryn Yutzey, Melissa Colbert, Margaret Kirby, Bjorn Olsen, Thomas Reid, George Nikas, Tariq Siddiqui, K. Lawson, Jonathan Cooke, J. E. Cook, Lee Niswander, Raymond Gasser, C. R. Ball, Donald R. Cahill, Lewis Williams, Y. Fukui, Stephan Carmichael, Ann Hirschfield, David Chan, Martin J. Cohn, R. Hunt, C. Ward Kischer, Stefan Mundlos, Herbert Steinbeisser, Richard Brand, Robb Krumlauf, Robert Arceci, Igor Dawid, Michael Gershon, Bruce Carlson, Colin Wendell-Smith, Jean Marx, M. Brueckner, John Saunders, Cynthia Loomis, E. L. Cardell, and John Fallon.

William J. Larsen, Ph.D.

Contents

Correlation of Timing Systems Used For Human Embryos (Weeks 1 Through 8)

Week	Day	Length (mm)[a]	Number of Somites	Carnegie Stage	Features (chapters in which features are discussed)[b]
1	1	0.1–0.15	—	1	Fertilization (1)
	1.5–3	0.1–0.2	—	2	First cleavage divisions occur (2–16 cells) (1)
	4	0.1–0.2	—	3	Blastocyst is free in uterus (1)
	5–6	0.1–0.2	—	4	Blastocyst hatches and begins implanting (1, 2)
2	7–12	0.1–0.2	—	5	Blastocyst fully implanted (1, 2)
	13	0.2	—	6	Primary stem villi appear (2); primitive streak develops (3)
3	16	0.4	—	7	Gastrulation commences; notochordal process forms (3)
	18	1–1.5	—	8	Primitive pit forms (3); neural plate and neural groove appear (3, 4)
	20	1.5–2.5	1–3	9	Caudal eminence and first somites form (3); neuromeres appear in presumptive brain vesicles (4, 13); primitive heart tube is forming (7); vasculature begins to develop in embryonic disc (8)
4	22	2–3.5	4–12	10	Neural folds begin to fuse; cranial end of embryo undergoes rapid flexion (4, 13); pulmonary primordium appears (6); myocardium forms and heart begins to pump (7); hepatic plate appears (9); first two pharyngeal arches and optic sulci begin to form (12)
	24	2.5–4.5	13–20	11	Primordial germ cells begin to migrate from wall of yolk sac (1); cranial neuropore closes (4); buccopharyngeal membrane ruptures (12); optic vesicles develop (12); optic pit begins to form
	26	3–5	21–29	12	Caudal neuropore closes (4); cystic diverticulum and dorsal pancreatic bud appear (9); urorectal septum begins to form (9, 10); upper limb buds appear (11); pharyngeal arches 3 and 4 form (12)
	28	4–6	30+	13	Dorsal and ventral columns begin to differentiate in mantle layer of spinal cord and brain stem (4, 13); septum primum begins to form in heart (7); spleen appears (9); ureteric buds appear (10); lower limb buds appear (11); otic vesicle and lens placode appear (12); motor nuclei of cranial nerves appear (13)
5	32	5–7	—	14	Spinal nerves begin to sprout (5); semilunar valves begin to form in heart (7); lymphatics and coronary vessels appear (8); greater and lesser stomach curvatures and primary intestinal loop form (9); metanephros begins to develop (10); lens pit invaginates into optic cup; endolymphatic appendage appears (12); secondary brain vesicles begin to form; cerebral hemispheres become visible (13)

[a]Length is the greatest length of embryo.

[b]Timing of some events will differ slightly in some embryos.

Correlation of Timing Systems Used For Human Embryos (Weeks 1 Through 8)

Week	Day	Length (mm)[a]	Number of Somites	Carnegie Stage	Features (chapters in which features are discussed)[b]
5	33	7–9	—	15	Atrioventricular valves and definitive pericardial cavity begin to form (7); cloacal folds and genital tubercle appear (10); hand plate develops (11); lens vesicle forms and invagination of nasal pit creates medial and lateral nasal processes (12); sensory and parasympathetic cranial nerve ganglia begin to form; primary olfactory neurons send axons into telencephalon (13)
6	37	8–11	—	16	Muscular ventricular septum begins to form (7); gut tube lumen becomes occluded (9); major calyces of kidney begin to form and kidneys begin to ascend; genital ridges appear (10); foot plate forms on lower limb bud (11); pigment appears in retina; auricular hillocks develop (12)
	41	11–14	—	17	Bronchopulmonary segment primordia appear (6); septum intermedium of heart is complete (7); subcardinal vein system forms (8); minor calyces of kidney are forming (10); finger rays are distinct (11); nasolacrimal groove forms (12); cerebellum begins to form (13); melanocytes enter epidermis; dental laminae form (14)
7	44	13–17	—	18	Skeletal ossification begins (4, 11); Sertoli cells begin to differentiate in the male gonad (10); elbows and toe rays appear (11); intermaxillary process and eyelids form in face (12); thalami of diencephalon expand (13); nipples and first hair follicles appear (14)
	47	16–18	—	19	Septum primum fuses with septum intermedium in heart (7); urogenital membrane ruptures (10); trunk elongates and straightens (15)
8	50	18–22	—	20	Primary intestinal loop completes initial counterclockwise rotation (9); in males, paramesonephric ducts begin to regress and vasa deferentia begin to form (10); upper limbs bend at elbows (11)
	52	22–24	—	21	Pericardioperitoneal canals close (6); hands and feet approach each other at the midline (11)
	54	23–28	—	22	Eyelids and auricles are more developed (12)
	56	27–31	—	23	Chorionic cavity is obliterated by the growth of the amniotic sac (6); definitive superior vena cava and major branches of the aortic arch are established (8); lumen of gut tube is almost completely recanalized (9); primary teeth are at cap stage (14)

[a]Length is the greatest length of embryo.

[b]Timing of some events will differ slightly in some embryos.

(Columns 1 through 5 from O'Rahilly R, Müller F. 1987. Developmental Stages in Human Embryos. Carnegie Institute, Washington, D.C., Publ. No. 637, with permission.)

1

Gametogenesis, Fertilization, and the First Week

Origin of the Germ Line; Meiosis; Gametogenesis in the Male and Female; the Menstrual Cycle; Fertilization; Cleavage

Human embryos begin development following the fusion of definitive male and female gametes during fertilization. This first chapter of *Essentials of Human Embryology* will, therefore, begin with a description of **gametogenesis** in males and females, including the cytoplasmic and nuclear processes that form the **haploid male** and **female germ cells;** the spermatozoon and the definitive oocyte. Then, the process of **fertilization,** by which the **diploid zygote** is formed, will be discussed, followed by a description of the first cell divisions or **cleavages** that form the embryonic **blastocyst,** which is **transported** through the oviduct to **implant** within the wall of the uterine cavity.

Historically, an understanding of the **cellular** and **biochemical mechanisms** that underlie the early developmental processes of human embryos has provided a basis for the diagnosis and treatment of human reproductive problems and congenital disease. For example, our understanding of the early stages of human gamete and zygote formation has provided strategies for the development of contraceptive techniques, while clinical procedures to manipulate human male and female gametes have been developed to assist reproduction in infertile couples. More recently, the explosive development of **molecular** and **genetic** methods of studying mammalian development is creating a new field of **mammalian molecular embryology,** which may have an even greater impact on clinical practice. For example, the techniques of Southern blotting, in situ hybridization and chromosome banding have expanded our understanding of the causes of abnormalities arising from chromosomal defects, such as Down syndrome (see below) or from mutations like those that give rise to diseases like Huntington's chorea, neurofibromatosis (see Ch. 2), spina bifida (Ch. 4), Hirschsprung's disease (see Ch. 5), cystic fibrosis, and surfactant B deficiency (see Ch. 6). An exciting new technology involving the manipulation of the mouse genome in transgenic animals is providing unparalleled insight into the function of regulatory genes that control normal human development. In addition, transgenic technology is also producing useful models for the study of human congenital disease.

At the very least, these new cellular and molecular techniques will lead to the creation of useful diagnostic tools; however, an understanding of the basis of disease and the identification of afflicted individuals is usually necessary for development of new therapies. Several therapies have already been successfully developed, and others are on the horizon. Applications to Clinical Practice sections at the end of each chapter will briefly review recent basic and clinical research that improves our understanding of the normal development of the early embryo and leads to practical applications in clinical diagnosis and treatment.

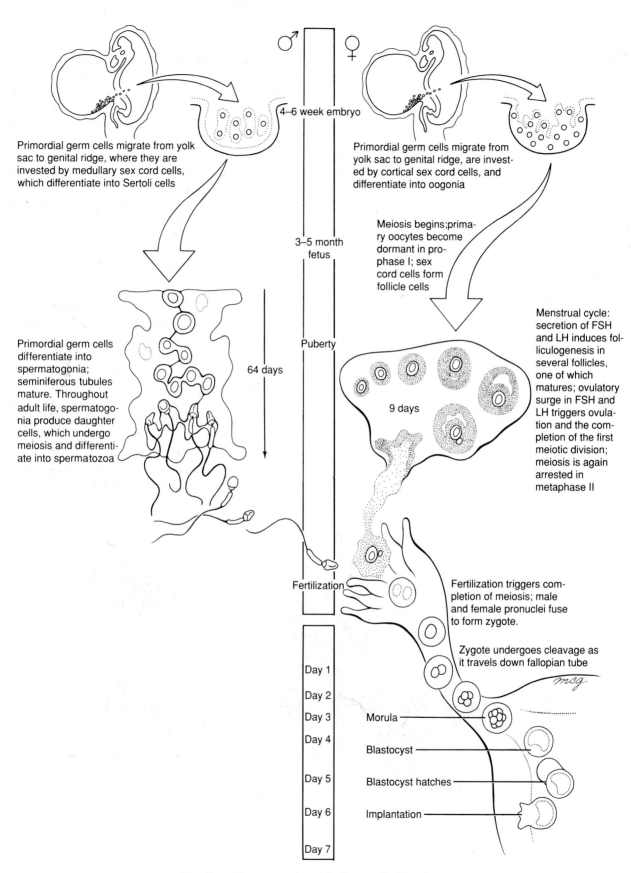

Timeline. Gametogenesis and the first week of development.

The germ cells arise within the embryo proper

The primordial germ cells originate within the primary ectoderm of the embryo and then migrate into the yolk sac

Cells that give rise to the **gametes** in both male and female mammals (including humans) originate within the primary ectoderm of the embryo during the second week of development (see Chs. 2 and 3). They then detach from the ectoderm and migrate by amoeboid movement into an extraembryonic structure called the **yolk sac.** At first they may be distinguished within a mass of extraembryonic mesoderm at the caudal end of the embryo and then within the endoderm of the yolk sac wall (Fig. 1-1A). These cells are called the **primordial germ cells,** and their lineage constitutes the **germ line.** Primordial germ cells can easily be recognized during their migration because of their distinctive pale cytoplasm and ovoid shape and because they specifically stain intensely with reagents that localize the enzyme alkaline phosphatase.

During the fourth week, the primordial germ cells migrate back into the posterior body wall of the embryo

Between 4 and 6 weeks, the primordial germ cells migrate by ameboid movement from the yolk sac to the wall of the gut tube and from the gut tube via the mesentery to the dorsal body wall (Fig. 1-1B). In the dorsal body wall, these cells come to rest on either side of the midline in the loose mesenchymal tissue just deep to the epithelial lining of the coelomic cavity. Most of the primordial germ cells populate the region of the body wall adjacent to the tenth thoracic vertebral level that will form the gonads (see Ch. 10). The primordial germ cells continue to multiply by mitosis during their migration. A few cells may become stranded along the route of migration or at inappropriate sites in the dorsal body wall. Occasionally, stray germ cells of this type give rise to a type of tumor called a **teratoma.**

The germ cells induce the formation of the gonads in the dorsal body wall

The differentiation of the gonads is described in detail in Chapter 10. When the germ cells arrive in the presumptive gonad region, they stimulate cells of the adjacent coelomic epithelium and mesonephros (embryonic kidney) to proliferate and form compact strands of tissue called **primitive sex cords** (Fig. 1-1C; see also Fig. 10-14). The proliferating sex cords create a swelling just medial to each mesonephros on either side of the vertebral column. These swellings, the **genital ridges,** represent the primordial gonads. The sex cords invest the primordial germ cells and give rise to the tissues that will nourish and regulate the development of the maturing sex cells

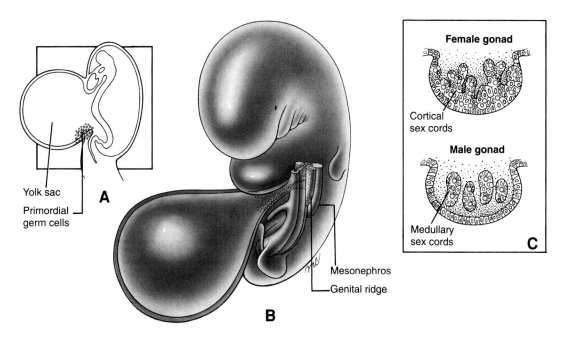

Fig. 1-1. **(A)** The primordial germ cells differentiate in the endodermal layer of the yolk sac at 4 to 6 weeks of development and migrate to the dorsal body wall. **(B)** Between 6 and 12 weeks, the primordial germ cells induce formation of the genital ridges. **(C)** Sex cord cells differentiate and invest the primordial germ cells. In females, the sex cords of the cortical region survive and become the ovarian follicle cells; in males, the medullary sex cords survive and become the Sertoli cells of the seminiferous tubules.

— the **ovarian follicles** in the female and the **Sertoli cells** of the **germinal epithelium (seminiferous epithelium)** of the **seminiferous tubules** in the male (Fig. 1-1C).

Gametogenesis is the process of meiosis and cytodifferentiation that converts germ cells into mature male and female gametes

The timing of gametogenesis is different in males and females

In both males and females, the primordial germ cells undergo further mitotic divisions within the gonads and then commence **gametogenesis,** the process that converts them to mature male and female gametes (**spermatozoa** and **definitive oocytes,** respectively). The timing of these processes differs in the two sexes, however (see timeline and Fig. 1-2).

The process of gametogenesis in the male and female (called **spermatogenesis** and **oogenesis,** respectively) are discussed in detail later in this chapter.

Meiosis halves the number of chromosomes and DNA strands in the sex cells

Although the timing of meiosis is very different in the male and female, the basic chromosomal events of the process are the same in the two sexes. Like all normal somatic (non-germ) cells, the primordial germ cells contain 23 pairs of chromosomes, or a total of 46. One chromosome of each pair is obtained from the maternal gamete and the other from the paternal gamete (see below). These chromosomes contain the **deoxyribonucleic acid (DNA)** that encodes virtually all the information required for the development and functioning of the organism. Of the total complement of 46 chromosomes, 22 pairs consist of matching, homologous chromosomes called **autosomes.** The remaining two chromosomes are called the **sex chromosomes** because they determine the sex of the individual. There are two kinds of sex chromosomes, X and Y. Individuals with two X chromosomes (XX) are genetically female; individuals with one X and one Y chromosome (XY) are genetically male. The

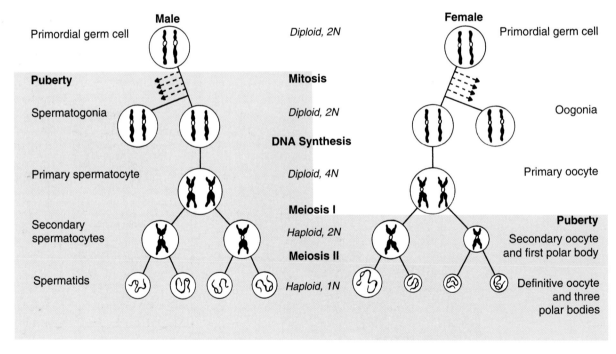

Fig. 1-2. Nuclear maturation of germ cells in meiosis in the male and female. In the male, the primordial germ cells remain dormant until puberty, when they differentiate into spermatogonia and commence mitosis. Throughout adulthood, the spermatogonia produce primary spermatocytes, which undergo meiosis and spermatogenesis. Each primary spermatocyte yields four spermatozoa. In the female, the primordial germ cells differentiate into oogonia, which undergo mitosis and then commence meiosis as primary oocytes during fetal life. The primary oocytes remain arrested in prophase I until stimulated to resume meiosis during a menstrual cycle. Each primary oocyte yields one definitive oocyte and three polar bodies.

mechanisms underlying sex determination are discussed in detail in Chapter 10.

Two designations that are often confused are the **ploidy** of a cell and its **N number.** *Ploidy* refers to the number of copies of each *chromosome* present in a cell nucleus, whereas the *N number* refers to the number of copies of each unique double-stranded *DNA molecule* in the nucleus. Each chromosome contains one or two molecules of DNA at different stages of the cell cycle (whether mitotic or meiotic), so the ploidy and N number of a cell do not always coincide. Somatic cells and primordial germ cells have two copies of each kind of chromosome and hence are called **diploid.** Mature gametes, in contrast, have just one copy of each kind of chromosome and are called **haploid.** Haploid gametes with one DNA molecule per chromosome are said to be **1N.** In some stages of the cell cycle, diploid cells also have one DNA molecule per chromosome and hence are **2N.** During the earlier phases of meiosis or mitosis, however, each chromosome of a diploid cell has two molecules of DNA, and so the cell is **4N.**

Meiosis, unlike mitosis, is a specialized process of cell division that occurs only in the germ line. In **mitosis** (normal cell division), a diploid, 2N cell undergoes a single division to yield two diploid, 2N daughter cells. In meiosis, a diploid germ cell undergoes two successive, qualitatively different nuclear and cell divisions to yield four haploid, 1N offspring. In males the cell divisions of meiosis are equal and yield four identical spermatozoa. In females, however, the meiotic cell divisions are dramatically unequal and yield a single, massive, haploid definitive oocyte and three minute, nonfunctional, haploid **polar bodies.**

Occasionally, an error during meiosis yields a gamete with an abnormal number of somatic or sex chromosomes. Some of these chromosomal anomalies and their effects on embryonic development are discussed in the Clinical Applications section at the end of this chapter.

The first meiotic division involves DNA replication and recombination and yields two haploid 2N daughter cells. The preliminary step in meiosis, as in mitosis, is the replication of each chromosomal DNA molecule, thus converting the diploid cell from 2N to 4N. This event marks the beginning of gametogenesis. In the female the oogonium is now called a **primary oocyte** and in the male the spermatogonium is now called a **primary spermatocyte** (Fig. 1-2). Once the DNA replicates, each chromosome consists of two parallel strands or **chromatids** joined together at a structure called the **centromere.** Each chromatid contains a single DNA molecule.

In the next step, called **prophase,** the chromosomes condense into compact, double-stranded structures. During the late stages of prophase, the double-stranded chromosomes of each homologous pair match up, centromere

to centromere, to form a joint structure called a **chiasma.** Chiasma formation makes it possible for the two homologous chromosomes to exchange large segments of DNA by a process called **crossing over.** The resulting **recombination** of the genetic material on homologous maternal and paternal chromosomes is largely random and therefore increases the genetic variability of the future gametes. As mentioned above, the primary oocyte enters a phase of meiotic arrest during the first meiotic prophase.

During **metaphase,** the four-stranded chiasma structures are organized on the equator of a spindle apparatus similar to the one that forms during mitosis, and during **anaphase** one double-stranded chromosome of each homologous pair is distributed to each of the two daughter nuclei. During the first meiotic division the centromeres of the chromosomes do not replicate, and therefore the two chromatids of each chromosome remain together. The resulting daughter nuclei thus are haploid but 2N: they contain the same amount of DNA as the parent germ cell but half as many chromosomes. After the daughter nuclei form, the cell itself divides (undergoes **cytokinesis**). The first meiotic cell division produces two **secondary spermatocytes** in the male and a **secondary oocyte** and a **first polar body** in the female (Fig. 1-2).

In the second meiotic division, the double-stranded chromosomes divide, yielding four haploid 1N daughter cells. No DNA replication occurs during the second meiotic division. The 23 double-stranded chromosomes condense during the second meiotic prophase and line up during the second meiotic metaphase. The chromosomal centromeres then replicate, and during anaphase the double-stranded chromosomes pull apart into two single-stranded chromosomes, one of which is distributed to each daughter nucleus. In males, the second meiotic cell division produces two **definitive spermatocytes or spermatids** (i.e., a total of four from each germ cell entering meiosis). In the female, the second meiotic cell division, like the first, is radically unequal, producing a large **definitive oocyte** and another diminutive polar body. The first polar body may simultaneously undergo a second meiotic division to produce a third polar body (Fig. 1-2).

In the female, the oocyte enters a second phase of meiotic arrest during the second meiotic metaphase before the replication of the centromeres. Meiosis does not resume unless the cell is fertilized.

Spermatogenesis begins at puberty and continues throughout adult life

Now that meiosis has been described, it is possible to investigate and compare the specific processes of spermatogenesis and oogenesis. At puberty, the testes begin to secrete greatly increased amounts of the steroid hormone

testosterone. This hormone has a multitude of effects. In addition to stimulating the development of many secondary sex characteristics, it triggers the growth of the testes, the maturation of the seminiferous tubules, and the commencement of spermatogenesis.

Under the influence of testosterone, the Sertoli cells within the solid **testis cords** differentiate into a system of seminiferous tubules (see Ch. 10). The dormant primordial germ cells resume development, divide several times by mitosis, and then differentiate into spermatogonia. These spermatogonia are located immediately under the basement membrane surrounding the seminiferous tubules, where they occupy pockets between the Sertoli cells (Fig. 1-3A). Each spermatogonium is connected to the adjacent Sertoli cells by specialized membrane junctions. In addition, all the Sertoli cells are joined to each other by dense bands of intercellular membrane junctions that completely surround each Sertoli cell and thus isolate the trapped spermatogonia from the tubule lumen.

Male germ cells are translocated to the seminiferous tubule lumen during spermatogenesis

The cells that will undergo spermatogenesis arise by mitosis from the spermatogonia. These cells are gradually translocated between the Sertoli cells from the basal to the luminal side of the seminiferous epithelium while spermatogenesis takes place (Fig. 1-3A). During this migratory phase, the recruited primary spermatocytes pass without interruption through both meiotic divisions, producing first two secondary spermatocytes and then four spermatids. The spermatids undergo the dramatic changes that convert them into mature sperm while they complete their migration to the lumen. This process of sperm cell differentiation is called **spermiogenesis.**

The Sertoli cells are also instrumental in spermiogenesis

The Sertoli cells participate intimately in the differentiation of the gametes. Maturing spermatocytes and spermatids are connected to the surrounding Sertoli cells not only by tight junctions and gap junctions but also by unique cytoplasmic processes called **tubulobulbar complexes** that extend into the Sertoli cells. The cytoplasm of the developing gametes shrinks dramatically during spermiogenesis; these tubulobulbar complexes are thought to provide a mechanism by which the excess cytoplasm is transferred to the Sertoli cells. As cytoplasm is removed, the spermatids undergo the dramatic changes in shape and internal organization that transform them into spermatozoa. Finally, the last connections with the Sertoli cells break, releasing the spermatozoa into the tubule lumen. This final step is called **spermiation.**

As shown in Figure 1-3B, a spermatozoon consists of a **head,** a **midpiece,** and a very long **tail.** The head contains the condensed nucleus and is capped by an apical vesicle filled with hydrolytic enzymes. This vesicle, the **acrosome,** plays an essential role in fertilization (see below). The midpiece contains large, helical mitochondria and generates the power for swimming. The tail contains the microtubules that form part of the propulsion system of the spermatozoon.

Errors in spermatogenesis or spermiogenesis are not at all uncommon. Examination of a sperm sample will reveal spermatozoa with abnormalities such as small, narrow, or piriform (pear-shaped) heads, double or triple heads, acrosomal defects, and double tails.

Continual waves of spermatogenesis occur throughout the seminiferous epithelium

Spermatogenesis takes place continuously from puberty to death. Gametes are produced in synchronous waves in each local area of the germinal epithelium, although the process is not synchronized throughout the seminiferous tubules. In many different mammals, the clone of spermatogonia derived from each spermatogonial stem cell populates a local area of the seminiferous tubules and displays synchronous spermatogenesis. That may be the case in humans as well. About four waves of synchronously differentiating cells can be observed in a given region of the human tubule epithelium at any time. Ultrastructural studies provide some evidence that these waves of differentiating cells remain synchronized because of incomplete cytokinesis throughout the series of mitotic and meiotic divisions between the division of a spermatogonium and the formation of spermatids. Instead of fully separating, the daughter cells produced by these divisions remain connected by slender cytoplasmic bridges that could allow passage of small signal molecules or metabolites (Fig. 1-3A).

In the human male, each cycle of spermatogenesis takes about 64 days. Spermatogonial mitosis occupies about 16 days, the first meiotic division takes about 8 days, the second meiotic division takes about 16 days, and spermiogenesis requires about 24 days.

Spermatozoa undergo a terminal step of functional maturation called capacitation

During its journey from the seminiferous tubules to the ampulla of the oviduct, a sperm cell undergoes a process of functional maturation that prepares it to fertilize an oocyte. Sperm produced in the seminiferous tubules are stored in the lower part of the **epididymis,** a special coiled duct connected to the **vas deferens** near its origin in the testis. During ejaculation, the sperm are propelled through the vas deferens and urethra and are mixed with nourish-

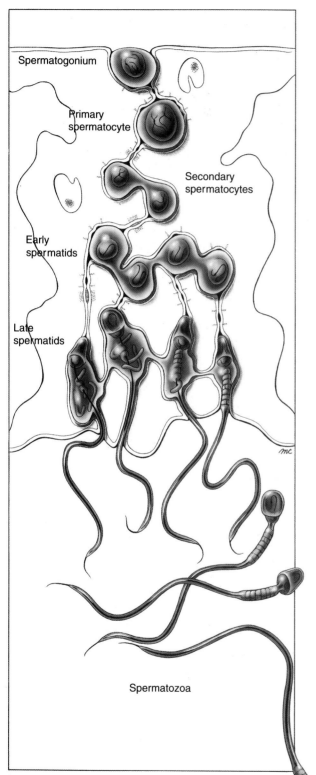

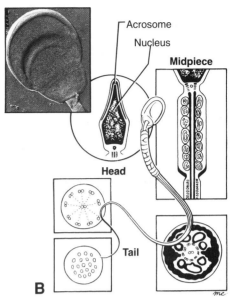

Fig. 1-3. (A) A schematic section through the seminiferous tubule wall. The spermatogonium just under the outer surface of the tubule wall (basal side) undergoes mitosis to produce daughter cells, which may either continue to divide by mitosis (thus renewing the spermatogonial stem cell population) or commence meiosis as primary spermatocytes. As spermatogenesis and spermiogenesis occur, the differentiating cell is translocated between adjacent Sertoli cells to the tubule lumen. The daughter spermatocytes and spermatids remain linked by cytoplasmic bridges. The entire clone of spermatogonia derived from each primordial germ cell is linked by cytoplasmic bridges. **(B)** Structure of the mature spermatozoan. The head contains the nucleus capped by the acrosome; the midpiece contains coiled mitochondria; the tail contains propulsive microtubules. The inset micrograph shows a piece of a human sperm. (Fig. B photo courtesy of Dr. Daniel S. Friend.)

ing secretions from the **seminal vesicles, prostate,** and **bulbourethral glands** (see Ch. 10 for further discussion of these structures). As many as 200 million spermatozoa may be deposited in the vagina by a single ejaculation, but only a few hundred succeed in navigating through the cervix, uterus, and oviduct and into its expanded ampullar region. In the **ampulla,** sperm survive and retain their capacity to fertilize an oocyte for 1 to 3 days.

Capacitation is defined as the final step of sperm maturation consisting primarily of changes in the acrosome that prepare it to release the enzymes required to penetrate the zona pellucida, a shell of glycoprotein surrounding the oocyte (see below). Capacitation is thought to take place within the female genital tract and to require contact with the secretions of the oviduct. Spermatozoa used in in vitro fertilization procedures are artificially capacitated.

Oogenesis is discontinuous and begins during fetal life

The total number of primary oocytes is produced in the ovaries by 5 months of fetal life

As mentioned earlier, the female germ cells undergo a series of mitotic divisions after they are invested by the sex cord cells and then differentiate into oogonia (Fig. 1-2). By 12 weeks of development, a proportion of the several million oogonia in the genital ridges enters the first meiotic prophase and then almost immediately becomes dormant. The nucleus of these dormant primary oocytes, containing the partially condensed prophase chromosomes, becomes very large and watery and is referred to as a **germinal vesicle.** The germinal vesicle is thought to protect the DNA during the long period of meiotic arrest.

Each primary oocyte becomes tightly enclosed by a single-layered, squamous capsule of epithelial **follicle cells** derived from the sex cord cells. This capsule and its enclosed primary oocyte constitute a **primordial follicle.** By 5 months, the number of primordial follicles in the ovaries peaks at about 7 million. Most of these follicles subsequently degenerate. By birth only 700,000 to 2 million remain and by puberty, only about 400,000.

The hormones of the female cycle control folliculogenesis, ovulation, and the condition of the uterus

After a girl reaches menarche (female puberty), monthly cycles in the secretion of hypothalamic, pituitary, and ovarian hormones control a **menstrual cycle,** which has the purpose of producing each month a single female gamete and a uterus in a condition to receive a fertilized embryo. This cycle consists of the monthly maturation of (usually) a single oocyte and its enclosing follicle, the concurrent proliferation of the uterine endometrium, the process of ovulation by which the oocyte is released, the continued development of the follicle into an endocrine corpus luteum, and, finally — unless a fertilized ovum implants in the uterus and begins to develop — the sloughing of the uterine endometrium and the involution of the corpus luteum. This entire cycle takes about 28 days.

The menstrual cycle is considered to begin with **menstruation** (also called the **menses**), the shedding of the degenerated uterine endometrium from the previous cycle. On about the fifth day of the cycle (the fifth day after the beginning of menstruation), an increase in secretion by the hypothalamus of the brain of a small peptide hormone, **gonadotropin-releasing hormone (GnRH),** stimulates the pituitary gland to increase its secretion of two **gonadotropic hormones (gonadotropins): follicle-stimulating hormone (FSH) and luteinizing hormone (LH)** (Fig. 1-4). Increased secretion of GnRH by the hypothalamus is also the event that initiates the first menstrual cycle at menarche. The rising levels of pituitary gonadotropins regulate later phases of **folliculogenesis** in the ovary and the **proliferative phase** in the uterine endometrium.

About 5 to 12 primary follicles resume development each month

Prior to a particular cycle and independent of pituitary gonadotropins, the cells of the single-layered follicular epithelium of a small group of primordial follicles thicken from squamous to cuboidal (Fig. 1-5). These follicles are now called **primary follicles.** The follicle cells and the oocyte jointly secrete a thin layer of acellular material, composed of only a few types of glycoprotein, onto the surface of the oocyte. Although this layer, the **zona pellucida,** appears to form a complete physical barrier between the follicle cells and the oocyte (Fig. 1-6A), actually it is penetrated by thin extensions of the follicle cells that are connected to the oocyte cell membrane by gap junctions and intermediate cell junctions (Fig. 1-6B). These extensions and their membrane junctions remain intact until just before ovulation and probably convey both developmental signals and metabolic support to the oocyte. The epithelium of 5 to 12 of these primary follicles then proliferates to form a multilayered capsule around the oocyte (Figs. 1-4 and 1-5). They are now called **growing follicles.** At this point, some of the growing follicles cease to develop and eventually degenerate, whereas a few continue to enlarge in response to rising levels of FSH, mainly by taking up fluid and developing a central fluid-filled cavity called the **antrum.** These follicles are called **antral** or **vesicular follicles.** At the same time, the connective tissue of the ovarian stroma surrounding each of these follicles differentiates into two layers, an inner layer called the **theca interna** and an outer layer called the

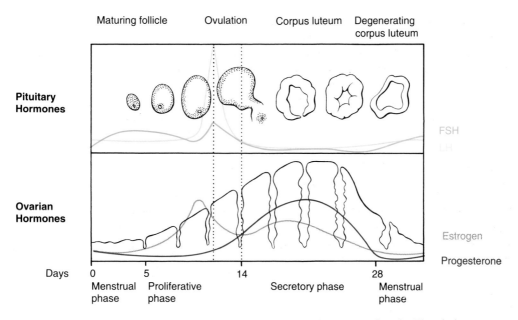

Fig. 1-4. Ovarian, endometrial, and hormonal events of the menstrual cycle. The pituitary hormones FSH and LH directly control the ovarian cycle and also control the production of estrogens and progesterone by the responding follicles and corpus luteum of the ovary. These ovarian hormones in turn control the cycle of the uterine endometrium.

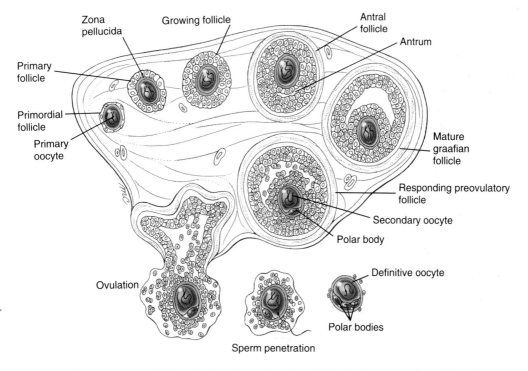

Fig. 1-5. Schematic depiction of folliculogenesis and ovulation in the ovary. Five to 12 primordial follicles initially respond to the rising levels of FSH and LH, but only one matures. In response to the ovulatory surge in LH and FSH, the oocyte of this mature graafian follicle resumes meiosis, and the follicle ovulates. The final steps of meiosis take place only if the released oocyte is penetrated by a sperm.

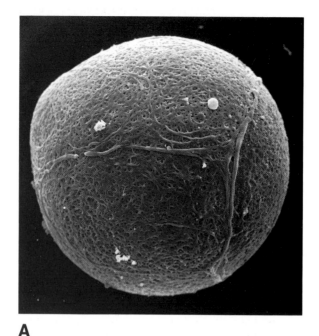

A

Cumulus
cells

Cumulus
cell process

Oocyte
surface

B

Fig. 1-6. **(A)** Scanning electron micrograph of the zona pellucida after removal of the cumulus cells. The zona consists of protein and muco-polysaccharide and forms a barrier that the sperm can penetrate only by means of its acrosomal enzymes. **(B)** Scanning electron micrograph of the oocyte surface and cumulus oophorus, with the zona pellucida digested away. The cumulus cells maintain contact with the oocyte via thin cell processes that penetrate the zona pellucida and form gap junctions and intermediate junctions with the oocyte cell membrane. (Fig. A from Phillips DM, Shalgi R. 1980. Surface architecture of the mouse and hamster zona pellucida and oocyte. J Ultrastruct Res 72:1, with permission. Fig. B photo courtesy of Dr. David Phillips.)

theca externa. These two layers become vascularized, in contrast to the follicle cells, which do not.

A single follicle becomes dominant and the rest degenerate

Eventually one of the growing follicles gains primacy and continues to enlarge by absorbing fluid, while the remainder of the follicles recruited during the cycle degenerate (undergo **atresia**). The oocyte, surrounded by a small mass of follicle cells called the **cumulus oophorus,** increasingly projects into the expanding antrum but remains connected to the layer of follicle cells that lines the antral cavity and underlies the basement membrane of the follicle. This layer is called the **membrana granulosa.** The large, swollen follicle is now called a **mature vesicular follicle** or **mature graafian follicle** (Fig. 1-5). At this point the oocyte still has not resumed meiosis.

Various theories have been proposed for the mechanism that selectively stimulates folliculogenesis in a few follicles

The reason why only 5 to 12 primordial follicles commence folliculogenesis each month, and why, of this group, all but one eventually degenerate is not well understood. One theory suggests that follicles become progressively more sensitive to the stimulating effects of FSH as they advance in development. Follicles that are slightly more advanced simply on a random basis would therefore respond more acutely to FSH and would be favored. Another theory proposes that the selection process is regulated by a complex system of feedback between the pituitary and ovarian hormones and growth factors.

The resumption of meiosis and ovulation are stimulated by an ovulatory surge in the levels of FSH and LH

On about day 13 or 14 of the menstrual cycle (at the end of the proliferative phase of the uterine endometrium), the levels of FSH and LH suddenly rise very sharply (Fig. 1-4). This **ovulatory surge** in the pituitary gonadotropins stimulates the primary oocyte of the remaining mature graafin follicle to resume meiosis. This response can be observed visually about 15 hours after the beginning of the ovulatory surge in FSH and LH, when the membrane of the swollen germinal vesicle (nucleus) of the oocyte breaks down (Fig. 1-7). By 20 hours, the chromosomes are lined up in metaphase. Cell division to form the secondary oocyte and first polar body rapidly ensues. The secondary oocyte promptly begins the second meiotic division but, about 3 hours before ovulation, is arrested at the second meiotic metaphase.

The cumulus oophorus expands in response to the ovulatory surge in LH and FSH. Just at the same time that the germinal vesicle breaks down, the cumulus cells surrounding the oocyte lose their cell-to-cell connections and disaggregate (Fig. 1-5). As a result, the oocyte and a mass of loose cumulus cells detach into the antral cavity. Over the next few hours, the cumulus cells secrete an abundant extracellular matrix, consisting mainly of hyaluronic acid, which causes the cumulus cell mass to expand severalfold. This process of **cumulus expansion** may play a role in several processes, including the regulation of meiotic progress and ovulation. In addition, the mass of matrix and entrapped cumulus cells that accompanies the ovulated oocyte may play a role in the transport of the oocyte in the oviduct, in fertilization, and in the early development of the zygote.

Ovulation depends on the breakdown of the follicle wall. The process of **ovulation** (the expulsion of the secondary oocyte from the follicle) is similar to an inflammatory response. The cascade of events that culminates in ovulation is believed to be initiated by the secretion of histamine and prostaglandins, well-known inflammatory mediators. Within a few hours after the ovulatory surge of FSH and LH, the follicle becomes more vascularized and is visibly pink and edematous in comparison with nonresponding follicles. The follicle is displaced to the surface of the ovary, where it forms a bulge (Fig. 1-5). As ovulation approaches, the projecting wall of the follicle begins to thin, resulting in the formation of a small, nipple-

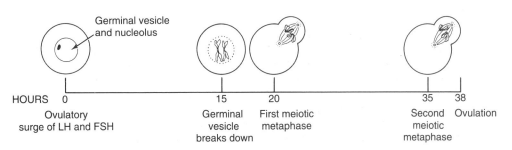

Fig. 1-7. Timing of meiotic events during the ovarian cycle.

shaped protrusion called the **stigma.** Finally, a combination of tension produced by smooth muscle cells in the follicle wall plus the release of collagen-degrading enzymes and other factors by fibroblasts in the region causes the follicle to rupture. The rupture of the follicle is not explosive: the oocyte, accompanied by a large number of investing cumulus cells bound in the hyaluronic acid matrix and by some follicular fluid, is slowly extruded onto the surface of the ovary. Ovulation occurs about 38 hours after the beginning of the ovulatory surge of FSH and LH.

The sticky mass formed by the oocyte and cumulus is actively scraped off the surface of the ovary by the fimbriated mouth of the oviduct (Fig. 1-8). The cumulus-oocyte complex is then moved into the ampulla of the oviduct by the synchronized beating of the cilia on the oviduct wall. Within the ampulla, the oocyte may remain viable for as long as 24 hours before it loses its capacity to be fertilized.

The ruptured follicle forms the endocrine corpus luteum. After ovulation, the membrana granulosa cells of the ruptured follicular wall begin to proliferate and give rise to the **luteal cells** of the **corpus luteum** (Figs. 1-5 and 1-8). As described below, the corpus luteum is an endocrine structure that secretes steroid hormones that maintain the uterine endometrium in a condition ready to receive an embryo. If no embryo implants in the uterus, the corpus luteum degenerates after about 14 days and is converted to a scarlike structure called a **corpus albicans.**

Estrogens and progesterone secreted by the follicle control the uterine events of the menstrual cycle

Beginning on day 5 of the menstrual cycle, the thecal and follicle cells of responding follicles secrete steroid **estrogens.** These hormones in turn cause the endometrial lining of the uterus to proliferate and undergo remodeling. This **proliferative phase** begins at about day 5 of the cycle and is complete by day 9 (Fig. 1-4).

After ovulation occurs, thecal cells in the wall of the corpus luteum continue to secrete estrogens, and the **luteal cells** that differentiate from the remaining follicle cells also begin to secrete high levels of a related steroid hormone, **progesterone.** Luteal progesterone stimulates the uterine endometrial layer to thicken further and to form glandular structures and increased vasculature. Unless an embryo implants in the uterine lining, this **secretory phase** of endometrial differentiation lasts about 13 days (Fig. 1-4). At that point (near the end of the menstrual cycle), the corpus luteum shrinks and the levels of progesterone fall. The developed endometrium, which is dependent on progesterone, degenerates and begins to slough. The 4- to 5-day **menstrual phase,** during which the endometrium is sloughed (along with about 35 ml of blood and the unfertilized oocyte), is conventionally taken as the start of the next cycle.

At fertilization, the sperm nucleus enters the oocyte, the oocyte completes meiosis, and the pronuclei of the two mature gametes fuse

Fertilization is a complex interaction between sperm and oocyte

If viable spermatozoa encounter an ovulated oocyte in the ampulla of the oviduct, they surround it and begin forcing their way through the cumulus mass (Fig. 1-9A). When a spermatozoon reaches the tough zona pellucida surrounding the oocyte, it binds in a human-specific interaction with a glycoprotein sperm receptor molecule in the zona (ZP3) and then the acrosome is induced to release degradative en-

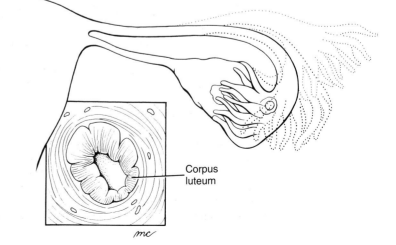

Corpus luteum

Fig. 1-8. The ovulated oocyte clings to the surface of the ovary by the gelatinous cumulus oophorus and is actively scraped off by the fimbriated oviduct mouth. After ovulation, the membrana granulosa layer of the ruptured follicle proliferates to form the endocrine corpus luteum.

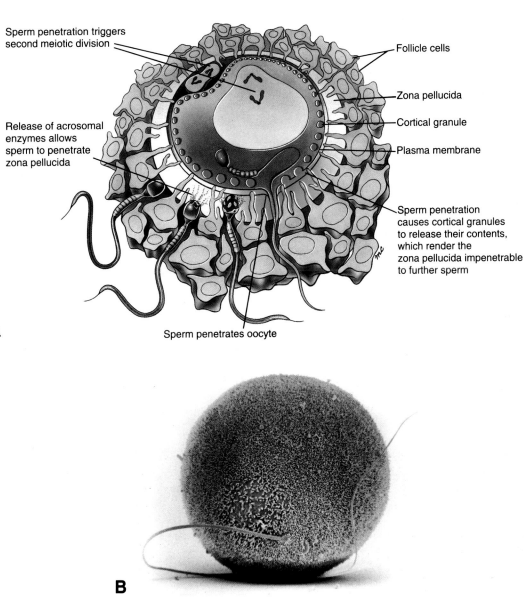

Sperm penetration triggers
second meiotic division

Follicle cells

Zona pellucida

Cortical granule

Plasma membrane

Release of acrosomal
enzymes allows
sperm to penetrate
zona pellucida

Sperm penetration
causes cortical granules
to release their contents,
which render the
zona pellucida impenetrable
to further sperm

Sperm penetrates oocyte

A

B

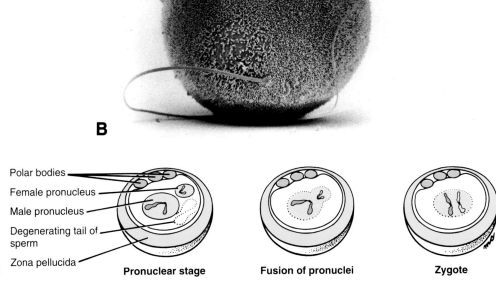

Polar bodies

Female pronucleus

Male pronucleus

Degenerating tail of
sperm

Zona pellucida

C

Pronuclear stage　　**Fusion of pronuclei**　　**Zygote**

Fig. 1-9. Fertilization. (**A**) Spermatozoa wriggle through the cumulus mass and release their acrosomal enzymes on contact with the zona pellucida. The acrosomal enzymes dissolve the zona pellucida and allow the sperm to reach the oocyte. As soon as the membranes of the sperm and oocyte fuse, the cortical granules of the oocyte release their contents, which cause the zona pellucida to become impenetrable to further sperm. The entry of the sperm nucleus into the cytoplasm induces the oocyte to complete the second meiotic diffusion. (**B**) Scanning electron micrograph showing a human sperm fusing with a hamster oocyte that has been enzymatically denuded of the zona pellucida. The ability of a man's sperm to penetrate a denuded hamster oocyte is often used as a clinical test of sperm activity. (**C**) The events of zygote formation. After the oocyte completes meiosis, the female pronucleus and the larger male pronucleus fuse to form the diploid nucleus of the zygote. (Fig. B photo courtesy of Dr. David Philips.)

zymes that allow the sperm to penetrate the zona pellucida. When a spermatozoon successfully penetrates the zona pellucida and reaches the oocyte, the cell membranes of the two cells fuse (Fig. 1-9A, B). This event immediately causes thousands of small **cortical granules** located just beneath the oocyte cell membrane to release their contents into the **perivitelline space** between the oocyte and the zona pellucida. The substance released from the cortical granules interact with the zona pellucida in such a way as to alter the sperm receptor molecules, causing the zona to become impenetrable by additional spermatozoa. This mechanism prevents **polyspermy,** or the fertilization of the oocyte by more than one spermatozoon.

The fusion of the spermatozoon cell membrane with the oocyte membrane also causes the oocyte to resume meiosis. The oocyte completes the second meiotic metaphase and rapidly proceeds through anaphase, producing another polar body. The first polar body simultaneously completes its second meiotic division. Disregarding the presence of the sperm, the oocyte is now considered to be a **definitive oocyte.**

The chromosomes of the oocyte and sperm are then respectively enclosed within **female** and **male pronuclei.** These pronuclei fuse with each other to produce the single, diploid, 2N nucleus of the fertilized **zygote** (Fig. 1-9C). This moment of zygote formation may be taken as the beginning or zero time point of embryonic development.

During the first days of development, the zygote travels down the oviduct and undergoes cleavage

Cleavage subdivides the zygote without increasing its size

Within 24 hours after fusion of the pronuclei, the zygote embarks on a regulated series of mitotic cell divisions called **cleavage** (Fig. 1-10). These divisions are not accompanied by cell growth, so they subdivide the large zygote into many smaller daughter cells called **blastomeres,** while the embryo as a whole does not change in size and remains enclosed in the zona pellucida. The first

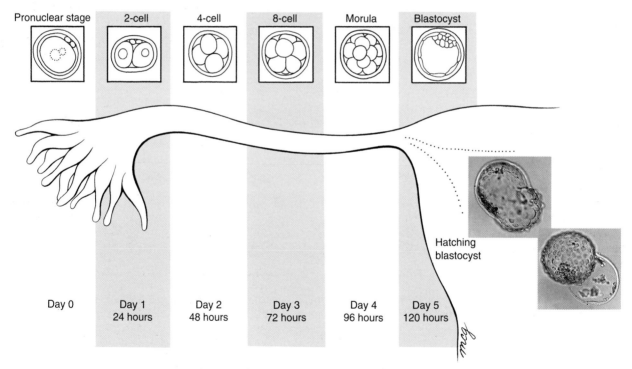

Fig. 1-10. Cleavage and transport down the oviduct. Fertilization occurs in the ampulla of the oviduct. During the first five days, the zygote undergoes cleavage as it travels down the oviduct and enters the uterus. On day 5, the blastocyst hatches from the zona pellucida and is then able to implant in the uterine endometrium. (From Boatman DE. 1987. In vitro growth of nonhuman primate pre- and peri-implantation embryos. p. 273. In Bavister BD (ed): The Mammalian Preimplantation Embryo. Plenum, New York, with permission. Photo courtesy of Drs. Barry Bavister and D.E. Boatman.)

cleavage division divides the zygote along a plane at right angles to its equator and in line with the polar bodies. Subsequent cleavage divisions become somewhat asynchronous. The second division, which is complete at about 40 hours after fertilization, produces four equal blastomeres. By 3 days, the embryo consists of 6 to 12 cells, and by 4 days, it consists of 16 to 32 cells. By the 32-cell stage, the embryo has the appearance of a small mulberry and is therefore called a **morula** (from Latin *morum,* mulberry).

The segregation of blastomeres into embryoblast and trophoblast precursors occurs in the morula

The cells of the morula will give rise not only to the embryo proper and its attached membranes, but also to the placenta and related structures. The cells that will follow these different developmental paths become segregated during cleavage. Starting at the eight-cell stage of development, the originally round and loosely adherent blastomeres begin to flatten, developing an inside-outside polarity that maximizes cell-to-cell contact among the blastomeres at the center of the mass. As differential adhesion develops, the outer surfaces of the cells become convex and their inner surfaces become concave. This reorganization, called **compaction,** involves the activity of cytoskeletal elements and adhesion of the blastomeres.

The development of differential adhesion between different groups of blastomeres also results in the segregation of some cells to the center of the morula and others to the outside. It is believed that the third- or fourth-generation blastomeres that divide earliest may be the ones displaced to the center of the morula. These centrally placed blastomeres are now called the **inner cell mass,** while the blastomeres at the periphery constitute the **outer cell mass.** Some exchange occurs between these groups. However, in general, the inner cell mass gives rise to most of the embryo proper and is therefore called the **embryoblast.** The outer cell mass is the primary source for the membranes of the placenta and is therefore called the **trophoblast** (see Ch. 2).

The morula develops a fluid-filled cavity and is transformed into a blastocyst

By 4 days of development, the morula, consisting now of about 30 cells, begins to absorb fluid. This fluid is thought to be taken up at first into intracellular vacuoles within the blastomeres, but then begins to collect between the cells. Meanwhile, specialized cell-to-cell junctions called **tight junctions** and **gap junctions** begin to develop between many blastomeres, especially those of the outer cell mass. As a result of tight junction formation between cells of the outer cell mass, the fluid that continues

to enter the morula collects mainly between the cells of the inner cell mass. As the hydrostatic pressure of this fluid increases, a large cavity called the **blastocyst cavity** forms within the morula (Fig. 1-10). The embryoblast cells (inner cell mass) then form a compact mass at one side of this cavity, and the outer cell mass or trophoblast is organized into a thin, single-layered epithelium. The embryo is now called a **blastocyst.** The side of the blastocyst containing the inner cell mass is called the **embryonic pole** of the blastocyst, and the opposite side is called the **abembryonic pole.**

The blastocyst implants in the uterine wall on about day 6

The blastocyst hatches from the zona pellucida before implanting

The morula reaches the uterus between 3 and 4 days of development. By day 5, the blastocyst hatches from the clear zona pellucida by enzymatically boring a hole in it and squeezing out (Fig. 1-10). The blastocyst is now naked of all its original investments and can interact directly with the endometrium.

Very soon after arriving in the uterus, the blastocyst becomes tightly adherent to the uterine lining (Fig. 1-11). The adjacent cells of the endometrial stroma respond to its presence and to the progesterone secreted by the corpus luteum by differentiating into metabolically active, secre-

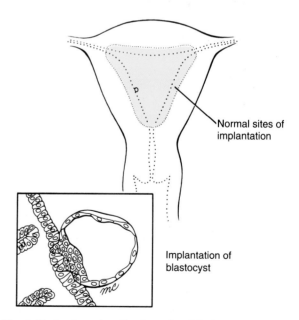

Fig. 1-11. Implantation. On about day 6.5 after fertilization, the trophoblast cells at the embryonic pole of the blastocyst proliferate to produce the syncytiotrophoblast, which is able to invade the uterine lining. The colored area indicates the normal sites of implantation in the uterine wall.

Normal sites of implantation

Implantation of blastocyst

tory cells called **decidual cells.** This response is called the **decidual reaction** (see Fig. 15-1). The endometrial glands in the vicinity also enlarge, and the local uterine wall becomes more highly vascularized and edematous. It is thought that the secretions of the decidual cells and endometrial glands include growth factors and metabolites that support the growth of the implanting embryo.

The uterine lining is maintained in a favorable state and kept from sloughing partly by the progesterone secreted by the corpus luteum. In the absence of an implanted embryo, the corpus luteum normally degenerates after about 13 days. If an embryo implants, however, the cells of the trophoblast produce the hormone **human chorionic gonadotropin (hCG),** which supports the corpus luteum and thus maintains the supply of progesterone (**maternal recognition of pregnancy**). The corpus luteum continues to secrete sex steroids for 11 to 12 weeks of embryonic development, after which the placenta itself begins to secrete large amounts of proges-

terone and the corpus luteum slowly involutes, becoming a corpus albicans.

Implantation in an abnormal site results in an ectopic pregnancy

Occasionally, a blastocyst implants in the peritoneal cavity, on the surface of the ovary, within the oviduct, or at an abnormal site in the uterus. The epithelium at these abnormal sites responds to the implanting blastocyst with increased vascularity and other supportive changes, so that the blastocyst is able to survive and commence development. These **ectopic pregnancies** often threaten the life of the mother since the blood vessels that form at the abnormal site are apt to rupture as a result of the growth of the embryo and placenta. The ectopic nature of a pregnancy is often revealed by symptoms of abdominal pain and/or vaginal bleeding. Surgical intervention may be required to remove the developing embryo.

APPLICATIONS TO CLINICAL PRACTICE

Chromosome anomalies may result in congenital malformations

Many human **congenital malformations** result from chromosomal abnormalities that arise during the process of meiosis. For example, chromosomes may be improperly segregated so that the resulting male or female gamete contains two copies (instead of one) of a given chromosome. When this abnormal gamete combines with a normal gamete from the opposite sex at fertilization, the resulting zygote then contains three copies of that chromosome (**trisomy**) or a total of 47 chromosomes rather than the normal human karyotype of 46 chromosomes (Fig. 1-12). Such trisomies may occur because the **homologous** (like) chromosomes of a given pair do not properly separate during the first or second meiotic division (**nondisjunction;** Fig. 1-12). Alternatively, a copy of one chromosome may become physically connected to a different chromosome during meiosis (**translocation;** Fig. 1-12), to produce a trisomic embryo. These events may occur during the first or second meiotic division.

A common and viable trisomy in humans is **Down syndrome,** which results from the presence of three copies of chromosome 21 in each cell (**trisomy 21;** Fig. 1-12). Individuals with Down syndrome exhibit a spectrum of anomalies including characteristic facial features (facies), mental retardation, and heart defects (particularly **endocardial cushion defect;** see Ch. 7). The incidence of Down syndrome is higher in older mothers (over 35).

Typically the chromosomal complement or **karyotype** of the fetus is determined by removal and examination of sloughed fetal cells from amniotic fluid (**amniocentesis**) or by biopsy of the placental villi (**chorionic villus sampling**). Identification of the extra chromosome as maternal or paternal in origin was originally based on karyotyping analysis that compared banding patterns of the extra chromosome 21 with chromosome 21 of the mother and father. These early studies concluded that about 70 to 75 percent of Down syndrome occurred as a consequence of nondisjunction in the mother. By the late 1980s, however, more sensitive karyotype analysis increased this frequency to 80 percent, while by the early 1990s an even more sensitive molecular technique (Southern blot analysis of DNA polymorphisms) provided evidence that as much as 95 percent of Down syndrome arises through nondisjunction in the maternal germ line. Trisomy 21 may also arise through abnormal mitosis during early cleavage divisions. In this case, only the daughter cells arising from the initially trisomic cell will contain the extra copy of chromosome 21 while other cells of the body will possess the normal human chromosome complement of 46 chromosomes. This individual comprises a **mosaic** of normal diploid and trisomic cells and is therefore called a **chimera.** If trisomic cells become incorporated only into the germ line, the individual may exhibit no visible evidence of Down syn-

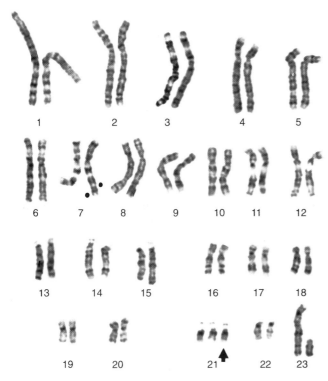

Fig. 1-12. Karyotype of a male with trisomy 21, causing Down syndrome. (Courtesy of Dr. Shirly Soukup).

drome but may pass this condition onto offspring. It should be noted that other viable trisomies occur in humans, including trisomies 8, 13, and 17, which each exhibit their own characteristic spectrum of abnormalities.

The acquisition of an extra chromosome by one gamete during meiosis is complemented by the loss of a chromosome from one of its sister gametes. The resulting chromosome-deficient gamete therefore contains only 22 chromosomes, and, if it combines with a normal gamete at fertilization, the resulting zygote contains only 45 chromosomes—22 pairs of chromosomes plus one copy of the chromosome that was missing from the abnormal gamete. Such a condition is called a **monosomy.** Typically, monosomic embryos are not viable. An exception, however, is in **Turner syndrome,** which occurs in embryos containing only one X chromosome. Their chromosome complement or **karyotype** is 45:XO. The discovery of the Turner syndrome karyotype along with the **Kleinfelter syndrome** karyotype (47:XXY) led to an initial understanding of the mechanism of sex determination in humans. While it was known by the late 1950s that female somatic cells contained two X chromosomes and that male somatic cells contained an X and a Y chromosome, it could not be determined whether male development resulted from the presence of a single Y chromosome or from a single X chromosome and whether female development resulted

from the absence of a Y chromosome or the presence of two X chromosomes. However, since Turner syndrome is typified by a single X chromosome and no Y chromosome and female development, while Kleinfelter syndrome is characterized by two X chromosomes and a single Y chromosome and male development, it was evident that male development in humans is determined by the presence of a Y chromosome and that female development is determined by absence of a Y chromosome. The molecular basis for sex determination is described in Applications to Clinical Practice in Chapter 10.

Knowledge of the cellular and molecular mechanisms of gametogenesis, fertilization, and ovulation is the basis for development of contraceptive strategies in humans

In these last decades of the twentieth century, the average number of children in American families is about two. In cultures that do not practice birth control, however, it is not uncommon for a healthy couple to produce as many as 10 to 20 children during their reproductive lifetime. Human behavior and reproductive physiology result in an astoundingly high reproductive efficiency, probably as a consequence of low survival rates, which typically occur in the absence of modern medical practice. Thus, with the advent of cures for infectious and nutritional diseases among others in the early part of the twentieth century and their increasing availability and application, contraception assumed an ever-increasing role in family planning.

Presently, six major forms of contraception are in common use or are being tested: (1) **barrier contraceptives,** such as the male and female condom, the diaphragm, cervical cap, and contraceptive sponge, which prevent mixing of the male and female gametes at intercourse; (2) **birth control pills,** which contain doses of estrogen and progestin typically varied over a 21-day cycle, preventing ovulation through disruption of the hormonal ovulatory stimulus; (3) **depot preparations** of medroxyprogesterone acetate (Depo-Provera), which continuously emit low antiovulatory levels of progesterone for a few months (intramuscular injection) to several years (subdermal capsules); (4) **nonmedicated intrauterine devices (IUDs)** consisting of a loop-shaped or T-shaped device, implanted in the uterus, which may interfere with the function of spermatozoa or oocytes; (5) the antiprogesterone compound **RU-486,** which, when taken within 8 weeks of the last menses, and typically in conjunction with prostaglandins, stimulates sloughing of the endometrium and the conceptus; and (6) **sterilization,** which in the male prevents the ejaculation of sperm by resection of the vas deferens and in the female, by ligation of the uterine tubes (oviducts) to prevent the mixing of gametes. All of these methods are characterized by specific advantages and disadvantages, and none, except the female condom, address the problem of sexually transmitted diseases (STDs). Some are considered morally objectionable or even illegal. For a variety of reasons, only 50 to 70 percent of women who begin to take "the pill" are still taking it a year later. In addition, the population explosion that continues in developing countries, the AIDs epidemic, concern about exposure to steroids, the relatively low efficacy of some contraceptive techniques, and concern about abortion have prompted research into development of safer and more effective methods of contraception.

The capacity to manipulate human gametes in culture has resulted in development of several techniques of alternate assisted reproduction

Infertility may occur in 15 to 30 percent of American couples. In males, the average sperm count has declined precipitously in recent years for unknown reasons. In females, pelvic inflammatory disease arising from infections of the genital tract may scar the oviducts. Diabetes is implicated in disruptions of ovulation and implantation in females, typically through disturbances of the hypothalamic-pituitary regulation of the ovarian and menstrual cycles.

Different forms of assisted reproduction may be used depending on the cause of infertility. For example, the technique of **in vitro fertilization and embryo transfer** is often used in cases of scarring of the oviducts. The woman's ovaries are induced to **superovulate,** typically by administration of human menopausal gonadotropin and pure follicle-stimulating hormone, sometimes combined with clomiphene citrate. Maturing oocytes are then harvested through a laparoscope. The oocytes are allowed to mature to the second meiotic metaphase and then fertilized with previously capacitated sperm, allowed to develop, and then inserted into the uterus at the 2- to 4-cell stage (or later). In cases where infertility occurs because of a deficiency in sperm motility and when the oviducts are normal, a technique called **gamete intrafallopian transfer (GIFT)** is often used. Harvested oocytes and precapacitated sperm are placed in the catheter of a laparoscope and introduced together into the ampulla of the oviduct where fertilization takes place. Further development is normal. In an alternative technique called **zygote intrafallopian transfer (ZIFT),** the oocytes are fertilized in vitro, and only fertilized pronuclear zygotes are introduced into the oviduct.

Manipulation of the mouse genome has led to development of several models of human congenital disease

Recently, new molecular and genetic techniques make it possible to insert specific DNA sequences into their correct locations in the mammalian genome. Thus transgenic animal models of human genetic diseases can readily be created by disabling specific genes. In addition, the ability to correct defective genes lays the groundwork to cure genetic disorders.

A transgenic animal is one whose genome has been altered by the integration of donor DNA sequences

Specific donor DNA sequences can be inserted into the mouse genome by directly injecting the DNA into the male pronucleus (at the pronuclear stage of zygote development). Sometimes the DNA is incorporated into the host chromosome and is expressed in the embryo or adult animal. Even more useful, however, is the targeting of the specific DNA sequence to a specific location in the host genome by a process called **homologous recombination.** In this approach, mouse blastocysts are grown in culture and the cells of the inner cell mass spontaneously erupt from the blastocyst. These **embryonic stem (ES) cells** are then suspended in medium containing many copies of the donor DNA. This mixture is subjected to an electric current that facilitates the movement of the donor DNA through the cell membrane, allowing the DNA to enter the nucleus and incorporate (in a small number of cases) into the desired target site in the genome. Appropriate marker genes and screening procedures are then used to clone the "targeted" ES cells.

To create transgenic mice containing the new DNA, groups of 8 to 12 targeted ES cells are injected into the cavity of normal mouse blastocysts, where they become incorporated into the inner cell mass and participate in formation of the embryo. The resulting blastocysts (called **injection chimeras** because of their formation from cells from two different sources) are then implanted into the uterus of a pseudopregnant mouse, where they develop normally. Depending on their location within the inner cell mass, the targeted ES cells may contribute to the development of virtually any tissue, and, when they contribute to the germ line, the donor genes can be passed on to offspring. Dominant donor genes may be expressed in the immediate offspring. However, if the donor genes are recessive, an inbreeding program is used to produce a homozygous strain that can express the gene. This strategy is typically required to produce a **null mutation** or **loss-**

of-function (knockout) transgenic animal in which both copies **(alleles)** of the specific gene are disabled. On the other hand, if multiple extra copies of a given gene have been incorporated into the germ line of the injection chimera, suitable **gain-of-function** transgenic animals may be found among the immediate offspring of the injection chimera.

These gene-targeting techniques are being used to develop animal models of several human congenital diseases including insulin-dependent diabetes mellitus, Hirschsprung's disease, cystic fibrosis, Lesch-Nyhan syndrome, surfactant B deficiency, and retinoblastoma. Moreover, the technique has served as a useful approach to the study of many genes that regulate various processes that underlie development of the mammalian embryo (see Ch. 3). Less advanced is the application of gene-targeting methodologies to the actual correction of genetic disorders by insertion of the normal gene (see Ch. 15).

2

The Second Week

Development of the Bilaminar Germ Disc and
Establishment of the Uteroplacental Circulation

SUMMARY

Implantation of the blastocyst into the uterine wall occurs at the end of the first week of development. By then, the embryo is a sphere comprised of a single layered outer cell mass or **trophoblast** and cells derived from the inner cell mass at one pole called the **embryoblast.** The trophoblast and embryoblast have decidedly different fates; the former will develop into the placenta and the latter, the embryo proper (see Ch. 1). As the embryoblast implants, it quickly differentiates into two layers to form the placenta during the second week.

The second week is often called "the week of twos" since many of the processes characteristic of the second week occur in twos. As noted, the embryoblast splits into two layers, the epiblast and the hypoblast. Placental development is also characterized by several twosomes: (1) the trophoblast differentiates into the cellular trophoblast or cytotrophoblast and the syncytial trophoblast or syncytiotrophoblast. (2) The blastocyst cavity undergoes two transformations as it is successively lined by two new layers derived from the hypoblast; the first transformation converts the blastocyst cavity to the primary yolk sac or exocoelomic cavity, while the second transformation results in its conversion to the secondary or definitive yolk sac. (3) Two new cavities are formed, the amniotic cavity and the chorionic cavity. (4) Two populations of extraembryonic mesoderm are formed, one associated with the yolk sac and the other associated with the cytotrophoblast.

The diagnosis of chromosome abnormalities (such as trisomy 21; see Ch. 1) can be determined through biopsy of placental structures derived from the embryonic trophoblast called **chorionic villi** (chorionic villus sampling) or by cytogenetic or karyotypic analysis of embryonic cells sloughed into the amniotic cavity (amniocentesis). These procedures are often performed on women over the age of 35 because of the increased incidence of Down syndrome in babies of older mothers (see Applications to Clinical Practice in Ch. 1). In addition, an unusual conceptus may develop consisting of the placenta only. These are called **hydatidiform moles.** While such conceptuses are typically aborted spontaneously, pieces of tissue may remain and invade the uterine wall, sometimes becoming malignant. Examination of this phenomenon led to the important discovery that the paternal chromosomes largely direct the early development of the placenta of the embryo proper. The molecular basis for these differences in activities of maternal and paternal chromsomes appears to involve transient molecular changes in the maternal and paternal DNA, a phenomenon called **genomic imprinting** (see Applications to Clinical Practice). It is also known that genomic imprinting and the parental origin of specific mutated genes determines the time of onset and severity of several inherited congenital diseases.

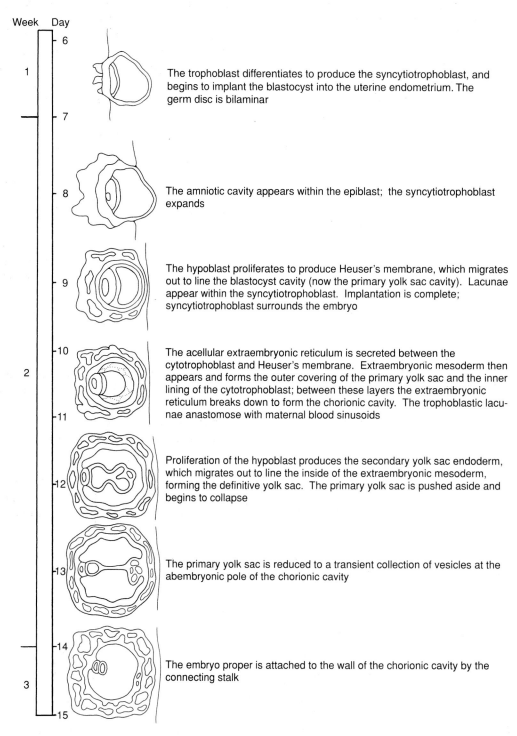

Week Day

1
- 6

The trophoblast differentiates to produce the syncytiotrophoblast, and begins to implant the blastocyst into the uterine endometrium. The germ disc is bilaminar

- 7

- 8

The amniotic cavity appears within the epiblast; the syncytiotrophoblast expands

- 9

The hypoblast proliferates to produce Heuser's membrane, which migrates out to line the blastocyst cavity (now the primary yolk sac cavity). Lacunae appear within the syncytiotrophoblast. Implantation is complete; syncytiotrophoblast surrounds the embryo

2
-10

The acellular extraembryonic reticulum is secreted between the cytotrophoblast and Heuser's membrane. Extraembryonic mesoderm then appears and forms the outer covering of the primary yolk sac and the inner lining of the cytotrophoblast; between these layers the extraembryonic reticulum breaks down to form the chorionic cavity. The trophoblastic lacunae anastomose with maternal blood sinusoids

-11

-12

Proliferation of the hypoblast produces the secondary yolk sac endoderm, which migrates out to line the inside of the extraembryonic mesoderm, forming the definitive yolk sac. The primary yolk sac is pushed aside and begins to collapse

-13

The primary yolk sac is reduced to a transient collection of vesicles at the abembryonic pole of the chorionic cavity

-14

The embryo proper is attached to the wall of the chorionic cavity by the connecting stalk

3
-15

Timeline. The second week of development.

The syncytiotrophoblast helps implant the embryo in the endometrium

The blastocyst adheres to the uterine wall at the end of the first week. Contact with the uterine endometrium induces the trophoblast at the embryonic pole to proliferate. Some of these proliferating cells lose their cell membranes and coalesce to form a syncytium called the **syncytiotrophoblast** (Fig. 2-1).

By contrast, the cells of the trophoblast, forming the wall of the blastocyst, retain their cell membranes and constitute the **cytotrophoblast.** The syncytiotrophoblast increases in volume throughout the second week as cells detach from the proliferating cytotrophoblast at the embryonic pole and fuse with the syncytium (Figs. 2-2 and 2-3).

Between days 6 and 9, the embryo becomes completely implanted in the endometrium. Hydrolytic enzymes secreted by the cytotrophoblast break down the extracellular matrix between the endometrial cells, and active processes extending from the cytotrophoblast penetrate between the separating endometrial cells (Figs. 2-1 and 2-2). The expanding syncytiotrophoblast gradually envelops the blastocyst, and by day 9, the blastocyst is blanketed by a thick layer of syncytiotrophoblast (Fig. 2-3). The small hole marking the point in the endometrial epithelium where the blastocyst implanted is sealed by a plug of acellular material called the **coagulation plug.**

The embryoblast splits into epiblast and hypoblast

Even before implantation occurs, cells of the embryoblast begin to differentiate into two layers. By day 8, the embryoblast consists of a distinct external layer of columnar cells called the **epiblast** or **primary ectoderm** and an internal layer of cuboidal cells called the **hypoblast** or **primary endoderm** (Fig. 2-2). An extracellular basement membrane is laid down between the two layers immediately after they become distinct. The resulting two-layered embryoblast is called the **bilaminar germ disc.**

The amniotic cavity develops within the epiblast

The first new cavity to form during the second week — the **amniotic cavity** — appears on day 8 as fluid begins to collect between cells of the epiblast (Fig. 2-2). A layer of epiblast cells is gradually displaced toward the embryonic pole by the accumulating fluid and differentiates into a thin membrane separating the new cavity from the cytotrophoblast. This membrane is the **amniotic membrane,** and the new cavity is the **amnion** (Fig. 2-3). The cells that form the amniotic membrane are called **amnioblasts.** The amniotic cavity expands steadily; by the eighth week the amnion encloses the entire embryo (see Fig. 6-12).

The formation of the yolk sac and chorionic cavity is not fully understood

The hypoblast gives rise to the extraembryonic endoderm that lines the primary yolk sac

On day 8, cells at the periphery of the newly formed hypoblast migrate out over the inner surface of the cytotrophoblast, becoming flattened. By day 12, these cells

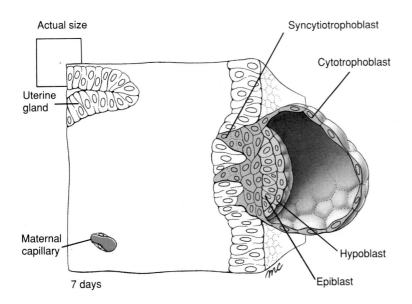

Actual size

Uterine gland

Maternal capillary

7 days

Syncytiotrophoblast

Cytotrophoblast

Hypoblast

Epiblast

Fig. 2-1. At 7 days, the newly hatched blastocyst contacts the uterine endometrium and begins to implant. The trophoblast at the embryonic pole of the blastocyst proliferates to form the invasive syncytiotrophoblast, which insinuates itself among the cells of the endometrium and begins to draw the blastocyst into the uterine wall. The germ disc is bilaminar, consisting of hypoblast and epiblast layers.

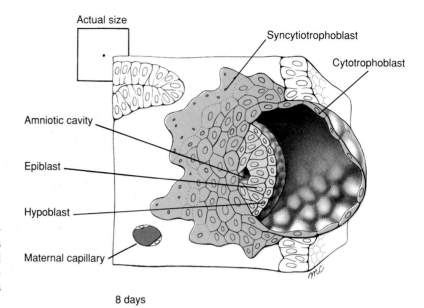

Actual size

Amniotic cavity

Epiblast

Hypoblast

Maternal capillary

Syncytiotrophoblast

Cytotrophoblast

8 days

Fig. 2-2. By 8 days, the amniotic cavity has appeared within the epiblast, and some epiblast cells begin to differentiate into the amnioblasts that will form the amniotic membrane. Implantation continues, and the growing syncytiotrophoblast expands to cover more of the blastocyst.

form a thin membrane of **extraembryonic endoderm** completely lining the former blastocyst cavity (Fig. 2-4A). This membrane is called the **exocoelomic membrane** or **Heuser's membrane,** and the former blastocyst cavity is now called the **primary yolk sac** or **exocoelomic cavity.** As soon as the primary yolk sac forms, a thick, loosely reticular layer of acellular material called the **extraembryonic reticulum** is secreted between Heuser's membrane and the cytotrophoblast (Fig. 2-4A).

The chorionic cavity is produced in conjunction with the development of the extraembryonic mesoderm

A distinctive population of **extraembryonic mesoderm** cells appears within the extraembryonic reticulum on about day 12 or 13. The extraembryonic mesoderm cells arise from the epiblast at the caudal end of the bilaminar germ disc and migrate out to form two layers, one

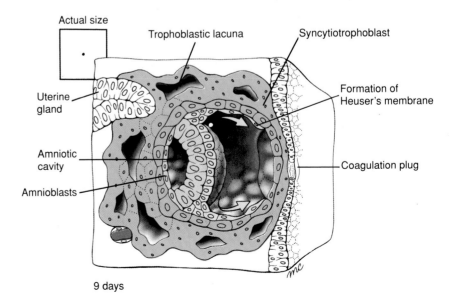

Actual size

Uterine gland

Amniotic cavity

Amnioblasts

Trophoblastic lacuna

Syncytiotrophoblast

Formation of Heuser's membrane

Coagulation plug

9 days

Fig. 2-3. By 9 days, the embryo is completely implanted in the uterine endometrium. The amniotic cavity is expanding, and the hypoblast has begun to proliferate and migrate out over the cytotrophoblast to form Heuser's membrane. Trophoblastic lacunae appear in the syncytiotrophoblast, which now completely surrounds the embryo. The point of implantation is marked by a transient coagulation plug in the endometrial surface.

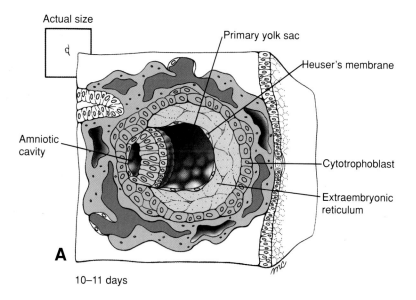

Actual size

Primary yolk sac

Heuser's membrane

Amniotic cavity

Cytotrophoblast

Extraembryonic reticulum

A

10–11 days

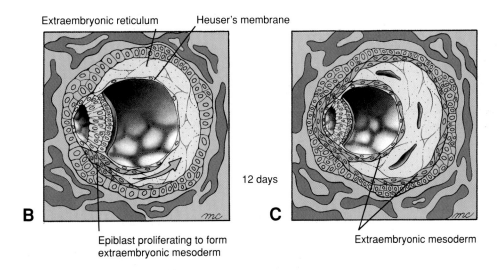

Extraembryonic reticulum   Heuser's membrane

B

Epiblast proliferating to form extraembryonic mesoderm

12 days

C

Extraembryonic mesoderm

Fig. 2-4. The extraembryonic mesoderm is formed in the middle of the second week. **(A)** On days 10-11, an acellular extraembryonic reticulum forms between Heuser's membrane and the cytotrophoblast. At the same time, the trophoblastic lacunae begin to anastomose with maternal capillaries and become filled with blood. **(B)** On days 11 and 12, the extraembryonic reticulum is rapidly invaded by extraembryonic mesoderm. According to the theory illustrated here, the extraembryonic mesoderm originates from the epiblast. Other theories hold that it arises from the cytotrophoblast or hypoblast. **(C)** By day 12, the extraembryonic mesoderm becomes organized to form a layer coating the outside of Heuser's membrane and a layer lining the inside of the cytotrophoblast. Lacunae appear in the extraembryonic reticulum between these layers and will coalesce to form the chorionic cavity. Heuser's membrane and its overlying layer of extraembryonic mesoderm constitute the primary yolk sac.

coating the outer surface of Heuser's membrane and the other lining the inner surface of the cytotrophoblast (Fig. 2-4B). The extraembryonic reticulum trapped between the two layers of extraembryonic mesoderm then breaks down and is replaced by fluid, forming the chorionic cavity (Figs. 2-4C and 2-5A).

As the chorionic cavity expands during the second week, the growth and migration of the extraembryonic mesoderm gradually separate the amnion from the cytotrophoblast. By day 13, the embryonic disc with its dorsal amnion and ventral yolk sac is suspended in the chori-

onic cavity solely by a thick stalk of mesoderm called the **connecting stalk** (Fig. 2-6).

The definitive yolk sac is formed by a new wave of cells that migrate from the hypoblast and displace Heuser's membrane

By day 12, cells of the hypoblast again begin to proliferate and migrate outward (Fig. 2-5A). As this new wave of cuboidal cells spreads out over the inner surface of the

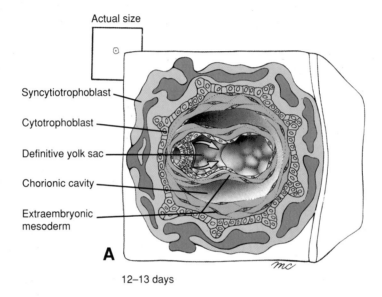

Actual size

Syncytiotrophoblast

Cytotrophoblast

Definitive yolk sac

Chorionic cavity

Extraembryonic mesoderm

A

12–13 days

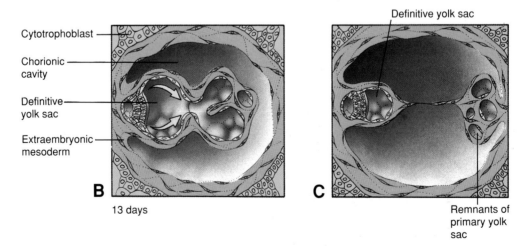

Cytotrophoblast

Chorionic cavity

Definitive yolk sac

Extraembryonic mesoderm

B

13 days

Definitive yolk sac

C

Remnants of primary yolk sac

Fig. 2-5. (**A**) On day 12, a second wave of proliferation in the hypoblast produces a new membrane that migrates out over the inside of the extraembryonic mesoderm, pushing the primary yolk sac in front of it. This new layer becomes the endodermal lining of the definitive (secondary) yolk sac. (**B, C**) As the definitive yolk sac develops on day 13, the primary yolk sac breaks up and is reduced to a collection of vesicles at the abembryonic end of the chorionic cavity.

extraembryonic mesoderm, the old primary yolk sac is pushed away toward the abembryonic pole, disintegrating into a collection of **exocoelomic vesicles** (Fig. 2-5B). By day 13, these exocoelomic vesicles can be seen lying at the abembryonic pole (Figs. 2-5C and 2-6). The space that constituted the blastocyst cavity and then the primary yolk sac thus becomes the **secondary** or **definitive yolk sac.**

The extraembryonic mesoderm forming the outer layer of the definitive yolk sac wall is a major site of **hematopoiesis** (blood formation), and the endoderm lining the yolk sac wall may produce serum proteins. The definitive yolk sac may also play a limited role in the metabolism of embryonic nutrients. The germ cells originating in the epiblast of the bilaminar germ disc first migrate to the yolk sac and then into the posterior body wall. After the fourth week, the yolk sac is rapidly overgrown by the developing embryonic disc. The yolk sac normally disappears before birth, but rarely it persists in the form of a digestive tract anomaly called a **Meckel's diverticulum** (see Ch. 9).

The uteroplacental circulatory system begins to develop during the second week

During the first week of development, the embryo obtains nutrients and eliminates wastes by simple diffusion. The growth of the embryo rapidly makes a more efficient method of exchange imperative. This need is filled by the **uteroplacental circulation** — the system by which maternal and fetal blood flowing through the **placenta** come into close contact and exchange gases and metabolites by diffusion. This system begins to form on day 9 as vacuoles called **trophoblastic lacunae** open within the syncytiotrophoblast (Fig. 2-3). Maternal capillaries near the syncytiotrophoblast then expand to form **maternal sinusoids** that rapidly anastomose with the trophoblastic lacunae (Figs. 2-4A and 2-7A). Between days 11 and 13, as these anastomoses continue to develop, the cytotrophoblast proliferates locally to form extensions that grow into the overlying syncytiotrophoblast (Figs. 2-5A and 2-7A). The growth of these protrusions is thought to be induced by the underlying newly formed extraembryonic mesoderm. These extensions of cytotrophoblast grow out into the blood-filled lacunae, carrying with them a covering of syncytiotrophoblast. The resulting out-growths are called **primary stem villi** (Fig. 2-7A).

It is not until day 16 that the extraembryonic mesoderm penetrates the core of the primary stem villi, thus transforming them into **secondary stem villi** (Fig. 2-7B). By the end of the third week, this villous mesoderm has given rise to blood vessels that connect with the vessels forming in the embryo proper, thus establishing a working uteroplacental circulation. Villi containing differentiated blood vessels are called **tertiary stem villi** (Fig. 2-7C). As can be seen from Figure 2-7C, the gases, nutrients, and wastes that diffuse between the maternal and fetal blood must cross four tissue layers: the endothelium of the villus capillaries, the loose connective tissue in the core of the villus, a layer of cytotrophoblast, and a layer of syncytiotrophoblast. The endothelial lining of the maternal blood vessels does not invade the trophoblastic lacunae. Further differentiation of the placenta and stem villi during fetal development is discussed in Chapter 15.

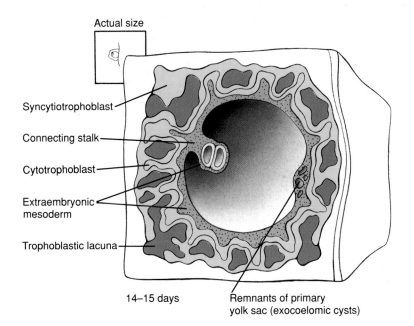

Actual size

Syncytiotrophoblast

Connecting stalk

Cytotrophoblast

Extraembryonic mesoderm

Trophoblastic lacuna

14–15 days

Remnants of primary yolk sac (exocoelomic cysts)

Fig. 2-6. By the end of the second week, the definitive yolk sac loses contact with the remnants of the primary yolk sac (exocoelomic cysts), and the bilaminar germ disc with its dorsal amnion and ventral yolk sac is suspended in the chorionic cavity by a thick connecting stalk.

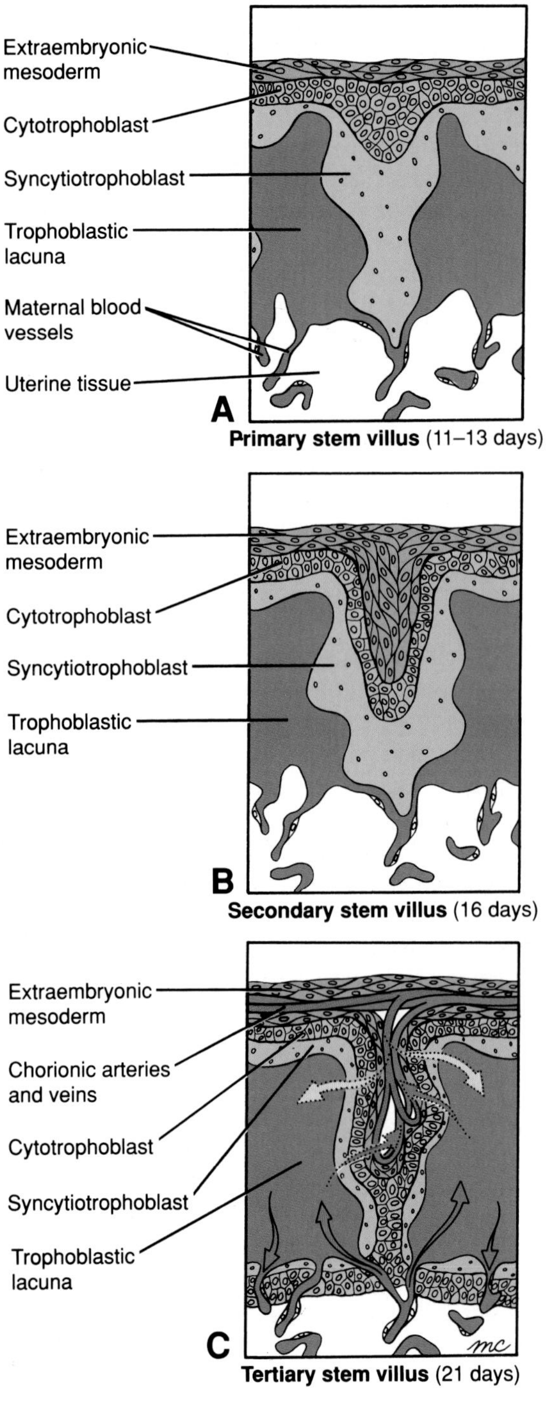

Fig. 2-7. Formation of the chorionic villi. (**A**) The primary stem villi appear on days 11-13 as cytotrophoblastic proliferations that bud into the overlying syncytiotrophoblast. (**B**) By day 16, the extraembryonic mesoderm begins to proliferate and invade the center of each primary stem villus, transforming each into a secondary stem villus. (**C**) By day 21, the mesodermal core differentiates into connective tissue and blood vessels, forming the tertiary stem villi.

APPLICATIONS TO CLINICAL PRACTICE

Hydatidiform mole

Approximately 0.1 to 0.5 percent of pregnancies result in **complete hydatidiform moles,** in which the fetus is entirely missing and only a placenta is present. Many swollen chorionic stem villi develop within the mass (Fig. 2-8) because embryonic vessels fail to form, resulting in the pooling of fluid taken up from the maternal circula-

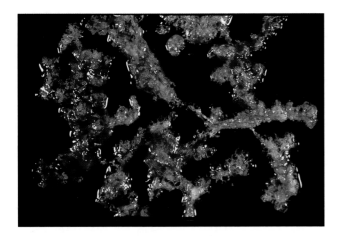

Fig. 2-8. This complete hydatidiform mole has been "dissected" to show the clear swollen villi characteristic of these structures. (Photo courtesy of Dr. Tariq Siddiqi.)

tion within the villi. These villi are often detected by ultrasound. Typically, the patient presents with symptoms of hypertension, edema, and vaginal bleeding.

Cells of complete moles carry 46 chromosomes but all of them are paternal in origin, apparently as a consequence of spontaneous loss of the female pronucleus, accompanied by dispermic fertilization or an initial division of the male pronucleus in the absence of cytokinesis (division of the zygote; Fig. 2-9). The fact that most of these moles are characterized by a 46,XX rather than a 46,XY karyotype argues for the most common origin of complete moles by the latter mechanism.

In some cases, a pregnancy may be characterized by partial embryo development and patchy regions of placenta with swollen chorionic stem villi. These conceptuses are called **partial hydatidiform moles** and are characterized by a 69,XXX, 69,XXY, or 69,XYY **triploid karyotype** (Fig. 2-10). The symptoms of partial moles are not as severe as those of complete moles and in some unusual cases have resulted in the birth of a nonviable triploid fetus.

While both complete and partial moles tend to abort spontaneously, they are often surgically removed after diagnosis. In either case, some of the molar tissue may remain, resulting in a condition called **persistent trophoblastic disease.** This molar tissue, like the placenta of a normal pregnancy, secretes the peptide hormone human chorionic gonadotropin (hCG), and so the presence or absence of residual molar tissue may be monitored by measurements of blood levels of hCG with standard radioimmunoassay or ELISA of this hormone. This is important since the residual trophoblastic tissue may form an **invasive mole** or **metastatic choriocarcinoma.** While these conditions were usually fatal as little as 20 years ago, both are now successfully treated with chemotherapy with high rates of success.

The different functions of the male and female chromosomes in early embryonic development implied by the development of hydatidiform moles have been dramatically demonstrated in experiments with mouse embryos. For example, the female pronucleus may be removed with a small pipette and replaced with another male pronucleus. The resulting diploid zygote, when implanted into the uterus of a pseudopregnant mother, forms a de-

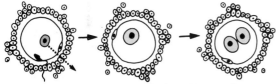

An oocyte is inseminated by a single sperm and the female pronucleus is lost

The single male pronucleus divides to form two haploid nuclei, which combine to form a diploid nucleus

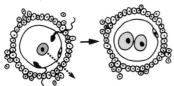

An oocyte is inseminated by two sperm and the female pronucleus is lost

The two male pronuclei combine to form a diploid nucleus

Fig. 2-9. Formation of complete hydatidiform mole. A complete mole is produced when an oocyte that has lost its female pronucleus acquires two male pronuclei. Two mechanisms are shown.

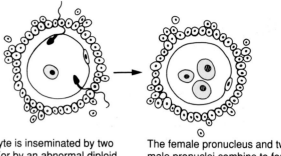

Fig. 2-10. A partial hydatidiform mole is produced when a normal oocyte acquires two male pronuclei (or a diploid male pronucleus).

An oocyte is inseminated by two sperm (or by an abnormal diploid sperm)

The female pronucleus and two male pronuclei combine to form a triploid nucleus

fective placenta with swollen stem villi, much like the human hydatidiform mole. Conversely, the male pronucleus can be removed and replaced with another female pronucleus. In this case, implantation of the resulting diploid zygote into a pseudopregnant mother results in development of an embryo with dramatically reduced placental membranes. These embryos never survive to term. In both types of conceptuses, at least one X chromosome must be present for any development to occur, but the type of conceptus does not depend on the presence or absence of X or Y chromosomes. In all cases the karyotype may be either 46,XX or 46,XY. Indeed, the type of conceptus formed in these mouse experiments depends only on the parental source of the chromosomes. A normal diploid conceptus consisting of both embryo and placenta must contain chromosomes from the mother and father; a diploid conceptus consisting only of the placenta contains only paternal chromosomes, and a diploid conceptus consisting of the embryo only contains only maternal chromosomes.

Genomic imprinting

Molecular analyses of inserted transgenes (see Applications to Clinical Practice in Ch. 1) and of normal endogenous genes have shown that differing activities of certain genes in the male and female genomes during early development are dependent on a process called **genomic imprinting.** Apparently the activities of these genes are related to the degree of **methylation** of their DNA. It has been shown that methylation may lead to gene silencing or, in other cases, to gene activation. Overall, female DNA is more highly methylated than the DNA of the male genome. It has been shown that sites of methylation are cytosine bases that immediately precede guanosine bases and that differential "imprinting" of the DNA takes place during the early development of the gametes. The oogonia, for example, contain one haploid chromosomal complement expressing the male pattern of methylation. However, this male DNA is reprogrammed to express the female pattern of methylation during early stages of oogenesis. Likewise, the reprogramming of maternal DNA to the male pattern occurs within the male germ cells during early stages of spermatogenesis.

Only a handful of imprinted genes have been described, including H19, IGF2, IGF2r, and MASH2, but it is thought that as many as 100 or 200 may exist. So far, it is apparent that these imprinted genes typically function in the regulation of intrauterine growth of the embryo and fetus. Interestingly, imprinting does not occur in oviparous (egg-laying) vertebrates, and so these observations have led to the speculation that the biological significance of genomic imprinting may be related to the regulation of the natural competition between mother and fetus for common nutritional resources during development in placental organisms.

Whether or not this is the case, genomic imprinting has clear significance to the inheritance of congenital disease in humans. For example, a deletion in a specific region of chromosome 15 (15q11–q13) causes Prader-Willi syndrome when the chromosome is inherited from the father but causes a phenotypically distinct condition, Angleman syndrome, when inherited from the mother. In addition, it has long been known that the severity and age of onset of several genetic diseases differ depending on the parent from whom the mutated gene is inherited. These diseases include Huntington's chorea, spinocerebellar ataxia, myotonic dystrophy, neurofibromatoses I and II, and a type of Wilms' tumor (see Applications to Clinical Practice in Ch. 10).

3

The Third Week

Gastrulation, Formation of the Trilaminar Germ Disc, and Initial Development of the Somites and Neural Tube

SUMMARY

During the third week of human development, the bilaminar germ disc is converted to a trilaminar germ disc by a process of **gastrulation** whereby epiblast cells migrate through a region called the **primitive streak** to form a middle layer or **mesoderm** of the embryo. In addition, gastrulation replaces the hypoblast with a new layer derived from the epiblast, namely, the **secondary** or **definitive endoderm,** and the epiblast is transformed into the **definitive ectoderm.** Gastrulation also initiates development of the basic vertebrate body plan. For example, mesoderm that forms in the midline gives rise to the **notochord,** while mesoderm just adjacent to the notochord forms the paraxial mesoderm. The paraxial mesoderm segments by first forming **somitomeres** and then **somites,** which give rise to the **myotomes,** the **sclerotomes,** and the **dermatomes.** These somitic derivatives form skeletal muscle, vertebrae, and dermal components, respectively (see Ch. 4). The **intermediate mesoderm** forms just lateral to the paraxial mesoderm and later gives rise to the urinary system (see Ch. 10), while the most lateral mesoderm, the **lateral plate mesoderm,** contributes to formation of the body wall and to somatic and visceral peritoneum. Moreover, formation of the mesoderm initiates a series of **inductive interactions** between itself and the adjacent endoderm and ectoderm. For example, the mesoderm induces ectoderm to form the central nervous system, and the endoderm induces mesoderm to form the cardiovasculature system. All of these processes proceed epigenetically (i.e., by the gradual evolution of complex from simple structures).

This **epigenetic development** of the human embryo is regulated by **cascades** of **gene expression.** At first, a class of **switch** or **selector genes,** called **maternal effect genes** (encoded within the oocyte), initiate development of the embryonic axes through expression of transcription and growth factors, which then activate a class of genes called **zygotic genes.** Some of the zygotic genes, like the *Hox* **genes** express transcription factors in specific combinations within specific parts of the embryo to direct development in that region by activating downstream genes that encode the enzymes and protein building blocks of the definitive cells and tissues of the body. Many specific developmental processes like the process of gastrulation are controlled by specific cascades of regulatory gene expression. In this case, maternal effect genes activate zygotic genes critical to establish and organize the primitive streak. These genes, in turn, activate genes that regulate the behavior of epiblast cells that bring about their involution and ingress to form the definitive endoderm and mesoderm. Indeed, disruptions of some of these genes (by mutation or teratogens) may result in human congenital abnormalities characterized by the underdevelopment of specific mesodermal structures (see Applications to Clinical Practice, below).

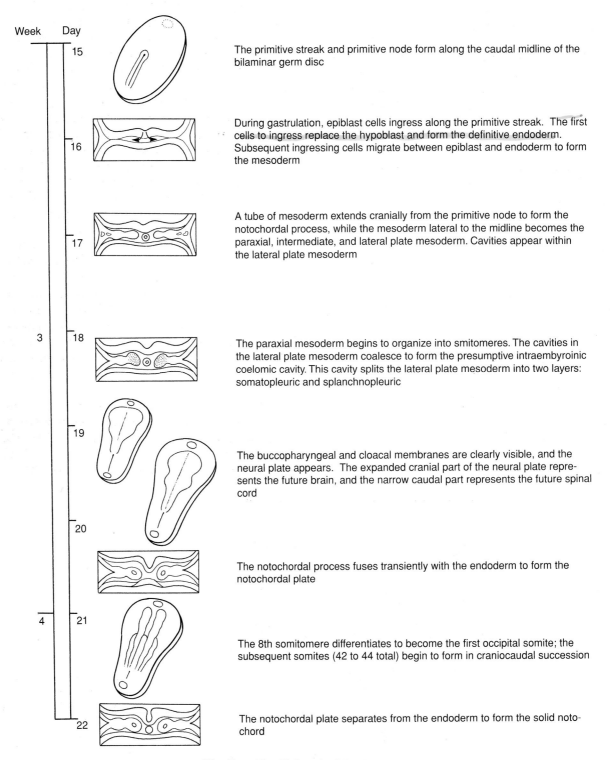

Week	Day	
	15	The primitive streak and primitive node form along the caudal midline of the bilaminar germ disc
	16	During gastrulation, epiblast cells ingress along the primitive streak. The first cells to ingress replace the hypoblast and form the definitive endoderm. Subsequent ingressing cells migrate between epiblast and endoderm to form the mesoderm
	17	A tube of mesoderm extends cranially from the primitive node to form the notochordal process, while the mesoderm lateral to the midline becomes the paraxial, intermediate, and lateral plate mesoderm. Cavities appear within the lateral plate mesoderm
3	18	The paraxial mesoderm begins to organize into smitomeres. The cavities in the lateral plate mesoderm coalesce to form the presumptive intraembyroinic coelomic cavity. This cavity splits the lateral plate mesoderm into two layers: somatopleuric and splanchnopleuric
	19	The buccopharyngeal and cloacal membranes are clearly visible, and the neural plate appears. The expanded cranial part of the neural plate represents the future brain, and the narrow caudal part represents the future spinal cord
	20	The notochordal process fuses transiently with the endoderm to form the notochordal plate
4	21	The 8th somitomere differentiates to become the first occipital somite; the subsequent somites (42 to 44 total) begin to form in craniocaudal succession
	22	The notochordal plate separates from the endoderm to form the solid notochord

Timeline. The third week of development.

The primitive streak appears at the beginning of the third week

On about day 15 of development, a faint groove appears along the longitudinal midline of the germ disc (Fig. 3-1). Over the course of the next day, this groove becomes deeper and elongates to occupy about half the length of the embryo. On day 16, a deeper depression surrounded by a slight mound of epiblast appears at the presumptive cranial end of the groove, near the center of the germ disc. This groove is called the **primitive groove,** the depression is called the **primitive pit,** and the mound surrounding it is called the **primitive node.** The entire structure is the **primitive streak.**

The future head will form at the end of the germ disc near the primitive pit, and the surface of the epiblast in the region adjacent to the midline will form the dorsal surface of the embryo. The appearance of the primitive streak establishes the longitudinal axis and thus the bilateral symmetry of the future adult. Thus, the fundamental cranial/caudal, left/right, and ventral/dorsal axes of the body are established early in the third week of development.

The definitive endoderm and intraembryonic mesoderm form by gastrulation through the primitive streak

On day 16, the epiblast cells near the primitive streak begin to proliferate, flatten, and lose their connections with each other (Fig. 3-2). These flattened cells develop long, footlike processes called **pseudopodia,** which allow them to migrate through the primitive streak into the space between the epiblast and the hypoblast. This process of involution and ingress is called **gastrulation.** Some of the ingressing epiblast cells invade the hypoblast and displace its cells, so that the hypoblast is completely replaced by a new layer of cells, the **definitive endoderm** or **entoderm** (Fig. 3-2). The definitive endoderm gives rise to the lining of the future gut and gut derivatives.

Starting on day 16, some of the epiblast cells migrating through the primitive streak diverge into the space between the epiblast and the definitive endoderm to form a third germ layer, the **intraembryonic mesoderm** (Fig. 3-2). Some of these mesoderm cells migrate laterally or cranially, whereas others are deposited on the midline near their site of entry (Figs. 3-2 and 3-3). The cells that migrate through the primitive pit and come to rest on the midline form two structures: first the **prechordal plate,** a compact mass of mesoderm cranial to the primitive pit, and then a dense midline tube called the **notochordal process** (see Fig. 3-6). On either side of the midline the mesoderm cells spread out to form a loose sheet that remains distinct from the epiblast and the endoderm (see Figs. 3-6 and 3-7).

When the intraembryonic mesoderm and definitive endoderm have formed, the epiblast takes on a new name, the **ectoderm.** The three definitive layers of the **trilaminar germ disc** — the ectoderm, mesoderm, and definitive endoderm — thus are all derived from the epiblast.

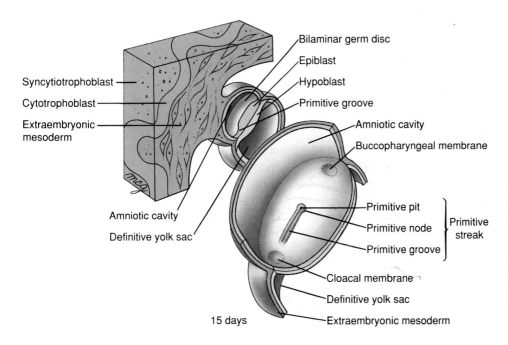

Syncytiotrophoblast
Cytotrophoblast
Extraembryonic mesoderm

Bilaminar germ disc
Epiblast
Hypoblast
Primitive groove
Amniotic cavity
Buccopharyngeal membrane

Amniotic cavity
Definitive yolk sac

Primitive pit
Primitive node   Primitive streak
Primitive groove

Cloacal membrane
Definitive yolk sac
Extraembryonic mesoderm

15 days

Fig. 3-1. View of the dorsal surface of the bilaminar germ disc through the sectioned amnion and yolk sac. The inset at the upper left shows the relation of the embryo to the wall of the chorionic cavity. The primitive streak, now one day old, occupies 50 percent of the length of the germ disc. The buccopharyngeal and cloacal membranes are present.

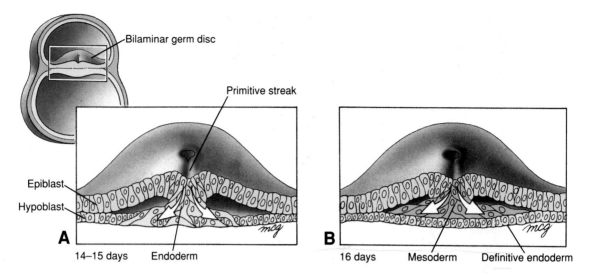

Fig. 3-2. Germ discs sectioned through the region of the primitive streak, showing gastrulation. **(A)** On days 14 and 15, the ingressing epiblast cells replace the hypoblast to form the definitive endoderm. **(B)** The epiblast that ingresses on day 16 migrates between the endoderm and epiblast layers to form the intraembryonic mesoderm.

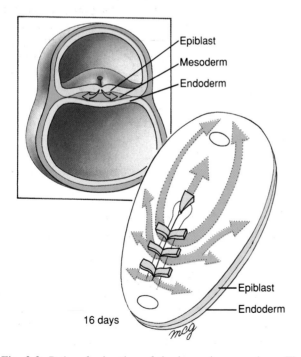

Fig. 3-3. Paths of migration of the ingressing mesoderm. The epiblast cells that ingress through the primitive node migrate directly cranially to form the prechordal plate and notochordal process. The cells that ingress through the primitive groove migrate to form the mesoderm lying on either side of the midline.

The primitive streak retreats and disappears, and the caudal eminence gives rise to caudal structures of the body

On day 16, the primitive streak spans about half the length of the embryo. As gastrulation proceeds, however, it regresses caudally, becoming gradually shorter (Fig. 3-4). By day 22, the primitive streak represents about 10 to 20 percent of the embryo's length; by day 26, it disappears.

The fate of gastrulating epiblast cells can be predicted from their site of origin

It is thought that somewhat different regions of the primitive streak are responsible for producing the extraembryonic mesoderm, the various subpopulations of the intraembryonic mesoderm, and the definitive endoderm. Indeed, cell tracing and cell lineage studies make it possible to construct a **fate map** showing the developmental destinies of specific regions of the epiblast (Fig. 3-5). It appears that the most caudal region of the streak produces the extraembryonic mesoderm; the midregion of the streak produces the mesoderm that migrates to the lateral parts of the germ disc; and the cranial regions of the streak produce the mesoderm that comes to rest on and adjacent to the midsagittal axis, as well as the definitive endoderm.

The notochord is produced by cells that ingress through the primitive node

Just caudal to the newly formed prechordal plate, the primitive node sprouts a hollow mesodermal tube, the **notochordal process.** This tube grows in length as cells pro-

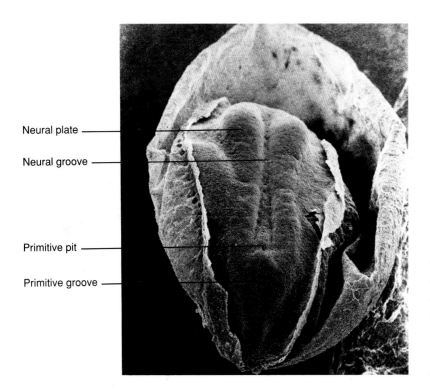

Neural plate

Neural groove

Primitive pit

Primitive groove

Fig. 3-4. Scanning electron micrograph showing the ectodermal surface of a trilaminar germ disc comparable to a 19-day human embryo (cranial end at the top). The neural plate and neural groove are discussed at the end of this chapter and in Chapter 4. (From Tamarin A. 1983. Stage 9 macaque embryos studied by electron microscopy. J Anat 137:765, with permission.)

liferating in the region of the primitive node add on to its proximal end and as the primitive streak regresses (Fig. 3-6). When the notochordal process is completely formed on about day 20, several structural transformations take place that convert it from a hollow tube to a solid rod (Fig. 3-7). First, the ventral floor of the tube fuses with the underlying endoderm. The tube then unzippers ventrally, starting in the region of the primitive pit. The yolk sac cavity thus transiently communicates with the amniotic cavity

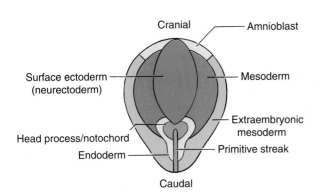

Fig. 3-5. Fate map of the epiblast of a mouse/embryo, showing the zones of epiblast that ingress through the primitive streak and form the major structures of the trilaminar germ disc. This map was deduced on the basis of cell lineage studies, in which epiblast cells were injected with tracer molecules and their labeled descendants later located. (Modified from Lawson KA, Peterson R. 1992. Clonal analysis of cell fate during gastration and early neurulation in the mouse. Symp. 165. John Wiley and Sons, New York, with permission.)

through an opening at the primitive pit called the **neurenteric canal** (Fig. 3-7B). The unzippering of the tube floor converts the **notochordal process** to a flattened, midventral bar of mesoderm called the **notochordal plate** (Fig. 3-7A, B). It is not until day 22 to 24 that the notochordal plate completely detaches from the endoderm and retreats back into the mesoderm-containing space between ectoderm and endoderm, changing as it does so into a solid cylinder called the **notochord** (Fig. 3-7C).

The rudiments of the vertebral bodies initially coalesce around the notochord, the notochord gives rise to the nucleus pulposus at the center of the vertebral discs. However, in early childhood the nucleus pulposus cells of notochordal origin degenerate and are replaced by adjacent mesodermal cells.

Mesoderm is excluded from the buccopharyngeal and cloacal membranes

During the third week of development, two faint depressions appear in the ectoderm, one at the cranial end of the embryo adjacent to the prechordal plate and the other at the caudal end behind the primitive streak. Late in the third week, the ectoderm in these areas fuses tightly with the underlying endoderm, excluding the mesoderm and forming a bilaminar membrane. The cranial membrane is called the **buccopharyngeal membrane,** and the caudal membrane is the **cloacal membrane.** The buccopharyngeal and cloacal membranes later become the blind ends of the gut tube. The buccopharyngeal membrane breaks

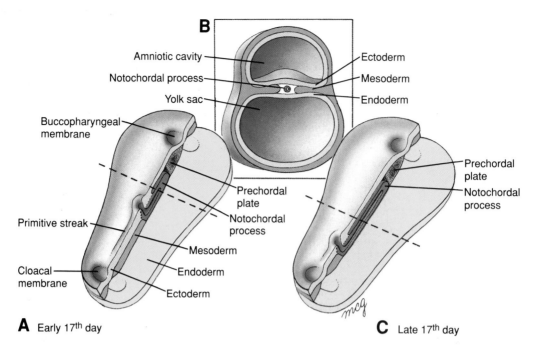

Fig. 3-6. Formation of the notochordal process and prechordal plate mesoderm. **(A, C)** Stages showing the hollow notochordal process growing cranially from the walls of the primitive pit. Note the changes in the relative length of the notochordal process and primitive streak as the embryo grows. Also note the fusion of ectoderm and endoderm in the buccopharyngeal and cloacal membranes. **(B)** Cross section of the germ disc at the level indicated by the dotted line.

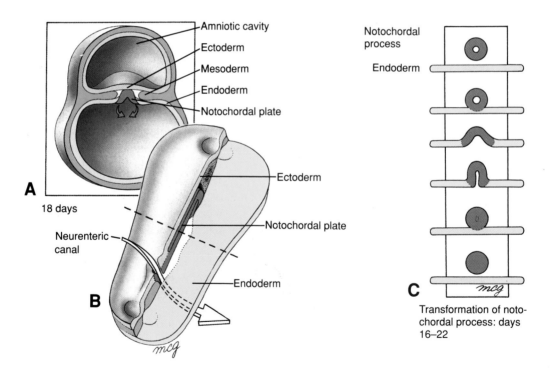

Fig. 3-7. The process by which the hollow notochordal process is transformed into a solid notochord between days 16 and 22. **(A, B)** First, the ventral wall of the notochordal process has begun to fuse with the endoderm to form the notochordal plate. As shown in Fig. B, this process commences at the caudal end of the notochordal process and proceeds cranially (the dotted line marks the level of section A). An open neurenteric canal is briefly created between the amniotic cavity and the yolk sac cavity. **(C)** The stages by which the notochordal process becomes the notochordal plate and then the notochord.

down in the fourth week to form the opening to the oral cavity, whereas the cloacal membrane disintegrates later, in the seventh week, to form the openings of the anus and the urinary and genital tracts (see Chs. 9 and 10).

Paraxial, intermediate, and lateral plate mesoderm are formed by cells migrating laterally from the primitive streak

As the primitive streak regresses during the third week, the mesoderm cells that migrated laterally from it begin to condense into rod- and sheetlike structures on either side of the notochord (Fig. 3-8). This process commences at the cranial end of the embryo and proceeds posteriorly, continuing throughout the third and fourth weeks. The mesoderm lying immediately on either side of the notochord forms a pair of cylindrical condensations called the **paraxial mesoderm.** A less pronounced pair of cylindrical condensations, the **intermediate mesoderm,** forms just lateral to the paraxial mesoderm. The remainder of the lateral mesoderm forms a flattened sheet and is called the **lateral plate mesoderm.**

The **paraxial mesoderm** differentiates into the axial skeleton, voluntary musculature, and part of the dermis of the skin. The **intermediate mesoderm** produces the uri-

nary system and parts of the genital system (see Ch. 10). Starting on day 17, the **lateral plate mesoderm** splits into two layers: a ventral layer associated with the endoderm and a dorsal layer associated with the ectoderm (Fig. 3-8C). The layer adjacent to the endoderm gives rise to the mesothelial covering of the visceral organs (viscera) and hence is called the **splanchnopleuric mesoderm** (from the Greek *splanchnon,* viscera). The layer adjacent to the ectoderm gives rise to the inner lining of the body wall, to parts of the limbs, and to most of the dermis and hence is called the **somatopleuric mesoderm** (from the Greek *soma,* body).

The paraxial mesoderm develops into somitomeres and then into somites

As soon as it forms, the cells of the paraxial mesoderm begin to form a series of rounded, whorl-like structures called **somitomeres.** Scanning electron microscopic analyses on embryos of animals ranging from fish to mice show that somitomeres first appear as a faint segmentation in the most cranial paraxial mesoderm, just on either side of the notochordal plate, at a stage corresponding to the 18th or 19th day of human development (Fig. 3-9). Formation of

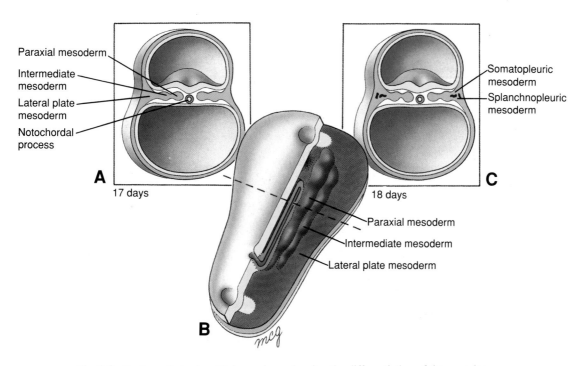

Fig. 3-8. Sections through a 17-day embryo showing the differentiation of the mesoderm on either side of the midline. **(A)** Early on day 17, the mesoderm has begun to differentiate into paraxial, intermediate, and lateral plate mesoderm. **(B)** Sagittal cutaway showing the rod-like condensations of paraxial and intermediate mesoderm. The dotted line marks the plane of the two transverse sections. **(C)** Later on day 17, the lateral plate begins to vacuolate to form the rudiment of the intraembryonic coelom.

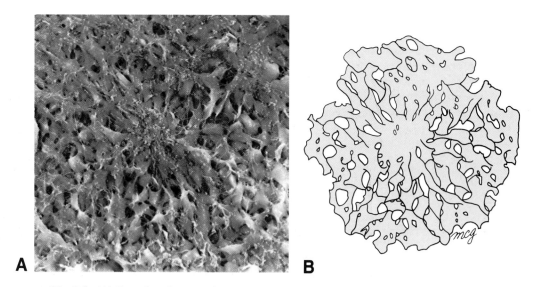

Fig. 3-9. (A) Scanning electron micrograph and (B) matching sketch of a somitomere. The concentric architecture of these structures is easiest to discern in stereophotographs. (Photo courtesy of Dr. Antone Jacobson.)

somitomeres continues throughout the third and fourth weeks, starting with several pairs in the cranial region and proceeding through the cervical, thoracic, lumbar, sacral, and coccygeal regions (Fig. 3-10).

Most of the somitomeres develop further to form discrete blocks of segmental mesoderm called **somites** (Figs. 3-11 and 3-12). In all species studied, however, the first seven pairs of somitomeres do not go on to form somites.

These seven pairs of somitomeres eventually give rise to the striated muscles of the face, jaw, and throat.

The first somites appear on day 20 in the region of the future base of the skull

The eighth, ninth, and tenth pairs of somitomeres differentiate into the first, second, and third pairs of **somites** on

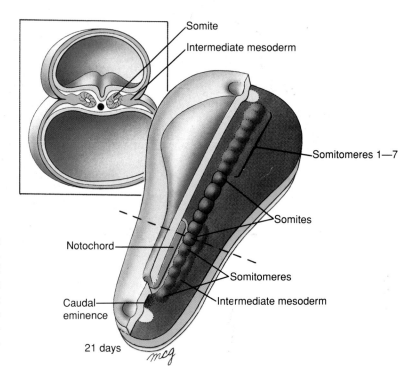

Fig. 3-10. Sections through a 21-day embryo. The cranial and caudal portions of the paraxial mesoderm have become organized into somitomeres, and the four occipital and first two cervical somitomeres have differentiated into somites. The seven most cranial somitomeres never become somites. The dotted line indicates the level of the transverse section. At this level, the lateral plate mesoderm contains the rudiment of the intraembryonic coelom.

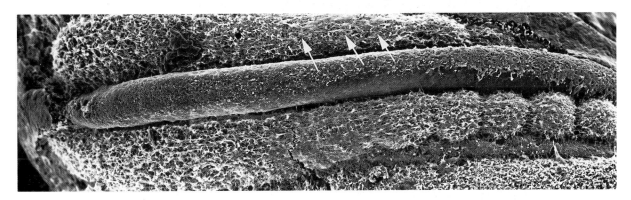

Fig. 3-11. Scanning electron micrograph of an embryo with the ectoderm removed to show somites and, more caudally, the paraxial mesoderm that has not yet segmented. Arrows indicate the region of somitomere formation. (From Bellairs R. 1986. The primitive streak. Anat Embryol 174:1, with permission.)

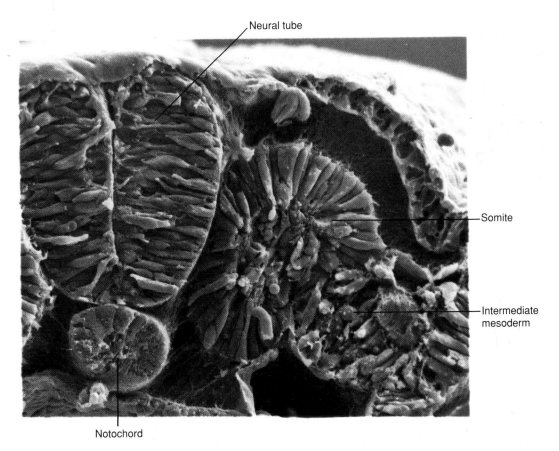

Fig. 3-12. Scanning electron micrograph of a transversely sectioned embryo showing a somite and the intermediate mesoderm. Note also the notochord and the developing neural tube. (Photo courtesy of Dr. Kathryn Tosney.)

day 20 (Fig. 3-10). The rest of the somites form in cranio-caudal progression at a rate of about three or four a day, finishing on about day 30. In the human, approximately 42 to 44 pairs of somites form, flanking the notochord from the occipital (skull base) region to the embryonic tail. The caudalmost several somites eventually disappear, however, giving a final count of approximately 37 pairs.

The somites establish the segmental organization of the body

The somites give rise to most of the axial skeleton, including the vertebral column and part of the occipital bone of the skull; to the voluntary musculature of the neck, body wall, and limbs; and to part of the dermis of the neck and trunk.

The first four pairs of somites form in the occipital region. These somites contribute to the development of the occipital part of the skull; to the bones that form around the nose, eyes, and inner ears; to the extrinsic ocular muscles; and to muscles of the tongue (see Ch. 12). The next eight pairs of somites form in the **cervical** region. The most cranial cervical somite also contributes to the occipital bone, and others form the cervical vertebrae and associated muscles as well as part of the neck dermis. The next 12 pairs, the **thoracic somites,** form thoracic vertebrae; the musculature and bones of the thoracic wall; part of the thoracic dermis; and part of the abdominal wall. Cells from cervical and thoracic somites also invade the upper limb buds to form the limb musculature (see Ch. 11).

Caudal to the thoracic somites, the five **lumbar somites** form abdominal dermis, the abdominal muscles, and the lumbar vertebrae, and the five **sacral somites** form the sacrum with its associated dermis and musculature. Cells from lumbar somites invade the lower limb buds to form the leg musculature. Finally, the three **coccygeal somites** that remain after degeneration of the caudalmost somites form the coccyx.

The axial mesoderm induces the overlying ectoderm to form the neural plate

The first event in the formation of the future central nervous system is the appearance on day 18 of a thickened **neural plate** in the epiblast along the midsagittal axis cranial to the primitive pit (Figs. 3-13 and 3-14). The neural plate develops in response to **inducing substances** secreted by the underlying axial mesodermal structures, that is, by the prechordal plate and the cranial portion of the notochordal plate (see the Applications to Clinical Practice section in Ch. 4). These substances diffuse to the overlying epiblast cells, in which they activate specific genes that cause the cells to differentiate into a thick plate of columnar, pseudostratified **neuroepithelial cells (neurectoderm).** The neural plate appears first at the cranial end of the embryo and differentiates craniocaudally. The neural plate is broad cranially and tapered caudally. The expanded cranial portion gives rise to the brain. Even at this very early stage of differentiation, the presumptive brain is visibly divided into three regions, the future forebrain, midbrain, and hindbrain (Fig. 3-14). The narrow caudal portion of the neural plate, which overlies the notochord and is flanked by the developing somites, gives rise to the spinal cord (Figs. 3-13 and 3-14).

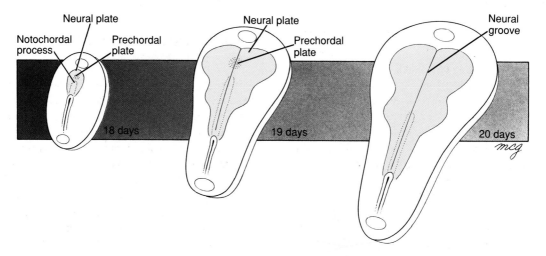

Fig. 3-13. A schematic sequence showing how the neural plate grows and changes proportions between day 18 and day 20. The primitive streak shortens only slightly, but it occupies a progressively smaller proportion of the length of the embryonic disc as the neural plate and embryo grow.

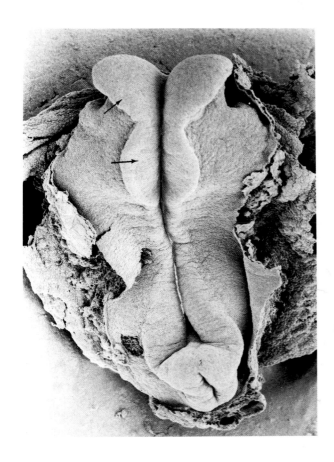

Fig. 3-14. Scanning electron micrograph of an embryo comparable to a 20-day human embryo. The neural plate is clearly visible, and the expansions that will become the major subdivisions of the brain are apparent (arrows). Only a small region of the primitive streak remains. The primitive streak will disappear on day 25. (From Tamarin A. 1983. Stage 9 macaque embryos studied by electron microscopy. J Anat 137:765, with permission.)

APPLICATIONS TO CLINICAL PRACTICE

A spectrum of malformations affecting diverse organ systems has been characterized as "caudal dysplasia syndrome"

In 1961, Duhamel described a constellation of malformations he called **caudal regression.** Affected individuals exhibited (1) flexion and outward rotation of the lower extremities, (2) lumbar and sacral vertebral malformations, (3) imperforate anus, (4) renal agenesis, and (5) agenesis of the internal genital organs except for the gonads. The most extreme condition, characterized by fusion of the lower extremities, was called **sirenomelia** (Fig. 3-15). Since it is unlikely that the reduction in caudal structures in these malformations is a consequence of formation and resorption, it has been suggested that the syndrome should be called **caudal dysplasia, caudal agenesis,** or **sacral agenesis** rather than caudal regression. In some cases, these defects are associated with more cranial malformations. One of these associations is called the **VATER association** because it includes the following anomalies: **V**ertebral defects, **A**nal atresia, **T**reacheal-**E**sophageal fistula, and **R**enal defects. An extension of this association, the **VACTERL association** also includes **C**ardiovascular anomalies and **L**imb defects.

Caudal dysplasia may result from gastrulation disruptions

The spectrum of anomalies evident in this condition has been attributed to failure of sufficient mesoderm formation during the process of gastrulation. Indeed, irradiation of the primitive streak in experimental animals or treatment of the animal with insulin during gastrulation results in malformations similar to those that characterize human caudal dysplasia. Moreover, the study of two mouse mutants, **brachyuric** and **anuric mice,** implicate disruption of a gene that functions during gastrulation, namely, the *T/t* or **brachyury complex.** These mice, which harbor mutations of the T/t complex, are characterized by varying degrees of loss of caudal structures similar to those exhibited in human caudal dysplasia. During the embryonic development of anuric or brachyuric mice, it is apparent that the notochord fails to separate from the

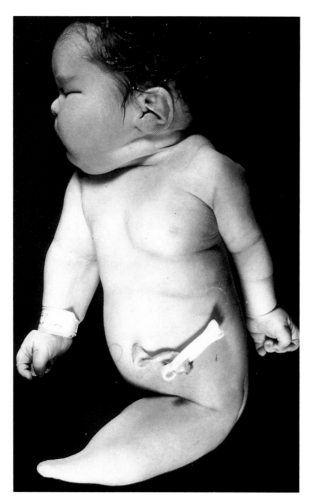

Fig. 3-15. Sirenomelia. Severe reduction of the caudal structures has resulted in fusion of the lower extremity limb buds. (Photo courtesy of Children's Hospital Medical Center, Cincinnati, OH.)

endoderm or secondarily fuses with the neural tube, suggesting that the brachyury gene product may function in cell adhesion.

Experimental studies of the *T/t* or brachyury gene implicate its product in the process of gastrulation

A useful technique in the study of gene expression in embryos is **in situ hybridization.** Tissues of interest are incubated with radiolabeled antisense "probes," which are copies of short specific basepair sequences complementary to the RNA or DNA characterizing the particular gene. The labeled antisense RNA or DNA binds to the appropriate sequence of the specific messenger RNA expressed by that gene and can be localized using the technique of **autoradiography.** In this method, the whole tissue or a tissue section is overlaid with a photographic emulsion, placed in the dark, and then developed. The presence of silver grains then reveals the location of the antisense probe, and the specific cells that bind it can then be identified with appropriate staining or phase microscopic techniques. When gastrulating embryos are analyzed with probes specific for the brachyury gene product, the label is first found in newly formed mesoderm just adjacent to the primitive streak. As mesoderm formation continues, the label becomes more concentrated in the developing notochord. Finally, as the vertebrae form, the brachyury gene product is found only within the nucleus pulposus.

This indirect evidence is supported by **transgenic animal studies** (see Applications to Clinical Practice in Ch. 1). When null mutants (knockouts) of the brachyury gene are produced, notochord development is disrupted and the body axis fails to lengthen. Interestingly, however, the cranial region of these animals is relatively normal. In contrast, knockout of another gene, called *lim-1*, results in disruption of **prechordal mesoderm** formation, and in these otherwise relatively normal animals the entire head is missing. Results such as these support the idea that **synergistic** or **antagonistic interactions** of different regulatory genes control complex developmental processes like gastrulation, and, indeed, a growing body of literature now implicates a variety of genes in the regulation of this process.

In particular, it appears that it is the interaction of two such classes of factors that control the process of gastrulation as well as other developmental processes, namely, **dorsalizing factors** and **ventralizing factors.** Dorsalizing factors like *lim-1* tend to be expressed in more dorsocranial regions of the embryo, while ventralizing factors like brachyury tend to be expressed in more ventrocaudal regions of the embryo. Other dorsalizing factors active in the process of gastrulation include the genes **goosecoid, nodal, noggin,** and **chordin,** and the growth factor **activin.** Ventralizing factors in addition to brachyury include **bone morphogenetic protein-4, basic fibroblast growth factor,** and **glycogen synthase kinase-3.**

Molecular genetic studies are becoming increasingly relevant to the study of human congenital disease

It should be apparent that mammalian embryos, including those of humans, utilize many of the genetic regulatory mechanisms that control morphogenetic mechanisms in ancestral organisms. In fact, mammals have even adapted many ancient regulatory schemes to regulate developmental processes that are novel to their development. It is now also obvious that disruption of these regulatory genes by mutation, abnormal meiosis, or actions of environmental or therapeutic teratogens produce congenital malformations in humans. As a consequence, an understanding of the molecular biology of human developmental genetics is becoming more relevant to the diagnosis (e.g., surfactant B deficiency, Ch. 6), prevention (e.g., fetal alcohol syndrome, Ch. 12), and treatment of human congenital disease (e.g., hydatidiform mole, Ch. 2)

4

The Fourth Week

Differentiation of the Somites and the Nervous System; Segmental Development and Integration

S U M M A R Y

The fourth week of human development is characterized by dramatic morphogenetic transformations that create the rudimentary vertebrate body form. These include the following:

1. The **somites** complete their segmentation and differentiate into **myotomes, sclerotomes,** and **dermatomes,** which, in turn, initiate muscle and vertebrae formation and differentiation of the dermis.

2. During the latter part of the third week and the early part of the fourth week, the prechordal plate and notochord induce formation of the **neural tube** by the process of **neurulation.** The neural tube is the precursor of the **brain** and **spinal cord,** which develop through inductive interactions with the notochord and surface ectoderm.

3. **Motor neurons** send axons out from the neural tube to form motor nerve fibers of the spinal nerves.

4. As this occurs, **neural crest cells** detach from the lateral folds of the neural plate and migrate to diverse locations of the body, initiating development of **sensory** and **autonomic nerves,** the adrenal medulla, melanocytes of the skin, some of the coverings of the central nervous system, the dermis and membrane bones of the head and neck, the facial skeleton, and other vital structures.

5. The initially flattened embryo **folds laterally** and **cephalocaudally** to generate the primitive three-dimensional vertebrate body form. This process of folding is thought to be driven by the overgrowth of dorsal structures such as the somites and the neural tube over the stagnating ventral yolk sac.

Much has recently been learned about the regulation of these processes at the genetic level, providing encouragement for the possibility that new diagnoses and therapies for significant human congenital conditions like **spina bifida** may be on the horizon. For example, initiation of the process of somite segmentation appears to require the action of **fibroblast growth factors,** while the segmentation process per se is under control of regulatory genes of the *Wnt* family that express **cell surface-associated molecules.** Coordination of somite segmentation along the longitudinal axis and from side to side is controlled by a gene homologous to a fruitfly **notch** gene, which again encodes a protein active in cell cohesion. On the other hand, differentiation of specific body segments is regulated by segment-specific **combinatorial codes** of *HOX* **gene expression.** The specific differentiation of the myotomes, sclerotomes, and dermatomes is controlled by regulatory genes that express other transcription factors, growth factors, and extracellular matrix proteins.

It is now known that spina bifida may occur through the mutation or disruption of some of these regulatory genes as occurs in several animal models exhibiting neural tube defects. The molecular dissection of processes of vertebrae and neural tube induction in experimental animals may lead to discovery of other genetic causes of spina bifida.

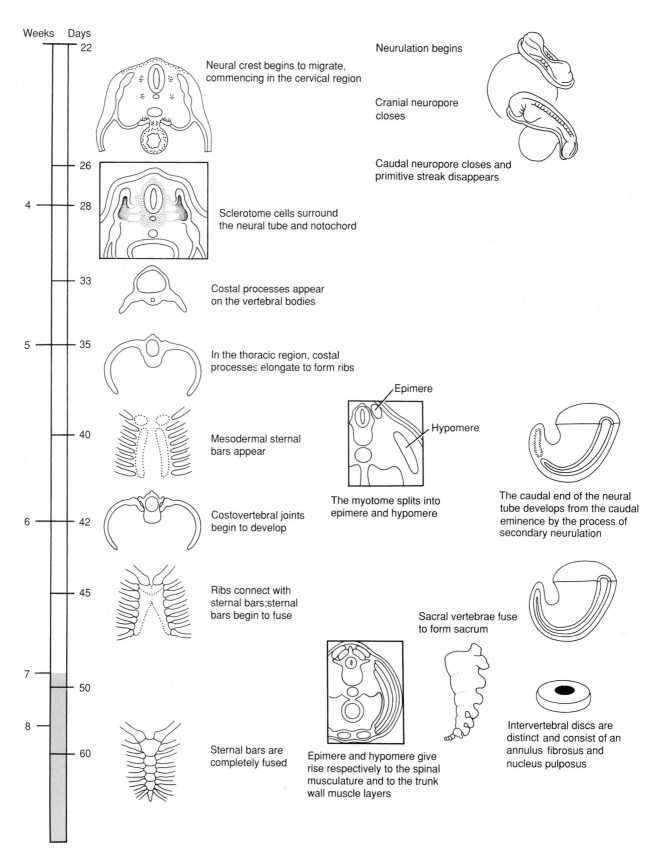

Timeline. Development of the somites and the neural tube.

The somites differentiate into sclerotome, myotome, and dermatome

The sclerotome cells surround the notochord and neural tube

Shortly after forming, each somite separates into subdivisions that give rise to specific mesodermal components. The first of these subdivisions to appear are the **sclerotomes,** which will develop into the vertebrae. The sclerotomes arise as follows. Each newly formed somite develops a central cavity that becomes occupied by a population of loose **core cells** (Fig. 4-1). The somite then ruptures on its medial side, and the core cells, plus some additional cells from the ventromedial wall of the somite, form the **sclerotome.** The ventral portion of the sclerotome surrounds the notochord and forms the vertebral body. The dorsal portion of the sclerotome surrounds the neural tube and forms the vertebral arch.

A number of spinal defects are caused by abnormal induction of the sclerotomes and the neural tube. Defective induction of vertebral bodies on one side of the body may result in a severe **scoliosis** (lateral bending of the spinal column), which must be surgically corrected. A range of defects, called **spina bifida, myeloschisis,** and **anencephaly,** are caused by abnormal development of the neural tube and vertebral arches (see Applications to Clinical Practice).

The segmental sclerotomes split and recombine to form intersegmental vertebral rudiments. The spinal nerves develop **segmentally;** that is, each spinal nerve emerges at the same level as the corresponding somite. Since the vertebral arches completely enclose the neural tube during the period when the spinal nerves sprout, one may wonder how the spinal nerves escape from the developing vertebral canal. A related question is why eight cervical sclerotomes produce seven cervical vertebrae, whereas in the rest of the vertebral column there is a one-to-one correspondence of sclerotomes to vertebrae.

The answer to these questions is that the sclerotomes split and recombine to produce vertebral rudiments that lie **intersegmentally.** Figure 4-2 illustrates this process. As the sclerotome surrounds the notochord and neural tube, it splits into a cranial half and a caudal half, and the caudal half of each sclerotome fuses with the cranial half of the succeeding sclerotome. The resulting composite structures surround the notochord and neural tube and thus produce vertebrae that lie intersegmentally.

Seven cervical vertebrae form from eight cervical somites because the cranial half of the first cervical sclerotome fuses with the caudal half of the fourth occipital sclerotome and contributes to the formation of the base of the skull (Fig. 4-3). The caudal half of the first cervical sclerotome then fuses with the cranial half of the second cervical sclerotome to form the first cervical vertebra (the atlas), and so on down the spine. The eighth cervical sclerotome

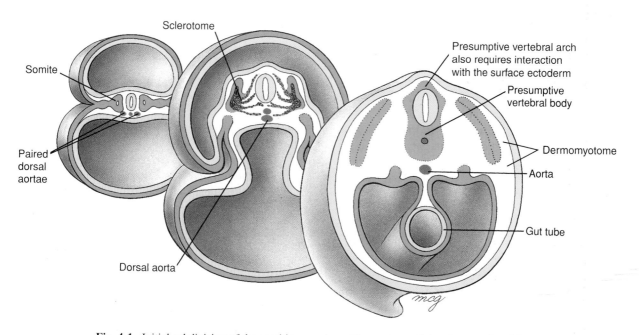

Fig. 4-1. Initial subdivision of the somitic mesoderm. The ventromedial and core cells of the somite, constituting the sclerotome, migrate toward the midline of the embryo to enclose the neural tube and notochord, where they subsequently form the vertebral arches and vertebral bodies, respectively. The remaining dorsolateral cells of the somite form the dermomyotome.

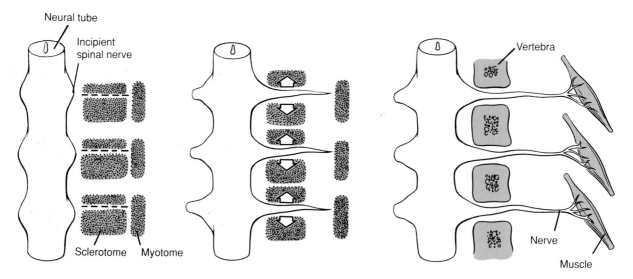

Fig. 4-2. Recombining of the sclerotomes to form vertebrae. Each sclerotome splits into cranial and caudal segments. As the segmental spinal nerves grow out to innervate the myotomes, the cranial segment of each sclerotome recombines with the caudal segment of the next superior sclerotome to form a vertebral rudiment.

thus contributes its cranial half to the seventh cervical vertebra and its caudal half to the first thoracic vertebra.

As a result of sclerotomal resegmentation, the segmental spinal nerves exit between the vertebrae. It is important to remember, however, that even though there are seven cervical vertebrae, there are eight cervical spinal nerves: the first spinal nerve exits between the base of the skull and the first cervical vertebra, and thus the eighth spinal nerve exits above the first thoracic vertebra. From this point onward, each spinal nerve exits just below the vertebra of the same number (Fig. 4-3).

The fibrous intervertebral discs form between the vertebral bodies at segmental levels (Fig. 4-4). The original core of each disc, the **nucleus pulposus,** is composed of cells of notochordal origin, whereas the surrounding **annulus fibrosus** develops from sclerotomal cells that are left in the region of sclerotome splitting during resegmentation.

The ribs develop from costal processes of the developing thoracic vertebrae. Small lateral mesenchymal condensations called **costal processes** develop in association with the vertebral arches of all the developing neck and trunk vertebrae (Fig. 4-5A). Concomitantly, the slightly more dorsal transverse processes grow laterally along the dorsal side of each costal process. Only in the thoracic region, however, do the distal tips of the costal processes lengthen to form ribs. The ribs begin to form and lengthen on day 35. The first seven ribs connect ven-

trally to the sternum via **costal cartilages** by day 45 and are called **true ribs.** The five lower ribs do not articulate directly with the sternum and are called **false ribs.** The ribs develop as cartilaginous precursors that later ossify, a process of **endochondral ossification.** Primary ossification centers appear near the angle of each rib in the sixth week, and further ossification occurs in a distal direction. Secondary ossification centers develop in the tubercles and heads of the ribs during adolescence.

The costal processes of the cervical vertebrae give rise to the lateral boundary, and the transverse processes give rise to the medial boundary of the foramina transversaria that transmit the vertebral arteries. In the lumbar region, the costal processes become the transverse processes of the lumbar vertebrae. The costal processes of the first two or three sacral vertebrae contribute to the development of the lateral sacral mass or ala of the sacrum.

The sternum develops from a pair of longitudinal mesenchymal condensations, the **sternal bars,** that form in the ventrolateral body wall (Fig. 4-5B). As the most cranial ribs make contact with them in the seventh week, the sternal bars meet along the midline and begin to fuse. Fusion commences at the cranial end of the sternal bars and progresses caudally, finishing with the formation of the xiphoid process in the ninth week. Like the ribs, the sternal bones ossify from cartilaginous precursors. The sternal bars ossify in craniocaudal succession from the fifth month until shortly after birth, producing the definitive bones of the sternum: the manubrium, the body, and the xiphoid process.

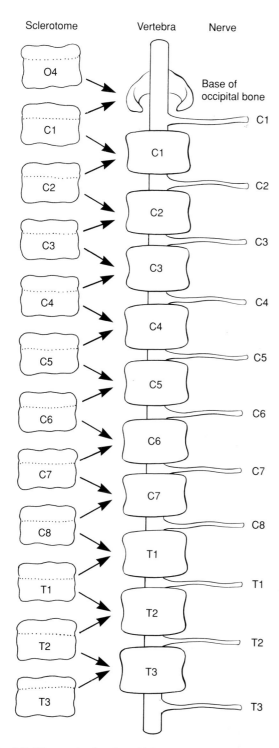

Fig. 4-3. The mechanism by which the cervical region develops eight cervical nerves but only seven cervical vertebrae. Each somite induces a ventral root to grow out from the spinal cord. When the sclerotomes recombine, however, the cranial half of the first sclerotome fuses with the occipital bone of the skull. In the thoracic, lumbar, and sacral regions, the number of spinal nerves matches the number of vertebrae.

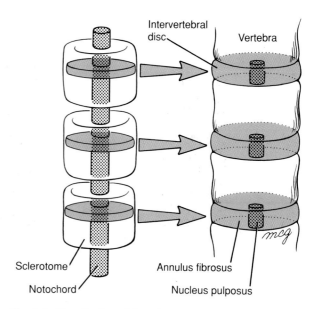

Fig. 4-4. Contribution of the sclerotome and notochord to the intervertebral disc. When the sclerotome splits, cells remaining in the plane of splitting coalesce to form the annulus fibrosus of the disc, and the notochordal cells enclosed by this structure differentiate to form the nucleus pulposus of the disc. The regions of the notochord enclosed by the developing vertebral bodies degenerate and disappear.

The myotomes and dermatomes develop at segmental levels

The portion of the somite that is translocated laterally while the sclerotome remains in its original medial location is called the **dermomyotome.** This structure quickly separates into two structures: a **dermatome** and a **myotome** (Fig. 4-6). The dermatomes with lateral plate mesoderm contribute to the dermis (including fat and connective tissue) of the neck, the back, and the ventral and lateral trunk.

The myotomes differentiate into myogenic (muscle-producing) cells. Each myotome splits into two structures: a dorsal **epimere** and a ventral **hypomere.** The epimeres give rise to the deep epaxial muscles of the back, including the erector spinae and transversospinalis groups. The hypomeres form the hypaxial muscles of the lateral and ventral body wall in the thorax and abdomen (Fig. 4-6). These include three layers of intercostal muscles in the thorax, the homologous three layers of the abdominal musculature (the external oblique, internal oblique, and transversus abdominis), and the rectus abdominis muscles that flank the ventral midline. The rectus column is usually limited to the abdominal region, but occasionally it develops on either side of the

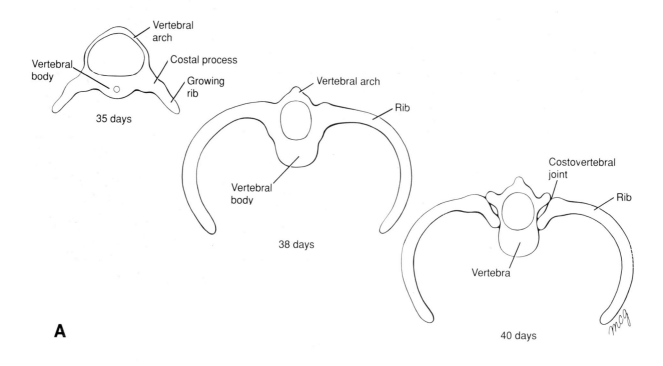

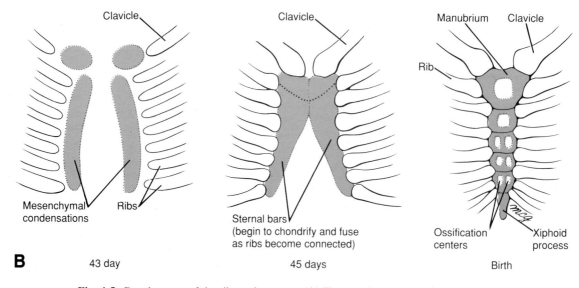

Fig. 4-5. Development of the ribs and sternum. **(A)** The costal processes of the vertebrae in the thoracic region begin to elongate in the fifth week to form ribs. Late in the sixth week, the costovertebral joints form and separate the ribs from the vertebrae. **(B)** Paired mesenchymal condensations called sternal bars form within the ventral body wall at the end of the sixth week. These bars quickly fuse together at their cranial ends while their lateral edges connect with the distal ends of the growing ribs. The sternal bars then zipper together in a craniocaudal direction. Ossification centers appear within the sternum as early as 60 days, but the xiphoid process does not ossify until birth.

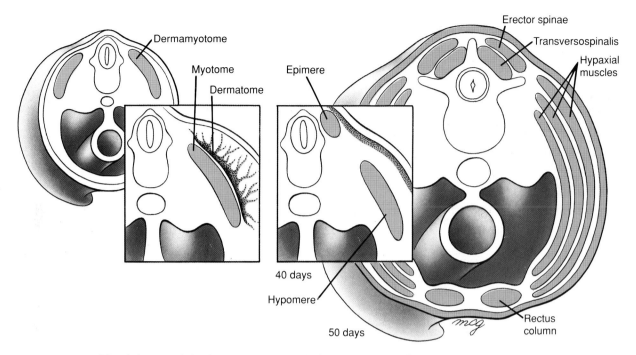

Fig. 4-6. Fate of the dermomyotome. Each dermomyotome splits into a dorsolateral dermatome and a myotome. Dermatome cells migrate to the surface ectoderm of the corresponding segmental region, where they collaborate with lateral plate mesoderm to form the dermis. Each myotome splits first into a dorsal epimere and ventral hypomere. The epimere forms deep muscles of the back. In the thoracic region, the hypomere splits into three layers of anterolateral muscles; in the abdominal region, a fourth ventral segment also differentiates and forms the rectus abdominis muscle.

sternum as a sternalis muscle. In the cervical region, hypaxial myoblasts form the strap muscles of the neck, including the geniohyoid, scalene, and infrahyoid muscles. In the lumbar region, the hypomeres form the quadratus lumborum muscles. Somitic myoblasts also invade the developing limb buds and give rise to the limb musculature (see Ch. 11).

Surprisingly, it appears that myotomes do not contribute to the formation of the tendons and internal connective tissue of the body wall muscles. Cell marking experiments indicate that these structures arise from somatopleuric lateral plate mesoderm.

The neural plate differentiates into brain and spinal cord regions and folds to form the neural tube

The future spinal cord and the divisions of the brain are apparent in the neural plate at the beginning of the fourth week

By the beginning of the fourth week, the neural plate consists of a broad cranial portion that will give rise to the brain and a narrow caudal portion that will give rise to the spinal cord. On about day 22, the cephalic end of the embryo begins to flex sharply ventrally (Fig. 4-7). This flexure marks the site of the future mesencephalon or midbrain and therefore is called the **mesencephalic flexure.** The portion of the future brain cranial to the mesencephalic flexure becomes the **prosencephalon** or forebrain, and the portion caudal to the flexure becomes the **rhombencephalon** or hindbrain. Even at this early stage of differentiation, the rhombencephalon is divided into segments by faint constrictions. These segments are called **neuromeres** or, more specifically, **rhombomeres** (see Applications to Clinical Practice in Chapter 12).

On day 22 (eight pairs of somites), the narrow caudal portion of the neural plate — the future spinal cord — represents only about 25 percent of the length of the neural plate. As somites continue to develop, however, the spinal cord region lengthens faster than the cephalic neural plate. By day 23 or 24 (12 and 20 pairs of somites, respectively), the future spinal cord occupies about 50 percent of the length of the neural plate, and by day 26 (25 pairs of somites), it occupies about 60 percent.

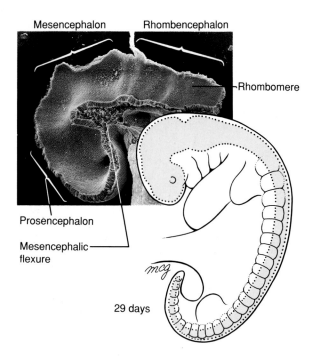

Fig. 4-7. The anlage of the central nervous system, the neural tube, is present by the end of the fourth week. It is formed by the process of neurulation described at the end of Chapter 3. Even at this early stage, the primary vesicles of the brain, two of its three flexures, and the rhombomeric subdivisions of the hindbrain can be identified. (Photo courtesy of Drs. Antone Jacobson and Patrick Tam.)

Formation of the neural tube begins on day 22 at the level of the first five somites

One of the most important events of the fourth week is the conversion of the neural plate into a **neural tube** by a process called **neurulation.** Neurulation commences as the neural plate begins to crease ventrally along its midline. This crease develops along the midline neural groove (see Ch. 3). The neural groove, which develops in response to induction by the closely apposed notochord, acts as a hinge region, and the two thick neural folds rotate around it like the leaves of a closing book (Fig. 4-8). The neural folds become concave as they rotate, so that the lateral lips of the folds meet dorsally to form a tube enclosing a **neural canal.** As the lips of the neural tube fuse, the junction between the neuroepithelium and the adjacent surface ectoderm is pulled dorsally, and the opposing margins of surface ectoderm also meet and fuse. As soon as the surface ectoderm fuses, the neural tube separates from it and sinks into the posterior body wall.

Closure of the neural tube proceeds bidirectionally, ending with closure of the cranial and caudal neuropores

The lips of the neural folds first make contact on day 22 in the area of the first five somites (Figs. 4-9 and 4-10). The newly formed neural canal communicates with the amniotic cavity at either end through large openings called the **cranial** and **caudal neuropores.** The neural folds may initially fuse at several separate points in the occipital region, but the small intervening openings rapidly fill in to produce a continuous canal. As neurulation continues, the cranial and caudal neuropores diminish in size. The cranial neuropore finally closes on day 24, and the caudal neuropore closes on day 26. Closure of the cranial neuropore is bidirectional, and final closure occurs in the area of the future forebrain. Closure of the caudal neuropore is strictly craniocaudal and finishes at the level of the second sacral segment (the level of somite 31).

The caudalmost portion of the neural tube is formed by secondary neurulation

The neural tube formed by closure of the caudal neuropore terminates at somite 31. How do the more caudal portions of the neural tube — the inferior sacral and coccygeal levels — form? Recall from Chapter 3 that gastrulation through the regressing primitive streak produces the mesodermal caudal eminence by day 20. Both experimental studies and the examination of human embryos support the hypothesis that it is the caudal eminence, rather than the neural plate, that gives rise to the caudal neural tube and to the caudal extension of the spinal cord coverings (Fig. 4-11). This process is called **secondary neurulation.** First a central mass of pluripotent tissue within the caudal eminence forms a solid **neural cord.** This cord then cavitates along its central axis, and the newly formed lumen joins with the neural canal. The formation of the caudal end of the neural tube is completed by about 8 weeks of development. The caudal extension of the dural and pial components of the spinal cord coverings, the filum terminale, is formed later by regression of the caudalmost part of the neural tube. The caudal eminence also produces the somites at the most inferior levels of the embryo.

Neural crest cells originate in the neural folds, migrate to specific locations in the body, and give rise to numerous structures

Neural crest cells detach from the lips of the neural folds during neurulation

The **neural crest** is a special population of cells that arises along the lateral margins of the neural folds. Dur-

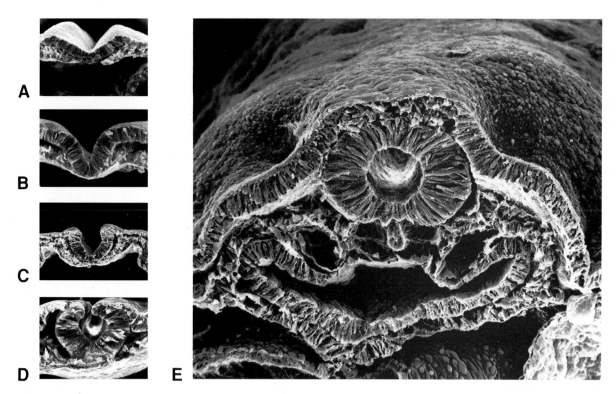

Fig. 4-8. Neurulation. **(A–C)** Neurulation begins in the occipitocervical region as the neural plate is thrown into neural folds. **(D)** The lateral edges of the neural folds meet in the midline and fuse while simultaneously detaching from the surface ectoderm. **(D, E)** These detaching edges of surface ectoderm then fuse with each other to enclose the neural tube completely. (Figs. A to D from Schoenwolf GC. 1982. On the morphogenesis of the early rudiments of the developing central nervous system. Scanning Microsc 1:289, with permission. Fig. E photo courtesy of Dr. Kathryn Tosney.)

ing neurulation, these cells detach from the neural plate and migrate to many locations in the body, where they differentiate into a remarkable variety of structures (Fig. 4-12; see also Fig. 4-14, below). This unusual tissue type first arose during the early evolution of the vertebrates.

Neural crest cells differentiate first in the mesencephalic zone of the neural folds and later in more cranial and caudal regions. In the spinal cord portion of the neural tube, the neural crest cells detach as the lateral lips of the tube fuse. Thus, detachment and migration of these neural crest cells occurs in a craniocaudal wave, beginning on day 22 at the cranial end of the spinal cord neural tube (Fig. 4-13A). Some neural crest is produced in the spinal cord neural tube even after the caudal neuropore closes on day 26. In contrast, the cephalic neural crest cells associated with the developing brain begin to detach and migrate before closure of the cranial neuropore, even while the neural folds are still widely open.

Cell tracing studies are used to study neural crest migration

The migration routes of the crest cells from various parts of the neural plate have been mapped by cell tracing studies in bird and mouse embryos (Figs. 4-12 and 4-13B). Figure 4-14 summarizes the structures derived from neural crest cells originating at various levels of the neural plate.

The cephalic neural crest forms structures of the head and neck

When the cephalic neural crest cells migrate away from the neural folds, they travel through the space just deep to the ectoderm and within the loose mesenchyme of the head and neck. Crest cells from different levels of the cephalic neural plate are trapped at specific sites, where they differentiate to form appropriate structures. Whether and to what extent the fate of a crest cell either is prede-

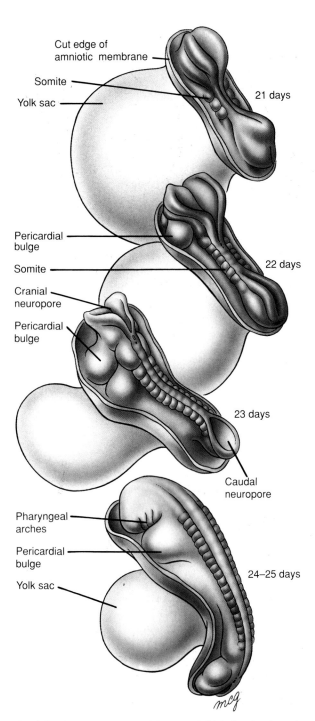

Cut edge of
amniotic membrane

Somite

Yolk sac

21 days

Pericardial
bulge

Somite

22 days

Cranial
neuropore

Pericardial
bulge

23 days

Caudal
neuropore

Pharyngeal
arches

Pericardial
bulge

Yolk sac

24–25 days

Fig. 4-9. The lateral edges of the neural folds first begin to fuse in the occipitocervical region on day 22, leaving the cranial and caudal neuropores open at each end. The neural tube increases in length as it zippers up both cranially and caudally, and the neuropores become progressively smaller. The cranial neuropore closes on day 24, and the caudal neuropore closes on day 26.

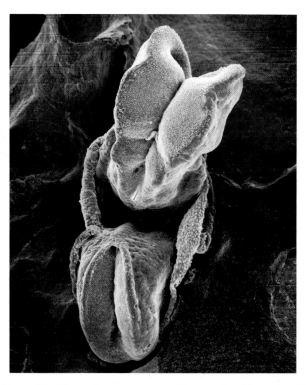

Fig. 4-10. This embryo is comparable to a day 22 or day 23 human embryo. The cranial and caudal neuropores are both open. (Photo courtesy of Dr. T. H. Shepard.)

termined before the crest cell leaves the neural fold or is determined by cues along the route of migration and at the site of differentiation is a major topic of neural crest research (see Chs. 12 and 13 and the Applications to Clinical Practice of Ch. 5).

Neural crest cells from the mesencephalon and caudal prosencephalon regions give rise to the parasympathetic ganglion of cranial nerve III, connective tissue around the developing eyes and optic nerves, to the muscles of the pupil and ciliary body in the optic globe, and to the head mesenchyme cranial to the level of the mesencephalon (see Chs. 12 and 13). Neural crest gives rise to the pia mater and arachnoid of the occipital region; the dura mater is thought to arise largely from paraxial mesoderm.

Neural crest cells from the mesencephalon and rhombencephalon regions also give rise to structures in the developing **pharyngeal arches** of the head and neck (see Ch. 12 and the Applications to Clinical Practice section in this chapter). These structures include cartilaginous rudiments of several bones of the nose, face, middle ear, and neck. The mesencephalon and rhombencephalon crest cells form the dermis, smooth muscle, and fat of the face, dermal bones of the skull, and ventral neck and the odontoblasts of the developing teeth. The rhombencephalon neural crest also contributes some of the cranial nerve ganglia (see Ch. 13).

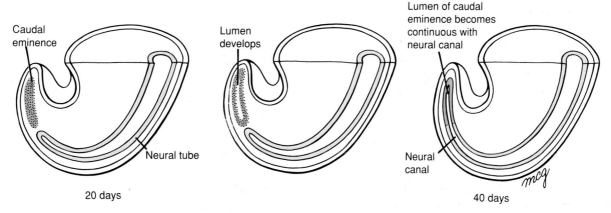

Fig. 4-11. Formation of the neural tube inferior to the second sacral level by secondary neurulation. Mesoderm invading this region during gastrulation condenses into a solid rod called the caudal eminence, which later develops a lumen. At the end of the sixth week, this structure fuses with the neural tube.

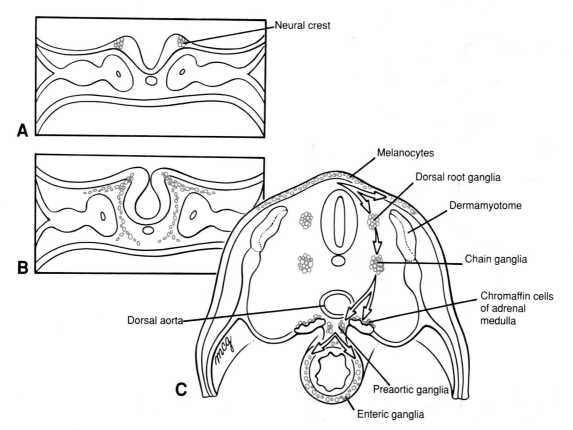

Fig. 4-12. Neural crest cells arising at the lateral edges of the neural plate detach during neurulation and migrate throughout the embryo to form many different tissues.

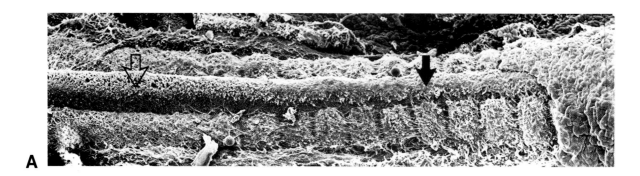

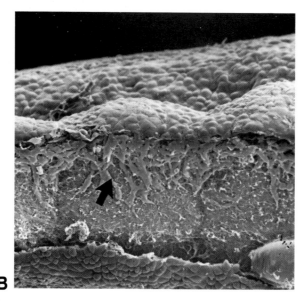

Fig. 4-13. (A) This scanning micrograph illustrates the craniocaudal sequence of release of neural crest cells from the neural tube. At this stage of development, neural crest cells have already begun to migrate from the neural tube in more cranial regions (solid arrow) but have not yet separated from the neural tube in more caudal regions (open arrow). **(B)** High magnification scanning electron micrograph showing neural crest cells migrating onto the surface of the somite. Their migration paths become segmental as they approach the boundary between the sclerotome and the dermomyotome. (Fig. A from Tosney K. 1978. The early migration of neural crest cells in the trunk region of the avian embryo. Dev Biol 62:317, with permission. Fig. B from Tosney K. 1988. Somites and axon guidance. Scanning Microsc 2:427, with permission.)

Occipital and spinal neural crest also produce major components of the peripheral nervous system

The peripheral nervous system of the neck, trunk, and limbs includes the following three types of peripheral neurons: the peripheral sensory neurons, the cell bodies of which reside in the dorsal root ganglia, and the parasympathetic and sympathetic peripheral motor neurons, the cell bodies of which reside, respectively, in the sympathetic and parasympathetic ganglia. All three types of peripheral neurons, plus their associated glia, are derived from neural crest cells. This chapter describes the origin of these structures; their further development is covered in Chapter 5.

The dorsal root ganglia are derived from spinal neural crest. Some of the neural crest cells arising from the spinal neural tube come to rest in the space between the dorsal neural tube and the developing somites, where they aggregate to form small clumps in register with the somites (Fig. 4-12). These clumps then differentiate into the segmental **dorsal root ganglia** of the spinal nerves, which

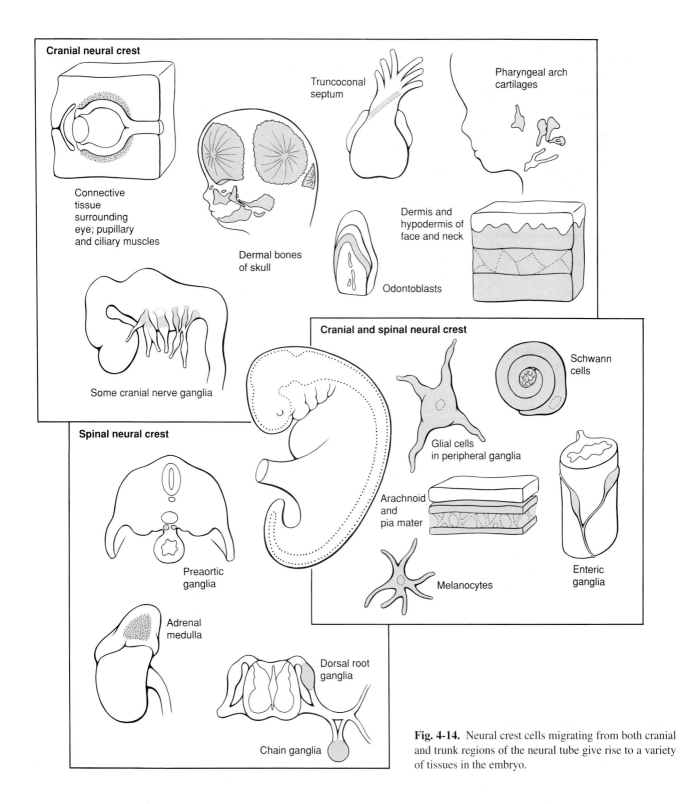

Fig. 4-14. Neural crest cells migrating from both cranial and trunk regions of the neural tube give rise to a variety of tissues in the embryo.

house the sensory neurons that conduct impulses to the spinal cord from end organs in the viscera, body wall, and extremities. Experiments with the quail-chick chimera system demonstrate that most of the cells in each ganglion are derived from the neural crest originating at the correspond-

ing level, although some may originate in neural crest adjacent to the caudal portion of the preceding somite.

It has been demonstrated that migrating neural crest cells prefer to travel through the cranial half of the sclerotomes. Experimental evidence also indicates that the survival and differentiation of the dorsal root ganglion anlagen may depend on a small protein, **brain-derived neural growth factor (BDNF),** which is secreted by the adjacent neural tube.

A pair of dorsal root ganglia develops at every segmental level except the first cervical and the second and third coccygeal levels (Figs. 4-12, 4-13B, and 4-15). Thus, there are 7 pairs of cervical, 12 thoracic, 5 lumbar, 5 sacral, and 1 coccygeal pair of dorsal root ganglia. The first pair of cervical dorsal root ganglia (adjacent to the second cervical somite) appears on day 28, and the others form in craniocaudal succession over the next few days.

Postganglionic parasympathetic neurons of the viscera are derived from the occipitocervical and sacral neural crests. Some peripheral motor neurons of the "two-neuron" parasympathetic autonomic nervous system arise from neural crest cells that migrate into the walls of the developing viscera, such as the heart, stomach, and bladder. The cell bodies of these neurons reside in the peripheral **parasympathetic ganglia,** which provide parasympathetic motor innervation of the adjacent viscera. Crest cells originating from the occipitocervical region of the neural tube (the "vagal region") migrate in the gut wall mesenchyme to innervate all regions of the gut tube from the esophagus to the rectum. The parasympathetic ganglion cells in the most inferior regions of the gut, however, have a dual origin: some arise from the occipitocervical neural crest, but others arise from the sacral neural crest.

The peripheral parasympathetic ganglia in the wall of the gut tube and its derivatives (collectively called **enteric ganglia**) may be connected to the central nervous system by axons that course either in the vagus nerve (cranial nerve X) or in pelvic splanchnic nerves from sacral levels 2, 3, and 4. The parasympathetic system is active during periods of relaxation and stimulates the visceral organs to carry out their routine functions of housekeeping and digestion. Because the proximal neurons of the system are located in the cranial and sacral regions of the central nervous system, the parasympathetic system is called a **craniosacral system** (see Ch. 5).

The sympathetic chain ganglia are innervated by preganglionic sympathetic thoracolumbar fibers. Some spinal cord neural crest cells migrate to a zone just ventral

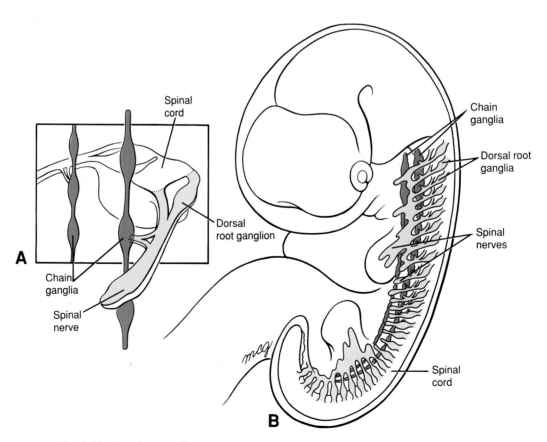

Fig. 4-15. Neural crest cells produce chain ganglia and dorsal root ganglia at almost every spinal segment.

to the future dorsal root ganglia, where they form a series of condensations that develop into the **chain ganglia** of the sympathetic autonomic system (Figs. 4-12C, 4-15). In the thoracic, lumbar, and sacral regions, one pair of chain ganglia forms in register with each pair of somites. In the cervical region, however, only three larger chain ganglia develop, and the coccygeal region has only a single chain ganglion, which forms at the first coccygeal level. Quail-chick cell marking experiments indicate that the neural crest cells that give rise to the chain ganglia originate along the corresponding level of the neural tube. Unlike the dorsal root ganglia, the chain ganglia do not depend on BDNF for survival, but they may depend on other growth factors such as **insulinlike growth factor.**

The neurons that develop in the chain ganglia become the peripheral neurons of the two-neuron sympathetic system. The sympathetic system provides autonomic motor innervation to most of the same structures as the parasympathetic system and exerts control over involuntary functions such as heartbeat, glandular secretions, and intestinal movements. By and large, however, the sympathetic system is activated during conditions of "fight or flight" and therefore has effects opposite to those of the parasympathetic system. Like the parasympathetic system, the sympathetic system consists of "two-neuron" pathways: the viscera are innervated by axons from the peripheral sympathetic neurons, which in turn receive axons from central sympathetic motor neurons in the spinal cord. These central sympathetic motor neurons are located at all 12 thoracic levels and at the first 2 lumbar levels. For that reason, the sympathetic system (central and peripheral) is called a **thoracolumbar system.**

Not all peripheral sympathetic neurons are located in the chain ganglia. The peripheral ganglia of some specialized sympathetic pathways develop from neural crest cells that congregate next to major branches of the dorsal aorta (Fig. 4-12C and see Ch. 5). One pair of these **prevertebral** or **preaortic ganglia** originates from the cervical neural crest and forms at the base of the celiac artery. Other, more diffuse ganglia develop in association with the superior mesenteric artery, the renal arteries, and the inferior mesenteric artery. These are formed by thoracic and lumbar neural crest cells.

The spinal cord neural crest forms a variety of non-neuronal structures in the body

Spinal neural crest cells in humans form the inner and middle meningeal coverings of the spinal cord (the pia mater and arachnoid, respectively), as well as glial cells of the ganglia derived from the spinal neural crest (Fig. 4-14). Some of the neural crest cells may differentiate into Schwann cells, which form the myelin sheaths (neuri-

lemma) of peripheral nerves. Spinal neural crest cells also differentiate into the neurosecretory chromaffin cells of the adrenal medulla and into neurosecretory cells of the heart and lungs. The neural crest also gives rise to the melanocytes (pigment cells) of the skin and contributes to the outflow tracts of the heart (see Ch. 7).

The neurons, glia, and ependyma of the central nervous system differentiate from the nerve epithelium adjacent to the neural canal

Neuroblasts appear in the rhombencephalic region on day 24

Cytodifferentiation of the neural tube commences in the rhombencephalic region just after the occipitocervical neural folds fuse and proceeds cranially and caudally as the tube zippers up. The precursors of most of the cell types of the future central nervous system — the neurons, some types of glial cells, and the ependymal cells that line the central canal of the spinal cord and the cerebral ventricles of the brain — are produced by proliferation in the layer of neuroepithelial cells that immediately surrounds the neural canal (Fig. 4-16). This layer of proliferating cells is called the **ventricular layer** of the differentiating neural tube. The first wave of cells produced in the ventricular layer consists of the **neuroblasts,** which will give rise to the neurons of the central nervous system. These neuroblasts migrate peripherally to establish a second layer, the **mantle layer** (Fig. 4-16A, C). This neuron-containing layer develops into the gray matter of the central nervous system. The neuronal processes that sprout from the mantle layer neurons grow peripherally to establish a third layer, the **marginal layer,** which contains no neuronal cell bodies and becomes the white matter of the central nervous system.

Glioblasts and ependymal cells are produced after the formation of neuroblasts ceases

As soon as the neuroepithelial layer lining the neural canal ceases to produce neuroblasts, it begins to produce a new cell type, the **glioblast** (Fig. 4-16A). These cells differentiate into a variety of types of glial cells, including **astrocytes** and **oligodendrocytes.** The glia provides metabolic and structural support to the neurons of the central nervous system. Finally, the neuroepithelial layer differentiates in place to produce the specialized **ependymal cells** that line the cerebral ventricles and the central canal of the spinal cord (Fig. 4-16A, C). Elaborations of the ependyma are responsible for producing the cerebrospinal fluid (CSF), which fills the cerebral ventricles,

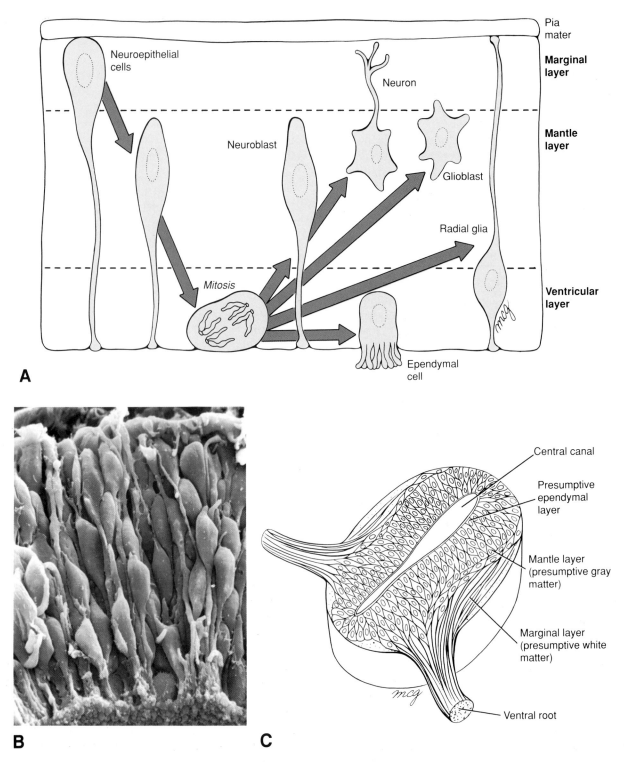

A

B

C

Fig. 4-16. Cytodifferentiation of the neural tube. **(A, B)** Neuroepithelial cells within the primitive neural tube elongate just before mitosis. Initial waves of mitosis and differentiation form first the neuroblasts, which will become the neurons of the central nervous system. **(A, C)** As neurons form, the neural tube becomes stratified into a ventricular layer (adjacent to the neural canal), a mantle layer (containing neuronal cell bodies), and a marginal layer (containing nerve fibers). Subsequent waves of mitosis and differentiation produce the glioblasts, which form several types of supporting cells of the central nervous system. The radial glia may provide pathways for neuroblast migration within the developing neural tube. (Fig. A modified from Rakic P. 1982. Early developmental events: cell lineages, acquisition of neuronal positions, and areal and laminar development. Neurosci Res Prog Bull 20:439, with permission. Fig B photo courtesy of Dr. Kathryn Tosney.)

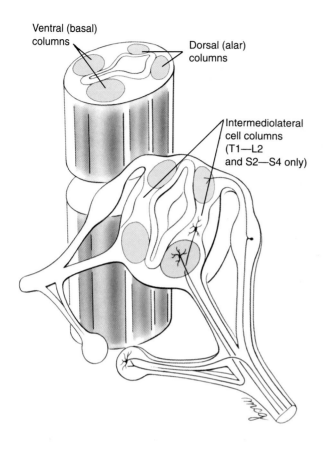

Ventral (basal) columns

Dorsal (alar) columns

Intermediolateral cell columns (T1—L2 and S2—S4 only)

Fig. 4-17. Neurons within the mantle layer of the neural tube become organized into two ventral motor (basal) columns and two dorsal sensory (alar) columns throughout most of the spinal cord and hindbrain. Intermediolateral cell columns also form at spinal levels T1–L2 and S2–S4.

the central canal of the spinal cord, and the subarachnoid space that surrounds the central nervous system. The CSF is under pressure and thus provides a fluid jacket that protects and supports the brain.

Dorsal and ventral columns begin to form in the mantle layer of the spinal cord at the end of the fourth week

Starting at the end of the fourth week, the neuroblasts in the mantle layer of the spinal cord become organized into four columns that run the length of the cord: a pair of **dorsal** or **alar columns** and a pair of **ventral** or **basal columns** (Fig. 4-17). Laterally, the alar and basal columns are separated by a groove called the **sulcus limitans;** dorsally and ventrally they are separated by acute thinnings of the neural tissue called, respectively, the **roof plate** and the

floor plate. The cells of the ventral columns become the **somatic motor neurons** of the spinal cord and innervate somatic motor structures such as the voluntary (striated) muscles of the body wall and extremities. The cells of the dorsal columns develop into **association neurons,** which will interconnect the motor neurons of the ventral columns with neuronal processes that soon grow into the cord from the sensory neurons of the dorsal root ganglia. In most regions of the cord — at all 12 thoracic levels, at lumbar levels L1 and L2, and at sacral levels S2 through S4 — the neuroblasts in more dorsal regions of the basal columns segregate to form distinct **intermediolateral cell columns** (Fig. 4-17). The thoracic and lumbar intermediolateral cell columns contain the central autonomic motor neurons of the sympathetic system, whereas the intermediolateral cell columns in the sacral region contain central autonomic motor neurons of the parasympathetic system.

APPLICATIONS TO CLINICAL PRACTICE

Vertebral development is specified by *HOX* genes

Evidence of the segmental development of the human trunk is revealed by the segmental organization of the vertebral column, the segmental spinal nerves, the segmental organization of striated musculature (particularly in the thorax), and the segmental arrangement of the blood supply of the trunk. While the development of individual segments is similar, differences along the trunk's longitudinal axis are obvious. For example, design of the cervical vertebrae facilitate their functions as a mobile pedestal for the head. The less flexible thoracic region is characterized by ribs, which serve as protection for thoracic vital organs and in respiration. The massive lumbar vertebrae and the sacrum support the trunk and locomotion.

The developmental mechanism by which these differences in morphology arise requires the segment-specific expression of a family of genes called *HOX* genes. In humans, there are four clusters of these genes, which are derived from ancesters common to the well-studied *Homc* cluster of homeotic genes in the fruitfly *Drosophila* (Fig. 4-18). The most cranial expression of each *Hox* gene in mammalian embryos typically occurs at approximate boundaries between specific somites (boundaries of *Hom-c* expression occur at segmental boundaries in fruitfly embryos), resulting in unique combinations of *HOX* gene expression within virtually every segment of the trunk (Fig. 4-18). Thus, it has been suggested that the *HOX* genes (as postulated for the *Homc* genes by Edward Lewis) may specify segment diversity through a **combinatorial code** of *HOX* gene expression.

Disruption of *HOX* gene expression may be the basis for a class of human congenital disease

Evidence for disrupted expression of *HOX* genes in some congenital malformations of the vertebral column in humans is provided by transgenic mouse studies in which specific *Hox* genes are either "knocked out" or expressed in ectopic locations in gain-of-function mutants. By so changing the combinatorial code of a given somite, the particular segment's developmental identity is altered to one similar to that of the segment normally expressing that code. Such a transformation is called a **homeotic transformation.** For example, a null mutation of *Hoxc-8* leads to the transformation of the first lumbar vertebra to a "14th thoracic" vertebra possessing a rib

(the mouse normally has 13 thoracic vertebrae; Fig. 4-19). Similarly, a null mutation of *Hoxa-4* results in transformation of the third cervical vertebra to one reminiscent of the second and the seventh to one more like the sixth. Conversely, a gain-of-function transgenic mouse in which *Hoxa-7* is expressed in regions cranial to its normal cranial boundary at the third thoracic vertebra results in transformation of the first cervical vertebra to one that looks like the second and the second to one more similar to the third. Interestingly, an extra atavistic (a structure in a contemporary organism recalling a characteristic present in a remote ancestor) cervical vertebra similar to the **proatlas** of reptiles appears just cranial to the former atlas. Similar effects are produced by the ectopic application of **retinoic acid,** suggesting that the effect of this teratogen on development in humans may be mediated, in part, by disruptions of the retinoic acid-sensitive *HOX* genes (see Applications to Clinical Practice of Chs. 11 and 12). Moreover, while the mechanism in humans is not understood, it is possible that disruptions of *HOX* gene expression may underlie the vertebral homeotic transformations characterized by the development of cervical or lumbar ribs.

The neural tube, vertebrae, striated muscles, and dermis arise through a complex interactive inductive cascade

Induction of the notocord, neural tube, somite, and surface ectoderm appears to require antagonistic and/or synergistic interactions of **dorsalizing** and **ventralizing factors** similar to those that underlie development of the primitive streak and production of mesoderm and endoderm (see Applications to Clinical Practice section of Ch. 3). Initially, the notochord acts as an **inducing tissue** by secreting a small peptide, homologous to the *Drosophila* hedgehog peptides called **sonic hedgehog (Shh).** This ventralizing signal induces the **responding tissue,** the presumptive floor plate of the neural tube, to differentiate and to synthesize Shh as well (Fig. 4-20). These enhanced signals then result in expression of floor plate-specific proteins like FP1, FP2, and SC1. Meanwhile, dorsalizing signals from the surface ectoderm induce the expression of genes like *Pax-3* and *Pax-7,* neural crest cell markers, the antigen AC4, and cellular retinoic acid-binding protein (CRABP) within the dorsal neural tube.

Shh produced by the notochord and ventral neural tube also induces the ventromedial region of the somite to form the sclerotome, which specifically expresses sclero-

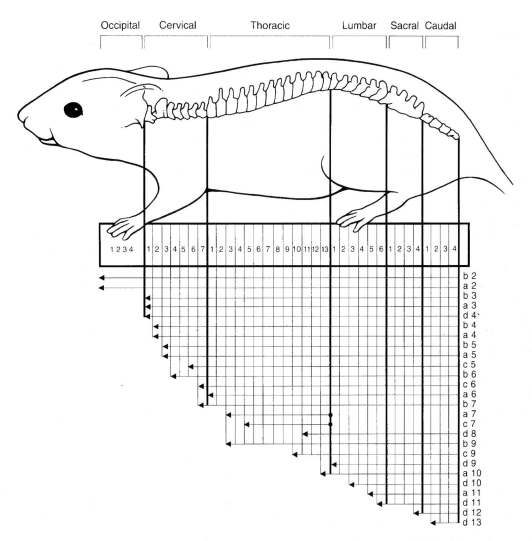

Fig. 4-18. Cranial expression boundaries of *Hox* genes in mice (b2–d13) parallel their sequence on the chromosomes and sensitivities to retinoic acid (see also Fig. 3-17). The resulting distribution creates specific combinatorial codes that specify development of individual somites or small groups of adjacent somites. It is not possible, however, to determine whether cranial expression boundaries occur precisely between somites or between the recombined caudal and cranial halves of the sclerotomes (prevertebrae) or both, at different times. (From Hunt P, Krumlauf R. 1992. *Hox* codes and positional specification in vertebrate embryonic axes. Annu Rev Cell Biol 8:227, with permission.)

tome marker genes such as *M-twist* and *Pax-1*. Meanwhile, the surface ectoderm and dorsal neural tube together induce development of the dermomyotome through signaling of the dorsolateral somite with extracellular matrix proteins of the *Wnt* gene family. As a consequence, the presumptive myotome expresses the muscle-specific markers N-*myc* and myogenin, and the presumptive dermatome expresses the dermatome-specific markers *gMHox* and *dermo-1*. It is likely that the interaction of these ventralizing and dorsalizing signals is required for

the full range of somite differentiation in ventral, dorsal, and intermediate regions.

Mutations of regulatory genes that control vertebrae and spinal cord development underlie the pathogenesis of some neural tube defects in humans

Approximately 400,000 infants are born worldwide with neural tube defects each year. Approximately 4,000

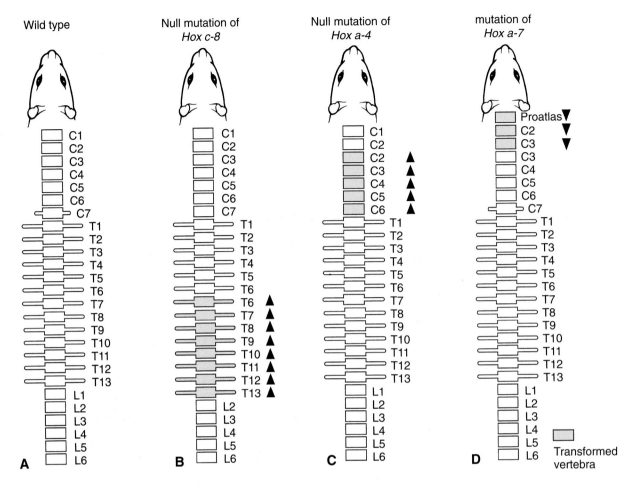

Fig. 4-19. Homeotic transformation of vertebral segments in loss-of-function and gain-of-function *Hox* genes in mice. Null mutations of *Hoxc-8* (compare **B** to **A**) and *Hoxa-4* (compare **C** to **A**) cranialize vertebrae within their normal expression domains. A gain-of-function mutation of *Hoxa-7* caudalizes vertebrae outside its normal expression domain (compare **D** to **A**). (Modified from Conlon RA. 1995. Retinoic acid and pattern formation in vertebrates. TIG 11:314, with permission.)

fetuses are affected in the United States annually; 2,500 are born, while 1,500 are aborted.

These defects, also generally called **spina bifida** or **spinal dysraphism,** range from mild to severe and typically result from a disruption of neural tube closure and/or vertebral arch development. In the mildest form, called **spina bifida occulta,** a single vertebral arch may fail to form with no significant defect of the spinal cord (Fig. 4-21A). In this case, the presence of the open vertebral arch may be revealed by a small dimple, a nevis, or a tuft of hair. In a more severe defect, called **meningocele,** two or more vertebral arches may be affected, leading to protrusion of the meninges onto the surface of the back (Fig. 4-21B). If neural tissue should also be contained within the sac, however, the malformation is called a **meningomye-**

locele (Fig. 4-21C, D). In the most severe cases, the neural tube may fail to close and to separate from the surface ectoderm, resulting in the presence of undifferentiated neural tissue exposed at the surface. In the case of failure of the cranial neural tube to close, this defect is called **anencephaly** or **craniorachischisis** (Fig. 4-21E). Babies born with this malformation may live for a few hours or a few days. Other, more caudal regions of the cranial neural tube may also be affected (4-21F). While the analogous defect of caudal spinal cord development, **myeloschisis,** is not always fatal, like the more severe cases of meningomyelocele, this condition is difficult to manage because of caudal spinal cord and nerve dysfunction.

In reviewing the description of neural tube and sclerotome induction in the paragraphs above, it would seem

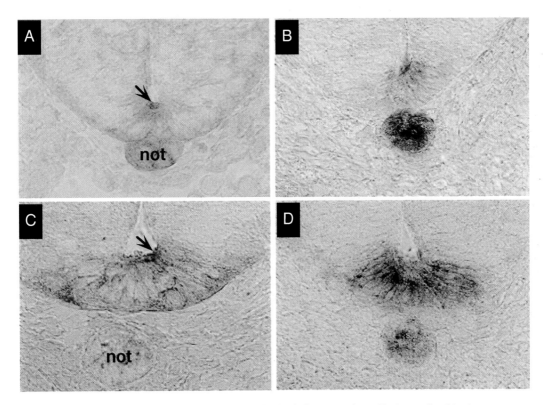

Fig. 4-20. Early expression of Shh mRNA in the 9-day postcoitum (dpc) notochord is shown by blue stain with in situ hybridization technique **(B)** while immunocytochemistry (light brown stain) shows Shh peptides in notochord and floor plate of neural tube **(A, B).** At later stage (9.5 dpc) the floor plate also transcribes Shh mRNA **(D)** and expresses Shh peptides **(C, D).** (Modified from Marti E, Takada R, Bumcrot DA, Sasaki H, McMahon A. 1995. Distribution of sonic hedgehog peptides in the developing chick and mouse embryo. Development 121:2537, with permission.)

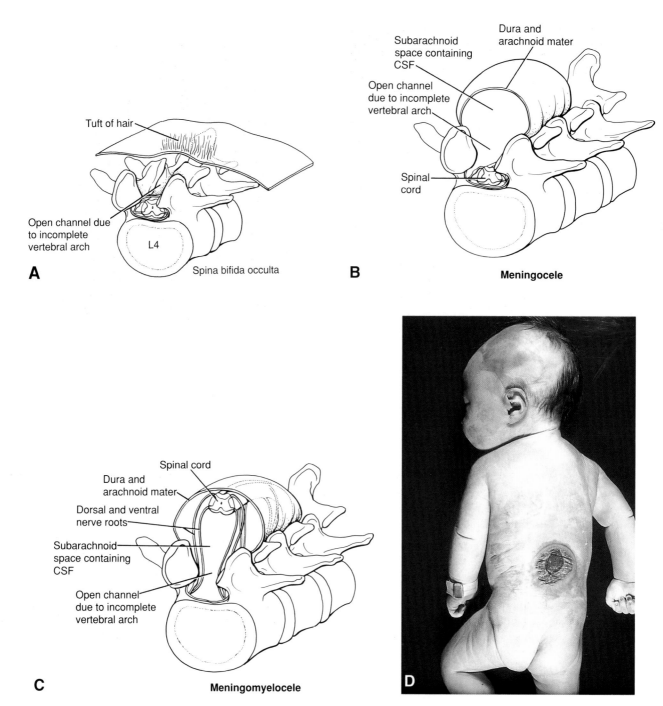

Fig. 4-21. **(A)** Spina bifida occulta may involve minor anomalies of neural arch formation and may not result in malformations of the neural tube. This condition often occurs in the midsacral region and may be revealed by a small dimple, tuft of hair, or nevus overlying the defective vertebra. Defective development of neural arches may result in formation of a cyst or cele. This cyst is called a meningocele if it includes dura and arachnoid only **(B)** or a meningomyelocele if it also contains meninges and a portion of the spinal cord and associated spinal nerves **(C)**. Meningomyelocele in newborn **(D)**. The spinal cord protrudes into the transparent meningeal sac (cele) in the lumbar region. (Photo courtesy of Children's Hospital Medical Center, Cincinnati, OH.) *(Figure continues.)*

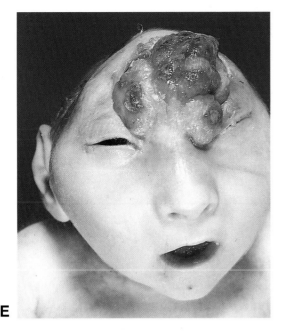

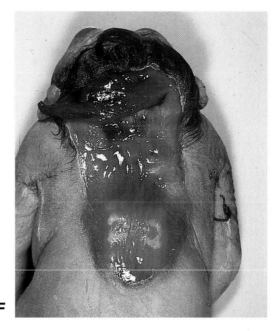

E

F

Fig. 4-21. *(Continued)* Anomalies resulting from failure of neurulation. **(E)** Although the neural folds may fail to neurulate in almost any region, the most frequent site is the cranial neuropore, resulting in the condition of craniorachischisis or anencephaly. **(F)** Occasionally, more caudal regions of the neural tube may fail to form and differentiate, as in this case of inionschisis. (Photos in Figs. E and F courtesy of Children's Hospital Medical Center, Cincinnati, Ohio.)

possible that neural tube defects could result from disruption of regulatory genes critical to normal development. Indeed, a well-described neural tube defect of the mouse called **splotch** suffers from a mutation of the regulatory gene *Pax-3.* More recently, it has been shown that one class of neural tube defects in humans, similar to those of the mouse splotch mutant called **Waardenburg type I syndrome** also results from mutation of *Pax-3.* Nonetheless it has been difficult to establish linkage between other familial neural tube defects and *Pax-3,* suggesting that other causes of neural tube defects may be more significant

in humans. A rare, autosomal recessive condition called **Meckel syndrome** and the autosomal dominant syndrome **Brachydactyly syndrome** may also exhibit craniorachischisis, but the identity of the genes have not been determined. Alternatively, several teratogens have also been correlated with spina bifida in humans, including valproic acid, maternal diabetes, and hyperthermia. It has also become apparent that disruption of folate metabolism may lead to spina bifida, and it has been recommended that the daily diet of pregnant mothers should include 0.4 mg of folic acid to reduce the risk of neural tube defects.

5

Development of the Peripheral Nervous System

Integration of the Developing Nervous System;
Innervation of Motor and Sensory End Organs

SUMMARY

The nervous system is comprised of complex networks of neuronal cell bodies and axons that carry information from peripheral sensory receptors to the central nervous system, which integrates, processes, and stores it and then returns motor impulses to various effectors of the body. The peripheral nervous system and its central pathways are traditionally divided into two systems. The somatic nervous system carries conscious sensations and innervates voluntary (striated) muscles of the body. The visceral nervous system controls most of the involuntary, visceral activities of the body through activities of its visceral sensory component and its motor component, which is called the autonomic nervous system. The autonomic system is comprised of two divisions, the parasympathetic system, which promotes visceral activities during periods of peace and relaxation, and the sympathetic system which controls the involuntary activities that occur during periods of stressful "fight or flight." Neurons that comprise the somatic and visceral nervous systems are formed from three embryonic tissues:

1. Neurons of the brain and spinal cord arise from the neuroepithelium of the neural tube itself.

2. Neural crest cells migrate from the lateral edges of the neural folds and aggregate to form the paired peripheral chain and prevertebral ganglia of the sympathetic system and the sensory dorsal root ganglia. Neural crest cells from forebrain, midbrain, and hindbrain contribute to formation of the cranial ganglia (see Ch. 13), and neural crest cells from the hindbrain migrate to the viscera to form the numerous scattered ganglia that constitute the peripheral parasympathetic ganglia of the trunk.

3. In the case of some cranial ganglia, neurons arise from ectodermal placodes (see Ch. 13).

The migration of neural crest cells that form the peripheral ganglia and the pathfinding behavior of neuronal growth cones that guide the axons that wire the scattered ganglia and end organs of the peripheral nervous system together are truly remarkable. Appropriate targeting of these structures requires the actions of attractants called tropic substances, the activities of trophic substances that ensure survival of specific elements along specific migration pathways and the contact guidance or chemoaffinity of the substrate. For example, the sclerotome provides a pathway for neural crest cells and guidance of motor axon growth cones from the ventral columns of the spinal cord, resulting in alignment of dorsal and ventral roots of the incipient spinal nerves.

Since many of the components of the peripheral nervous system arise through complex migrations of neural crest cells, the behavior of these cells is especially prone to perturbations resulting in congenital disease. Several such diseases, including Hirschsprung's disease, Waardenburg type 1 and Waardenburg type 2 syndromes, and piebaldism, are discussed in the Applications to Clinical Practice Section of this chapter. Other neural crest disruptions affect heart development (Ch. 7), while some result in craniofacial anomalies (Ch. 12).

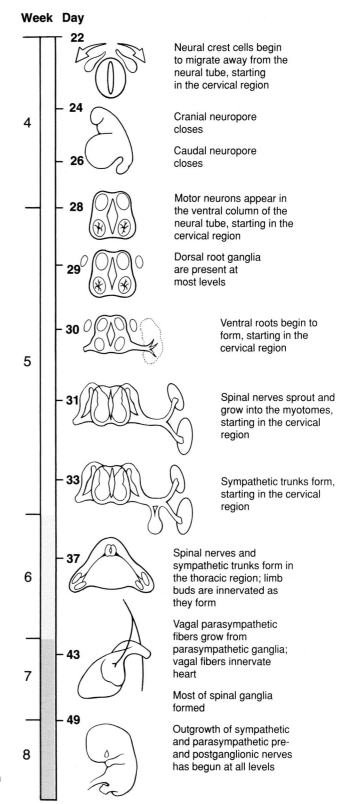

Week Day

22 Neural crest cells begin to migrate away from the neural tube, starting in the cervical region

4

24 Cranial neuropore closes

26 Caudal neuropore closes

28 Motor neurons appear in the ventral column of the neural tube, starting in the cervical region

29 Dorsal root ganglia are present at most levels

30 Ventral roots begin to form, starting in the cervical region

5

31 Spinal nerves sprout and grow into the myotomes, starting in the cervical region

33 Sympathetic trunks form, starting in the cervical region

37 Spinal nerves and sympathetic trunks form in the thoracic region; limb buds are innervated as they form

6

43 Vagal parasympathetic fibers grow from parasympathetic ganglia; vagal fibers innervate heart

7 Most of spinal ganglia formed

49 Outgrowth of sympathetic and parasympathetic pre- and postganglionic nerves has begun at all levels

8

Timeline. Development of the peripheral nervous system from the fourth to the eighth week.

Axons are guided to their targets by apical growth cones

As development proceeds, the sensory and motor neurons of the brain become interconnected in functional patterns, and axons grow out of the CNS and ganglia to innervate appropriate **target organs (end organs).** Axons travel to their target structures through the active locomotion of an apical structure called a **growth cone** (Fig. 5-1; see also Fig. 13-21). The growth cone, which moves by means of filopodia, guides the axon to its destination by sensing molecular markers that designate the correct route. This activity of the growth cone is called **pathfinding.** Once the growth cone reaches its target, it halts and forms a synapse. Somatic motor and sensory fibers synapse directly with their end organs. The axons of central autonomic neurons, in contrast, terminate in peripheral autonomic ganglia where they synapse with the peripheral neuron of the two-neuron autonomic pathway.

Numerous mechanisms have been proposed to explain the ability of neurons to establish correct connections with each other and with end organs. It has been suggested, for example, that at the appropriate time during development the end organ secretes either a **tropic substance** that attracts the correct growth cones or a **trophic substance** that supports the viability of the growth cones that happen to take the right path. Examples of tropic substances are **netrin-1** and **netrin-2.** These laminin-related proteins are implicated in the guidance of spinal cord **commissural axons** along a pathway from the dorsal cord to ventral floor plate cells. **Netrin** has also been implicated in the guidance of retinal axons. Examples of trophic substances include the brain-derived neural growth factor (BDNF) and insulin-like growth factor (IGF), molecules that support the viability of appropriately situated axons or neuronal cell bodies.

According to other theories, the growth cone may be guided by adhering to special guidance structures in the extracellular matrix. According to the **contact guidance theory,** the growing axon tip is guided by the physical orientation of molecules in the extracellular matrix. According to the somewhat different **chemoaffinity hypothesis,** the growth cone exhibits differential adherence to molecules that are specifically distributed in the extracellular matrix, such as fibronectin, laminin, and neural cell adhesion molecule (NCAM).

It is also likely that the first or **"pioneer"** growth cones to traverse a route establish a pathway that is used by later growing axons. This mechanism would account for the formation of nerves, in which many axons travel together.

Ventral column motor axons are the first to sprout from the spinal cord

The first axons to emerge from the spinal cord are produced by somatic motor neurons in the ventral gray columns. These fibers appear in the cervical region on about day 30 (Fig. 5-2), and others sprout in a craniocaudal wave down the spinal cord.

The ventral motor axons initially leave the spinal cord as a continuous broad band. As they grow toward the sclerotomes, however, they rapidly condense to form discrete segmental nerves. Although these axons will eventually synapse with muscles derived from the developing myotomes, their initial guidance apparently depends only on the sclerotomes and not on myotomal or dermatomal elements of the somite. Like neural crest cells, the ventral column axons prefer to migrate within the cranial portion of each sclerotome. As a result, these growing axons pass close to the dorsal root ganglion at each level.

The pioneer axons that initially sprout from the cord are soon joined by more ventral column motor axons, and the growing bundle is now called a **ventral root** (Fig. 5-2). At spinal levels T1 through L2, the ventral root is also joined by axons from the sympathetic motor neurons developing in the intermediolateral cell columns at these levels (Fig. 5-2).

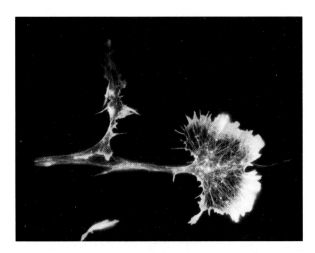

Fig. 5-1. Axonal growth cone. The nerve cell body is at the left. The actin filaments in the fan-shaped growth cone are stained with rhodamine-labeled phalloidin. Rhodamine is a fluorescent molecule, and phalloidin (the toxin in the poisonous green fungus *Amanita phalloides*) binds strongly to actin filaments. (From Bridgeman PC, Dailey ME. 1989. The organization of myosin and actin in rapid frozen nerve growth cones. J Cell Biol 108:95, with permission.)

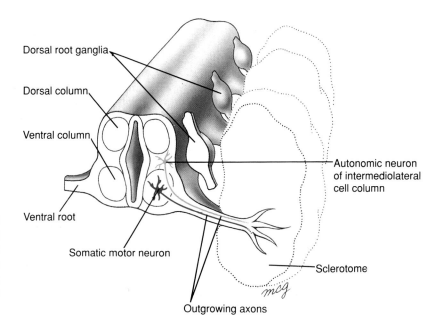

Fig. 5-2. Outgrowth of the ventral roots and formation of the dorsal root ganglia. Axons growing from ventral column motor neurons at each segmental level of the spinal cord are guided by the superior part of the sclerotome to form a ventral root. Dorsal root ganglia form in the same plane.

Somatic and autonomic motor fibers combine with sensory fibers to form spinal nerves

As the tip of each ventral root approaches its corresponding dorsal root ganglion, the neurons in the dorsal root ganglion begin to sprout axons. Each of these neurons has a branch that grows medially toward the dorsal column of the spinal cord and a branch that joins the ventral root and grows toward the periphery to innervate the end organ (Fig. 5-3). Collectively, the dorsal root ganglion plus the

rami (branches) that connect it to the spinal cord and the ventral root are called the **dorsal root.** The medially growing dorsal root fibers penetrate the dorsal columns of the spinal cord and synapse there with the developing **association neurons** (Fig. 5-3). These association neurons, in turn, sprout axons that either synapse with autonomic motor neurons in the intermediolateral cell columns or with somatic motor neurons in the ventral columns or else ascend to higher levels in the spinal cord in the form of **tracts.** The axons of some association neurons synapse with motor neurons on the same or **ipsilateral** side of the spinal cord,

Fig. 5-3. Once the ventral roots are formed, sensory neurons within each dorsal root ganglion sprout processes that grow into the neural tube to synapse with association neurons in the dorsal column. Other processes grow outward from the dorsal root ganglion to join the ventral root, forming a typical spinal nerve. The dorsal root ganglion and its fibers constitute the dorsal root. The axon of the association neuron in this illustration synapses with a motor neuron on the same side of the spinal cord at the same segmental level (axons may also display other patterns of connection; see text).

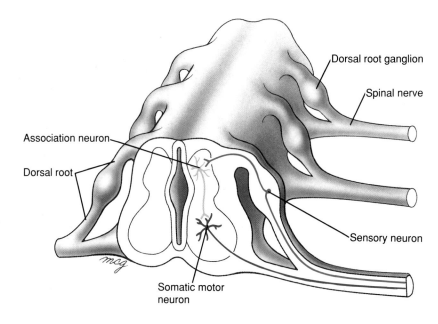

whereas others cross over to synapse with motor neurons on the opposite or **contralateral** side of the cord.

The mixed motor and sensory trunk formed at each level by the confluence of the dorsal and ventral roots is called a **spinal nerve** (Fig. 5-3). The sympathetic fibers that exit via the ventral roots at levels T1 through L2 soon branch from the spinal nerve and grow ventrally to enter the corresponding sympathetic chain ganglion (see Ch. 4) (Fig. 5-4). This branch is called a **white ramus.** Some of the sympathetic fibers carried in the white ramus synapse directly with a neuron in the chain ganglion (Fig. 5-4). This neuron becomes the second (peripheral) neuron in a two-neuron sympathetic pathway and sprouts an axon that grows to innervate the appropriate peripheral end organ. Because the peripheral autonomic neurons reside in ganglia, the axons of the central sympathetic neurons are called **preganglionic fibers,** and the axons of the peripheral sympathetic neurons are called **postganglionic fibers.** (This terminology is used for both sympathetic and parasympathetic pathways.)

Not all the preganglionic sympathetic fibers that enter a chain ganglion via the white ramus synapse there. The re-mainder pass onward and synapse in a more cranial or caudal chain ganglion or in one of the prevertebral ganglia (see Ch. 4).

The postganglionic fibers that originate in each chain ganglion form a small branch, the **gray ramus,** that grows dorsally to rejoin the spinal nerve which then grows toward the periphery (Fig. 5-4). Distal to the gray ramus, the spinal nerve thus carries sensory fibers, somatic motor fibers, and postganglionic sympathetic fibers.

Axons in the spinal nerves grow to very specific sites

The growth cones of the motor and sensory fibers carried by the spinal nerves grow to very specific targets in the body wall and extremities. Shortly after leaving the spinal column, each axon first chooses one of two routes, growing either dorsally toward the epimere or ventrally toward the hypomere. In consequence, the spinal nerve splits into two **primary rami.** The axons that direct their path toward the epimere form the **dorsal primary ramus,**

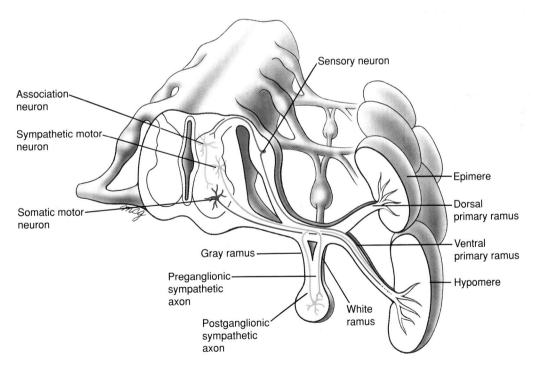

Fig. 5-4. Organization of spinal nerves and associated chain ganglia at levels T1–L2 and S2–S4. In this example, the preganglionic fiber growing from the intermediolateral cell column exits the spinal nerve through a white ramus and synapses with a neuron in the chain ganglion at the same level. The postganglionic fiber then exits through the gray ramus and re-joins the same spinal nerve. Each spinal nerve splits into a dorsal primary ramus and a ventral primary ramus, which innervate the segmental epimere and hypomere, respectively. Both rami contain motor, sensory, and autonomic fibers.

and the fibers that grow toward the hypomere form the **ventral primary ramus** (Fig. 5-4).

The axons of somatic motor fibers in the dorsal and ventral rami seek out specific muscles or bundles of muscle fibers and form synapses with the muscle fibers, whereas the postganglionic sympathetic motor fibers innervate the smooth muscle of blood vessels and the sweat glands and arrector pili muscles in the skin. The specific signals that guide the growth cones of motor fibers to their targets are not known, but it has been suggested that sympathetic fibers use the developing vascular system as a guide. Sensory axons grow somewhat more slowly than motor axons. For most of their length they follow the pathways established by the somatic and sympathetic motor fibers, but eventually they branch from the combined nerves and innervate sensory end organs such as muscle spindles, temperature and touch receptors in the dermis of the skin, and pressure sensors and chemoreceptors in the developing vasculature.

The pattern of somatic motor and sensory innervation is segmental

The motor and sensory nerves innervate the body wall and limbs in a pattern that is based on the segmental organization established by the somites (Fig. 5-2). For example, the intercostal muscles between a given pair of ribs are innervated by the spinal nerve that grows out at that level. The sensory innervation of the skin is also segmental: each dermatome is innervated by the spinal nerve growing out at the same level. The sensory component of each spinal nerve, however, also spreads into the adjacent dermatomes, so there is some overlap in dermatomal innervation (Fig. 5-5).

The pattern of sympathetic innervation is not entirely segmental

The sympathetic fibers traveling in the spinal nerves share the segmental distribution of the somatic motor and sensory fibers. Therefore, the segments of the body wall and extremities developing at levels T1 through L2 are innervated by postganglionic fibers originating from chain ganglia at the corresponding levels of the spinal cord. Another pattern, however, is required to provide sympathetic innervation to the remaining levels of the body wall and extremities, which correspond to cord levels lacking central sympathetic neurons. Recall from Chapter 4 that chain ganglia develop in the cervical, lower lumbar, sacral, and coccygeal regions in addition to the thoracic and upper lumbar regions. How do these ganglia receive central sympathetic innervation? The answer (as hinted earlier) is that some of the preganglionic sympathetic fibers that enter chain ganglia at levels T1 through L2 travel cranially or caudally to another chain ganglion before synapsing. Some of these ascending or descending fibers supply the chain ganglia outside of T1 through L2 (Fig. 5-6).

The postganglionic fibers from each chain ganglion enter the corresponding spinal nerve via a gray ramus. As a result, the spinal nerves at levels T1 through L2 have both white and gray rami, whereas all other spinal nerves have

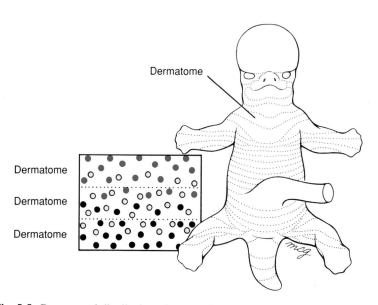

Fig. 5-5. Dermatomal distribution of sensory innervation. The sensory fibers of each spinal nerve innervate primarily receptors in the corresponding body segment or dermatome. The innervation of adjacent dermatomes shows some overlap, however, so that ablation of a dorsal root does not entirely obliterate sensation in the corresponding dermatome.

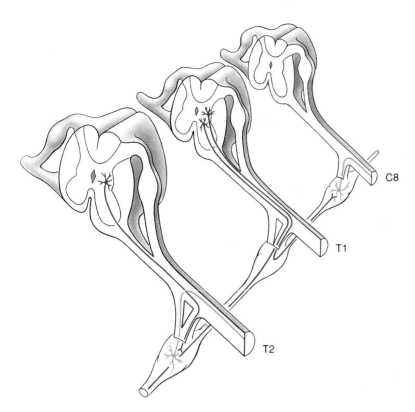

C8

T1

T2

Fig. 5-6. Preganglionic fibers growing from the intermediolateral cell column may synapse with a neuron in a chain ganglion at their own level, at a lower level, or at a higher level. This mechanism provides sympathetic innervation to spinal levels other than T1–L2. Spinal nerves developing at C1–C8, L3 and L5, S1–S5, and the first coccygeal nerve thus lack a white ramus.

just a gray ramus. The motor fibers linking chain ganglia to one another thus are exclusively preganglionic sympathetic fibers. These fibers, visceral afferent fibers, plus chain ganglia themselves, constitute the **sympathetic trunk.**

The head receives sympathetic innervation via the cervical chain ganglia while the heart, trachea, and lungs receive sympathetic innervation from cervical and thoracic chain ganglia

The sympathetic supply to the heart originates at cord levels T1 through T4 (Fig. 5-7). Some of the fibers from T1 travel up the sympathetic trunk to synapse in the three cervical chain ganglia — the **inferior cervical ganglion** (which is sometimes fused with the chain ganglion at T1 to form the **stellate ganglion**), the **middle cervical ganglion,** and the **superior cervical ganglion.** Postganglionic fibers from these ganglia join postganglionic fibers emanating directly from nerves T1 through T4 to form the cardiac nerves, which innervate the heart muscle.

The sympathetic supply to the head originates at cord levels T1 through T4 and reaches the head exclusively via the sympathetic trunk. The preganglionic fibers synapse in the superior cervical ganglion, and the postganglionic fibers arising here follow blood vessels to the various structures in the head that receive sympathetic innervation, such as the lacrimal glands, the dilator pupillae muscles of the iris, and the nasal and oral mucosa.

Postganglionic sympathetic fibers exiting directly from chain ganglia associated with levels T1 through T4 or from cervical ganglia innervated by preganglionic fibers originating at cord levels T1 to T4 also innervate the trachea and lungs.

The preganglionic sympathetic fibers that supply the gut terminate in the prevertebral ganglia

The preganglionic sympathetic fibers destined to supply the gut arise from cord levels T5 through L2 and enter the corresponding chain ganglia. Instead of synapsing, however, they immediately leave via **splanchnic nerves,** which emerge directly from the chain ganglia (Fig. 5-7). These splanchnic nerves innervate the various prevertebral ganglia, which in turn send postganglionic fibers to the visceral end organs. The pattern of distribution is as follows.

Fibers from levels T5 through T9 come together to form the **greater splanchnic nerves** serving the **celiac ganglia.**

Fibers from T10 and T11 form the **lesser splanchnic nerves** serving the **aorticorenal ganglia.**

Fibers from T12 alone form the **least splanchnic nerves** serving the superior mesenteric ganglia.

Fibers from L1 and L2 form the **lumbar splanchnic nerves** serving the **inferior mesenteric ganglia.**

Recall from Chapter 4 that the prevertebral ganglia develop next to major branches of the descending aorta. The

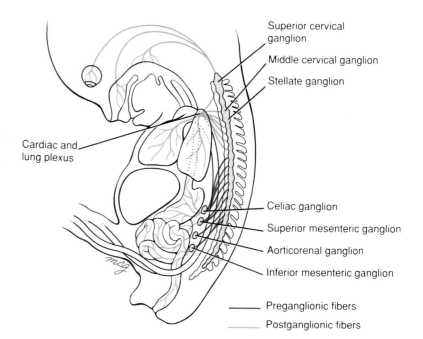

Fig. 5-7. Some postganglionic sympathetic fibers do not join with spinal nerves. Postganglionic fibers emanating from cervical and thoracic chain ganglia follow blood vessels to structures in the head and pharynx and to the heart and lungs. The splanchnic nerves are preganglionic fibers that pass directly out of the chain ganglia at levels T5 to L2 to innervate neurons within the celiac, superior, mesenteric, aorticorenal, and inferior mesenteric ganglia. Postganglionic fibers from these ganglia grow out along blood vessels to innervate their visceral end organs.

postganglionic sympathetic axons from the prevertebral ganglia grow out along these arteries and thus come to innervate the same tissues that the arteries supply with blood (Fig. 5-7). Thus, the postganglionic fibers from the celiac ganglia innervate the *foregut* region vascularized by the celiac artery – that is, the portion of the foregut from the abdominal esophagus through the duodenum to the entrance of the bile duct. Similarly, fibers from the superior mesenteric ganglia innervate the **midgut** (the remainder of the duodenum, the jejunum, and the ileum) plus the ascending colon and about two-thirds of the transverse colon. The aorticorenal ganglia innervate the kidney and suprarenal gland, and the inferior mesenteric ganglia innervate the **hindgut,** including the distal one-third of the transverse colon, the descending and sigmoid colons, and the upper two thirds of the anorectal canal.

The parasympathetic system has long preganglionic fibers and short postganglionic fibers

Recall from Chapter 4 that the parasympathetic ganglia, unlike the sympathetic ganglia, form close to the organs they are destined to innervate and therefore produce only short postganglionic fibers. The central neurons of the two-cell parasympathetic pathways reside either in one of four motor nuclei in the brain (associated with cranial nerves III, VII, IX, and X) or in the intermediolateral regions of the sacral cord at levels S2 through S4. The cranial nuclei supply the head and the viscera superior to

the hindgut, whereas the sacral neurons supply the viscera inferior to this point (Fig. 5-8).

The preganglionic parasympathetic fibers associated with cranial nerves III, VII, and IX travel to parasympathetic ganglia located near the structures to be innervated, where they synapse with the second neuron of the pathway. Organs receiving parasympathetic innervation in this way include the dilator pupillae muscles of the eye, the lacrimal and salivary glands, and glands of the oral and nasal mucosa (see Ch. 13). In contrast, the preganglionic parasympathetic fibers associated with cranial nerve X join with somatic motor and sensory fibers to form the vagus nerve. Some branches of the vagus serve structures in the head and neck, but other parasympathetic and sensory fibers within the nerve continue into the thorax and abdomen, where the parasympathetic fibers synapse with secondary neurons in numerous small parasympathetic ganglia embedded in the walls of target organs such as the heart, liver, adrenal cortex, kidney, gonads, and gut. The preganglionic vagal fibers therefore are very long, whereas the postganglionic fibers that penetrate the target organs are short.

The parasympathetic preganglionic fibers arising in the sacral cord emerge from the ventral rami of the cord and join together to form the **pelvic splanchnic nerves.** These nerves ramify throughout the pelvis and lower abdomen, innervating ganglia embedded in the walls of the descending and sigmoid colon, rectum, ureter, prostate, bladder, urethra, and phallus. The postganglionic fibers from these ganglia innervate smooth muscle or glands in the target organs (Fig. 5-8).

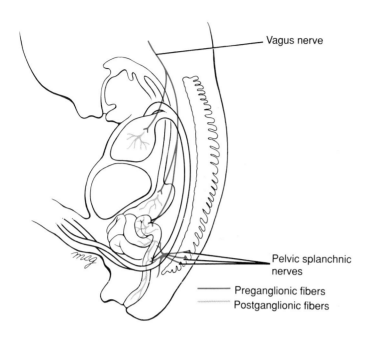

Fig. 5-8. The vagus nerve and pelvic splanchnic nerves provide preganglionic parasympathetic innervation to ganglia embedded in the walls of visceral organs. The preganglionic fibers originating at cord levels S2 through S4 issue from the cord at those levels and then branch off to form pelvic splanchnic nerves, which innervate the parasympathetic ganglia of the target viscera. The postganglionic parasympathetic fibers are relatively short.

APPLICATIONS TO CLINICAL PRACTICE

Hirschsprung's disease is a clinically important disease of the neural crest

One in 5,000 infants is afflicted with a condition called **Hirschsprung's** disease or congenital megacolon, which is characterized by dilation of a segment of the gastrointestinal tract, most typically regions of the colon. The passage of meconium is usually delayed in afflicted infants, who may also exhibit constipation, vomiting, and abdominal distention. The disease was first described by Hirschsprung in 1888, but controversy surrounded its pathogenesis until the 1940s. It was thought that the dilated region of the bowel was the primary site of the defect and that the disease could be cured by resecting it. Swenson, however, used a barium enema to demonstrate that the dilated region of the bowel was a secondary symptom caused by obstruction and lack of peristalsis in the constricted colon segment distal to the dilation (Fig. 5-9). Swenson's method of removing this terminal region of the bowel or some variation of this technique remains the only effective treatment of the disease.

By the late 1940s it was found that the constricted non-peristaltic segment of the gastrointestinal tract in congenital megacolon lacked parasympathetic enteric ganglia. While microscopic studies of the lethal spotted *(ls)* mouse showed that the enteric ganglia were absent from this constricted segment, neurons containing the neurotrans-

mitter characteristic of parasympathetic ganglion cells were found adhering to the outside of this bowel segment but could not penetrate the gut wall.

Genetic studies of mice and humans suggest that congenital megacolon may arise through mutations of different genes

Normal development of enteric neurons requires the successful execution of several different processes, including (1) induction of neural crest cell differentiation and their release from the neural tube, (2) their migration and differential adhesion along specific pathways, (3) their penetration of the gut wall, and (4) their proliferation and differentiation to produce the functional neurons that characterize the enteric nervous system. It is therefore possible that defects in any of these developmental mechanisms could result in congenital megacolon, and several related studies of mice and humans provide evidence for this speculation.

As discussed in Chapter 4, the murine splotch mutant *(Sp)* harbors mutations of *Pax-3,* a gene resembling the paired-box *Drosophila* segmentation genes. In addition to the neural tube defects these mice exhibit, homozygotes of several well-described mutations of *Pax-3* also exhibit severe defects of neural crest cell migration, including hearing loss, pigmentation defects, and congenital mega-

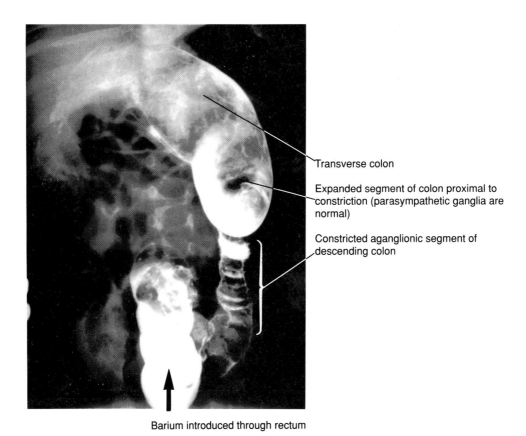

Transverse colon

Expanded segment of colon proximal to constriction (parasympathetic ganglia are normal)

Constricted aganglionic segment of descending colon

Barium introduced through rectum

Fig. 5-9. Radiograph after a barium enema showing the constricted inferior gastrointestinal tract of an individual with Hirschsprung's disease. The adjacent superior region of the tract with normal autonomic innervation is distended. (Photo courtesy of Children's Hospital Medical Center, Cincinnati, OH.)

colon. Humans with mutations of *PAX3* (Waardenburg type 1 syndrome; mapped to chromosome 2q) also exhibit congenital megacolon. It is thought that this mutation may disrupt the differentiation and release of neural crest cells from the lateral edges of the neural folds.

Mutations of *PAX3,* however, do not explain all of the heritable forms of congenital megacolon in humans. Indeed, the *ret* proto-oncogene (mapped to chromosome 10q11.2), has also been implicated in some human forms of Hirschsprung's disease, which involves disruption of a domain similar to the cell-adhesion molecule cadherin, suggesting that this mutation may affect the migratory behavior of neural crest cells.

Finally, it has been shown that certain human patients with Hirschsprung's disease harbor mutations of a gene encoding the endothelin receptor. A similar mutation is shared by the piebald lethal *(sl)* mouse, which also exhibits congenital megacolon. Since the lethal spotted mouse discussed above is characterized by mutations of the endothelin-3 ligand gene, it is likely that these forms of congenital megacolon arise from abnormal development of the termi-

nal part of the gut, preventing the normal penetration of neural crest cells to form the enteric ganglia.

Transgenic animals and several spontaneous mutants provide insight into several neural crest cell-related congenital conditions

Transgenic knockouts of the endothelin ligand gene *(Edns)* or of the endothelin receptor gene *(Ednrb)* result in mice with congenital megacolon like that which occurs by spontaneous mutation of these genes in mice and humans described above. On the other hand, transgenic knockouts of genes encoding retinoic acid receptor proteins result in the disruption of neural crest migration and associated defects of heart septation (see Ch. 7).

In addition, a staggering array of spontaneous mutations of genes that affect neural crest cell differentiation, migration, and survival in mice have been described. For example, white-spotting *(w)* and Steel *(sl)* mutants harbor disruptive mutations of genes that encode c-kit receptor and the ligand for this receptor, c-kit ligand, respectively. The c-kit ligand is an apparent trophic substance required for survival of the neural crest cells that give rise to melanocytes. Studies with these animals show that if the appropriate migratory pathway does not express a functional receptor, then disruptions of pigmentation occur. Likewise, the Patch mutation *(Ph)* of the alpha subunit of platelet-derived growth factor ($PDGF_{2\alpha}$) disrupts the development of non-neuronal derivatives of the neural crest while the kreisler mutant *(kr)* exhibits wide-ranging craniofacial defects attributed to disruption of *Hox* genes and the migration and differentiation of neural crest cells (see Ch. 12). Thus, genetic studies, along with classic explantation, ablation, and cell marking experiments, are contributing to a growing body of information that is rapidly expanding our understanding of the diversity of pathogenetic mechanisms responsible for neural crest-related congenital disease.

6

Embryonic Folding

Folding of the Embryo and Formation of the Body Cavities and Mesenteries; Development of the Lungs

SUMMARY

During the fourth week, the embryo undergoes a process of **embryonic folding,** converting it from a flat trilaminar germ disc to a three-dimensional embryo. This process is facilitated by rapid growth of the neural tube and somites over the stagnating yolk sac and vitelline duct, resulting in folding under of the lateral, cephalic, and caudal edges of the embryo. As opposite edges of the ectoderm, mesoderm, and endoderm are pulled together along the ventral midline, three concentric tubes are created; (1) the outer investing ectoderm, (2) the mesodermal muscles and connective tissues of the body wall, and (3) the inner endodermal gut tube. In addition, the lateral cavities created by vacuolization of the lateral plate mesoderm (see Ch. 3) merge to form a single cavity between the outer splanchnopleuric lining of the gastrointestinal viscera and the inner somatopleuric lining of the body wall. This **intraembryonic coelomic cavity** is then partitioned into four cavities. First, during folding, the cranial mesodermal **septum transversum** swings caudally and ventrally to the boundary of the presumptive thorax and abdomen. This incomplete partition, however, leaves two posterolateral **pericardioperitoneal canals** between the superior **primitive pericardial cavity** and the inferior **peritoneal cavity.** Then during the fifth week, the primitive pericardial cavity is partitioned into a ventral **definitive pericardial cavity** and two dorsal **pleural cavities** by a pair of coronal **pleuropericardial folds.** Finally, the pericardioperitoneal canals are closed by transverse **pleuroperitoneal membranes.**

Often, one of the pleuroperitoneal membranes may fail to form, allowing herniation of abdominal organs into the pleural cavity. This condition, called **congenital diaphragmatic hernia,** is a common cause of human **pulmonary hypoplasia** often leading to **respiratory insufficiency** at birth and to death. Insufficient amniotic fluid or **oligohydramnios** may also result in pulmonary hypoplasia as a consequence of compression of the fetal thoracic cavity. In addition, lung growth may be disrupted by intrinsic defects in the **branching morphogenesis** that converts the endodermal **lung bud** to the bronchi, bronchioles, and terminal sacs. However, the primary cause of respiratory insufficiency in **premature infants** is inadequate **pulmonary surfactant** production. This mixture of phospholipids and surfactant proteins is synthesized during the weeks before birth to reduce the surface tension of the film lining the alveoli to facilitate their inflation. In some cases, **surfactant replacement therapy** may prevent asphyxiation. Unfortunately, therapies for congenital **surfactant B deficiency disease,** a life-threatening consequence of mutations of the surfactant B gene, have not yet been developed. However, molecular studies, utilizing **in situ hybridization** and **transgenic animal** technologies are being used to examine the role of this gene as well as genes that underlie **cystic fibrosis** in the hope that **gene therapies** may be developed. In addition, these techniques are also being used to study the functions of many other regulatory genes and growth factors critical to normal pulmonary development.

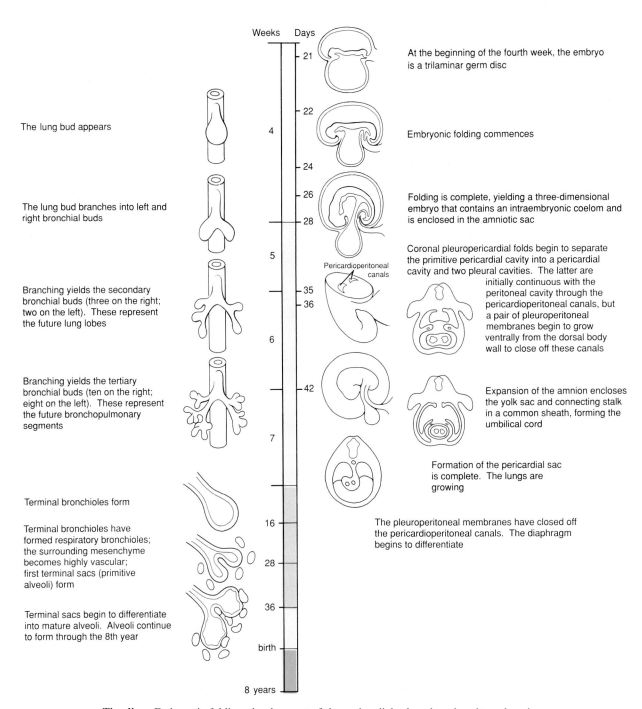

Weeks | Days

21 — At the beginning of the fourth week, the embryo is a trilaminar germ disc

The lung bud appears

4

22 — Embryonic folding commences

24

The lung bud branches into left and right bronchial buds

26 —
28 — Folding is complete, yielding a three-dimensional embryo that contains an intraembryonic coelom and is enclosed in the amniotic sac

5

Coronal pleuropericardial folds begin to separate the primitive pericardial cavity into a pericardial cavity and two pleural cavities. The latter are initially continuous with the peritoneal cavity through the pericardioperitoneal canals, but a pair of pleuroperitoneal membranes begin to grow ventrally from the dorsal body wall to close off these canals

Branching yields the secondary bronchial buds (three on the right; two on the left). These represent the future lung lobes

Pericardioperitoneal canals

35 —
36 —

6

Branching yields the tertiary bronchial buds (ten on the right; eight on the left). These represent the future bronchopulmonary segments

42 — Expansion of the amnion encloses the yolk sac and connecting stalk in a common sheath, forming the umbilical cord

7

Formation of the pericardial sac is complete. The lungs are growing

Terminal bronchioles form

Terminal bronchioles have formed respiratory bronchioles; the surrounding mesenchyme becomes highly vascular; first terminal sacs (primitive alveoli) form

16 — The pleuroperitoneal membranes have closed off the pericardioperitoneal canals. The diaphragm begins to differentiate

28 —

Terminal sacs begin to differentiate into mature alveoli. Alveoli continue to form through the 8th year

36 —

birth —

8 years —

Timeline. Embryonic folding, development of the pericardial, pleural, and peritoneal cavities, and development of the lungs.

The vertebrate body form arises through cephalocaudal and lateral flexion

Differential growth and active reshaping cause the embryo to fold

At the end of the third week, the embryo is a flat, ovoid, trilaminar disc. During the fourth week it grows rapidly, particularly in length, and undergoes a process of folding that generates the recognizable vertebrate body form (Figs. 6-1 and 6-2). Although some active remodeling of tissue layers takes place, the main force responsible for embryonic folding is the differential growth of various embryonic structures. During the fourth week, the embryonic disc and amnion grow vigorously, but the yolk sac hardly grows at all. Because the yolk sac is attached to the ventral rim of the embryonic disc, the expanding disc balloons into a three-dimensional, cylindrical shape. The developing notochord, neural tube, and somites stiffen the dorsal axis of the embryo, so most of the folding is concentrated in the thin, flexible outer rim of the disc. The cranial, caudal, and lateral margins of the disc fold completely under the dorsal axis structures and give rise to the ventral surface of the body. Since the embryo grows faster in length than in width, these reflections are deeper at the caudal and (especially) the cranial ends of the embryo than along the sides.

Cephalic folding may occur in response to the overgrowth and flexure of the cephalic neural plate

In preparation for folding, the broad, thick cephalic neural folds become elevated dorsally by proliferation and migration of the underlying head mesenchyme (**mesenchyme** is loose embryonic tissue). As the cephalic portion of the embryonic axis overgrows the yolk sac, the cephalic neural plate flexes sharply at specific levels (see Chs. 4 and 13).

As described in Chapter 3, the cranial rim of the germ disc—the thin area located cranial to the neural plate—contains the buccopharyngeal membrane, which represents the future mouth. Cranial to the buccopharyngeal membrane, a second important structure has begun to appear: the horseshoe-shaped **cardiogenic area,** which will give rise to the heart (see Ch. 7). The overgrowth and flexure of the cephalic neural plate cause the thin cranial rim of the disc to fold under, forming the ventral surface of the future face, neck, and chest (Fig. 6-1).

A second important structure that is brought into the future thorax by cephalic folding is the **septum transversum.** This structure appears on day 22 as a thickened bar of mesoderm lying between the cardiogenic area and the cra-

nial margin of the embryonic disc. Cephalic folding carries this bar ventrally and caudally until it is wedged between the cardiogenic region and the neck of the yolk sac (Fig. 6-1B, E; see also Fig. 6-5A). As described later in this chapter, the septum transversum forms the initial partition separating the coelom into thoracic and abdominal cavities and gives rise to part of the diaphragm and the ventral mesentery of the stomach and duodenum (see Ch. 9).

Caudal folding places the connecting stalk next to the yolk sac

Starting on about day 23, a similar process of folding commences in the caudal region of the embryo as the rapidly lengthening neural tube and somites overgrow the caudal rim of the yolk sac. The thin caudal rim of the germ disc, containing the cloacal membrane, folds under and becomes part of the ventral surface of the embryo (Fig. 6-1). When the caudal rim of the disc folds under the body, the connecting stalk (which connects the caudal end of the germ disc to the developing placenta) is carried cranially until it merges with the neck of the yolk sac, which has begun to lengthen and constrict (Figs. 6-1 and 6-2). The root of the connecting stalk contains a slender endodermal hindgut diverticulum called the **allantois** (Fig. 6-1E).

The lateral edges of the germ disc fuse along the ventral midline

Simultaneously with cephalocaudal flexion, the right and left sides of the embryonic disc flex sharply ventrally, constricting and narrowing the neck of the yolk sac (Fig. 6-1C). At the head and tail ends of the embryo, these lateral edges of the germ disc are pulled together, resulting in continuity of all three germ layers from one side of the embryo to the other (Fig. 6-1E). As a result, the ectoderm of the original germ disc covers the entire surface of the three-dimensional embryo except for the future **umbilical region,** where the yolk sac and connecting stalk emerge. The ectoderm, along with contributions from the dermatomes, lateral plate mesoderm, and neural crest, will eventually produce the skin (see Ch. 14).

Folding of the endoderm creates the gut tube

The endoderm of the trilaminar germ disc is destined to give rise to the lining of the gastrointestinal tract. When the cranial, caudal, and lateral edges of the embryo fold under the embryo, the superior and inferior portions of the endoderm are converted into blind-ending tubes—the future **foregut** and **hindgut.** At first, the central **midgut** region remains broadly open to the yolk sac (Fig. 6-1A, B). However, as the gut tube forms, the neck of the yolk sac is gradually constricted, reducing its communi-

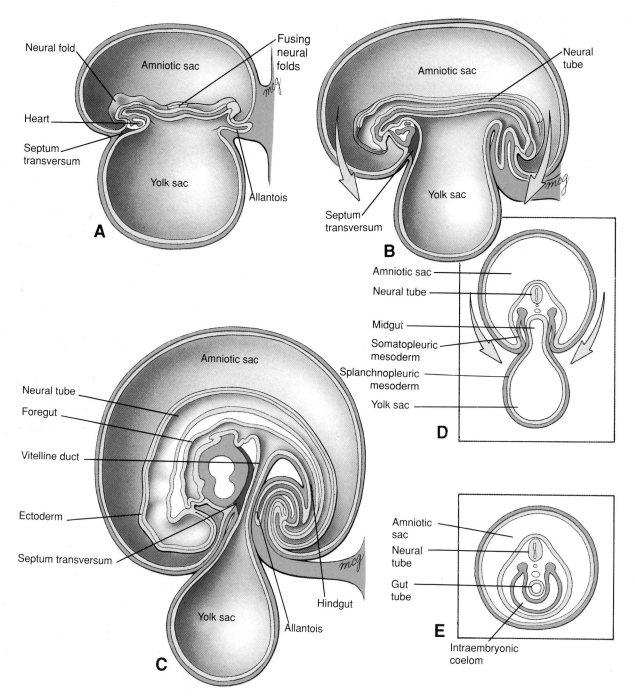

Fig. 6-1. The process of cephalocaudal and lateral folding that transforms the embryo from a flat disc to a three-dimensional vertebrate body form. As folding occurs, the embryo grows more rapidly than the yolk sac, the cavity of which remains continuous with the developing gut tube through the narrowing vitelline duct. The septum transversum forms cranial to the cardiogenic area in the germ disc (**A**) and is translocated to the future lower thoracic region through the folding of the cranial end of the embryo (**B, C**). The allantois and connecting stalk combine with the yolk sac and vitelline duct through the folding of the caudal end of the embryo (**A–C**). Fusion of the ectoderm, mesoderm, future coelomic cavities, and endoderm from opposite sides is prevented in the immediate vicinity of the vitelline duct (**D**) but not in more cranial and caudal regions (**E**).

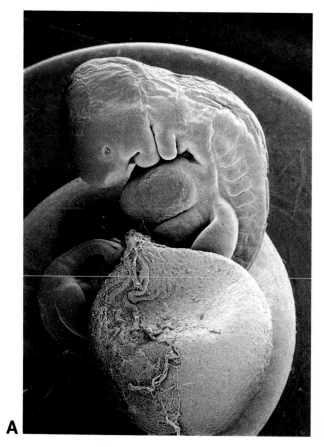

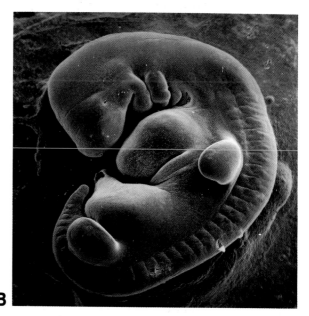

Fig. 6-2. **(A)** The form of this embryo is characteristic of a 4-week human embryo just subsequent to the folding process. Note the relatively large definitive yolk sac. **(B)** A three-dimensional incipient human form is apparent in this 5-week embryo. The yolk sac has been removed. (Fig. A scanning electron micrograph courtesy of Dr. Arnold Tamarin.)

cation with the midgut. By the end of the sixth week, the gut tube is fully formed and the neck of the yolk sac has been reduced to a slim stalk called the **vitelline duct** (Fig. 6-1C). The cranial end of the foregut is capped by the buccopharyngeal membrane, which ruptures at the end of the fourth week to form the mouth. The caudal end of the hindgut is capped by the cloacal membrane, which will rupture during the seventh week to form the orifices of the anus and urogenital system (see Ch. 10).

Folding of the embryo converts the intraembryonic coelom into a closed cavity

The intraembryonic coelom, its serosal lining, and the mesenteries are products of the lateral plate mesoderm

As described in Chapter 3, the lateral plate mesoderm splits into two layers: the **somatopleuric mesoderm,** which adheres to the ectoderm, and the **splanchnopleuric meso-**

derm, which adheres to the endoderm. The space between these layers is originally open to the chorionic cavity. When the folds of the embryo fuse along the ventral midline, however, this space is enclosed within the embryo and becomes the **intraembryonic coelom** (Figs. 6-1D, E and 6-3). The two layers of the lateral plate mesoderm become the **serous membranes** lining this cavity: the somatopleuric mesoderm lines the inside of the body wall and the splanchnopleuric mesoderm invests the visceral organs derived from the gut tube.

The dorsal mesentery suspends the abdominal gut tube within the coelom

When the coelom first forms, the gut is broadly attached to the dorsal body wall (Figs. 6-1E and 6-3A). In the region of the future abdominal viscera (from the abdominal esophagus to the most proximal part of the future rectum), however, mesenchyme within this region of attachment gradually disperses during the fourth week, resulting in

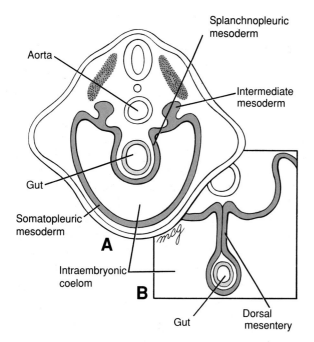

Fig. 6-3. Formation of the dorsal mesentery. The primitive gut tube initially hangs from the posterior body wall by a broad bar of mesenchyme (**A**), but in regions inferior to the septum transversum this connection thins out to form a membranous dorsal mesentery composed of reflected peritoneum (**B**).

formation of a thin, bilayered **dorsal mesentery** that suspends the abdominal viscera in the coelomic cavity (Fig. 6-3B). Because the abdominal gut tube and its derivatives are suspended in what will later become the peritoneal cavity, they are referred to as **intraperitoneal** viscera. This term is traditional and rather loose; strictly, there is nothing in the peritoneal cavity itself except serous fluid and, in women, a monthly ovulated oocyte.

Retroperitoneal organs are not suspended by mesentery. In contrast to the intraperitoneal location of most of the gut tube and its derivatives, some of the visceral organs develop in the body wall and are separated from the coelom by a covering of serous membrane (Fig. 6-4A). These organs are said to be **retroperitoneal**. It is important to realize that the designation *retroperitoneal* means that an organ is located behind the peritoneum from a viewpoint inside the peritoneal cavity—not that it is necessarily located in the dorsal body wall. Thus, the kidneys are retroperitoneal, and so is the bladder, which develops in the ventral body wall (Fig. 6-4A).

Parts of the gut tube adhere to the body wall during development and become secondarily retroperitoneal. To complicate the intraperitoneal/retroperitoneal distinc-

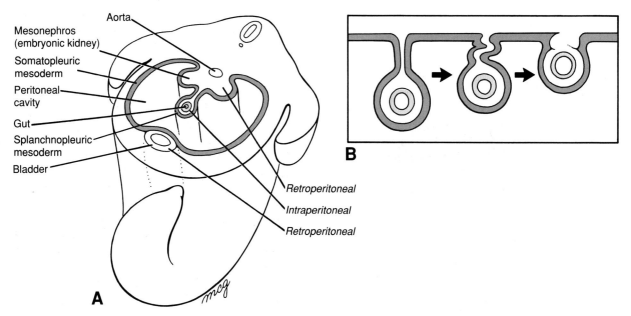

Fig. 6-4. The distinction between intraperitoneal, retroperitoneal, and secondarily retroperitoneal positions of the viscera. (**A**) Viscera suspended within the peritoneal cavity by a mesentery are called intraperitoneal, whereas organs embedded in the body wall and covered by peritoneum are called retroperitoneal. (**B**) The mesentery suspending some intraperitoneal organs disappears as both mesentery and organ fuse with the body wall. These organs are then called secondarily retroperitoneal.

tion further, some parts of the gut tube that are initially suspended by mesentery later become fused to the body wall, thus taking on the appearance of retroperitoneal organs (Fig. 6-4B). These organs, which include the ascending and descending colon, the duodenum, and the pancreas, are said to be **secondarily retroperitoneal.**

The formation of the pericardial sac and diaphragm between 5 and 7 weeks subdivides the coelom into four cavities

The septum transversum partially separates the thoracic and abdominal cavities

The septum transversum forms a transverse (horizontal) partition that partially separates the coelomic cavity into superior (thoracic) and inferior (abdominopelvic) portions (Figs. 6-1B, C, and 6-5). The superior cavity contains the developing heart and is called the **primitive pericardial cavity,** whereas the inferior cavity is the future **peritoneal cavity.** The septum transversum is attached ventrally and laterally to the body wall and dorsally to the mesenchyme associated with the foregut. However, the peritoneal and primitive pericardial cavities communicate through two large dorsolateral openings, the **pericardioperitoneal canals** (Fig. 6-5).

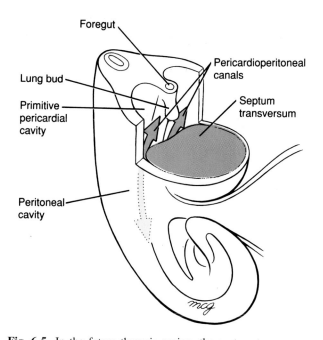

Fig. 6-5. In the future thoracic region, the septum transversum forms a ventral partition partially separating the intraembryonic coelomic cavity into a primitive pericardial cavity superiorly and a peritoneal cavity inferiorly. These cavities remain in continuity through the posterior pericardioperitoneal canals (arrows).

Caudal translocation of the septum transversum is accompanied by elongation of the phrenic nerves

During the fourth and fifth weeks, the continued folding and differential growth of the embryonic axis cause a gradual caudal displacement of the septum transversum. The ventral edge of the septum finally becomes fixed to the anterior body wall at the 7th thoracic level, and the dorsal connection to the esophageal mesenchyme becomes fixed at the 12th thoracic level. Meanwhile, myoblasts (muscle cell precursors) differentiate within the septum transversum. These cells, which will form part of the future diaphragm muscle, are innervated by spinal nerves at a transient, cervical level of the septum transversum—that is, by fibers from the spinal nerves of cervical levels 3, 4, and 5 (C3, C4, C5). These fibers join together to form the paired **phrenic nerves,** which elongate as they follow the migrating septum caudally.

The pericardial sac is formed by pleuropericardial folds that grow from the lateral body wall in a coronal plane

During the fifth week, the pleural and pericardial cavities are divided from each other by **pleuropericardial folds** that originate along the lateral body walls in a coronal plane (Fig. 6-6). These septae appear at the beginning of the fifth week as broad folds of mesenchyme and pleura that grow medially toward each other between the heart and the developing lungs (Fig. 6-6A, B). At the end of the fifth week, the folds meet and fuse with each other and with the foregut mesenchyme, thus subdividing the primitive pericardial cavity into three compartments: a fully enclosed, ventral **definitive pericardial cavity** and two dorsolateral **pleural cavities** (Fig. 6-6C). The latter are still continuous with the peritoneal cavity through the pericardioperitoneal canals. (The term *pericardioperitoneal canal* is retained even though the canal now provides communication between the pleural cavities and the peritoneal cavity.)

As the tips of the pleuropericardial folds grow medially toward each other and fuse, their roots migrate toward the ventral midline (Fig. 6-6B, C).

The pleuropericardial folds are three-layered, consisting of body wall mesenchyme sandwiched between two layers of somatopleuric mesoderm. The thin definitive pericardial sac retains this threefold composition, consisting of inner and outer serous membranes (the inner **parietal pericardium** and the outer **mediastinal pleura**) separated by a delicate filling of mesenchyme-derived connective tissue, the **fibrous pericardium.** The phrenic nerves, which originally run through the portion of the body wall mesenchyme incorporated into the pleuropericardial folds, course through the fibrous pericardium of the adult.

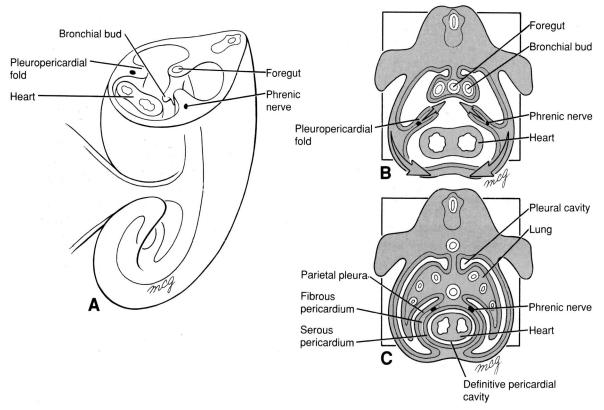

Fig. 6-6. Subdivision of the primitive pericardial cavity. **(A)** During the fifth week, coronal pleuropericardial folds grow out from the lateral body wall toward the midline, where they fuse with each other and with mesoderm associated with the esophagus. Simultaneously, the roots of these folds migrate ventrally so that they ultimately originate from the ventral body wall. **(B)** The phrenic nerves initially embedded in the body wall are swept into these developing partitions. **(C)** The pleuropericardial folds with their associated serous membrane form the pericardial sac and transform the primitive pericardial cavity into a definitive pericardial cavity and right and left pleural cavities.

Pleuroperitoneal membranes growing from the posterior and lateral body wall seal off the pericardioperitoneal canals

At the beginning of the fifth week, a pair of transverse membranes, the **pleuroperitoneal membranes,** arise along an oblique line connecting the root of the 12th rib with the tips of ribs 12 through 7 (Fig. 6-7A). These membranes grow ventrally to fuse with the posterior margin of the septum transversum, thus sealing off the pericardioperitoneal canals. Closure of the canals is complete by the seventh week (Fig. 6-7B). The membranes are called *pleuroperitoneal membranes* because they do not contact the septum transversum until after the pericardial sac is formed; thus, they separate the definitive pleural cavities from the peritoneal cavity.

The left pericardioperitoneal canal is larger than the right and closes later. This difference may account for the fact that congenital diaphragmatic hernias of the ab-

dominal viscera are more common on the left side than on the right.

The diaphragm is a composite of four embryonic structures

The definitive musculotendinous diaphragm incorporates derivatives of four embryonic structures: (1) the septum transversum, (2) the pleuroperitoneal membranes, (3) paraxial mesoderm of the body wall, and (4) esophageal mesenchyme (Fig. 6-8). Some of the myoblasts that arise in the septum transversum emigrate into the pleuroperitoneal membranes, pulling their phrenic nerve branches along with them. Most of the septum transversum gives rise to the nonmuscular **central tendon** of the diaphragm (Fig. 6-8).

The bulk of the **diaphragm muscle** within the pleuroperitoneal membranes is innervated by the phrenic nerve. The outer rim of diaphragmatic muscle, however,

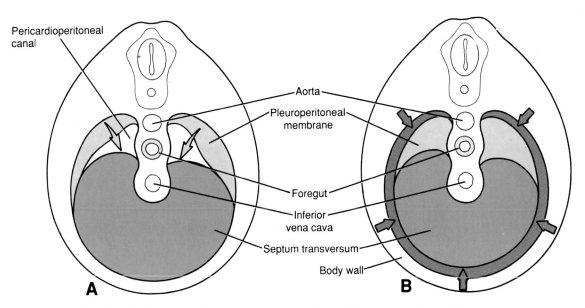

Fig. 6-7. (A, B) Closure of the pericardioperitoneal canals. Between weeks 5 and 7, a pair of horizontal pleuroperitoneal membranes grow from the posterior body wall to meet the posterior edge of the septum transversum, thus closing the pericardioperitoneal canals. These membranes form the posterior portions of the diaphragm and completely seal off the pleural cavities from the peritoneal cavity.

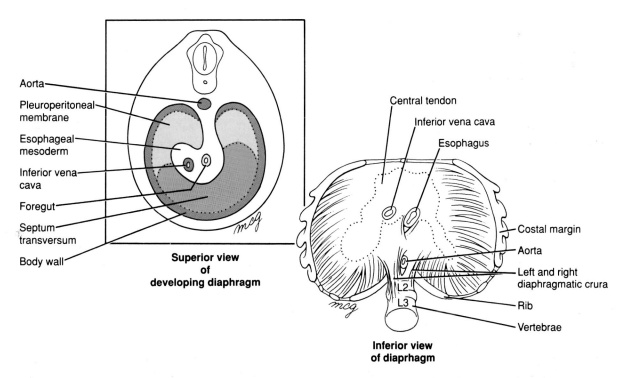

Fig. 6-8. Formation of the diaphragm. The definitive diaphragm is a composite structure including elements of the septum transversum, pleuroperitoneal membranes, and esophageal mesenchyme, as well as a rim of body wall mesoderm.

arises from a ring of body wall paraxial mesoderm (Fig. 6-7B) and is therefore innervated by spinal nerves from thoracic spinal levels T7 through T12. Finally, mesenchyme associated with the foregut at vertebral levels L1 through L3 condenses to form two muscular bands, the **right** and **left crura** of the diaphragm, which originate on the vertebral column and insert into the dorsomedial diaphragm (Fig. 6-8). The right crus originates on vertebral bodies L1 through L3, and the left crus originates on vertebral bodies L1 and L2.

The lungs begin to develop in the fourth week and begin to mature just before birth

The respiratory tree originates as a foregut diverticulum that undergoes a controlled series of branchings

The first rudiment of the lung, a keel-shaped ventral outpouching of the endodermal foregut called the **respiratory diverticulum** or **lung bud,** appears on day 22 (Fig. 6-9). The lung bud begins to grow ventrocaudally through the mesenchyme surrounding the foregut. On days 26 to 28, it undergoes a first bifurcation, splitting into right and left **primary bronchial buds** (Fig. 6-9). These buds are the rudiments of the two lungs. Between weeks 5 and 28, they branch an additional 16 times to generate the respiratory trees of the lungs. Experiments suggest that the pattern of branching of the lung endoderm is regulated by the surrounding mesenchyme. The stages of development of the lungs are summarized in Table 6-1.

The stem of the respiratory tree proximal to the first bifurcation becomes the trachea and larynx, and the stems of the right and left primary bronchial buds become the right and left primary bronchi. The next round of branching, which occurs early in the fifth week, yields three **secondary bronchial buds** on the right side and two on the left (Fig. 6-9). These buds give rise to the lung lobes: three in the right lung and two in the left lung. During the sixth week, another round of branching yields about 10 tertiary bronchi on both sides; these become the bronchopulmonary segments of the mature lung (Fig. 6-9).

By week 16, after about 14 more branchings, the respiratory tree produces small branches called **terminal bron-**

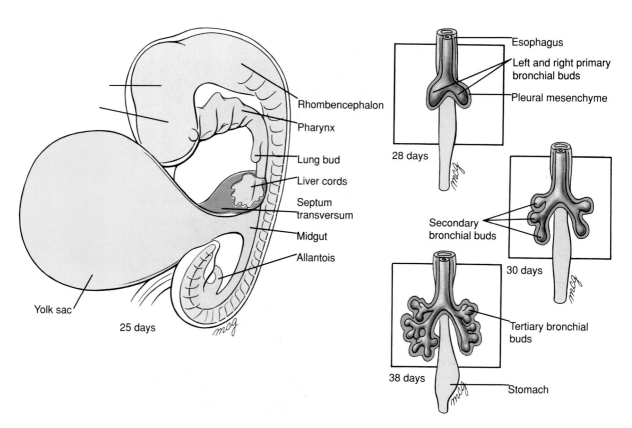

Fig. 6-9. Development of the lung buds. The lung bud first appears as an evagination of the foregut on day 22 and bifurcates into two primary bronchial buds between day 26 and day 28. Early in the fifth week, the right bronchial bud branches into three secondary bronchial buds while the left bronchial bud branches into two. By the sixth week, secondary bronchial buds branch into tertiary bronchial buds (usually about 10 on both sides) to form the bronchopulmonary segments.

Table 6-1.   Stages of human lung development

STAGE OF DEVELOPMENT	PERIOD	EVENTS
Embryonic	26 days to 6 weeks	The lung bud arises as a ventral outpouching of the foregut endoderm and undergoes three initial rounds of branching, producing the primordia successively of the two lungs, the lung lobes, and the bronchopulmonary segments.
Pseudoglandular	6 to 16 weeks	The respiratory trees of the lungs undergo 14 more generations of branching, resulting in the formation of terminal bronchioles.
Canalicular	16 to 28 weeks	Each terminal bronchiole divides into two or more respiratory bronchioles. The respiratory vasculature begins to develop.
Saccular	28 to 36 weeks	The respiratory bronchioles subdivide to produce terminal sacs (primitive alveoli). Terminal sacs continue to be produced until well into childhood.
Alveolar	36 weeks to term	The alveoli mature.

(Modified from Langston C, Kida K, Reed M, Thurlbeck WM. 1984. Human lung growth in late gestation in the neonate. Am Rev Respir Dis *129:607, with permission.)*

chioles (Fig. 6-10). Between 16 and 28 weeks, each terminal bronchiole divides into two or more **respiratory bronchioles,** and the mesodermal tissue surrounding these structures becomes highly vascularized (Fig. 6-10). By week 28, the respiratory bronchioles begin to sprout a final generation of stubby branches (Fig. 6-10). These branches develop in craniocaudal progression, appearing first at more cranial terminal bronchioles. By week 36, the first-formed wave of terminal branches are invested in a dense network of capillaries and are called **terminal sacs (primitive alveoli)** (Fig. 6-10). Limited respiration is possible at this point, but the alveoli are still so few and immature that

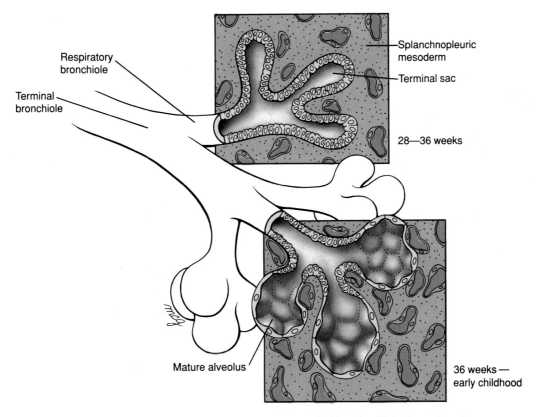

Fig. 6-10. Maturation of the lung tissue. Terminal sacs (primitive alveoli) begin to form between weeks 28 and 36 and begin to mature between 36 weeks and birth. Only 5 to 20 percent of all terminal sacs produced by the age of 8 years, however, are formed prior to birth.

infants born at this age often die of respiratory insufficiency (see Applications to Clinical Practice). Additional terminal sacs continue to form and differentiate in craniocaudal progression both before and after birth, possibly until as late as 8 years. About 20 to 70 million terminal sacs are formed in each lung before birth; the total number in the mature lung is 300 to 400 million. Continued thinning of the squamous epithelial lining of the terminal sacs begins just before birth, resulting in the differentiation of these primitive alveoli into mature alveoli (Fig. 6-10).

The lung is a composite of endodermal and mesodermal tissues. The endoderm of the lung bud gives rise to the mucosal lining of the bronchi and to the epithelial cells of the alveoli. The vasculature of the lung and the muscle and cartilage supporting the bronchi are derived from the foregut splanchnopleuric mesoderm, which covers the bronchi as they grow out from the mediastinum into the pleural space.

The umbilical cord is formed when the connecting stalk and vitelline duct are bound together by the expanding amnion

As the embryo grows and folds, the amnion keeps pace, expanding until it encloses the entire embryo except for the umbilical area where the connecting stalk and yolk sac emerge (Fig. 6-11). Between the fourth and eighth weeks,

an increase in the production of amniotic fluid causes the amnion to swell until it completely takes over the chorionic space (Fig. 6-12). When the amnion contacts the chorion, the layers of extraembryonic mesoderm covering

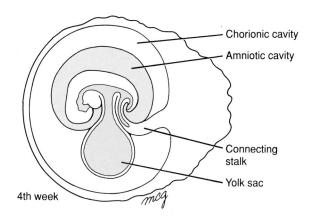

4th week

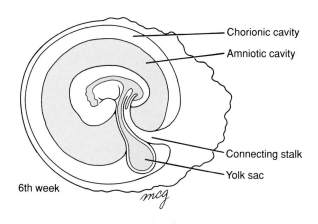

6th week

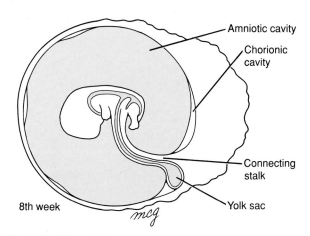

8th week

Fig. 6-12. The rapidly expanding amniotic cavity fills with fluid and obliterates the chorionic cavity between weeks 4 and 8.

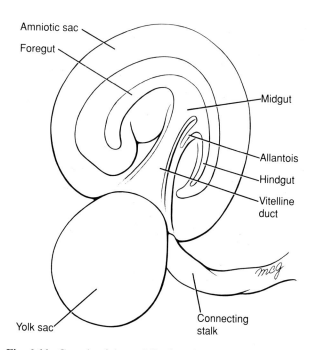

Fig. 6-11. Genesis of the umbilical cord. The folding of the embryo and the expansion of the amniotic cavity bring the connecting stalk and yolk sac together to form the umbilical cord. As the amnion continues to grow, a layer of amniotic membrane gradually encloses the umbilical cord.

the two membranes fuse loosely. The chorionic cavity thus disappears except for a few rudimentary vesicles.

After embryonic folding is complete, the amnion takes origin from the **umbilical ring** surrounding the roots of the vitelline duct and connecting stalk. The progressive expansion of the amnion therefore creates a tube of amniotic membrane that encloses the connecting stalk and the vitelline duct (Figs. 6-11 and 6-12). This composite structure is now called the **umbilical cord.** As the umbilical cord lengthens, the vitelline duct narrows and the pear-shaped body of the yolk sac remains within the umbilical sheath. Normally both the yolk sac and the vitelline duct disappear by birth.

The main function of the umbilical cord is to circulate blood between the embryo and the placenta. Umbilical arteries and veins develop in the connecting stalk to perform this function (see Ch. 8). The expanded amnion creates a roomy, weightless chamber in which the fetus can grow and develop freely.

APPLICATIONS TO CLINICAL PRACTICE

Clinically significant developmental anomalies of the lung may arise from extrinsic or indirect causes

Failure of the left pleuroperitoneal membrane to completely span the left pericardioperitoneal canal and evagination of abdominal contents into the pleural cavity is the single most common cause of pulmonary hypoplasia, occurring four to eight times more frequently than on the right side (Fig. 6-13). These **diaphragmatic hernias** may result from the fact that the left pericardioperitoneal canal is larger and/or that it normally closes later than the canal on the right. Rarely, surgical repair of the fetal diaphragm has allowed lung growth that then supports normal respiration (see Ch. 15). Thoracic compression and pulmonary hypoplasia may also result from reduced amniotic fluid or

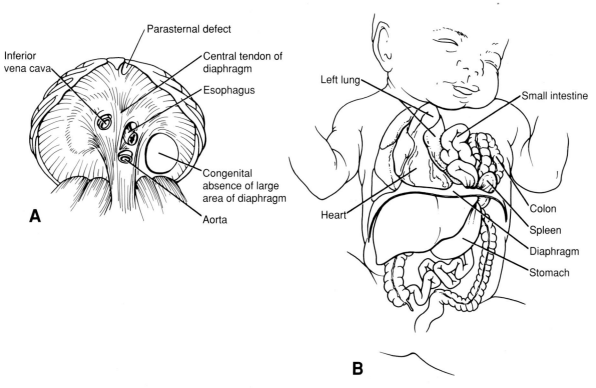

Fig. 6-13. Diaphragmatic hernia. This defect most often occurs through failure of the left pleuroperitoneal membrane to seal off the left pleural cavity completely from the peritoneal cavity. **(A)** Ventral view. **(B)** Abdominal contents may herniate through the patent pericardioperitoneal canal, preventing normal development of the lung on that side.

oligohydramnios. Amniotic fluid levels are normally maintained by a balance between excretion of fetal urine into the amnion and the swallowing of fluid and its transfer to the mother via the placenta. Oligohydramnios may be caused by **bilateral renal agenesis** or by obstruction of the urinary tract. Excess amniotic fluid or **polyhydramnios** may occur in cases of **esophageal atresia** (Fig. 6-14), which often occurs with **tracheoesophageal fistula,** suggesting that both conditions may be caused by an anomaly of endodermal proliferation in the thoracic foregut. The chief danger of esophageal atresia is that the newborn baby may aspirate its first drink of fluid and drown.

Lung malformations may also arise from intrinsic causes

Anomalies of **branching morphogenesis** of the lungs result from failure of the lung bud or bronchial buds to branch. Inhibition of splitting and growth of the lung bud may result in **pulmonary agenesis** or total absence of the lungs. Failure of the bronchial buds to bifurcate and grow may result in defects ranging from a reduction in lung lobes or bronchial segments to a paucity of alveoli. In situ hybridization and transgenic animal studies have shown that normal branching morphogenesis is regulated by growth factors, extracellular matrix molecules, and transcription factors produced by regulatory genes. For example, branching during the **pseudoglandular stage** is regulated by epithelial growth factor (EGF), platelet-derived growth factor (PDGF), fibroblast growth factor (FGF), and thyroid transcriptional factor (TTF-1). FGF and EGF are also active in branching during the **saccular stage.** One study implicated FGF in branching by a **dominant-negative mutation** of the FGF receptor gene. A transgene consisting of the surfactant C promoter element (see below) and a mutant form of the FGF receptor that lacked a kinase sequence was constructed and incorporated into embryonic stem cells (see Ch. 1) that were used to create heterozygous founder mice. The transgene was only expressed in the airway epithelium because it included the surfactant C promoter element. Since development of functional FGF receptors requires dimerization of two normal FGF receptor monomers, dimerization between mutant monomers and endogenous wild-type monomers (produced by the normal allele) resulted in formation of inactive pulmonary FGF receptors. Branching of the respiratory tree was completely blocked, resulting in formation of elongated epithelial tubes incapable of supporting respiration (Fig. 6-15).

The lungs mature rapidly just prior to birth

As birth approaches, the lungs undergo several transformations that prepare them for breathing. The fluid filling the alveoli is absorbed, the defenses that will protect the lungs against invading pathogens and oxidative effects of the atmosphere are activated, and the surface area for alve-

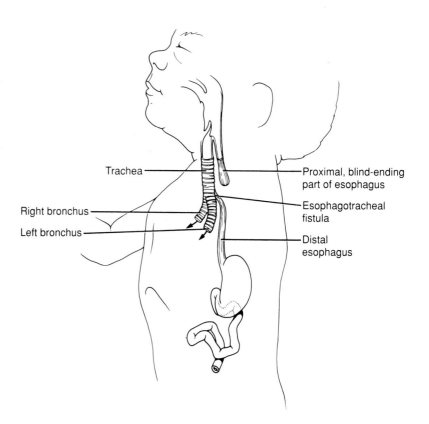

Fig. 6-14. This diagram of an infant with esophageal atresia and esophagotracheal fistula shows how the first drink of fluid after birth could be diverted into the newly expanded lungs (arrows).

Trachea —
Right bronchus —
Left bronchus —
Proximal, blind-ending part of esophagus
Esophagotracheal fistula
Distal esophagus

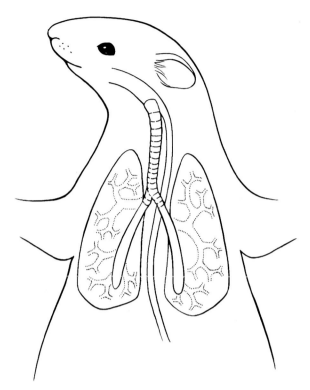

Fig. 6-15. Dominant-negative mutation of FGF receptor specifically expressed in the lungs results in inhibition of branching of the respiratory tree and formation of elongated epithelial tubes. (Modified from Peters K, Werner S, Liao X et al. 1994. Targeted expression of a dominant negative FGF receptor blocks branching morphogenesis and epithelial differentiation of the mouse lung. EMBO J. 13:3296, with permission.)

olar gas exchange greatly increases. These processes accelerate in the days preceding term delivery. In a premature birth, the status of the lungs usually determines whether the baby will live. Infants born between 32 weeks and term (38 weeks) have a good chance to live. Infants born before 28 weeks (end of the canalicular stage) cannot survive without intensive respiratory assistance and then often die.

Respiratory distress may result from failure to produce surfactant proteins

Efficient gas exchange within the alveoli only occurs if the barrier separating air from blood is thin; that is,

the alveoli are thin-walled, properly inflated, and not filled with fluid. The walls of the alveoli thin out just before birth. In addition, alveolar type II cells begin to secrete **pulmonary surfactant,** a mixture of phospholipids and surfactant proteins that reduces the surface tension of the air-alveolar interface, facilitating their inflation. Four surfactant proteins are synthesized by the alveolar type II cells (surfactants A, B, C, and D), and it appears that the primary cause of **respiratory distress syndrome** in **premature** infants is an inadequate production of surfactant. However, critically ill premature newborns have been successfully treated with **surfactant replacement therapy** since the 1970s, and now a variety of surfactant preparations are used, some derived from animal lungs or human amniotic fluid. It has been shown, however, that these preparations would be more effective if they included some of the normal surfactant proteins. Perhaps as it is learned how specific regulatory elements control their synthesis, strategies will be developed that stimulate premature infants to synthesize their own surfactant proteins. It is now known that **TTF-1** and hepatic nuclear factor-3 (HNF-3), tumor necrosis factor-α (TNF-α), glucocorticoids, and thyroxine play important roles in surfactant production.

Finally, a mutation of the surfactant B gene was found in babies exhibiting respiratory distress at term. Thus, while diagnosis of this **surfactant B deficiency syndrome** is possible, therapies for this variant of **pulmonary alveolar proteinosis** have not been developed. These infants die within the first year.

Cystic fibrosis is also studied with transgenic animal models

Mouse mutants in which the cAMP-stimulated chloride secretory activity of the cystic fibrosis gene is disrupted are created by homologous recombination. Current approaches to gene therapy of human cystic fibrosis are directed to the liposome- or adenovirus-mediated delivery of normal cystic fibrosis genes directly to the airway epithelial cells of afflicted infants and children.

7

Development of the Heart

Formation and Folding of the Primitive Heart Tube; Morphogenesis of the Heart Chambers and Valves; Development of the Cardiac Conduction System

The heart primordium forms within a **cardiogenic area** located cranial and lateral to the brain. At first, angioblasts in the splanchnopleuric mesoderm respond to inductive signals from the endoderm to form **lateral endocardial tubes,** and then during embryonic folding in the fourth week these vessels are translocated to the thoracic region, where they fuse to form the **primitive heart tube.** From week 5 to 8, the primitive heart tube undergoes folding, remodeling, and septation to form the four-chambered heart. Sinistral **looping** positions the regions of the heart tube that will form the primitive atria and ventricles and raises the inflow vessels to the level of the outflow tracts. As **remodeling** begins, the systemic venous circulation is diverted to the primitive right atrium so that the left atrium can be utilized for pulmonary venous return after birth. In addition, the **definitive right atrium** is formed by replacement of the primitive atrium by the right **sinus venosus,** while the **left sinus venosus** forms the **coronary sinus,** which then receives blood only from the wall of the heart. The **definitive left atrium** also forms as the left primitive atrium is replaced by incorporation of **pulmonary veins** that grew from its dorsal wall. The definitive left and right atria are then separated by the **septum primum** and **septum secundum,** the left and right ventricles and their outflow tracts are partitioned by **muscular** and **membranous ventricular septa,** and the left and right atrioventricular canals are formed by the **endocardial cushions.** Finally, **atrioventricular valves** are sculpted from the muscular ventricular walls, while the **aortic** and **pulmonary semilunar valves** are formed by the **truncoconal swellings** of the outflow tracts. Atrial and aortic-pulmonary shunts allow the entire heart to be utilized during gestation for systemic circulation, but their rapid closure at birth quickly creates distinct systemic and pulmonary circulations connected in series.

While most cardiac defects are **multifactorial** in origin, others arise from **single-gene mutations.** The latter include **familial cardiac hypertrophy** and **congenital long QT syndrome. Dextrocardia** or reverse looping of the heart may also be caused by single-gene mutations. Other malformations of the heart, including **atrial septal defects,** may be associated with chromosome anomalies such as trisomy 21. By far, the single most common life-threatening congenital cardiac anomaly is **ventricular septal defect.** This defect and related defects of the outflow tracts, including **persistent truncus arteriosus** and **tetralogy of Fallot,** may be caused by disruption of **neural crest cell migration.** These defects often occur with **craniofacial anomalies** and may arise from genetic causes or from the actions of teratogens like **retinoic acid.** Recent in situ hybridization and transgenic animal studies have implicated the disruption of regulatory genes and retinoic acid receptors among many other genes in normal cardiac development and congenital heart disease. These studies lay the groundwork for future diagnoses, preventative strategies, and therapies for the treatment of cardiac malformations.

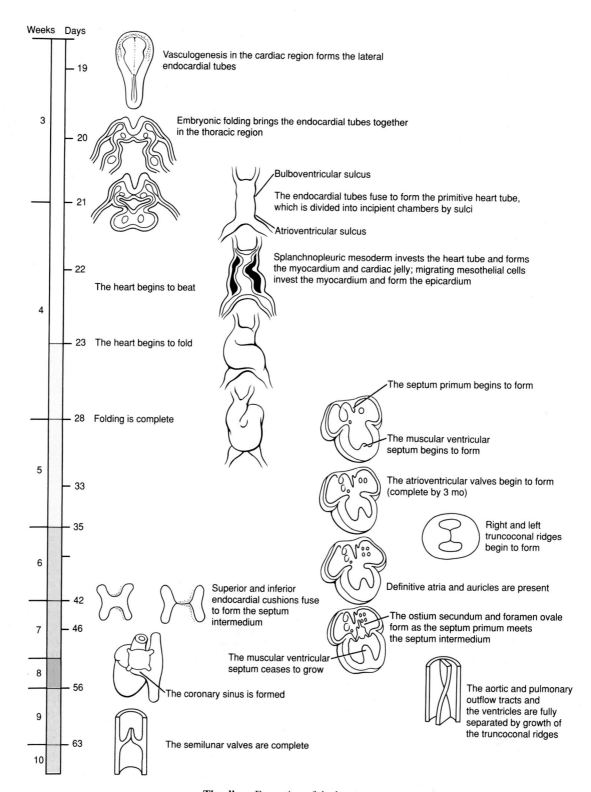

Weeks | **Days**

19 — Vasculogenesis in the cardiac region forms the lateral endocardial tubes

3

20 — Embryonic folding brings the endocardial tubes together in the thoracic region

Bulboventricular sulcus

21 — The endocardial tubes fuse to form the primitive heart tube, which is divided into incipient chambers by sulci

Atrioventricular sulcus

Splanchnopleuric mesoderm invests the heart tube and forms the myocardium and cardiac jelly; migrating mesothelial cells invest the myocardium and form the epicardium

22 — The heart begins to beat

4

23 — The heart begins to fold

The septum primum begins to form

28 — Folding is complete

The muscular ventricular septum begins to form

5

33 — The atrioventricular valves begin to form (complete by 3 mo)

35 — Right and left truncoconal ridges begin to form

6

Definitive atria and auricles are present

42 — Superior and inferior endocardial cushions fuse to form the septum intermedium

7   46 — The ostium secundum and foramen ovale form as the septum primum meets the septum intermedium

The muscular ventricular septum ceases to grow

8   56 — The coronary sinus is formed

The aortic and pulmonary outflow tracts and the ventricles are fully separated by growth of the truncoconal ridges

9

63 — The semilunar valves are complete

10

Timeline. Formation of the heart.

The lateral endocardial tubes develop in the cardiogenic region and fuse to form the primary heart tube

On day 19, a pair of vascular elements called the **endo-cardial tubes** begin to develop in the **cardiogenic region,** a horseshoe-shaped zone of splanchnopleuric mesoderm located cranial and lateral to the neural plate on the embryonic disc. These vessels form from splanchnopleuric mesoderm by a process called **in situ vesicle formation and fusion** or **vasculogenesis** (Fig. 7-1). Late in the third week, the cephalic and lateral folding of the embryo brings the two lateral endocardial tubes into the thoracic region (see Ch. 6), where they meet along the midline and fuse to form a single tube (Fig. 7-2). The fusion of the two tubes is facilitated by programmed cell death in their contacting surfaces.

The paired dorsal aortae of the primitive circulatory system form simultaneously with the lateral endocardial tubes

It is important to realize that many of the major vessels of the embryo develop at the same time as the endocardial tubes. The paired **dorsal aortae,** which form the primary outflow tract of the heart, develop in the dorsal mesenchyme of the embryonic disc on either side of the notochord and make their connection with the endocardial tubes before folding begins (Figs. 7-1 and 7-3). As the flexion and growth of the cephalic fold carries the endocardial tubes first into the cervical and then into the thoracic region (Figs. 7-3 and 7-4), the cranial ends of the dorsal aortae are pulled ventrally until they form a dorsoventral loop, the **first aortic arch** (Fig. 7-3D). A series of four more aortic arches will develop during the

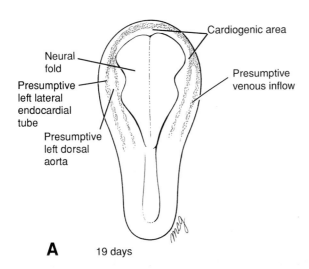

A   19 days

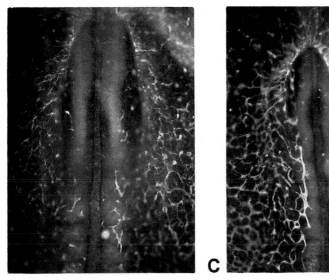

B

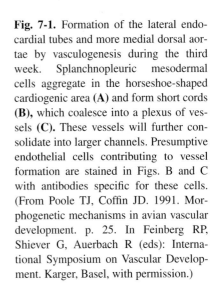

C

Fig. 7-1. Formation of the lateral endo-cardial tubes and more medial dorsal aortae by vasculogenesis during the third week. Splanchnopleuric mesodermal cells aggregate in the horseshoe-shaped cardiogenic area **(A)** and form short cords **(B),** which coalesce into a plexus of vessels **(C).** These vessels will further consolidate into larger channels. Presumptive endothelial cells contributing to vessel formation are stained in Figs. B and C with antibodies specific for these cells. (From Poole TJ, Coffin JD. 1991. Morphogenetic mechanisms in avian vascular development. p. 25. In Feinberg RP, Shiever G, Auerbach R (eds): International Symposium on Vascular Development. Karger, Basel, with permission.)

fourth and fifth weeks in connection with the pharyngeal arches (Fig. 7-5) (see Ch. 8).

The inflow to the heart is initially supplied by six vessels, three on each side (Fig. 7-5). Venous blood from the body of the embryo enters the heart through a pair of short trunks, the **common cardinal veins,** which are formed by the confluence of the paired **posterior cardinal veins** draining the trunk and the paired **anterior cardinal veins** draining the head region (Fig. 7-5). The yolk sac is drained by a pair of **vitelline veins,** and oxygenated blood from the placenta is delivered to the heart by a pair of **umbilical veins** (see Ch. 8).

A series of constrictions and expansions subdivide the primary heart tube

By day 21, a series of constrictions (**sulci**) and expansions appear in the presumptive heart tube (Fig. 7-6). Over the next 5 weeks, these expansions contribute to the various heart chambers. Starting at the inferior (inflow) end, the **sinus venosus** consists of the partially confluent left and right **sinus horns** into which the common cardinal veins drain. Cranial to the sinus venosus, the next two chambers are the **primitive atrium** and the **ventricle,** which are separated by the **atrioventricular sulcus.** The primitive atrium will give rise to parts of both atria, and the ventricle will give rise to most of the definitive left ventricle. The ventricle is separated from the next expansion, the **bulbus cordis,** by the **bulboventricular sulcus.** Because the inferior part of the bulbus cordis will form most of the **right ventricle,** this sulcus is also called the **interventricular sulcus.** The superior end of the bulbus cordis is also called the **conotruncus.** This region of the heart will form the distal outflow regions of the left and right ventricles, including the **conus cordis** and the **truncus arteriosus.** The truncus arteriosus eventually splits to form the **ascending aorta** and the **pulmonary trunk** and is connected at its superior end to a dilated expansion called the **aortic sac.** The aortic sac is continuous with the first aortic arch and, eventually, with the other four aortic arches. The aortic arches form major arteries that transport blood to the head and trunk (see Ch. 8).

Fig. 7-2. Cephalocaudal and lateral folding at the end of the third week quickly brings the lateral endocardial tubes into the ventral midline in the upper thoracic region **(A, B),** where they fuse to form the primitive heart tube **(C).** (Fig. C from Hurle JM, Icardo JM, Ojeda JL. 1980. Compositional and structural heterogeneity of the cardiac jelly of the chick embryo tubular heart: a TEM, SEM and histochemical study. J Embryol Exp Morphol 56:211, with permission.)

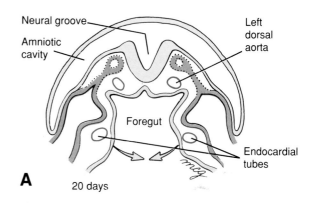

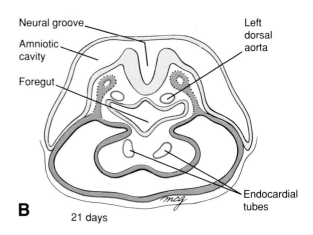

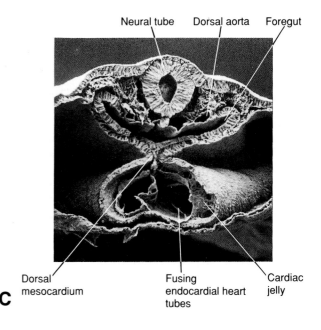

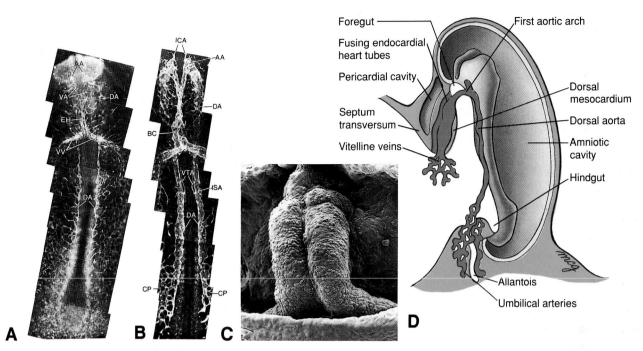

Fig. 7-3. Formation of embryonic vessels. **(A)** Vascular cords in the dorsal body wall form paired dorsal aortae (DA) both cranial and caudal to the embryonic heart tube (EH) developing in the ventral thoracic region. Vitelline veins (VV) are forming just caudal to the primitive heart tube, and the ventral region of the first aortic arch (VA) is forming just superior to the embryonic heart. The first aortic arch itself (AA) loops superiorly and dorsally to connect with the superior ends of the dorsal aortae (DA). **(B)** At a slightly later stage, the lateral endocardial tubes have fused and formed a distinct bulbus cordis (BC). The aortic arches (AA) loop dorsally to connect the superior end of the ventrally located heart with the superior ends of the dorsal aortae (DA). The dorsal aortae give off intersomitic arteries (ISA) and finally break up into capillary plexuses (CP). The third arch has begun to sprout internal carotid arteries (ICA). **(C)** Ventral view shows the fusing endocardial tubes within the primitive pericardial cavity. **(D)** Drawing shows the first aortic arches encircling the superior end of the foregut. Figs. A and B prepared as in Figure 7-1B, C. (Figs. A and B from Coffin JD, Poole TJ. 1988. Embryonic vascular development: immunohistochemical identification of the origin and subsequent morphogenesis of the major vessel primordia in quail embryos. Development 102:735, with permission. Fig. C from Icardo JM, Fernandez-Teran MA, Ojeda JL. 1990. Early cardiac structure and developmental biology. p. 3. In Meisami E, Timiras PS (eds): Handbook of Human Growth and Developmental Biology. Vol. 3. CRC Press, Boca Raton, with permission.)

Four layers become apparent in the wall of the primary heart tube

The primary heart tube consists initially of endothelium. By day 22, however, a thick mass of splanchnopleuric mesoderm invests the fused endocardial tubes and differentiates into two new layers: the **myocardium** or heart muscle and the **cardiac jelly,** a layer of thick acellular matrix that is secreted by the developing myocardium and separates it from the fused endocardial tubes (Fig. 7-7A). This structure, comprised of an endocardial tube, invested by cardiac jelly within a myocardial tube is called the primitive heart tube. The **serous epicardium (vis-**

ceral pericardium) is formed by a population of **mesothelial cells** that are independently derived from splanchnopleuric mesoderm and migrate onto the surface of the heart from the region of the sinus venosus or septum transversum (Fig. 7-7B). These epicardial cells also give rise to the coronary vessels of the heart.

The transverse pericardial sinus is formed by the rupture of the dorsal mesocardium

The primary heart tube is initially suspended in the primitive pericardial cavity by a **dorsal mesocardium (dorsal mesentery of the heart)** formed of foregut

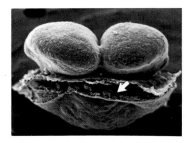
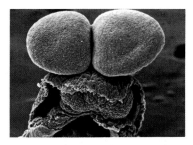
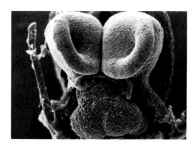

Fig. 7-4. Scanning electron micrographs showing how cephalic flexion translocates the developing endocardial tubes from a region just cranial to the neural plates to the thoracic region. (Arrow, cardiogenic region.) (From Kaufman MH. 1981. The role of embryology in teratological research, with particular reference to the development of the neural tube and the heart. J Reprod Fertil 62:607, with permission.)

splanchnopleuric mesoderm. This dorsal mesocardium promptly ruptures, however, leaving the heart suspended in the primitive pericardial cavity by its attached vasculature. The region of the ruptured dorsal mesocardium becomes the **transverse pericardial sinus** within the pericardial sac of the definitive heart (Fig. 7-8).

The heart tube loops to establish the spatial relationships of the future heart chambers

On day 23, the heart tube begins to elongate and simultaneously to loop. The bulbus cordis is displaced interiorly, ventrally, and to the right; the ventricle is displaced to the left; and the primitive atrium is displaced posteriorly and superiorly (Fig. 7-9). Looping is complete by day 28.

Considerable effort has gone into identifying the forces responsible for looping. It was at one time suggested that looping occurs simply because the heart tube outgrows the primitive pericardium; however, hearts excised from experimental animals and grown in culture demonstrate an intrinsic ability to loop. Some studies have suggested that the state of hydration of the cardiac jelly controls looping, but, when the jelly was removed enzymatically, looping was unaffected. Another suggestion is that looping is induced by the hemodynamic forces of circulating blood. Hemodynamic forces are certainly important in heart morphogenesis, but, again, cultured hearts loop cor-

Fig. 7-5. Schematic depiction of the embryonic vascular system in the middle of the fourth week. The heart has begun to beat and to circulate blood. The outflow tract of the heart now includes four pairs of aortic arches and the paired dorsal aortae that circulate blood to the head and trunk. Three pairs of veins—the umbilical, vitelline, and cardinal veins—deliver blood to the inflow end of the heart.

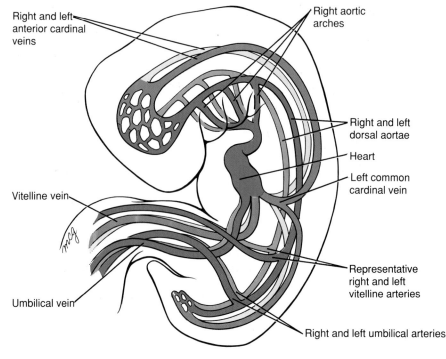
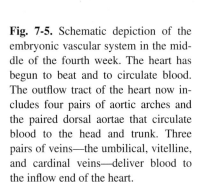

Right and left anterior cardinal veins

Right aortic arches

Right and left dorsal aortae

Heart

Left common cardinal vein

Vitelline vein

Umbilical vein

Representative right and left vitelline arteries

Right and left umbilical arteries

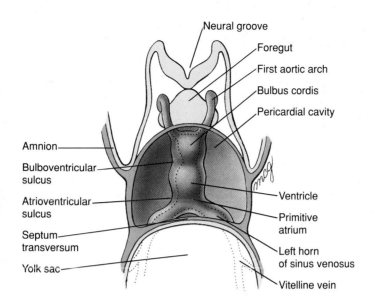

Fig. 7-6. As early as day 21, a series of visible constrictions and expansions divide the heart tube into primitive regions that will give rise to chambers of the adult heart.

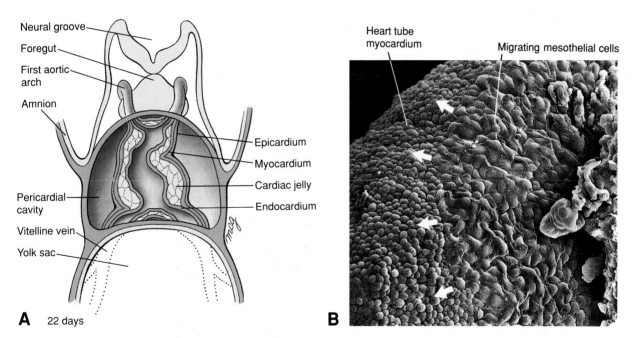

A 22 days

B

Fig. 7-7. Differentiation of the heart wall. **(A)** By 22 days, the primitive heart tube (the endocardium of the future heart) is invested by a layer of cardiac jelly, a layer of myocardial cells, and an epicardium. The myocardium is derived from a mass of splanchnopleuric mesoderm that encloses the primitive heart tube. The myocardium then secretes the extracellular cardiac jelly between itself and the primitive heart tube. **(B)** The epicardium is derived from a sheet of splanchnopleuric mesoderm that migrates from the region of the sinus venosus to cover the myocardium. (Fig. B from Ho E, Shimada Y. 1978. Formation of the epicardium studied with the scanning electron microscope. Dev Biol 66:579, with permission.)

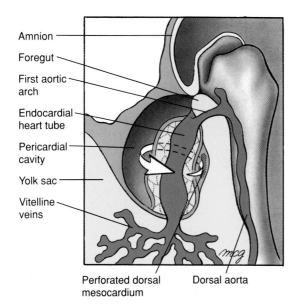

Amnion

Foregut

First aortic arch

Endocardial heart tube

Pericardial cavity

Yolk sac

Vitelline veins

Perforated dorsal mesocardium   Dorsal aorta

Fig. 7-8. Formation of the transverse and oblique coronary si-nuses of the definitive pericardial cavity by rupture of the dorsal mesocardium early in the fourth week.

rectly in the absence of blood flow. Looping may alterna-tively be caused by active migration or remodeling of my-ocytes or by controlled regional proliferation.

The result of looping is to bring the four presumptive chambers of the future heart into their correct spatial re-lation to each other. The remainder of heart develop-ment consists of the remodeling of these chambers and the development of the appropriate septa and valves be-tween them.

Coordinated remodeling of the bilaterally symmetrical heart tube and primitive vasculature produces the systemic and pulmonary circulations

At day 22, the heart and primitive circulatory system are bilaterally symmetrical: right and left cardinal veins drain the two sides of the body, and blood from the heart is pumped into right and left aortic arches and dorsal aor-tae. The paired dorsal aortae fuse from T4 to L4 in the fourth week to form a single midline dorsal aorta. The ve-nous system undergoes a complicated remodeling (de-tailed in Ch. 8) with the result that all the systemic venous blood drains into the right atrium through the newly formed superior and inferior venae cavae.

Starting at birth, the systemic and pulmonary circula-tions are wholly separate and are arranged in series. This arrangement would be impracticable in the fetus, how-ever, because oxygenated blood enters the fetus via the

umbilical vein and because little blood can flow through the collapsed lungs. The fetal heart chambers and outflow tracts therefore contain foramina and ducts that shunt the oxygenated blood entering the right atrium to the left ven-tricle and aortic arch, thus largely bypassing the pul-monary circulation. These shunts close at birth, abruptly separating the two circulations (see Ch. 8).

Remodeling of the heart tube commences as the venous inflow to the sinus venosus shifts to the right

The heart starts to beat on day 22, and by day 24 blood begins to circulate throughout the embryo. Venous return initially enters the right and left sinus horns via the com-mon cardinals (Fig. 7-10A). Within the next few weeks, however, the venous system is remodeled so that all the systemic venous blood enters the right sinus horn via the **superior** and **inferior venae cavae** (Fig. 7-10B, C). As venous inflow shifts to the right, the left sinus horn ceases to grow and is transformed into a small venous sac on the posterior wall of the heart (Fig. 7-10C). This structure gives rise to the **coronary sinus** and the small **oblique vein of the left atrium.** The coronary sinus will receive most of the blood draining from the coronary circulation of the heart muscle.

The left and right atria undergo extensive remodeling

The right sinus horn is incorporated into the right posterior wall of the primitive atrium

As the right sinus horn and the venae cavae enlarge to keep pace with the rapid growth of the rest of the heart, the right side of the sinus venosus is gradually incorpo-rated into the right posterior wall of the developing atrium, displacing the original right half of the primitive atrial wall ventrally and to the right (Figs. 7-10C and 7-11). The differential growth of the right sinus venosus also pulls the vestigial left sinus horn (the future coronary sinus) to the right. The portion of the atrium that consists of incorporated sinus venosus is now called the **sinus ve-narum,** while the original right side of the primitive atrium becomes a diminutive ventral flap of tissue called the **right auricle.** The auricle can be distinguished in the adult heart by the pectinate (comblike) trabeculation of its wall, which contrasts with the smooth wall of the sinus venarum.

Through this process of **intussusception** of the right sinus venosus, the openings or **ostia** of the superior and in-ferior venae cavae and future coronary sinus (former left horn of the sinus venosus) are pulled into the posterior wall

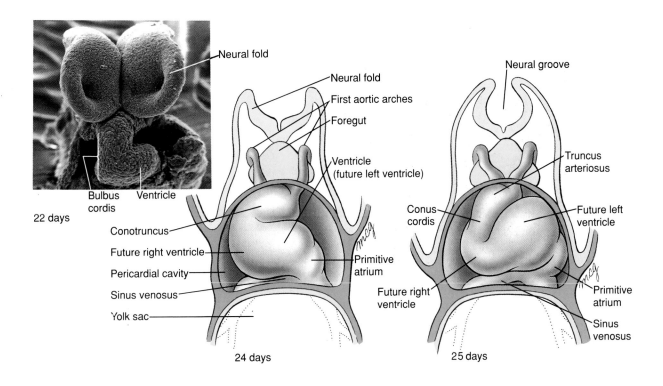

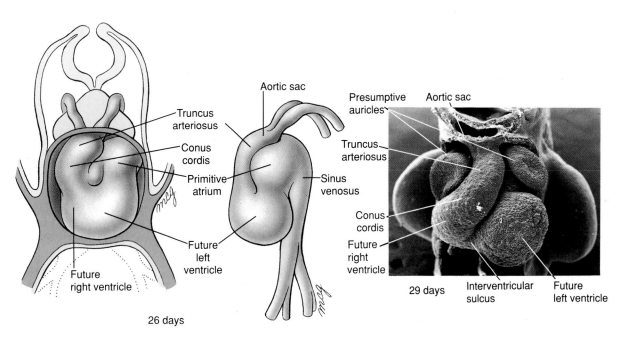

Fig. 7-9. Looping of the heart tube. The looping of the heart tube repositions the bulbus cordis anteriorly and to the right and shifts the ventricle to the left and the primitive atrium posteriorly and superiorly. The superior end of the bulbus cordis will form outflow regions of the right and left ventricles, while its inferior end will form most of the right ventricle. The ventricle will form most of the definitive left ventricle, and the primitive atrium will give rise to the rudimentary auricles of the heart. (Photos from Kaufman MH. 1981. The role of embryology in teratological research, with particular reference to the development of the neural tube and the heart. J Reprod Fertil 62:607, with permission.)

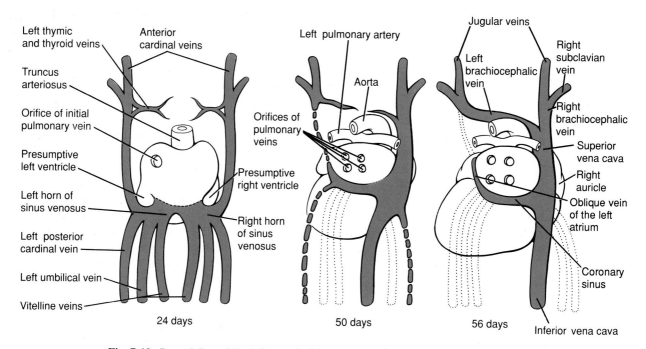

Left thymic and thyroid veins

Anterior cardinal veins

Truncus arteriosus

Orifice of initial pulmonary vein

Presumptive left ventricle

Left horn of sinus venosus

Left posterior cardinal vein

Left umbilical vein

Vitelline veins

24 days

Left pulmonary artery

Aorta

Orifices of pulmonary veins

Presumptive right ventricle

Right horn of sinus venosus

50 days

Jugular veins

Left brachiocephalic vein

Right subclavian vein

Right brachiocephalic vein

Superior vena cava

Right auricle

Oblique vein of the left atrium

Coronary sinus

56 days

Inferior vena cava

Fig. 7-10. Remodeling of the inflow end of the heart between weeks 4 and 8 so that all systemic blood flows into the future right atrium. The left sinus horn is reduced and pulled to the left. It loses its connection with the left anterior cardinal vein and becomes the coronary sinus that drains blood only from the heart wall. The left anterior cardinal vein becomes connected to the right anterior cardinal vein through an anastomosis of thymic and thyroid veins, which form the left brachiocephalic vein. A remnant of the right vitelline vein becomes the terminal segment of the inferior vena cava (see Ch. 8).

Fig. 7-11. Initial differentiation of the primitive atrium. During the fifth week, the primitive atrial tissue on the left and right sides is displaced anteriorly and laterally to form the trabeculated, rudimentary auricles of the adult heart. On the right side, the right sinus horn is incorporated into the posterior wall of the right side of the atrium as the smooth-walled sinus venarum, which will give rise to the definitive right atrium. Meanwhile, a single pulmonary vein sprouts from the left side of the primitive atrium and then branches twice to produce two right and two left pulmonary veins. The sinus venarum continues to expand within the posterior wall of the future right atrium.

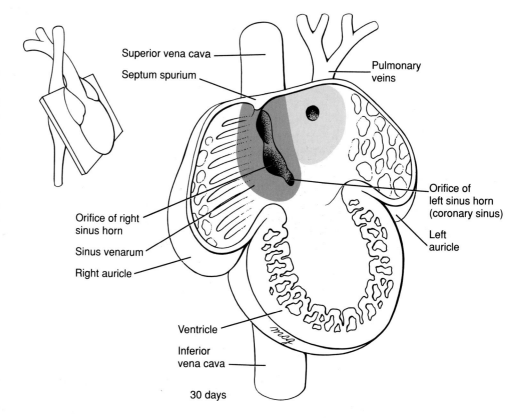

Superior vena cava

Septum spurium

Pulmonary veins

Orifice of left sinus horn (coronary sinus)

Left auricle

Orifice of right sinus horn

Sinus venarum

Right auricle

Ventricle

Inferior vena cava

30 days

of the definitive right atrium, where they form the **orifices of the superior and inferior venae cavae** and the **orifice of the coronary sinus** (Figs. 7-12 and 7-13). As this occurs, a pair of tissue flaps, the **left** and **right venous valves,** develops on either side of the three ostia. Superior to the sinuatrial orifices, the left and right valves join to form a transient septum called the **septum spurium.** The left valve eventually becomes part of the septum secundum, one of the septa that contribute to the separation of the definitive right and left atria (discussed below). The right venous valve, in contrast, remains intact and forms the **valve of the inferior vena cava** and the **valve of the coronary sinus.**

Superior to the valve of the inferior vena cava, a ridge of tissue called the **crista terminalis** now delimits the trabeculated right auricle from the smooth-walled sinus venarum (Fig. 7-13).

The trunk of the pulmonary venous system is incorporated into the posterior wall of the left atrium

While the right atrium is being remodeled during the fourth and fifth weeks, the left atrium undergoes a somewhat similar process. At the beginning of the fourth week, the primitive atrium sprouts a pulmonary vein (Fig. 7-11). This vein promptly branches into right and left pulmonary branches, which bifurcate again to produce a total of four pulmonary veins. These veins grow toward the lungs, where they anastomose with veins developing in the mesoderm investing the bronchial buds (see Ch. 6).

During the fifth week a process of intussusception incorporates the trunk and first two branchings of the pulmonary vein system into the posterior wall of the left side of the primitive atrium (Figs. 7-11 and 7-12), where they form the smooth wall of the definitive left atrium. The trabeculated left side of the primitive atrium is displaced ventrally and to the left, where it becomes the vestigial left auricle. As a result of this process, the pulmonary venous system opens into the atrium initially through a single large orifice, then transiently through two orifices, and finally through the four orifices of the definitive pulmonary veins (Fig. 7-13).

Septation of the atria and division of the atrioventricular canal begin in the fourth week, but right-to-left shunting of blood persists until birth

At the end of the fourth week, the septum primum begins to grow down from the atrial roof

On about day 26, while atrial remodeling is in progress, the roof of the atrium becomes depressed along

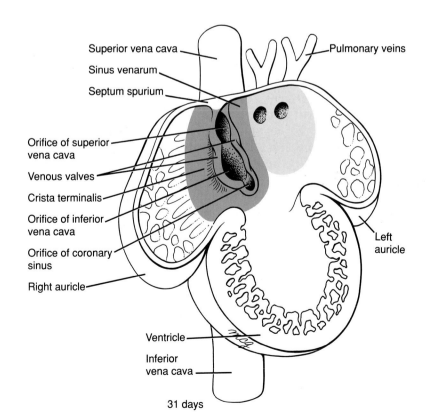

Fig. 7-12. Further differentiation of the atrium. Later in the fifth week, the pulmonary vein system begins to undergo intussusception into the posterior wall of the primitive atrium to form the definitive left atrium.

Superior vena cava

Sinus venarum

Septum spurium

Pulmonary veins

Orifice of superior vena cava

Venous valves

Crista terminalis

Orifice of inferior vena cava

Orifice of coronary sinus

Right auricle

Left auricle

Ventricle

Inferior vena cava

31 days

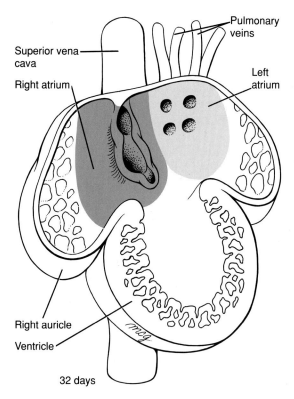

Fig. 7-13. Definitive formation of the left atrium. The first four pulmonary branches are incorporated into the posterior wall of the left side of the primitive atrium, completing the formation of the smooth-walled part of the future left atrium.

the midline by the overlying conotruncus. On day 28, this deepening depression produces a crescent-shaped wedge of tissue called the **septum primum** that begins to extend into the atrium from the superoposterior wall (Fig. 7-14). During the fifth week, the free edge of the septum primum grows caudally toward the atrioventricular canal, thus gradually separating the nascent right and left atria. The diminishing foramen between the atria is called the **ostium primum.**

The septum primum fuses with the septum intermedium

As the septum primum is growing downward, four expansions of tissue develop in the endocardium around the periphery of the atrioventricular canal (Fig. 7-14A). These thickenings are called the **left, right, superior,** and **inferior endocardial (atrioventricular) cushions.** The endocardium is induced to form the cushions by signals from the adjacent myocardium. At the end of the sixth week, the superior and inferior cushions meet and fuse, forming the **septum intermedium** that divides the common atrioventricular canal into **right** and **left atrioven-**

tricular canals (Figs. 7-15A, 7-16, and 7-17C). At the end of the sixth week, the growing edge of the septum primum fuses with the septum intermedium (Figs. 7-15A and 7-19D). This event obliterates the ostium primum.

Before the ostium primum closes, however, programmed cell death in an area near the superior edge of the septum primum creates small perforations that coalesce to form a new foramen, the **ostium secundum** (Fig. 7-15B). Thus, a new channel for right-to-left shunting opens before the old one closes.

An incomplete septum secundum forms next to the septum primum

While the septum primum is growing, a second crescent-shaped ridge of tissue appears on the ceiling of the right atrium, just adjacent to the septum primum (Fig. 7-15A). This **septum secundum** is thick and muscular, in contrast to the thin, membranous septum primum. The edge of the septum secundum grows posteroinferiorly, but it halts before it reaches the septum intermedium, leaving an opening called the **foramen ovale** near the floor of the right atrium (Fig. 7-16). Throughout the rest of fetal development, therefore, the blood that shunts from the right atrium to the left atrium passes through two staggered openings: the foramen ovale near the floor of the right atrium and the foramen secundum near the roof of the left atrium. This shunt closes at birth because the abrupt dilation of the pulmonary vasculature combined with the cessation of umbilical flow reverses the pressure difference between the atria and pushes the flexible septum primum against the more rigid septum secundum (see the discussion of changes in circulation at birth at the end of Ch. 8).

Extensive remodeling aligns the right and left atrioventricular canals with their respective atria and ventricles and the left and right ventricles with their future outflow tracts

Even after the heart tube finishes looping, the atrioventricular canal provides a direct pathway only between the future atrium and the future left ventricle (Fig. 7-17A). Moreover, the superior end of the presumptive right ventricle, but not the presumptive left ventricle, is initially continuous with the conus cordis and truncus arteriosus that will eventually give rise to both the aortic and pulmonary outflow tracts. The heart must therefore undergo a complicated remodeling to bring the developing right atrioventricular canal into line with its atrium and ventricle and simultaneously to provide the left ventricle with a direct outflow path through the conus cordis to the truncus arteriosus. This process is illustrated in Figure 7-17. It is thought that the apparent rightward movement of the

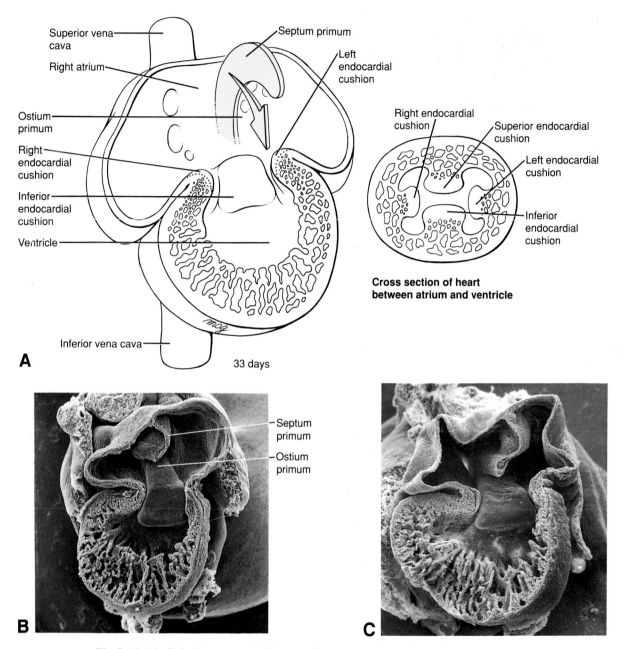

Fig. 7-14. (A–C) Initial septation of the atria. The septum primum forms from the roof of the atrial chamber during the fifth week and grows as a crescent-shaped wedge toward the atrioventricular canal. Simultaneously, the atrioventricular canal is being divided into right and left atrioventricular orifices by the growing superior and inferior endocardial cushions. (Figs. B and C from Icardo JM. 1988. Heart anatomy and developmental biology. Experientia 44:910, with permission.)

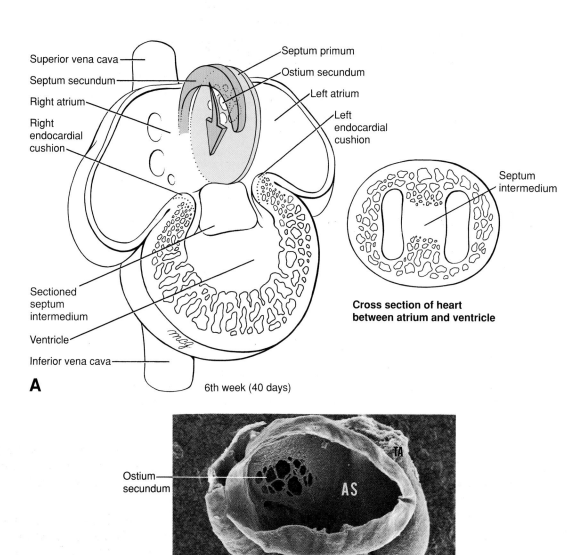

Fig. 7-15. Further septation of the atria. **(A)** During the sixth week, the thick septum secundum grows from the roof of the right atrium and the septum primum fuses with the superior and inferior endocardial cushions (septum intermedium). Before the ostium primum is obliterated, however, the ostium secundum forms by the coalescence of small ruptures in the septum primum. **(B)** Scanning electron micrograph showing the development of the ostium secundum. (Fig. B from Hendrix MJC, Morse DE. 1977. Atrial septation. I. Scanning electron microscopy in the chick. Dev Biol 57:345, with permission.)

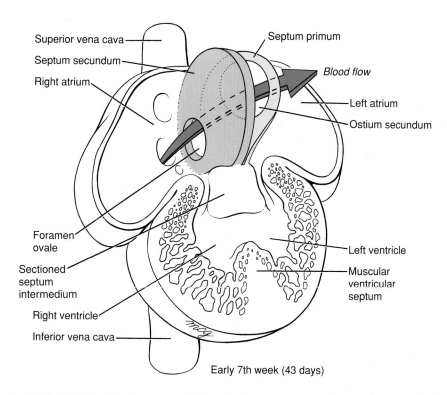

Superior vena cava

Septum secundum

Right atrium

Septum primum

Blood flow

Left atrium

Ostium secundum

Foramen ovale

Sectioned septum intermedium

Right ventricle

Inferior vena cava

Left ventricle

Muscular ventricular septum

Early 7th week (43 days)

Fig. 7-16. Definitive fetal separation of the atria. The septum secundum does not completely close, leaving a patent foramen ovale. During embryonic and fetal life, much of the blood entering the right atrium passes to the left atrium via the foramen ovale and ostium secundum.

canal may result wholly from the obliteration of the superior internal protrusion of the bulboventricular sulcus and the widening of the conotruncus. In addition, at the same time that the canal is shifting to the right, it is being divided into right and left canals by the growth of the superior and inferior endocardial cushions. Thus, by the time the common canal has split into right and left atrioventricular canals, they are correctly aligned with their respective atria and ventricles (Fig. 7-17C).

The repositioning that brings the presumptive left ventricle into line with the proximal portion of the truncus arteriosus is apparently due to several factors working in concert. The reduction of the bulboventricular flange by differential growth and the widening of the proximal part of the conus cordis partly effects this shift. A role also seems to be played by the left wall of the proximal end of the conus cordis, which is incorporated into the left ventricle and by the differential expansion of the right wall of the right ventricle and the left wall of the left ventricle (Fig. 7-17).

Both ventricles seem thus to be composite structures. The right ventricle is derived mainly from the most inferior part of the bulbus cordis and from the right wall of the conus cordis. In addition, part of the inlet region of the right ventricle, near the tricuspid atrioventricular valve, originates in the primitive ventricle and is carried over to the right ventri-

cle during the repositioning of the atrioventricular canal. The definitive left ventricle is derived from the primitive ventricle and from the left wall of the conus cordis.

Septation of the ventricles is coordinated with the formation of atrioventricular valves and septation of the outflow tracts

Starting at the end of the fourth week, a muscular ventricular septum incompletely separates the ventricles

At the end of the fourth week, the inferior part of the bulboventricular sulcus begins to protrude into the cardiac lumen along the interface between the presumptive right and left ventricular chambers (Figs. 7-17 and 7-18). This septum apparently forms as the growing walls of the right and left ventricle become more closely opposed to one another. However, the growth of this **muscular ventricular septum** halts in the middle of the seventh week before its leading edge meets the septum intermedium. This arrest of growth is crucial: if fusion occurred too soon, the left ventricle would be shut off from the ventricular outflow tract.

At the same time that the muscular ventricular septum is forming, the myocardium begins to thicken, and myocar-

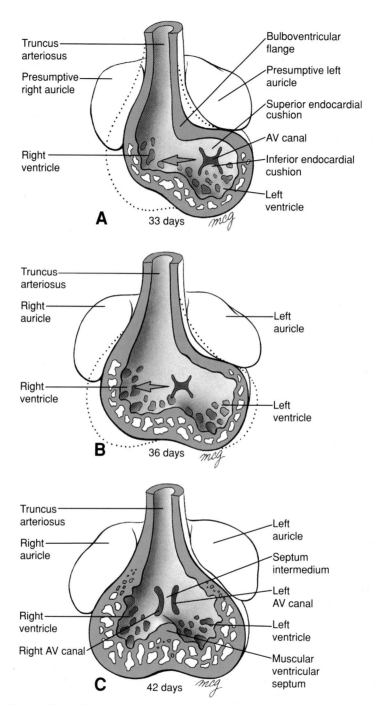

Fig. 7-17. (A–C) Realignment of the heart. As the septum intermedium forms during the fifth and sixth weeks, the heart is remodeled to align the developing left atrioventricular canal with the left atrium and ventricle and the right atrioventricular canal with the right atrium and ventricle.

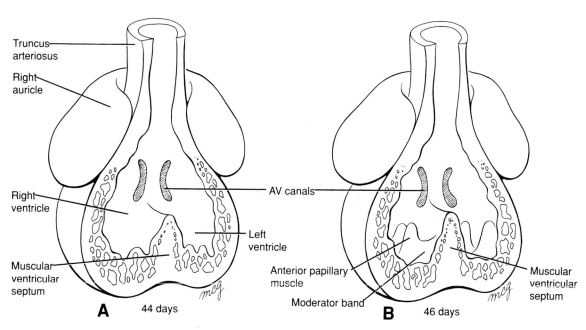

Fig. 7-18. (**A & B**) Initial septation of the ventricles. The muscular interventricular septum enlarges in the region of the interventricular sulcus between weeks 4 and 7. (See Fig. 7-17 for the completion of ventricular septation.)

dial ridges or **trabeculae** appear on the inner wall of both ventricles. The anterior portion of the muscular ventricular septum is trabeculated and is called the **primary ventricular fold** or **septum** (Fig. 7-18B). The posterior part of the septum is smooth walled and is called the **inlet septum** because of its proximity to the atrioventricular canals. On the right wall of the muscular ventricular septum, the boundary between the trabeculated primary fold and the inlet septum is marked by a constant, prominent trabeculation called the **septomarginal trabecula** or **moderator band** (Fig. 7-18B). This structure connects the muscular septum with the **anterior papillary muscle** that has begun to form as part of the right atrioventricular valve.

The atrioventricular valves are formed from the ventricular myocardium and prevent backflow of blood during systole

The atrioventricular valves begin to form between the fifth and eighth weeks. Undermining of the myocardium surrounding the left and right atrioventricular canals forms anterior and posterior **leaflets** or **cusps** on either side of both canals (Fig. 7-19). These valve leaflets are firmly rooted in the rim of the canals but are not thought to arise as differentiations of the adjacent endocardial cushions. The free edge of each leaflet is attached to the anterior and posterior ventricular walls by thin sinews called **chordae tendinae,** which insert into small hillocks of myocardium called **papillary muscles** (Fig. 7-19C, D).

The valve leaflets are designed so that they fold back to allow blood to enter the ventricles from the atria during diastole but shut to prevent backflow when the ventricles contract (Fig. 7-19D).

The left atrioventricular valve has only anterior and posterior leaflets and is called the **bicuspid valve (mitral valve).** The right atrioventricular valve usually (but not always) develops a third, small **septal cusp** during the third month and therefore is called the **tricuspid valve** (Fig. 7-19D).

The spiral prowth of the truncoconal septa results in the helical arrangement of the ascending aorta and pulmonary trunk

At the time when the muscular interventricular septum ceases to grow, the two ventricles communicate with each other through the interventricular foramen and also with the expanded base of the conus cordis (Fig. 7-20). Further septation of the ventricles and the outflow tract must occur in tight coordination if the heart is to function properly. Not surprisingly, a large proportion of cardiac defects are due to errors in this complex process.

The cardiac outflow pathway is divided into two by swellings or ridges that grow from the opposite walls of the conus cordis and truncus arteriosus and meet in the middle (Figs. 7-20 and 7-21A). These ridges are bulbous at first (see Fig. 7-21A) and fill much of the conotruncal lumen, but eventually they thin and fuse to form a septum that completely separates the right and left ventricular outflow pathways. The final division of the truncus arteriosus to form the **ascending aorta** and the **pulmonary trunk** is accomplished by a split that develops within the plane of the septum itself (Fig. 7-20).

It has been suggested that as many as three separate pairs of swellings (aortopulmonary complex, truncal septa, and conal septa) join to form the final septum. An alternative theory is that septation is accomplished by a single pair of **truncoconal swellings** that grow in both directions. In either case, it is clear that septation commences at the inferior end of the truncus arteriosus and proceeds superiorly and inferiorly.

Separation of the aortic and pulmonary outflow tracts becomes complete when the truncoconal swellings fuse with the inferior endocardial cushion and the muscular interventricular septum, thus completely separating the right and left ventricles. Growth of this **membranous ventricular septum** normally occurs between weeks 5 and 8; however, failure of complete fusion, resulting in a ventricular septal defect, is the most common congenital heart defect (see the Clinical Applications section of this chapter).

The swellings that separate left and right ventricular outflow tracts apparently arise in a spiral along the walls of the truncus arteriosus and the ventricular outflow tracts. As a result, the left and right ventricular outflow tracts and, eventually, the aorta and pulmonary trunk twist around each other in a helical arrangement (Fig. 7-20).

The truncus swellings also contribute to the semilunar valves in the aortic and pulmonary trunks

By the middle of the fifth week, a small tubercle or bulge appears on the tip of each truncus swelling at the inferior end of the truncus arteriosus (Fig. 7-21A). At this level, the truncus swellings are rooted in the right and left lateral walls of the truncus. When the swellings fuse together to separate the outflow tracts, these lateral tubercles are split in two, so that half of each is distributed into each of the resulting outflow tracts (Fig. 7-21B). Meanwhile, a second pair of tubercles develop on the anterior and posterior walls of the truncus at the same level. After septation, the tubercle on the anterior wall lies in the developing pulmonary channel, and the tubercle on the posterior wall lies in the developing aortic channel.

After septation, each outflow tract thus contains three tubercles laid out in a triangle: two formed from the split lateral tubercles and a third growing on the anterior or posterior truncal wall. These tubercles give rise to the cusps of the three-cusped **semilunar valves** that prevent backflow from the aorta and pulmonary trunk into the ventricles. The cup-shaped valve leaflets are formed by

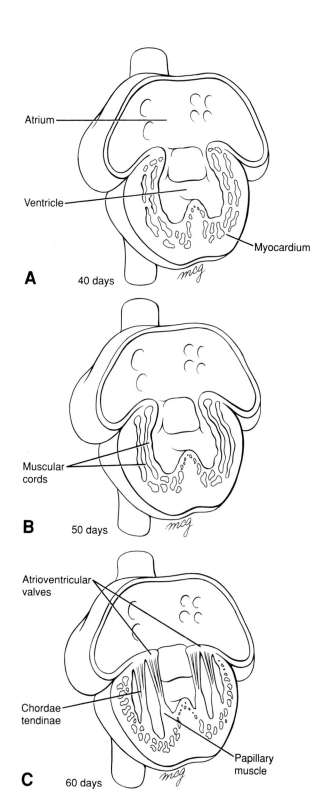

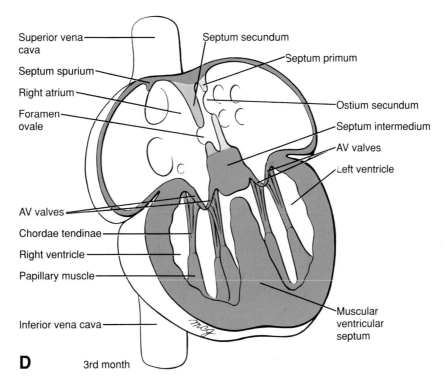

Fig. 7-19. (A–D) Development of the atrioventricular valves. The structures of the atrioventricular valves, including the papillary muscles, chordae tendinae, and cusps, are sculpted from the muscular walls of the ventricles. The definitive tricuspid valve within the right ventricle is not completely formed until the development of a septal cusp in the third month.

the excavation of truncal tissue inferior to the initial site of tubercle formation. As a result of this excavation, the bases of the leaflets migrate inferiorly during the maturation of the valves. This migration follows the spiral course of the outflow vessels, so the valves appear to rotate slightly during development (Fig. 7-21C). Development of the semilunar valves is complete by 9 weeks.

The pacemaker and conduction system form early to coordinate the beating of the heart

The heart is one of the few organs that has to function almost as soon as it is formed—it begins to beat and to propel blood through the embryo and placenta on day 22. The rhythmic waves of electrical depolarization (action potentials) that trigger the myocardium to contract are **myogenic**—that is, they arise spontaneously in the cardiac muscle itself and spread from cell to cell. The sympathetic and parasympathetic neural input to the heart modifies the heart rate but does not initiate beats. Myocytes removed from the primitive heart tube and grown in tissue culture will begin to beat in unison if they become connected to one another, and studies with voltage-

sensitive dyes indicate that cardiac myocytes may begin to produce rhythmic electrical activity even before the lateral endocardial tubes have fused.

In a normally functioning heart, the beat is initiated in a **pacemaker region** that has a faster rate of spontaneous depolarization than the rest of the myocardium. Moreover, the depolarization spreads from the pacemaker to the rest of the heart along specialized **conduction pathways** that control the timing of contraction of the various regions of the myocardium and thus ensure that the chambers will contract efficiently and in the right sequence. In the primitive heart tube, the ventricle seems to serve as the initial pacemaker. However, pacemaker activity is rapidly taken over by a cluster of pacemaking cells in the sinoatrial region, which are derived either from the right common cardinal vein or from the right sinus venosus. These cells form a distinct ovoid structure called the **sinoatrial node** (SAN) in the left venous valve.

Soon after the development of the SAN, cells in the superior endocardial cushion begin to form a secondary pacemaker center, the **atrioventricular node** (AVN), which receives impulses from the SAN and controls the beating of the two ventricles. The main conduction pathway between the SAN and the AVN runs through the

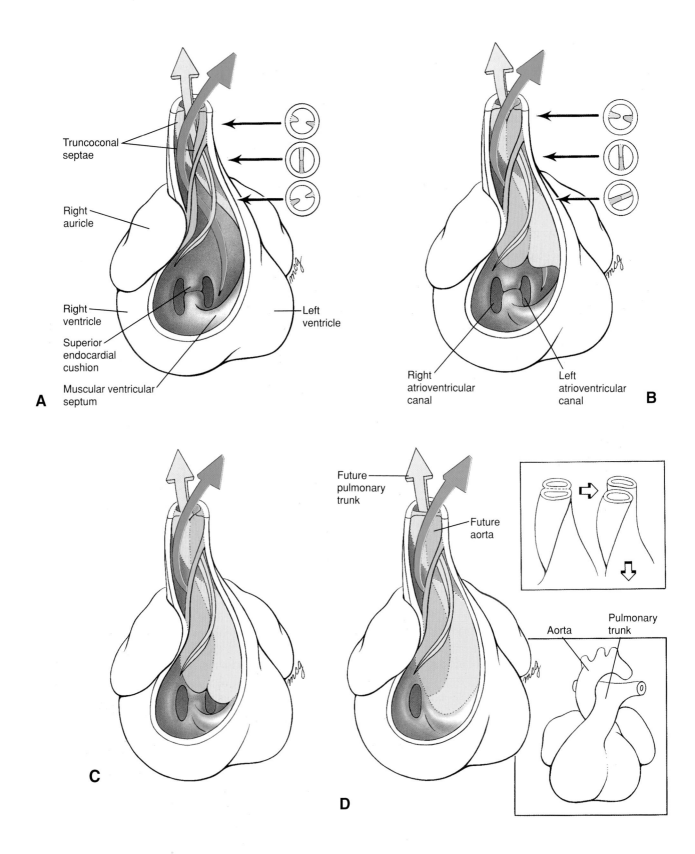

Truncoconal
septae

Right
auricle

Right
ventricle

Left
ventricle

Superior
endocardial
cushion

Muscular ventricular
septum

A

Right
atrioventricular
canal

Left
atrioventricular
canal

B

C

Future
pulmonary
trunk

Future
aorta

Aorta   Pulmonary
trunk

D

◀ **Fig. 7-20.** Septation of the cardiac outflow tract and final septation of the ventricles. Right oblique view. The anterolateral wall of the right ventricle has been removed to show the interior of the right ventricular chamber and the presumptive outflow tracts of both ventricles. **(A, B)** Starting in the fifth week, the right and left truncoconal swellings grow out from the walls of the common ventricular outflow tract at the junction of the truncus arteriosus and conus cordis. When they meet, they begin to zipper together superiorly and interiorly. **(C, D)** By the ninth week, the inferior regions of the truncoconal swellings have grown down onto the upper ridge of the muscular ventricular septum and onto the inferior endocardial cushion separating the right and left ventricular chambers. The truncoconal swellings have grown in a spiral configuration, separating the aortic and pulmonary outflow tracts from each other. (Modified from Steding G, Seidl W. 1980. Contribution to the development of the heart. Part I. Normal development. Thorac Cardiovasc Surg 28:386, with permission.)

crista terminalis, as mentioned earlier, although other pathways in the interatrial septum may also exist. The development of the AVN is accompanied by the appearance of a bundle of specialized conducting cells, the **bundle of His,** which sends one branch into the right ventricle and the other into the left ventricle within the septomarginal trabeculation or moderator band. This conduction path-

way must be carefully avoided during the repair of ventricular septal defects.

The detailed ontogeny of the cardiac conduction system is somewhat controversial. It has been suggested that most of the conduction pathway arises from cardiogenic mesoderm but that the sinus node may originate from the neural crest.

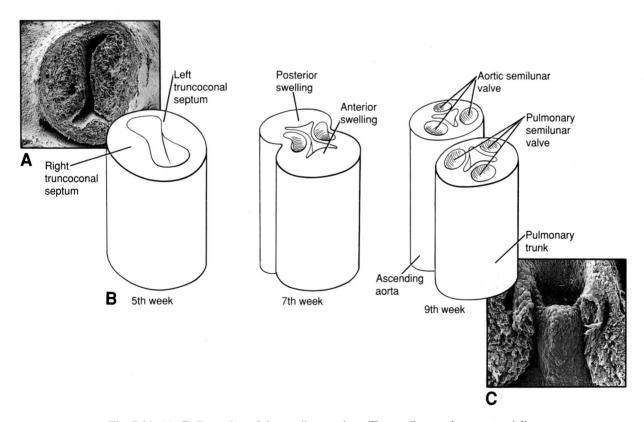

Fig. 7-21. **(A–C)** Formation of the semilunar valves. The semilunar valves are specializations of the right and left truncoconal swellings and two minor swellings. Note that the left and right truncoconal swellings each form right and left semilunar valves of the aorta and the pulmonary trunk. (Figs. A and C from Hurle JM, Colvee E, Blanco AM. 1980. Development of mouse semilunar valves. Anat Embryol 160:83, with permission.)

APPLICATIONS TO CLINICAL PRACTICE

Cardiovascular malformations are the most common type of life-threatening congenital defect

Congenital cardiac malformations account for about 20 percent of all congenital defects in liveborn infants. They occur in about 5 to 8 of every 1,000 live births, and the percentage in stillborn infants is probably even higher. Ventricular septal defects are the most common congenital cardiac malformation, although defects may involve almost any region of the heart. Like other congenital malformations, heart defects result from disturbances of normal developmental mechanisms. A few are associated with single-gene mutations; others result from chromosomal aberrations such as trisomies; yet others arise from the action of teratogens. Most cardiac malformations, however, are **multifactorial;** that is, they stem from the interaction of environmental influences with a poorly defined constellation of the individual's own genetic determinants.

Disruption of virtually any step in heart development may result in clinically significant cardiac malformations

An error in almost any step of heart development from formation of the primitive heart tube to septation of the outflow tracts may result in a cardiac defect. For example, **dextrocardia** occurs when the primitive heart tube loops to the right instead of to the left (Fig. 7-22) and is often accompanied by reversal in the organization of all organs,

a condition called **situs inversus.** Several genes that regulate situs, including heart tube looping have been identified in experimental animals (see Applications to Clinical Practice section of Ch. 9). Mutations of the gene encoding the gap junction protein connexin 43 also disturb the looping of the primitive heart tube in humans in an autosomal recessive syndrome. Transgenic knockout of the connexin 43 gene in mice, however, does not affect heart tube looping but disrupts development of the outflow tract resulting in death at birth.

In about 6 of 10,000 live births, the septum secundum is too short to completely cover the ostium secundum, so an **atrial septal defect** may persist after birth. The massive shunting of blood from the left to the right atrium may be asymptomatic in the newborn, but may lead to enlargement of the right ventricle and pulmonary trunk with ensuing heart failure. Atrial septal defect is associated with almost all documented autosomal and sex chromosome aberrations and is a characteristic of several partial and complete trisomies, including trisomy 21.

Atrioventricular septal defect (endocardial cushion defect) arises from failure of the superior and inferior (atrioventricular) cushions to fuse, leading to incomplete closure of the septum primum and ventricular septum. **Congestive heart failure in infancy** may result if significant left-to-right shunting of blood occurs. This defect can be surgically corrected.

Valvular defects may affect either the atrioventricular or mitral valves. In **Ebstein's disease,** the tricuspid valve balloons into the right ventricle, blocking access of blood

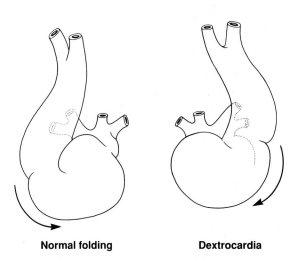

Normal folding **Dextrocardia**

Fig. 7-22. In dextrocardia, the folding of the heart tube is reversed from the normal sinistral folding, producing a heart that is normal in form but is a mirror image of the normal heart.

to the pulmonary orifice and allowing blood to regurgitate into the right atrium. As a result, right atrial blood shunts to the left atrium through a persistent foramen ovale. Blood reaches the pulmonary circulation through the left ventricle, aorta, and persistent truncus arteriosus. This causes the left ventricle to enlarge while the right ventricle becomes hypoplastic. This condition tends to cause **cyanosis** (inadequate oxygenation of the blood) in the newborn and can be surgically corrected.

Disruptions of neural crest cell migration and differentiation result in ventricular septal defects and defects in septation of the outflow tracts. These may occur together or as isolated defects. **Ventricular septal defects** account for 25 percent of all cardiac abnormalities in live infants and occurs as an isolated defect in 12 of 10,000 live births. A ventricular septal defect can occur because of (1) deficient development of the proximal truncoconal swellings, (2) failure of the muscular and membranous ventricular septa to fuse (Fig. 7-23), (3) endocardial cushion defect, and (4) excessive perforation of the muscular ventricular septum. A serious consequence of this defect is massive left-to-right shunting of blood and pulmonary hypertension after birth. Surgical repair of the defect in children usually results in rapid correction of the pulmonary blood pressure and reduction of the heart to normal size. In about 1 in 10,000 live births the truncoconal septa and ventricular membranous septum do not form at all, resulting in a **persistent truncus arteriosus** (Fig. 7-24A). In this condition, blood from both sides of the heart mix, and both body and lungs receive partially oxygenated blood. Untreated infants usually die within 2

years, but surgical correction, while difficult, is possible. In about 5 of 10,000 infants, the truncoconal septa do not spiral within the outflow tracts, resulting in a condition called **transposition of the great vessels,** in which the left ventricle empties into the pulmonary circulation and the aorta empties into the systemic circulation (Fig. 7-24B). It is not immediately fatal as long as deoxygenated systemic and oxygenated pulmonary blood can mix through a patent ductus arteriosus. Nonetheless, this condition is the leading cause of death in infants under 1 year old with cyanotic heart disease.

Tetralogy of Fallot arises through a pathogenetic cascade

In some cases, a primary malformation sets off a cascade of effects that leads to other malformations. An example is a condition described by Steno of Denmark in 1673 and first called *la maladie bleue* by Etienne-Louis Arthur Fallot in 1888. This syndrome, now called the **tetralogy of Fallot** is characterized by four classic malformations: (1) **pulmonary stenosis,** (2) **ventricular septal defect,** (3) rightward displacement of the aorta (sometimes called **overriding aorta**), and (4) **right ventricular hypertrophy** (Fig. 7-25). The primary defect is malalignment of the muscular outlet septum, which leads to pulmonary stenosis, disruption of normal fusion between the muscular and membranous ventricular septa, and rightward displacement of the aorta. These defects together raise the blood pressure within the right ventricle, resulting in its enlargement. Tetralogy of Fallot is the most

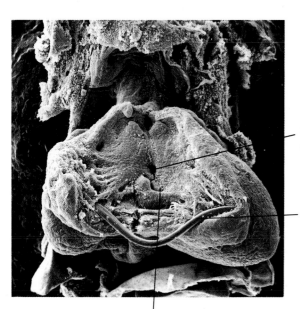

Ventricular septal defect

Pin holding ventricle open

Muscular ventricular septum

Fig. 7-23. Typical ventricular septal defect in a mouse fetus with trisomy 12. Failure of the membranous ventricular septum to fuse with the upper ridge of the muscular septum in this heart has resulted in a ventricular septal defect. (From Pexieder T. 1978. Development of the outflow tract of the embryonic heart. Birth Defects XIV:29, with permission.)

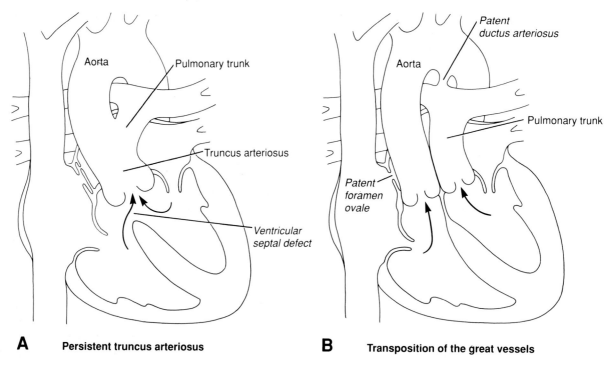

A   Persistent truncus arteriosus   **B**   Transposition of the great vessels

Fig. 7-24. **(A)** Persistent truncus arteriosus. Incomplete separation of aortic and pulmonary outflow tracts may accompany a ventricular septal defect when the right and left truncoconal septae fail to form. **(B)** Transposition of the great arteries results from failure of the truncoconal septae to spiral as they separate the aortic and pulmonary outflow tracts.

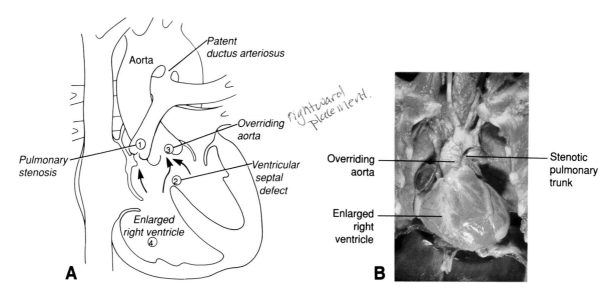

Fig. 7-25. Tetralogy of Fallot **(A)** Classically, tetralogy of Fallot is characterized by (1) stenosis (narrowing) of the pulmonary trunk, (2) ventricular septal defect, (3) overriding aorta, and (4) an enlarged right ventricle. A patent ductus arteriosus is also present, however. **(B)** The enlarged right ventricle and overriding aorta are obvious in this case of tetralogy of Fallot. (Fig. B photo courtesy of Children's Hospital Medical Center, Cincinnati, OH.)

common cyanotic congenital heart malformation, occurring in 10 of 10,000 liveborn infants. Infant survival depends on maintenance of a patent ductus arteriosus. The condition may be corrected surgically by relieving the obstruction of the pulmonary trunk and repairing the ventricular septal defect. Care must be exercised in suturing along the ventricular muscular septum, however, to avoid postoperative **complete right bundle branch block,** which may lead to fatal ventricular dysrhythmia.

Molecular-genetic studies are establishing the disruption of specific developmental mechanisms as causes of cardiac abnormalities

Human congenital cardiac conditions may arise from single-gene mutations that affect cardiac contractility. **Familial hypertrophic cardiomyopathy (FHC)** is an autosomal dominant disease characterized by thickening of the ventricular walls and interventricular septum, disorganization of the muscle fibrils, and formation of loose connective tissue. The disease may result in arrhythmias and pumping inefficiency leading to cardiac failure and **sudden death** in early adulthood. The genetic bases for the disease are mutations of the β-cardiac myosin heavy chain gene on chromosome 14 or of genes encoding other contractile proteins like troponin T and α-tropomyosin, suggesting that FHC is a **disease of the sarcomere.**

Congenital long QT syndrome is characterized by prolongation of the QT interval of the electrocardiogram,

fainting, and **sudden death.** It is an autosomal dominant disease resulting from disruptions of the *SCN5A, HERG,* and *KVLQT1* genes, which encode cardiac ion channels. While the molecular embryology of heart development is in its infancy, in situ hybridization and transgenic studies have also implicated numerous regulatory genes in cardiac development and congenital disease. For example, vertebrate homologs of the *Drosophila* gene **tinman,** called *Nkx-2.3* and *Nkx-2.5,* are expressed in the cardiogenic mesoderm of chicks, and a human homology has been mapped to chromosome 5q34. The paired-related homeobox genes *Prx-1* and *Prx-2* are expressed in the endocardial cushions and heart valves. Transgenic knockouts of *Sox-4* result in defects of the semilunar valves and the phenotype of **persistent truncus arteriosus.** Numerous "downstream" transcription factors that regulate differentiation of the myocardium have also been identified, including **Mef 2c, TEF-1, N-*myc*,** and members of the **GATA family.** *Nkx-2.5* regulates the process of looping and myosin expression, while *N-myc* and TEF-1 regulate differentiation and thickening of the myocardium. The role of **retinoic acid** in the pathogenesis of some of the cardiac defects that result from disruption of neural crest cell migration has been affirmed by **double retinoic acid receptor knockouts.** These animals exhibit persistent truncus arteriousus and double-outlet right ventricle. Similarly, spontaneous mutations of *Pax-3,* like **splotch** and transgenic knockouts of the **neurofibromatosis gene *NF-1*** result in disruptions of neural crest and cardiac anomalies such as ventricular septal defect.

8

Development of the Vasculature

*Vasculogenesis; Development of the Aortic Arches
and Great Arteries; Development of the Vitelline,
Umbilical, and Cardinal Venous Systems;
Development of the Coronary Circulation;
Circulatory Changes at Birth*

SUMMARY

In human embryos, the first blood vessels form within yolk sac mesoderm in conjunction with blood cells on day 17, a process called **blood island formation.** Blood vessels form in the embryo a day later, independently of blood cells. In the latter process, called **vasculogenesis,** mesodermal angioblastic cysts fuse to form networks of angioblastic cords that coalesce, grow, and invade embryonic tissues to form the arterial, venous, and lymphatic channels. Development of the **arterial system** commences as embryonic folding carries the endocardial tubes into the thorax, while their connections to the paired dorsal aortae form the first **aortic arches.** Remodeling of all five pairs of aortic arches forms the great vessels of the thorax and vessels of the head and neck. The paired dorsal aortae fuse below the level of the fourth thoracic segment to form a single median dorsal aorta that sprouts three main types of branches by the process of **angiogenesis:** (1) **ventral vitelline arteries** supply the gut and its derivatives; (2) **lateral arteries** supply retroperitoneal structures, including adrenal glands, kidneys, and gonads; and (3) dorsolateral **intersegmental arteries** serve the body wall, head and neck, limbs, and vertebral column. In addition, the paired **umbilical arteries** carry deoxygenated blood from the embryo to the placenta. The **primitive venous system** consists of (1) the **cardinal system,** which drains the head, neck, body wall, and limbs; (2) the **vitelline veins,** which drain the gut; and (3) the **umbilical veins,** which carry oxygenated blood from the placenta to the embryo. All three are bilateral at first, but are then remodeled; the left cardinal and vitelline veins regress, and those on the right form the great veins including the inferior and superior vena cava. In contrast, the right umbilical vein regresses, but its blood returns to the right side through the ductus venosus. **Lymphatics** also form by vasculogenesis but later than arterial and venous systems. **Coronary vessels** arise from the visceral epicardium of the heart.

Many anomalies including **double inferior vena cava** and **double superior vena cava** result from abnormal remodeling of the vasculature. The persistence of parts of the right dorsal aorta may result in **vascular rings** that constrict the esophagus and trachea. Retention of the right dorsal aorta and regression of the right fourth aortic arch may result in an **anomalous right subclavian** vein that passes posterior to the esophagus. **Coarctation of the aorta** may constrict the aorta proximal or distal to the ductus arteriosus, resulting in collateral arterial supplies to the trunk. Abnormal patterns of coronary vessel formation include development of a single coronary artery, which may result in **sudden death. Hemangiomas** may arise from single-gene mutations, chromosomal anomalies, or conditions like diabetes. They may be harmless or life-threatening depending on size and location. Current studies of vasculogenesis have significant clinical applications. The identification of angiogenic (vessel forming) and anti-angiogenic substances is the basis for therapies to inhibit the growth of **hemangiomas.** Similar anti-angiogenic strategies may be useful in therapies designed to reduce tumor growth, which depends on the proliferation of new vessels.

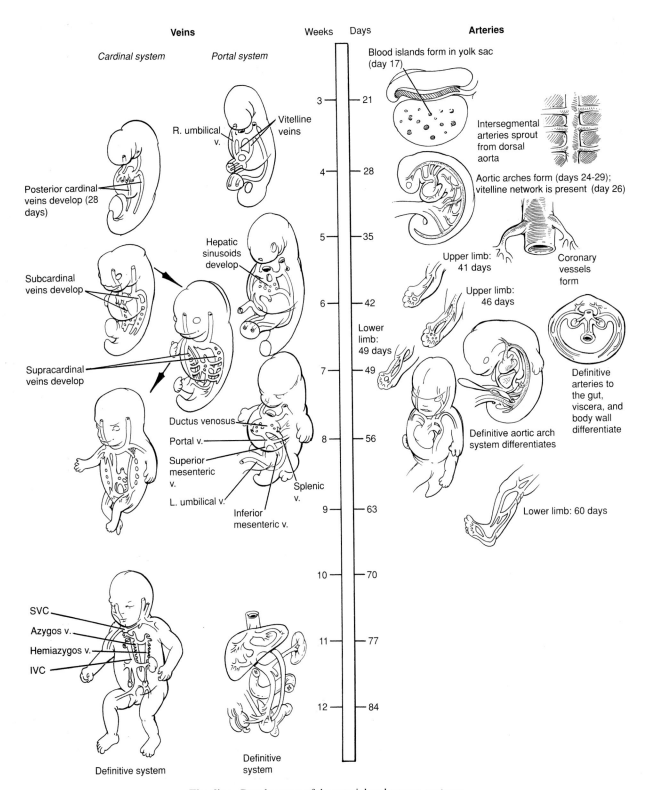

Veins   Weeks   Days   **Arteries**

Cardinal system   *Portal system*

Blood islands form in yolk sac (day 17)

R. umbilical v.

Vitelline veins

Intersegmental arteries sprout from dorsal aorta

Posterior cardinal veins develop (28 days)

Aortic arches form (days 24-29); vitelline network is present (day 26)

Hepatic sinusoids develop

Subcardinal veins develop

Upper limb: 41 days

Coronary vessels form

Upper limb: 46 days

Supracardinal veins develop

Lower limb: 49 days

Ductus venosus

Portal v.

Superior mesenteric v.

Splenic v.

L. umbilical v.

Inferior mesenteric v.

Definitive arteries to the gut, viscera, and body wall differentiate

Definitive aortic arch system differentiates

Lower limb: 60 days

SVC

Azygos v.

Hemiazygos v.

IVC

Definitive system

Definitive system

Timeline. Development of the arterial and venous systems.

The vasculature begins to form early in the third week

Vasculogenesis commences with the formation of blood islands in the extraembryonic mesoderm of the yolk sac, chorion, and connecting stalk

The first evidence of blood vessel formation can be detected in the splanchnopleuric mesoderm of the yolk sac on day 17, as mesodermal aggregations called **blood islands** develop next to the endoderm. Each blood island segregates into a core of embryonic **hemoblasts** surrounded by flattened **endothelial cells.** The hemoblasts differentiate into the first blood cells of the embryo, and the endothelial cells develop into blood vessel endothelium. These vessel precursors lengthen and interconnect, establishing an initial vascular network. By the end of the third week, this network completely vascularizes the yolk sac, the connecting stalk, and the chorionic villi (see Ch. 2).

Vasculogenesis in the embryo commences in the splanchnopleuric mesoderm and does not involve the formation of blood cells

On day 18, blood vessels begin to develop in the splanchnopleuric mesoderm of the embryonic disc. Inducing substances (see Applications to Clinical Practice) secreted by the underlying endoderm cause some cells of the splanchnopleuric mesoderm to differentiate into **angioblasts,** which develop into flattened endothelial cells that join together to form small vesicular structures called **angiocysts.** These angiocysts then coalesce into long tubes or vessels called **angioblastic cords** (Fig. 7-1B, C). The entire process is **in situ vesicle formation and fusion** or **vasculogenesis.** Angioblastic cords develop throughout the germ disc and coalesce to form a pervasive network of **angioblastic plexuses** that establish the initial configuration of the circulatory system of the embryo. This network grows and spreads throughout the embryo by three processes: (1) the continued formation and fusion of angiocysts; (2) **angiogenesis,** the budding and sprouting of new vessels from existing angioblastic cords; and (3) the intercalation of new mesodermal cells into the walls of existing vessels.

All types of embryonic mesoderm except the prechordal plate have been shown to be capable of vasculogenesis. The mesodermlike ectomesenchyme derived from the neural crest also cannot form blood vessels.

The origin of the stem cells that populate the embryonic hematopoietic organs is controversial

The yolk sac is the first supplier of blood cells to the embryonic circulation. Starting in the fifth week, however, the task of **hematopoiesis** (blood cell production) is taken over by a sequence of embryonic organs, including the liver, spleen, thymus, and, finally, the bone marrow. The source of the hematopoietic stem cells that populate these organs, however, remains an enigma.

Cell tracing studies show that the source of the hematopoietic stem cells (HSCs) that develop within the yolk sac is the primary ectoderm. As the erythroid burst-forming units and granulomacrophage progenitors within the yolk sac decline between the fourth and fifth weeks, however, they reciprocally increase in the liver. This suggests that the HSCs of the yolk sac migrate to the liver, where they establish nests of proliferating cells that eventually seed other hematopoietic organs of the embryo like the spleen, lymph nodes, and bone marrow. This view is further supported by the concomitant "switching" from embryonic to fetal hemoglobin isoforms that occurs with establishment of hepatic HSC proliferation. Nonetheless, an alternate hypothesis for the origin of the definitive HSCs of the adult hematopoietic organs describes their origin from the intraembryonic splanchnopleuric mesoderm in the region of the **a**orta, **g**onad, and **m**esonephros (the **AGM**). However, while this region appears to contain cells with hematopoietic capacity, their developmental relationships with blood cells of the yolk sac and liver remain to be determined.

The human aortic arches are remnants of the gill vasculature of fishes

The respiratory apparatus of the jawless fishes that gave rise to higher vertebrates consisted of a variable number of gill bars separated by gill slits (Fig. 8-1). Each of the gill bars of **branchial arches** is vascularized by an **aortic arch artery,** which arises as a branch of the ventral aorta (aortic sac).

In the human embryo, five pairs of mesenchymal condensations develop on either side of the pharynx, corresponding to bronchial arches 1, 2, 3, 4, and 6 of the early fish. The fifth arch never develops at all or appears briefly and then regresses. The mesodermal and endodermal components of the arches have been modified through evolution so that, in humans, they form structures of the lower face and neck and derivatives of the pharyngeal foregut. These structures are thus more appropriately called **pharyngeal arches** than branchial arches.

The human aortic arches arise in craniocaudal sequence and form a basket of arteries around the pharynx

As described in Chapter 7, the first pair of aortic arches is formed between day 22 and day 24, when the process of embryonic folding that carries the endocardial tubes

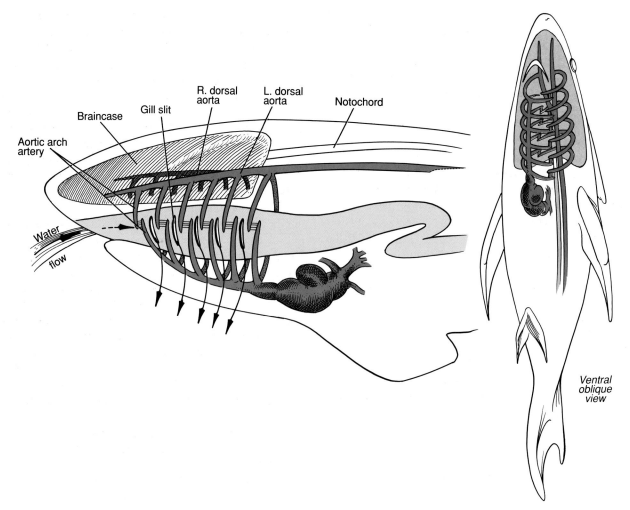

Fig. 8-1. Schematic view of the branchial arch artery system of a shark. The pharyngeal arch arteries of humans evolved from the branchial arch arteries of protochordates and fishes. The branchial arch arteries occupy the gill bars and thus enclose the pharynx like a basket. The arteries supply blood to the gills, which extract oxygen from water flowing through the gill slits.

into the future thorax also draws the cranial ends of the attached aortae into a dorsoventral loop (see Fig. 7-3). The resulting first pair of aortic arches lies in the thickened mesenchyme of the first pair of pharyngeal arches on either side of the developing pharynx (Fig. 8-2A). Ventrally, the aortic arch arteries arise from the **aortic sac,** an expansion at the cranial end of the truncus arteriosus. Dorsally, they connect to the left and right dorsal aortae. The dorsal aortae remain separate in the region of the aortic arches, but during the fourth week they fuse together from the fourth thoracic segment to the fourth lumbar segment to form a midline **dorsal aorta** (see Fig. 8-3B, below).

Between days 26 and 29, aortic arches 2, 3, 4, and 6 develop by vasculogenesis and angiogenesis within their re-

spective pharyngeal arches, incorporating angioblasts that migrate from the surrounding splanchnopleuric mesoderm.

The first two arches regress as the later arches form. The second aortic arch arises in the second pharyngeal arch by day 26 and grows to connect the aortic sac to the dorsal aortae. Simultaneously, the first pair of aortic arches regresses completely (except, possibly, for small remnants that may give rise to portions of the **maxillary arteries**) (Fig. 8-2A). On day 28, while the first arch is regressing, the third and fourth aortic arches appear. Finally, on day 29, the sixth arch forms, and the second arch regresses except for a small remnant that gives rise to part of the **stapedial artery** (Fig. 8-2B, C), which supplies blood to the primordium of the stapes bone in the developing ear (see Ch. 12).

Arches 3, 4, and 6 give rise to important vessels of the head, neck, and upper thorax

The third aortic arch becomes the common carotid and internal carotid arteries. By day 35, the segments of dorsal aorta connecting the third and fourth arch arteries disappear on both sides of the body, so that the cranial extensions of the dorsal aortae that supply the head receive blood entirely through the third aortic arches (Fig. 8-2B). The third arch arteries give rise to the right and left **common carotid arteries** (Fig. 8-2B, C) and also to the proximal portion of the right and left **internal carotid arteries.** The distal portion of the internal carotid arteries is derived from the cranial extensions of the dorsal aortae, and the right and left **external carotid arteries** sprout from the common carotids (Fig. 8-3C).

The fourth and sixth arches undergo asymmetric remodeling to supply blood to the upper extremities, dorsal aorta, and lungs. By the seventh week, the right dorsal aorta loses its connections with both the fused midline dorsal aorta and the right sixth arch, while remaining connected to the right fourth arch (Fig. 8-2C). Meanwhile it also acquires a branch, the **right seventh cervical intersegmental artery,** which grows into the right upper limb bud. The definitive **right subclavian artery** supplying the upper limb, therefore, is derived from (1) the right fourth arch, (2) a short segment of the right dorsal aorta, and (3) the right seventh intersegmental artery. The region of the aortic sac connected to the right fourth artery is modified to form the branch of the developing aorta called the **brachiocephalic artery** (Fig. 8-2C).

The left fourth aortic arch retains its connection to the fused dorsal aorta and with a small segment of the aortic sac becomes the **aortic arch** and the most cranial portion of the **descending aorta.** The remainder of the descending aorta, from the fourth thoracic level caudally, is derived from the fused dorsal aortae. The **left seventh intersegmental artery** sprouts directly from the left dorsal aorta and gives rise to the **left subclavian artery** supplying the left upper extremity (Fig. 8-2C).

The right and left sixth arches arise from the proximal end of the aortic sac, but further development is then asymmetrical (Fig. 8-2C). By the seventh week, the distal connection of the right sixth arch with the right dorsal aorta disappears. The left sixth arch, in contrast, remains complete, and its distal portion forms the **ductus arteriosus** that allows blood to shunt from the pulmonary trunk to the descending aorta throughout gestation. This bypass closes at birth and is later transformed into the **ligamentum arteriosum** that attaches the pulmonary trunk to the aorta (Fig. 8-2B, C).

As shown in Figure 8-2B, C, the asymmetrical development of the left and right sixth arches is responsible for the curious asymmetry of the **left and right recurrent laryngeal nerves,** which branch from the vagus. These nerves originally arise below the level of the sixth arch and cross under them to innervate intrinsic muscles of the larynx. During development, the larynx is translocated cranially relative to the aortic arches. The left recurrent laryngeal nerve becomes caught under the sixth arch on the left side and remains looped under the ligamentum arteriosum. Because the distal right sixth aortic arch disappears (and because no fifth arch develops), the right recurrent laryngeal nerve becomes caught under the fourth arch, which becomes the right subclavian artery.

The pulmonary arteries may initially arise from the fourth rather than the sixth aortic arch. Although the pulmonary arteries become connected to the sixth arch arteries and finally to the pulmonary trunk, several classic observations, as well as more recent quailchick chimera experiments, suggest that these arteries initially sprout from the fourth aortic arches. As these pulmonary artery sprouts grow toward the lungs, their roots make secondary contact with the sixth arches as they lose their connection to the fourth arches. In the lungs, their distal ends anastomose with the vasculature developing in the mesenchyme surrounding the bronchial buds (see Ch. 6).

The dorsal aorta develops ventral, lateral, and posterolateral branches

The vitelline arteries to the yolk sac give rise to the arterial supply of the gastrointestinal tract

The blood vessels that arise in the yolk sac wall differentiate to form the arteries and veins of the **vitelline system** (Fig. 8-3). As the yolk sac shrinks relative to the folding embryo, the right and left vitelline plexuses coalesce to form a number of major arteries that anastomose both with the vascular plexuses of the future gut and with the ventral surface of the dorsal aorta. These vessels eventually lose their connection with the yolk sac, becoming the arteries that supply blood from the dorsal aorta to the gastrointestinal tract.

Cranial to the diaphragm, about five pairs of these arteries usually develop and anastomose with the dorsal aorta at variable levels to supply the thoracic esophagus. Caudal to the diaphragm, three pairs of major arteries develop to supply specific regions of the developing abdominal gut. The fields of vascularization of these three arteries constitute the basis for dividing the abdominal gastrointestinal tract into three embryologic regions: the **abdominal foregut,** the **midgut,** and the **hindgut.**

The most superior of the three abdominal vitelline arteries, the **celiac artery,** initially joins the dorsal aorta at

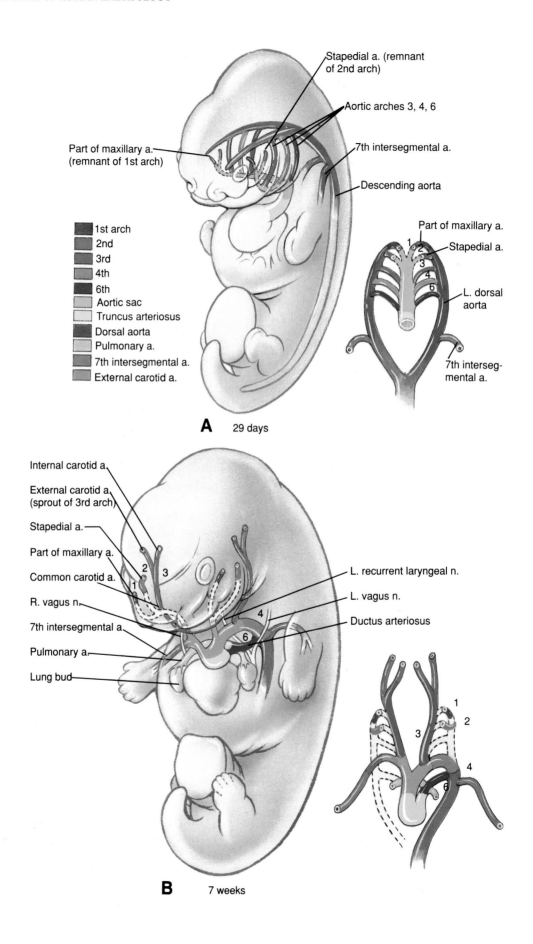

1st arch
2nd
3rd
4th
6th
Aortic sac
Truncus arteriosus
Dorsal aorta
Pulmonary a.
7th intersegmental a.
External carotid a.

Stapedial a. (remnant of 2nd arch)

Aortic arches 3, 4, 6

Part of maxillary a. (remnant of 1st arch)

7th intersegmental a.

Descending aorta

Part of maxillary a.

Stapedial a.

L. dorsal aorta

7th intersegmental a.

A   29 days

Internal carotid a.

External carotid a. (sprout of 3rd arch)

Stapedial a.

Part of maxillary a.

Common carotid a.

R. vagus n.

7th intersegmental a.

Pulmonary a.

Lung bud

L. recurrent laryngeal n.

L. vagus n.

Ductus arteriosus

B   7 weeks

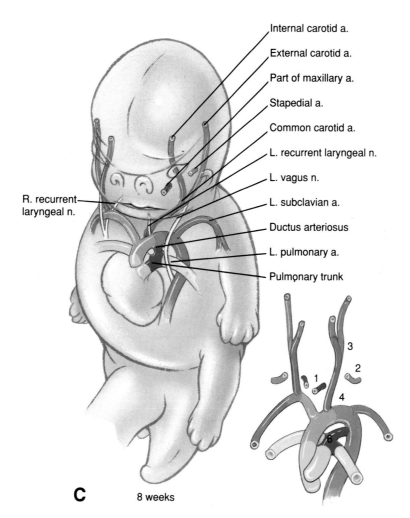

Internal carotid a.

External carotid a.

Part of maxillary a.

Stapedial a.

Common carotid a.

L. recurrent laryngeal n.

L. vagus n.

L. subclavian a.

Ductus arteriosus

L. pulmonary a.

Pulmonary trunk

R. recurrent laryngeal n.

C   8 weeks

Fig. 8-2. Development of the aortic arch system. **(A)** The five pairs of aortic arches that form in humans correspond to arches 1, 2, 3, 4, and 6 of evolutionary predecessors. The first arch is complete by day 24 but regresses as the second arch forms on day 26. The third and fourth arches form on day 28; the second arch degenerates as the sixth arch forms on day 29. **(B)** Development of the arches in the second month. Note that the structures arising from the first three pairs of aortic arches are bilateral, whereas arches 4 and 6 develop asymmetrically. The pulmonary arteries initially sprout from arch 4 and become secondarily reconnected to the roots of the sixth arches. **(C)** 8 weeks. Note the asymmetric development of the recurrent laryngeal branches of the vagus nerve, which innervate the laryngeal muscles. As the larynx is displaced superiorly relative to the arch system, the recurrent laryngeal nerves are caught under the most inferior remaining arch on each side. The right recurrent laryngeal therefore loops under the right subclavian artery, while the left recurrent laryngeal nerve loops under the ductus arteriosus.

the seventh cervical level. This connection subsequently descends to the twelfth thoracic level, and the celiac artery develops branches that vascularize not only the abdominal part of the foregut from the abdominal esophagus to the descending segment of the duodenum, but also the several embryological outgrowths of the foregut—the liver, pancreas, and gallbladder. The celiac artery also produces a large branch that vascularizes the spleen,

which is a mesodermal derivative of the dorsal mesogastrium (see Ch. 9). (The dorsal mesogastrium is the portion of the dorsal mesentery that suspends the stomach.)

The second abdominal vitelline artery, the **superior mesenteric artery,** initially joins the dorsal aorta at the second thoracic level; this connection later migrates to the first lumbar level. This artery supplies the developing midgut—the intestine from the descending segment of

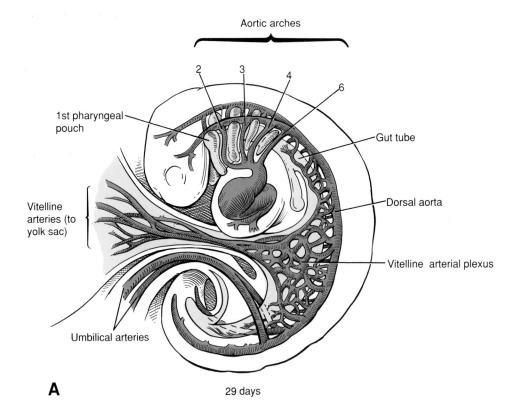

Aortic arches

2   3   4   6

1st pharyngeal
pouch

Vitelline
arteries (to
yolk sac)

Umbilical arteries

Gut tube

Dorsal aorta

Vitelline arterial plexus

A   29 days

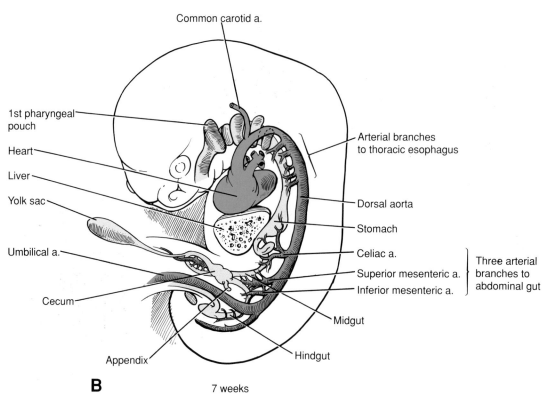

Common carotid a.

1st pharyngeal
pouch

Heart

Liver

Yolk sac

Umbilical a.

Cecum

Appendix

Arterial branches
to thoracic esophagus

Dorsal aorta

Stomach

Celiac a.

Superior mesenteric a.

Inferior mesenteric a.

Three arterial
branches to
abdominal gut

Midgut

Hindgut

B   7 weeks

Fig. 8-3. Development of the ventral aortic branches supplying the gut tube and derivatives. **(A)** In the fourth week, a multitude of vitelline arteries emerge from the ventral surfaces of the dorsal aortae to supply the yolk sac. **(B)** After the paired dorsal aortae fuse at the end of the fourth week, many of the vitelline channels disappear, reducing the final number to about five in the thoracic region and to three (the celiac, superior mesenteric, and inferior mesenteric arteries) in the abdominal region.

the duodenum to a region of the transverse colon near the left colic flexure.

The third and final abdominal vitelline artery, the **inferior mesenteric artery,** initially joins the dorsal aorta at the twelfth thoracic level and later descends to the third lumbar level. It supplies the hindgut: the distal portion of the transverse colon, the descending and sigmoid colon, and the rectum.

Lateral sprouts of the descending aorta vascularize the suprarenal glands, the gonads, and the kidneys

The suprarenal (adrenal) glands, gonads, and kidneys are all vascularized by lateral branches of the descending aorta. As shown in Figure 8-4, however, these three organs and their arteries have different developmental histo-

ries. The suprarenal glands form in the posterior body wall between the sixth and twelfth thoracic segments and become vascularized mainly by a pair of lateral aortic sprouts that arise at an upper lumbar level. The suprarenal glands also acquire branches from the renal artery and inferior phrenic artery, but the **suprarenal arteries** developing from these aortic sprouts remain the major supply to the glands. These glands and their aortic branches develop in place. The presumptive gonads become vascularized by **gonadal arteries** that arise initially at the tenth thoracic level. The gonads descend during development, but the origin of the gonadal arteries becomes fixed at the third or fourth lumbar level. As the gonads (especially the testes) descend further, the gonadal arteries elongate. The definitive kidneys, in contrast, arise in the sacral region and migrate upward to a lumbar site just below the suprarenal glands. As they migrate, they are vascularized

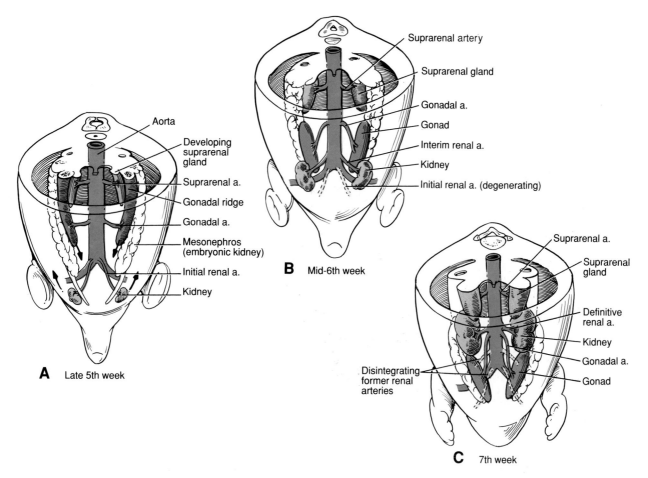

Fig. 8-4. Development of the lateral branches of the abdominal aorta. **(A)** Lateral sprouts of the dorsal aorta vascularize the suprarenal glands, the gonads, and the kidneys. During the sixth week, the gonads begin to descend while the kidneys ascend. **(B, C)** The gonadal artery lengthens during the migration of the gonad, but the ascending kidney is vascularized by a succession of new, more superior aortic sprouts. The suprarenal arteries remain in place.

by a succession of transient aortic sprouts that arise at progressively higher levels. Successive renal arteries thus degenerate and are replaced. The final pair of arteries in this series form in the upper lumbar region and become the definitive **renal arteries.** Occasionally, a more inferior pair of renal arteries persist as accessory renal arteries.

Intersegmental sprouts arise from the posterolateral surface of the descending aorta and vascularize the somite derivatives

At the end of the third week, small posterolateral sprouts arise from the dorsal aorta at the cervical through sacral levels and grow into the spaces between the developing somites (Fig. 8-5). In the cervical **thoracic** and **lumbar** regions, a dorsal branch of each of these intersegmental sprouts vascularizes both the developing neural tube and the epimeres that will form the deep muscles of the neck and back (Fig. 8-6A). Cutaneous branches of these arteries also supply the dorsal skin. The ventral branch of each of these intersegmental sprouts supplies the developing hypomeric muscles and associated skin. In the **thoracic** region, these ventral branches become the **intercostal arteries** and their cutaneous branches, whereas in the lumbar and sacral regions they become the **lumbar** and **lateral sacral arteries.** The short continuation of the dorsal aorta beyond its bifurcation into the common iliac arteries is called the **median sacral artery.**

In the cervical region, the intersegmental sprouts anastomose with each other to form a more complex pattern

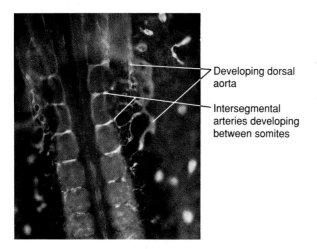

Fig. 8-5. Intersegmental arteries sprout from the dorsal aortae and penetrate between the somites as they grow toward the midline. (From Coffin D, Poole TJ. 1988. Embryonic vascular development: immunohistochemical identification of the origin and subsequent morphogenesis of the major vessel primordia of quail embryos. Development 102:735, with permission.)

of vascularization (Fig. 8-6B). The paired **vertebral arteries** arise from longitudinal branches that link together to form a longitudinal vessel and secondarily lose their intersegmental connections to the aorta. The **deep cervical, ascending cervical, superior intercostal, internal thoracic,** and **superior** and **inferior epigastric arteries** also develop from anastomoses of intersegmental arteries.

The umbilical arteries initially join the dorsal aortae but shift their origin to the internal iliac arteries

The right and left **umbilical arteries** develop in the connecting stalk in the early fourth week and are thus among the earliest embryonic arteries to arise. These arteries form an initial connection with the paired dorsal aortae in the sacral region (Fig. 8-3A). During the fifth week, however, these connections are obliterated, and the umbilical arteries develop a new junction with a pair of fifth lumbar intersegmental artery branches called the **internal iliac arteries.** The internal iliac arteries vascularize pelvic organs and (initially) the lower extremity limb bud. As discussed below, the fifth lumbar intersegmental arteries also give rise to the **external iliac arteries.** Proximal to these branches, the root of the fifth lumbar intersegmental artery is called the **common iliac artery** (see Fig. 8-8).

The arteries to the limbs are formed by remodeling of intersegmental artery branches

As indicated above, the arteries to the developing upper and lower limbs are derived mainly from the seventh cervical intersegmental artery and the fifth lumbar intersegmental artery, respectively. These arteries initially supply each limb bud by joining an **axial** or **axis artery** that develops along the central axis of the limb bud (Figs. 8-7 and 8-8). In the upper limb, the axis artery develops into the **brachial artery** of the upper arm and the **anterior interosseous artery** of the forearm. In the hand, a small portion of the axis artery persists as the **deep palmar arch.** The other arteries of the upper limb, including the **radial, median,** and **ulnar arteries,** develop partly as sprouts of the axis artery.

In the lower limb, in contrast, the axis artery—which arises as the distal continuation of the internal iliac artery—largely degenerates, and the definitive supply is provided almost entirely by the **external iliac artery** (Fig. 8-8). The axis artery persists as three remnants: the small **sciatic (ischiatic) artery,** which serves the sciatic nerve in the posterior thigh; a segment of the **popliteal artery;** and a section of the **popliteal** and **peroneal arteries** in the leg. Virtually all the other arteries of the lower limb develop as sprouts of the external iliac artery.

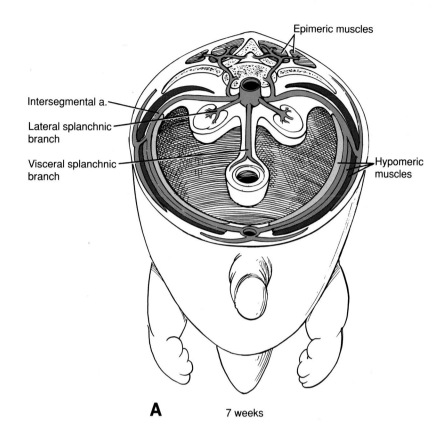

A   7 weeks

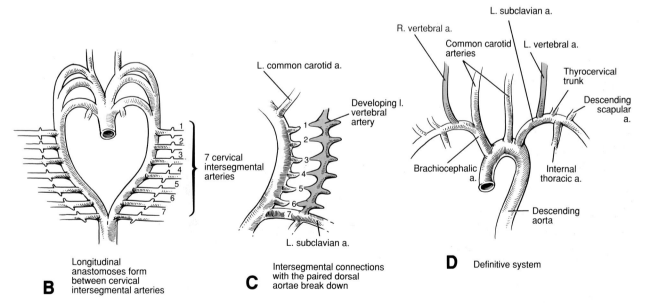

Fig. 8-6. Development of the arterial supply to the body wall. **(A)** Intersegmental artery system in the trunk region. Branches of the paired intersegmental arteries supply the posterior, lateral, and anterior body wall and musculature, the vertebral column, and the spinal cord. **(B–D)** The vertebral artery is formed from longitudinal anastomoses of the first through seventh cervical intersegmental arteries.

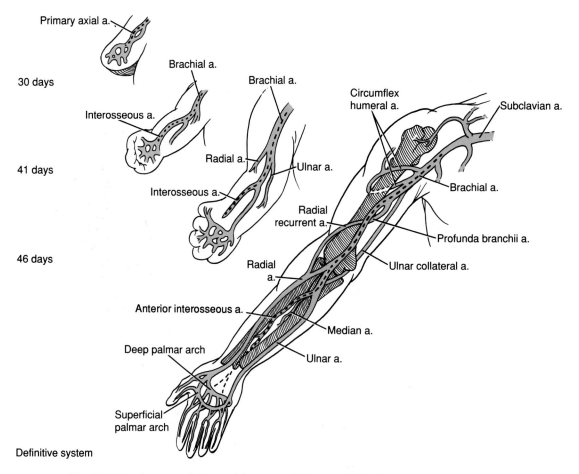

Fig. 8-7. Development of the arterial system of the upper limb. The seventh cervical inter-segmental arteries grow into the limb buds to form the axis arteries of the developing upper limbs. The axis artery gives rise to the subclavian, axillary, brachial, and anterior interosseous arteries and to the deep palmar arch. Other arteries of the upper extremity develop as sprouts of the axis artery.

The primitive embryonic venous system is divided into vitelline, umbilical, and cardinal systems

The vitelline system gives rise to the liver sinusoids, the portal system, and a portion of the inferior vena cava

Like the vitelline arteries, the vitelline veins arise from the capillary plexuses of the yolk sac and form part of the vasculature of the developing gut and gut derivatives. Initially, the vitelline system empties into the sinus horns of the heart via a pair of symmetrical **vitelline veins** (Fig. 8-9A). Right and left vitelline plexuses also develop in the septum transversum and connect to the vitelline veins (Fig. 8-9B). The vessels of these plexuses become surrounded by the growing liver cords and give rise to the **liver sinusoids,** a dense network of anastomosing venous

spaces. As the left sinus horn regresses to form the coronary sinus, the left vitelline vein also diminishes. By the third month, the left vitelline vein has completely disappeared in the region of the sinus venosus, and the blood from the left side of the abdominal viscera drains across to the right vitelline vein via a series of transverse anastomoses that have formed both within the substance of the liver and around the abdominal portion of the foregut (Fig. 8-9C).

After the left vitelline vein loses its connection with the heart, the blood from the entire vitelline system drains into the heart via the enlarged right vitelline vein (Fig. 8-9C). The *superior* portion of this vein (the portion between the liver and the heart) becomes the **terminal portion of the inferior vena cava** (IVC) (Fig. 8-10E). Meanwhile, a single oblique channel among the hepatic anastomoses becomes dominant and drains directly into the nascent IVC. As described below, this channel, the

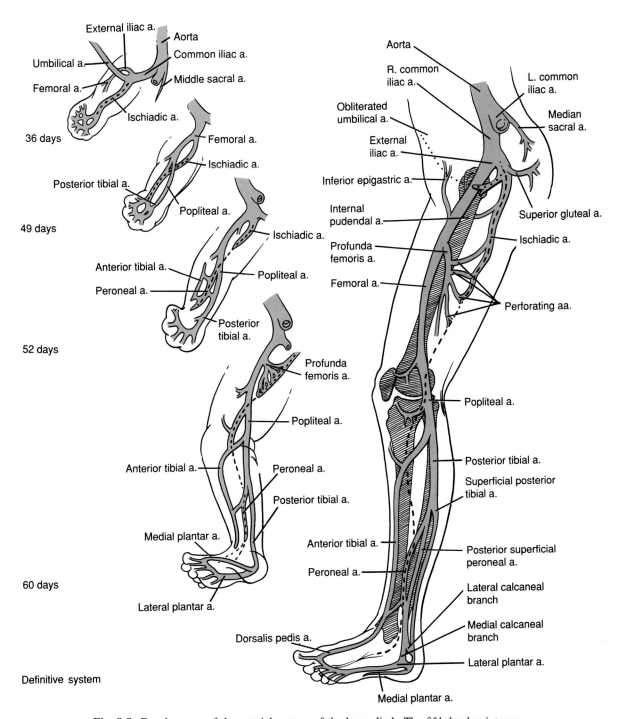

Fig. 8-8. Development of the arterial system of the lower limb. The fifth lumbar intersegmental artery forms the axis artery of the lower extremity. The only remnants of this vessel in the lower limb of the adult are the ischiatic artery, a small portion of the popliteal artery, and the peroneal artery.

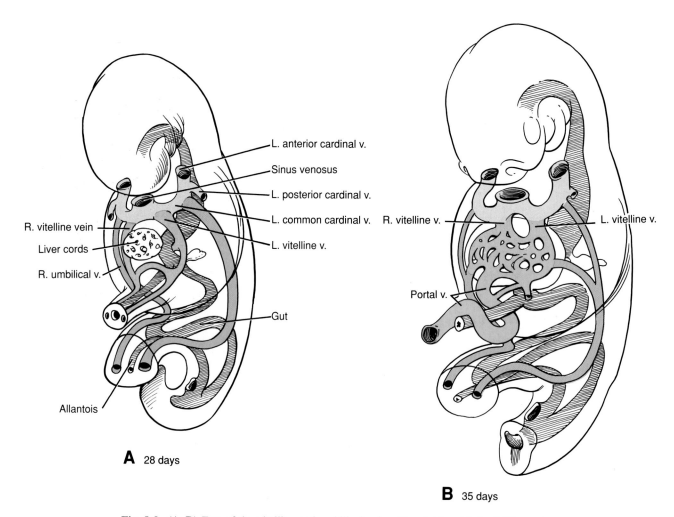

Fig. 8-9. (A–D) Fate of the vitelline and umbilical veins. The right and left vitelline veins form a portal system that drains blood from the abdominal foregut, midgut, and upper part of the anorectal canal. (*Figure continues.*)

ductus venosus, is crucial during fetal life because it receives oxygenated blood from the umbilical system and shunts it directly to the right atrium.

The vitelline veins inferior to the liver regress during the second and third months, with the exception of the portion of the right vitelline vein just inferior to the developing liver and a few of the proximal ventral left-to-right vitelline anastomoses (Fig. 8-9B). These veins become the main channels of the **portal system,** which drain blood from the gastrointestinal tract to the liver sinusoids. The segment of the right vitelline vein inferior to the liver becomes the **portal vein and the superior mesenteric vein** (Fig. 8-9C, D). Persisting branches collect blood from the abdominal foregut (including the abdominal esophagus, stomach, gallbladder, duodenum, and pancreas) and the midgut. Prominent left-to-right vitelline anastomoses are remodeled to deliver blood to the distal

end of the portal vein through two veins: the **splenic vein,** which drains the spleen, part of the stomach, and the greater omentum (see Ch. 9), and the **inferior mesenteric vein,** which drains the hindgut.

The right umbilical vein disappears and the left umbilical vein anastomoses with the ductus venosus

In contrast to the regression of the left vitelline vein, the *right* umbilical vein becomes completely obliterated during the second month, whereas the *left* umbilical vein persists (Fig. 8-9). Concurrently, however, the left umbilical vein loses its connection with the left sinus horn and forms a new anastomosis with the ductus venosus. Oxygenated blood from the placenta thus reaches the heart via the single umbilical vein and the ductus venosus. As

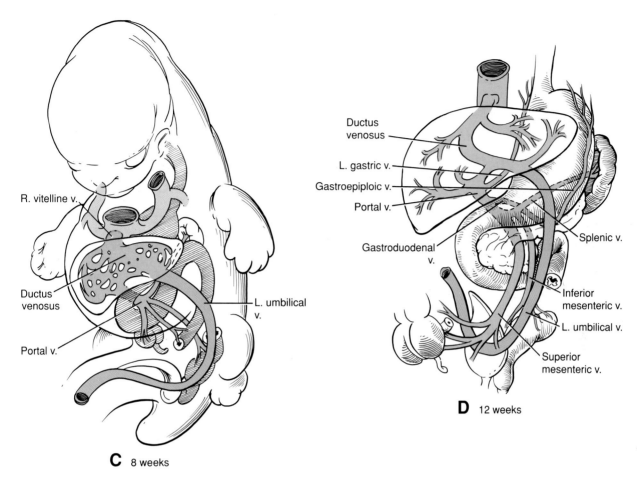

R. vitelline v.

Ductus venosus

Portal v.

L. umbilical v.

C 8 weeks

Ductus venosus

L. gastric v.

Gastroepiploic v.

Portal v.

Gastroduodenal v.

Splenic v.

Inferior mesenteric v.

L. umbilical v.

Superior mesenteric v.

D 12 weeks

Fig. 8-9 *(Continued).* The right umbilical vein disappears, but the left umbilical vein anastomoses with the ductus venosus in the liver, thus shunting oxygenated placental blood into the inferior vena cava and to the right side of the heart.

described at the end of this chapter, the ductus venosus constricts shortly after birth, eliminating this venous shunt through the liver.

The posterior cardinal system is augmented and then superseded by paired subcardinal and supracardinal veins

As shown in Figure 8-10A, the bilaterally symmetrical cardinal vein system that develops in the third and fourth weeks to drain the head, neck, and body wall initially consists of paired **posterior (inferior)** and **anterior (superior) cardinal veins,** which join near the heart to form the short **common cardinals** that empty into the sinus horns. The posterior cardinal veins are supplemented and later largely replaced by two additional pairs of veins, the **subcardinal** and **supracardinal** veins, which develop in the body wall medial to the posterior cardinal veins.

The subcardinal system drains structures of the median dorsal body wall, principally the kidneys and gonads. The left and right subcardinal veins sprout from the base of the posterior cardinals by the end of the sixth week and grow caudally in the median dorsal body wall (Fig. 8-10B). By the seventh and eighth weeks, these subcardinal veins become connected to each other by numerous median anastomoses and also form some lateral anastomoses with the posterior cardinals. However, the longitudinal segments of the left subcardinal vein soon regress, so that by the ninth week the structures on the left side of the body served by the subcardinal system drain solely through transverse anastomotic channels to the right subcardinal vein. Meanwhile, the right subcardinal vein loses its original connection with the posterior cardinal vein and develops a new anastomosis with the segment of the right vitelline vein just inferior to the heart to form the portion of the inferior vena cava between the liver and the kidneys (Fig. 8-10C–E). Through this re-

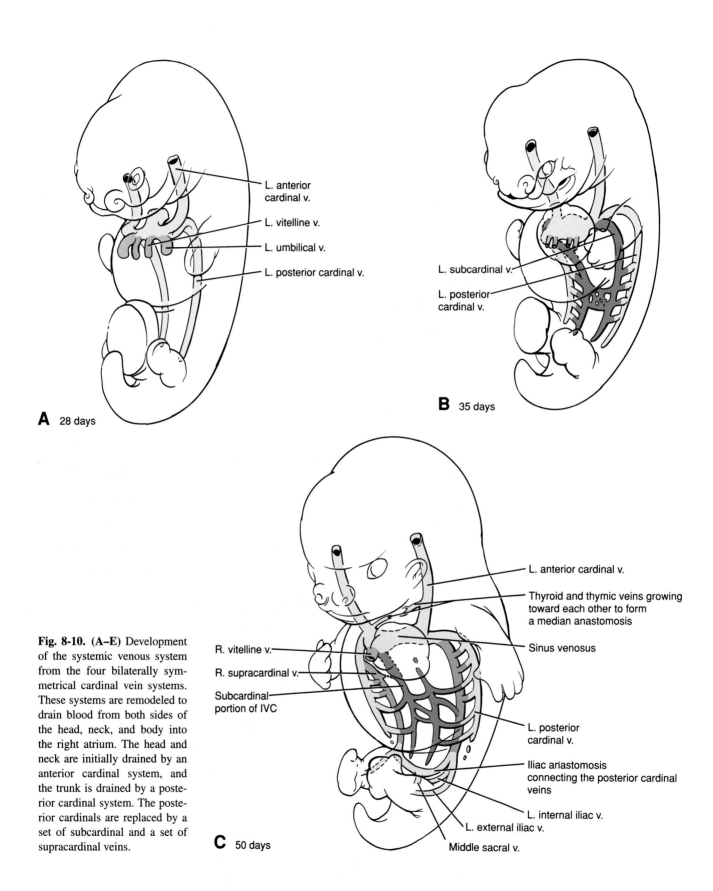

A   28 days

B   35 days

L. anterior
cardinal v.

L. vitelline v.

L. umbilical v.

L. posterior cardinal v.

L. subcardinal v.

L. posterior
cardinal v.

L. anterior cardinal v.

Thyroid and thymic veins growing
toward each other to form
a median anastomosis

Sinus venosus

R. vitelline v.

R. supracardinal v.

Subcardinal
portion of IVC

L. posterior
cardinal v.

Iliac anastomosis
connecting the posterior cardinal
veins

L. internal iliac v.

L. external iliac v.

Middle sacral v.

C   50 days

Fig. 8-10. (A–E) Development of the systemic venous system from the four bilaterally symmetrical cardinal vein systems. These systems are remodeled to drain blood from both sides of the head, neck, and body into the right atrium. The head and neck are initially drained by an anterior cardinal system, and the trunk is drained by a posterior cardinal system. The posterior cardinals are replaced by a set of subcardinal and a set of supracardinal veins.

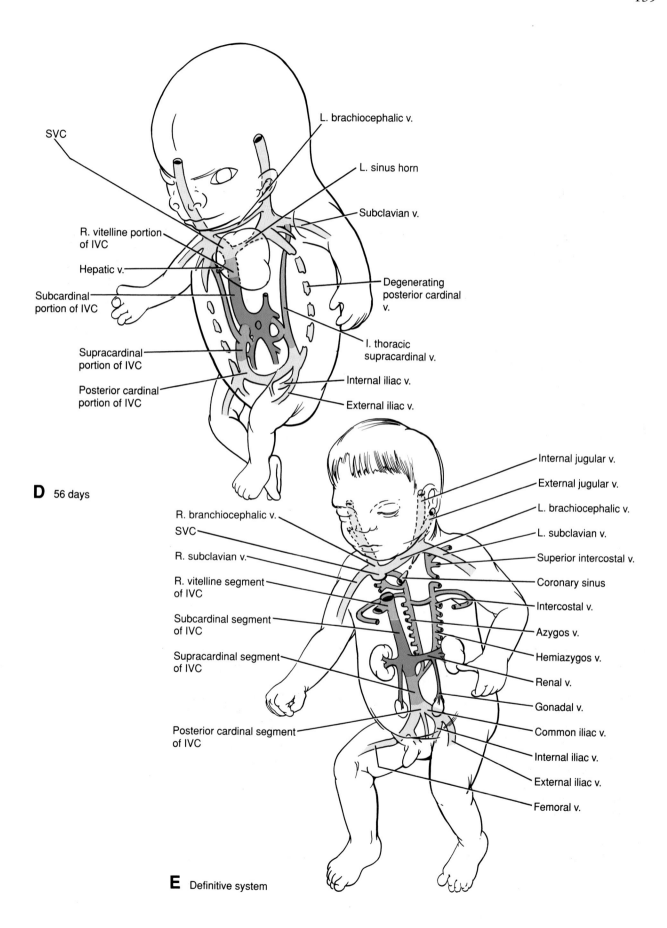

SVC

L. brachiocephalic v.

L. sinus horn

Subclavian v.

R. vitelline portion
of IVC

Hepatic v.

Subcardinal
portion of IVC

Degenerating
posterior cardinal
v.

Supracardinal
portion of IVC

l. thoracic
supracardinal v.

Internal iliac v.

Posterior cardinal
portion of IVC

External iliac v.

D 56 days

R. branchiocephalic v.

SVC

R. subclavian v.

R. vitelline segment
of IVC

Subcardinal segment
of IVC

Supracardinal segment
of IVC

Posterior cardinal segment
of IVC

Internal jugular v.

External jugular v.

L. brachiocephalic v.

L. subclavian v.

Superior intercostal v.

Coronary sinus

Intercostal v.

Azygos v.

Hemiazygos v.

Renal v.

Gonadal v.

Common iliac v.

Internal iliac v.

External iliac v.

Femoral v.

E Definitive system

modeling process, the organs originally drained by the right and left subcardinal veins ultimately empty into the right atrium via the IVC.

The supracardinal system gives rise to a portion of the IVC and to the azygos system draining the thoracic body wall. While the subcardinal system is being remodeled, a new pair of veins, the supracardinal veins, sprout from the base of the posterior cardinals and grow caudally just medial to the posterior cardinal veins (Fig. 8-10C). These veins drain the body wall via the segmental **intercostal veins,** thus taking over the function of the posterior cardinals.

While the supracardinals are developing, the posterior cardinals become obliterated over most of their length (Fig. 8-10C, D). The most caudal portions of the posterior cardinals (including a large median anastomosis) do persist, but lose their original connection to the heart and form a new anastomosis with the supracardinal veins. This caudal remnant of the posterior cardinals develops into the common iliac veins and the caudalmost, sacral portion of the IVC. The common iliac veins in turn sprout the internal and external iliac veins, which grow to drain the lower extremities and pelvic organs.

In the abdominal region, the remodeling of the supracardinal system commences with the obliteration of the inferior portion of the left supracardinal vein (Fig. 8-10D, E). The remaining abdominal segment of the right supracardinal vein then anastomoses with the right subcardinal vein to form a segment of the IVC just inferior to the kidneys.

The thoracic part of the supracardinal system drains the thoracic body wall via a series of **intercostal veins.** The thoracic portions of the supracardinals originally empty into the left and right posterior cardinals and are connected to each other by median anastomoses. However, the left thoracic supracardinal vein, called the **hemiazygos vein,** soon loses its connection with the left posterior cardinal vein and left sinus horn and subsequently drains into the right supracardinal system (Fig. 8-10E). The remaining portion of the inferior right supracardinal vein also loses its original connection with the posterior cardinal vein and makes a new anastomosis with the segment of the superior vena cava derived from the anterior cardinal vein (which, in turn, drains into the heart via a segment representing a small remnant of the right common cardinal vein). The right supracardinal vein is now called the **azygos vein.** Both the hemiazygos and the azygos veins now drain into the right atrium via the superior vena cava (Fig. 8-10E).

The definitive IVC is constructed from remnants of four separate systems. Figure 8-10E shows the sources of the four portions of the IVC. From superior to inferior, (1) the right vitelline vein gives rise to the terminal segment of the IVC; (2) the right subcardinal vein gives rise to a segment between the liver and the kidneys; (3) the right supracardinal vein gives rise to an abdominal segment inferior to the kidneys of the IVC; and (4) the right and left posterior cardinal veins plus the median anastomosis connecting them give rise to the sacral segment of the IVC.

Blood is drained from the head and neck by the anterior cardinal veins

The left and right anterior cardinal veins originally drain blood into the sinus horns via the right and left common cardinal veins (Fig. 8-10A–D). However, the proximal connection of the left anterior cardinal vein with the left sinus horn soon regresses, leaving only a small remnant lying directly on the heart, called the **oblique vein of the left atrium** (Fig. 8-10E; see also Ch. 7 and Fig. 7-10). This small remnant collects blood from the left atrial region of the heart and returns it directly to the coronary sinus, which is a vestige of the left sinus horn.

The cranial portions of the anterior cardinal veins in the developing cervical region give rise to the **internal jugular veins,** while capillary plexuses in the face become connected with these vessels to form the **external jugular veins.** Simultaneously, a median anastomosis connecting the left and right anterior cardinals develops from thymic and thyroid veins (Fig. 8-10C–E). Once the left anterior cardinal vein loses its connection with the heart, all the blood from the left side of the head and neck shunts over to the right anterior cardinal through this anastomosis. The **subclavian vein,** which coalesces from the venous plexus of the left upper limb bud, also empties into the proximal left anterior cardinal vein. The intercardinal anastomosis thus carries the blood from the left upper limb as well as the left head and is called the **left brachiocephalic vein** (Fig. 8-10C–E). The left brachiocephalic vein enters the right anterior cardinal at its junction with the **right brachiocephalic vein** draining the right upper limb bud. The small segment of right anterior cardinal vein between the junction of the right and left brachiocephalic veins and the right atrium becomes the **superior vena cava** (Fig. 8-10E). Thus, by the end of the eighth week, the definitive superior vena cava drains blood from (1) both sides of the head, (2) both upper limbs, and (3) the thoracic body wall (via the azygos vein).

The coronary vessels develop from blood islands deep to the epicardium

The first evidence of coronary vessel development is the appearance at the beginning of the fifth week of structures like blood islands just under the epicardium in the sulci of the developing heart. These vessels arise from cells of the epicardium. During the late fifth and sixth weeks, the capillary plexuses developing from these foci form connections both with **coronary veins** sprouting from the coronary sinus and with **coronary arteries** growing from the aorta. In fact, the coronary arteries actually sprout not directly from the aorta but rather from a pair of special aortic branches, the left and right **aortic sinuses,** that emerge from the aorta just above the two cusps of the semilunar valve (Fig. 8-11). It has been suggested that the developing capillary plexuses in the sulci induce the sprouting of the coronary veins and arteries.

The lymphatic system develops by mechanisms similar to those that produce the blood vessels

Like blood vessels, lymphatic channels arise by vasculogenesis and angiogenesis from splanchnopleuric mesodermal precursors. Lymphatics do not begin to appear until about the fifth week, however. By the end of the fifth week, a pair of enlargements, the **jugular lymph sacs,** develop and collect fluid from the lymphatics of the upper limbs, upper trunk, head, and neck (Fig. 8-12). In the sixth week, four additional lymph sacs develop to collect lymph from the trunk and lower extremities: the **retroperitoneal lymph sac,** the **cysterna chyli,** and the paired **posterior lymph sacs** associated with the junctions of the external and internal iliac veins.

The cysterna chyli initially drains into a symmetrical pair of thoracic lymphatic ducts that empty into the ve-

nous circulation at the junctions of the internal jugular and subclavian veins. During development, however, portions of both of these ducts are obliterated, and the definitive **thoracic duct** is derived from the caudal portion of the right duct, the cranial portion of the left duct, and a median anastomosis.

Dramatic changes occur in the circulatory system at birth

In the fetal circulation (Fig. 8-13A), oxygenated blood enters the body through the left umbilical vein. In the ductus venosus, this blood mixes with a small volume of deoxygenated portal blood and then enters the IVC, where it mixes with deoxygenated blood returning from the trunk and legs. In the right atrium, this stream of blood, still highly oxygenated, is largely shunted through the foramen ovale to the left atrium. The oxygenated blood entering the fetal right atrium from the inferior vena cava and the deoxygenated blood entering from the superior vena cava form hemodynamically distinct streams and undergo little mixing in the atrium.

In the left atrium, oxygenated blood from the right atrium mixes with the very small amount of blood returning from the lungs via the pulmonary veins. Little blood flows through the pulmonary circulation during fetal life because the vascular resistance of the collapsed fetal lungs is very high. The oxygenated blood in the left ventricle is then propelled into the aorta for distribution first to the head, neck, and arms and then, via the descending aorta, to the trunk and limbs. As blood enters the descending aorta, it mixes with the deoxygenated blood

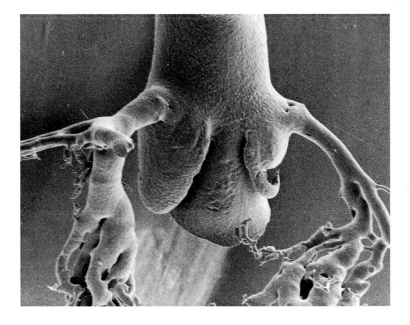

Fig. 8-11. Cast of the embryonic aorta, showing the coronary arteries sprouting from the aortic sinuses. (From Aikawa E, Kawano J. 1982. Formation of coronary arteries sprouting from the primitive aortic sinus wall of the chick embryo. Experientia 38:816, with permission.)

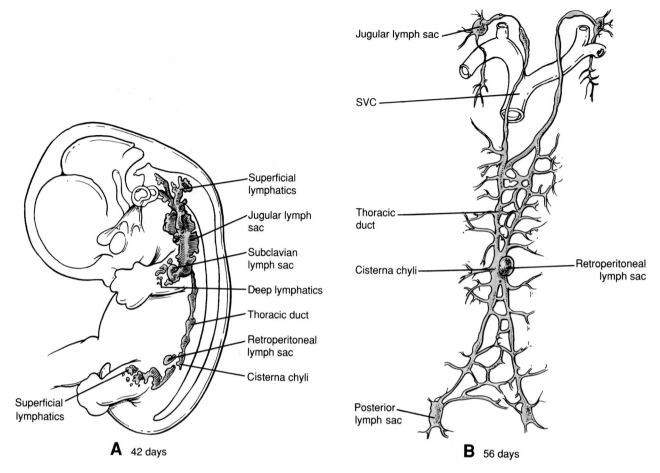

Fig. 8-12. Development of the lymphatic system. **(A)** Several lymph sacs and ducts develop by vasculogenesis and eventually drain fluid from tissue spaces throughout the entire body. **(B–D)** The single thoracic duct that drains the cisterna chyli and the posterior thoracic wall is derived from parts of the right and left thoracic ducts and their anastomoses.

shunted through the ductus arteriosus. This blood consists mainly of the blood entering the right atrium from the superior vena cava and expelled via the right ventricle and pulmonary trunk. Thus, the blood delivered to the head, neck, and arms by the fetal circulation is more highly oxygenated than the blood delivered to the trunk and lower limbs. After the descending aorta has distributed blood to the trunk and lower limbs, the remaining blood enters the umbilical arteries and returns to the placenta for oxygenation.

The fetal circulatory pattern functions throughout the birth process. As soon as the newborn infant takes its first breath, however, major changes convert the circulation to the adult configuration (Fig. 8-13B). As the alveoli fill with air, the constricted pulmonary vessels open and the resistance of the pulmonary vasculature drops precipitously. The opening of the pulmonary vessels is thought to be a direct response to oxygen, since hypoxia

in newborns can cause the pulmonary vessels to constrict. At the same time, spontaneous constriction (or obstetrical clamping) of the umbilical vessels cuts off the flow from the placenta.

The opening of the pulmonary circulation and the cessation of umbilical flow create changes in pressure and flow that cause the ductus arteriosus to constrict and the foramen ovale to close. When the pulmonary circulation opens, the resulting drop in pressure in the pulmonary trunk is thought to cause a slight reverse flow of oxygenated aortic blood through the ductus arteriosus. This increase in local oxygen tension apparently induces the ductus arteriosus to constrict. Constriction of the ductus arteriosus normally occurs within 10 to 15 hours after birth in infants born at term.

The initial closing of the foramen ovale, in contrast, is a strictly mechanical effect of the reversal in pressure between the two atria. The opening of the pulmonary vascu-

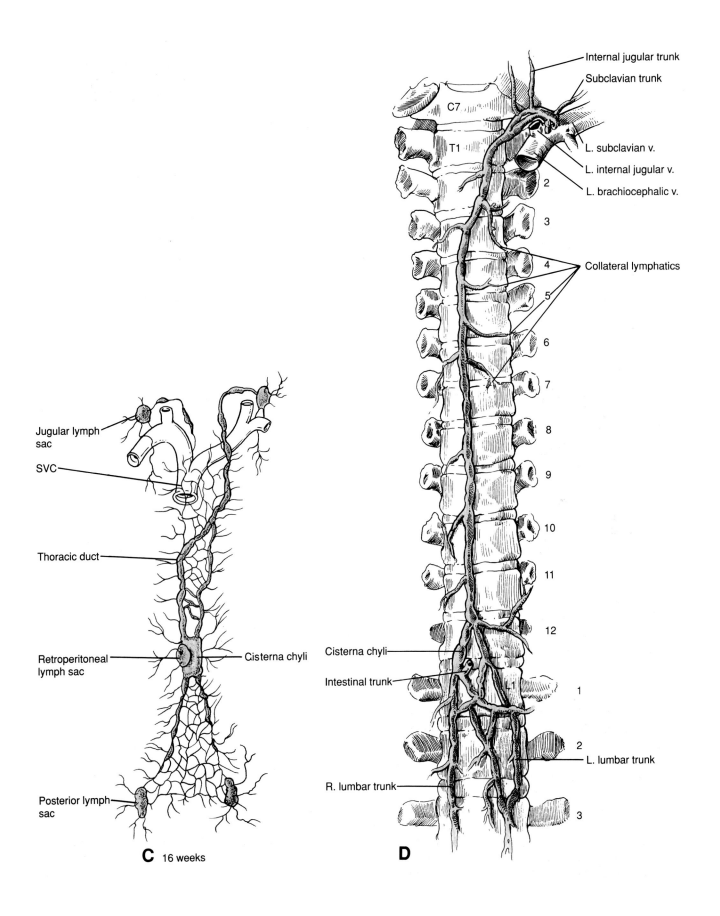

C   16 weeks

D

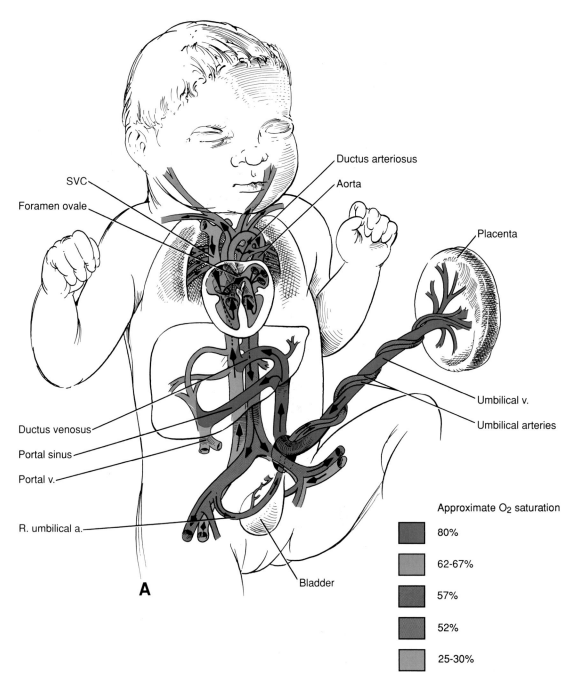

SVC

Foramen ovale

Ductus arteriosus

Aorta

Placenta

Ductus venosus

Portal sinus

Portal v.

R. umbilical a.

Umbilical v.

Umbilical arteries

Bladder

Approximate O₂ saturation

80%

62-67%

57%

52%

25-30%

A

Fig. 8-13. Conversion of the circulation from the fetal to the air-breathing pattern. At birth, the single circuit of the fetal circulation is rapidly converted to two circuits (pulmonary and systemic), arranged in series. **(A)** Pattern of blood flow in the fetus and placenta just before birth. **(B)** Pattern of blood flow just after birth.

lature and the cessation of umbilical flow reduce the pressure in the right atrium, whereas the sudden increase in pulmonary venous return raises the pressure in the left atrium. The resulting pressure change forces the flexible septum primum against the more rigid septum secundum,

functionally closing the foramen ovale. The septum primum and septum secundum normally fuse by about 3 months after birth.

In some individuals, the ductus venosus also closes soon after birth. Rapid constriction of the ductus venosus

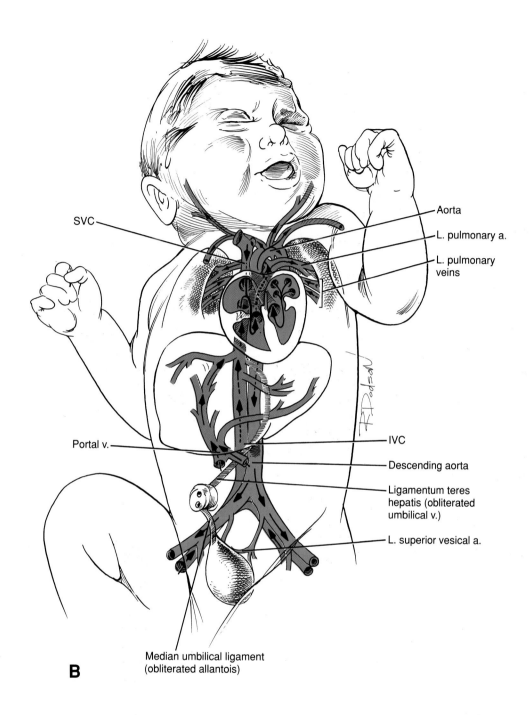

SVC

Aorta

L. pulmonary a.

L. pulmonary veins

Portal v.

IVC

Descending aorta

Ligamentum teres hepatis (obliterated umbilical v.)

L. superior vesical a.

B

Median umbilical ligament (obliterated allantois)

is not essential to the infant, however, because blood is no longer flowing through the umbilical vein.

Prostaglandins appear to play a role in maintaining the patency of the ductus venosus during fetal life, but the signal that brings about the apparently active constriction of this channel after birth is not understood. Nevertheless, the hepatic blood flow from the placenta is supplanted by a normal portal circulation within a few days of birth.

The fact that the patency of the ductus arteriosus is under hormonal control has important clinical conse-

quences. In term infants, as mentioned above, the ductus arteriosus apparently constricts in response to a rise in oxygen tension. During fetal life, however, the ductus is apparently kept patent by circulating prostaglandins. Infants that have cardiovascular malformations in which a patent ductus is essential to life may be treated with injections of prostaglandins to keep the ductus open until the malformation can be corrected surgically. Conversely, premature infants in which the ductus arteriosus does not constrict spontaneously are sometimes treated with prostaglandin inhibitors such as indomethacin.

APPLICATIONS TO CLINICAL PRACTICE

Many vascular anomalies arise from errors in remodeling of the great vessels

As described in this chapter, the bilaterally symmetrical vasculature undergoes a series of regressions and remodelings to produce the adult pattern of great arteries and veins. **Double inferior vena cava** arises when the caudal portion of the left supracardinal system fails to regress and forms an abnormal left IVC (Fig. 8-14A). If the left anterior cardinal persists, the result is a **double superior vena cava** (Fig. 8-14B). In the case of **situs inversus** (see Applications to Clinical Practice section of Ch. 9), left-right asymmetry of the vasculature may be completely reversed. Occasionally, instead of regressing, the right aorta persists, producing a **vascular ring** enclosing the esophagus and trachea (Fig. 8-15). In a related malformation, the superior portion of the right fourth aortic arch may regress, leaving the seventh intersegmental artery connected to its inferior stem (Fig. 8-16). The right subclavian artery thus connects with the descending aorta, passing posterior to the esophagus. As in the case of the vascular ring above, this **anomalous right subcla-** vian artery may result in **dysphagia** and difficulty in breathing.

Coarctation of the aorta results from a localized thickening of the aortic wall in the vicinity of the ductus arteriosus

Coarctation of the aorta is a congenital malformation occurring in 3 of 1,000 live births and is more common in males. It is, however, the most common cardiac anomaly in Turner syndrome. This anomaly may be triggered by teratogens or genetic factors and appears to be caused by abnormal proliferation of ectopic ductal tissue within the aortic arch. If the coarctation is **postductal,** blood cannot be delivered to the trunk and lower extremities unless collateral routes of circulation develop during embryonic and fetal life (Fig. 8-17). In the case of **preductal coarctation,** blood is delivered to the trunk and extremities during embryonic and fetal life via the pulmonary trunk, the ductus arteriosus, and descending aorta. After birth, however, when the ductus closes, collaterals similar to those developing in postductal coarctation may also develop in these individuals.

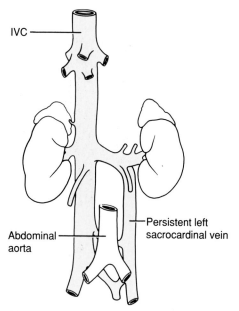

A Double inferior vena cava

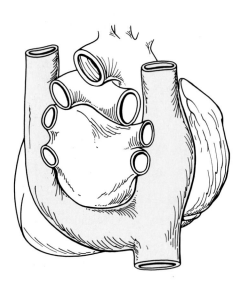

B Double superior vena cava

Fig. 8-14. Venous anomalies caused by failure of cardinal veins on the left to undergo normal regression. **(A)** Preservation of the left supracardinal vein inferior to the kidney may result in double inferior vena cava. **(B)** Preservation of the left anterior cardinal at the level of the heart may result in double superior vena cava. The anomalous left superior vena cava empties into the coronary sinus.

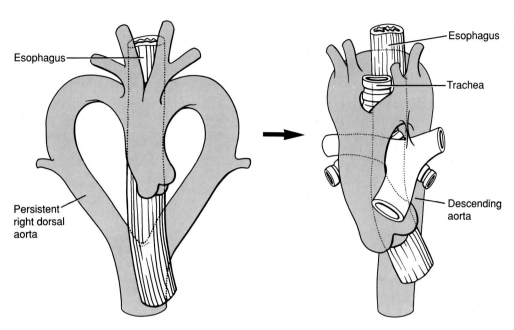

Fig. 8-15. A double aortic arch results from failure of the left dorsal aorta to regress in the region of the heart. Both the esophagus and trachea are enclosed in the resulting double arch.

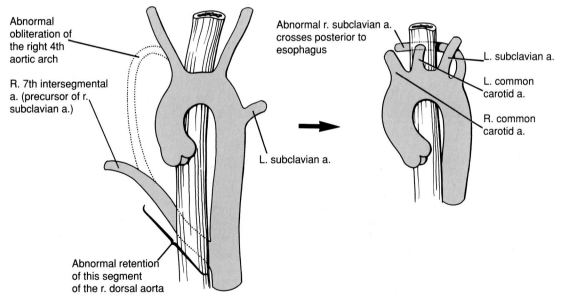

Fig. 8-16. Retention of the right dorsal aorta at the level of the seventh intersegmental artery coupled with abnormal regression of the right fourth aortic arch may result in an anomalous right subclavian artery that passes posterior to the esophagus.

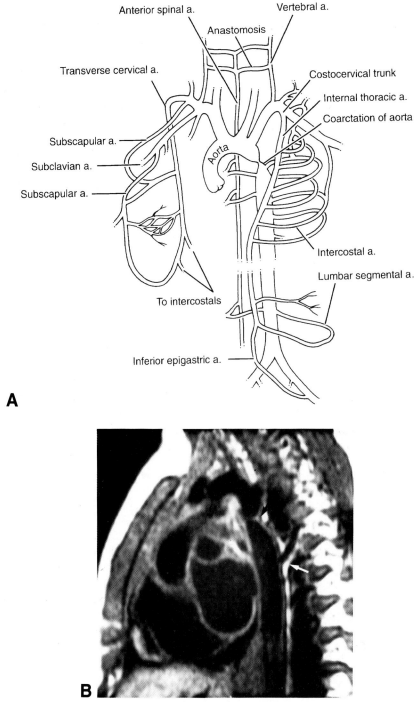

Fig. 8-17. Coarctation of the aorta. The aortic constriction partly or completely blocks the flow of blood into the descending aorta. The trunk and lower extremities receive blood through enlarged collaterals that develop in response to the block. **(A)** Diagram showing the constriction in the aorta (arrow). Collateral circulation developing in post ductal coarctation prior to birth may utilize internal thoracic arteries or the thyrocervical trunk to deliver blood to the descending aorta via segmental arteries of the trunk. (From Edwards JE, Mayo Clin Proc 23:333, 1948, with permission.) **(B)** Sagittal magnetic resonance imaging scan in lateral view showing the site of coarctation (black arrow) and a major collateral entering the descending aorta (white arrow). (Photo courtesy of Children's Hospital Medical Center, Cincinnati, OH.)

Abnormalities of the coronary circulation may result in myocardial ischemia and heart failure

In 30 to 50 percent of humans, the conal artery may branch directly from the ascending aorta rather than from the right coronary artery. More rarely, the **anterior descending** and **circumflex branches** of the left coronary artery may branch directly from the aorta. These variations are considered normal. Other variations, however, may cause sudden death in children and young adults. This may occur when one of the coronary arteries is absent or stenotic or when an excessive number of coronary arterial branches return their blood directly to the cardiac lumen, thus bypassing myocardial capillary beds. The need to understand normal and abnormal development of coronary arteries are clear: in the United States, **coronary angiography** is performed on nearly 1 million people each year, and as many as 300,000 individuals undergo **coronary angioplasty** or **coronary bypass surgery.**

Lymphedema may result from lymphatic hypoplasia

A congenital disorder of the lymphatic system is **herediatry lymphedema,** which may or may not be associated with other abnormalities. Swelling generally occurs in the legs, but in lymphedema in Turner syndrome blockage of lymphatic ducts may result in development of jugular cysts. These may disappear if lymphatic drainage improves during subsequent development.

Angiomas may result from excessive local vessel growth

Blood and lymphatic vessels are stimulated to grow into developing organs by **angiogenic factors.** If vessel growth is not inhibited at the proper time or is stimulated later in life, excessive vessel growth may produce a tangled mass. These tumors may range from the harmless capillary hemangioma (nevus vascularis) called **nevus flammeus** or **birthmark** to dangerous life-threatening vascular tumors in the skull that compress the central nervous system. Many of these tumors have a genetic basis, and some are associated with syndromes resulting from chromosomal anomalies.

Angiogenesis inhibitors or stimulators may serve as therapeutic agents

In addition to the excessive growth of vessels in angiomas, **neovascularization** occurs in many diseases of the child and adult. For example, the growth and enlargement of solid tumors may require the ingrowth of vessels to provide the tumor with oxygen and nutrients. Neovascularization of the retina, particularly in **diabetes,** is a cause of blindness. Neovascularization also occurs in **nasopharyngeal angiofibromas, atherosclerotic plaques,** in joints affected by **rhematoid arthritis,** and in a pathology of the dermis called **psoriasis. Angiogenesis inhibitors** have been considered in development of therapies for these conditions. In contrast, it has been suggested that **angiogenesis stimulators** might stimulate the development of new vasculature in myocardium following infarct or in the ulcerated gastrointestinal tract.

The activities of potential angiogenesis inhibitors and stimulators can be assayed in several experimental systems, including (1) intact cornea of the rabbit, rat, or mouse; (2) chorioallantoic membrane of the chick embryo; and (3) a layer of cultured endothelial cells. Stimulators of angiogenesis defined by these approaches include **angiogenin, basic fibroblast growth factor (bFGF),** and **transforming growth factor-β (TGF-β).** Potent anti-angiogenic factors include **staurosporine,** a fragment of the hormone **prolactin,** the **antitumor agent AGM-1470, interferon-α,** and the spasmolytic **thalidomide** (see Ch. 11). AGM-1470 reduces tumor volume and prolongs survival in animals with hemangioendothelioma. The antiangiogenic agent interferon-α_{2a} has shown promise in reducing the growth of corticosteroid resistant, life-threatening hemangiomas in human infants. A fruitful strategy in the search for angiogenic or anti-angiogenic factors is the analysis of tumors themselves. For example, growth of the Lewis lung tumor is associated with production of the circulating anti-angiogenic factor **angiostatin. Thrombospondin** and **glioma-derived inhibitory factor** are produced in association with the growth of neovascularized tumors. The study of tumor growth has also resulted in identification of a potent angiogenic factor called **vascular endothelial growth factor (VEGF),** which acts as an endothelial mitogen. Moreover, in situ hybridization has shown that VEGF plays an important role in development of the mouse embryonic vasculature as well; transcripts for VEGF are localized in endoderm, and transcripts for **flt-1,** a VEGF **receptor tyrosine kinase,** are localized within adjacent vessel-producing mesoderm. In addition, if VEGF is injected into embryos at the outset of vasculogenesis, neovascularization occurs in avascular areas and vessels fuse excessively. Hypervascularization is also observed in transgenic gain-of-function quail embryos in which VEGF is overexpressed. In contrast, organized blood vessels fail to form in null mutations of the VEGF receptor tyrosine kinase flk-1 and in transgenic mice bearing only a single normal allele for the gene encoding VEGF.

9

Development of the Gastrointestinal Tract

Development of the Stomach, Liver, Digestive Glands, and Spleen; Organization of the Mesenteries; Folding and Rotation of the Midgut; Septation of the Cloaca and Formation of the Anus

SUMMARY

Embryonic folding in the fourth week forms the primitive endodermal gut tube, consisting of a cranial blind-ended **foregut,** a **midgut** that opens into the yolk sac, and a caudal blind-ended **hindgut.** The foregut will form the thoracic and abdominal esophagus, stomach, and about half the duodenum; the midgut will form half the duodenum, the jejunum and ileum, ascending colon, and two-thirds of the transverse colon. The hindgut will form one-third of the transverse colon, the descending and sigmoid colons, and rectum. As discussed in Chapter 8, the network of vitelline arteries that initially vascularizes the yolk sac is reduced to a few branches that supply the developing gut as the yolk sac disappears: Four or five thoracic branches supply the thoracic esophagus, a **celiac artery** supplies the abdominal foregut, a **superior mesenteric artery** supplies the midgut, and the **inferior mesenteric artery** supplies the hindgut. The expanding fusiform stomach rotates in its longitudinal and dorsoventral axes. Meanwhile, endodermal buds sprout from the inferior end of the foregut to form the **liver, gallbladder,** and **pancreas.** The nearby **spleen** condenses from mesoderm, however, within the dorsal mesentery. The midgut and part of the hindgut elongate between the fourth and sixth weeks, forming a **primary intestinal loop** that rotates 90 degrees counterclockwise while it herniates through the umbilicus. It retracts and rotates another 180 degrees counterclockwise in the 10th week to produce definitive midgut and hindgut segments of the small and large intestines. Finally, the terminal hindgut expansion, the **cloaca,** is partitioned into a ventral **primitive urogenital sinus** and the posterior **rectum.** The distal one-third of the anorectal canal forms from an ectodermal invagination called the **anal pit.**

Several defects of gut development are related to disruptions of fusion of the ventral body wall or of normal gut rotation. For example, if the umbilical ring fails to close completely, the midgut may evaginate, resulting in an **omphalocele.** Failures in ventral midline fusion in other regions may result in evagination of the heart **(ectopia cordis)** or in **exstrophy of the bladder or cloaca.** Another anomaly involving eventration of parts of the gastrointestinal tract through a defect apparently produced by abnormal regression of the right umbilical vein is called **gastroschisis.** Several **rotational malformations** of the gut, including nonrotation, reversed rotation, and mixed rotation, may occur. These malrotations of the gut tend to produce clinical symptoms if gut segments twist around each other, compromising the blood supply or obstructing the gut lumen. Current studies of the mechanism by which the **handed asymmetry** of the gut and other organs is achieved implicate growth factors and unknown products of the single genes *iv* and *inv.* Interestingly, these latter genes predictably affect the symmetry of early expression of several growth factor genes with respect to the primitive streak as well as situs. Their postulated actions provide a model that explains how normal situs is established and how disruptions of this mechanism result in reversal of situs in mammals.

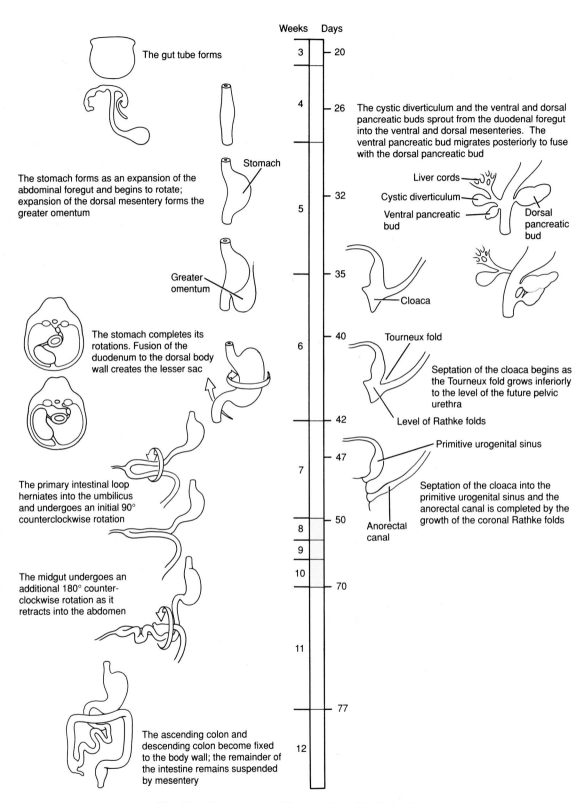

Weeks Days

3 — 20

The gut tube forms

4 — 26

The cystic diverticulum and the ventral and dorsal pancreatic buds sprout from the duodenal foregut into the ventral and dorsal mesenteries. The ventral pancreatic bud migrates posteriorly to fuse with the dorsal pancreatic bud

Stomach

The stomach forms as an expansion of the abdominal foregut and begins to rotate; expansion of the dorsal mesentery forms the greater omentum

5 — 32

Liver cords

Cystic diverticulum

Ventral pancreatic bud

Dorsal pancreatic bud

35

Greater omentum

Cloaca

6 — 40

The stomach completes its rotations. Fusion of the duodenum to the dorsal body wall creates the lesser sac

Tourneux fold

Septation of the cloaca begins as the Tourneux fold grows inferiorly to the level of the future pelvic urethra

42

Level of Rathke folds

47

Primitive urogenital sinus

7

The primary intestinal loop herniates into the umbilicus and undergoes an initial 90° counterclockwise rotation

Septation of the cloaca into the primitive urogenital sinus and the anorectal canal is completed by the growth of the coronal Rathke folds

8 — 50

Anorectal canal

9

10 — 70

The midgut undergoes an additional 180° counter-clockwise rotation as it retracts into the abdomen

11

77

The ascending colon and descending colon become fixed to the body wall; the remainder of the intestine remains suspended by mesentery

12

Timeline. Development of the gut tube and its derivatives.

Embryonic folding converts the trilaminar germ disc into a nested set of three-dimensional tubes

As described in Chapter 6, the cephalocaudal and lateral folding of the embryo in the third and fourth weeks converts the flat trilaminar germ disc into an elongated cylinder (Fig. 9-1). This cylinder consists of three concentric nested tubes. The outer tube is the ectoderm, which now covers the entire outer surface of the embryo, except in the umbilical region, where the yolk sac and connecting stalk emerge. The central tube is the endodermal **primary gut tube.** Separating these two layers is a tube of mesoderm, which encloses the coelom. Thus, the three germ layers bear the same fundamental topologic relation to each other after folding as they did in the flat germ disc.

The foregut, midgut, and hindgut are distinguished on the basis of arterial supply

When folding first forms the three-dimensional embryo, the gut tube consists of cranial and caudal blind ending tubes, the presumptive **foregut** and **hindgut,** and a central **midgut,** which still opens ventrally to the yolk sac. Cranially the foregut terminates in the **buccopharyngeal membrane;** caudally the hindgut terminates in the **cloacal membrane.** The neck of the yolk sac narrows until it becomes the slender **vitelline duct.** Table 9-1 shows the organs and structures that are ultimately derived from the three portions of the gut tube.

By convention, the boundaries of the foregut, midgut, and hindgut correspond to the territories of the three arteries that supply the abdominal gut tube. As described in Chapter 8, the gut tube and its derivatives are vascularized by unpaired ventral branches of the descending aorta that initially serve artery plexuses that arise on the yolk sac, spread to vascularize the gut tube, and anastomose with the dorsal aortae (see Fig. 8-3). About five definitive aortic branches supply the thoracic part of the foregut (the thoracic esophagus). Development of the pharyngeal part of the foregut will be discussed in Chapter 12. The remainder of the gut tube is served by three arteries: the **celiac trunk,** which supplies the abdominal foregut; the **superior mesenteric trunk,** which supplies the midgut; and the **inferior mesenteric artery,** which supplies the hindgut (see Fig. 8-3).

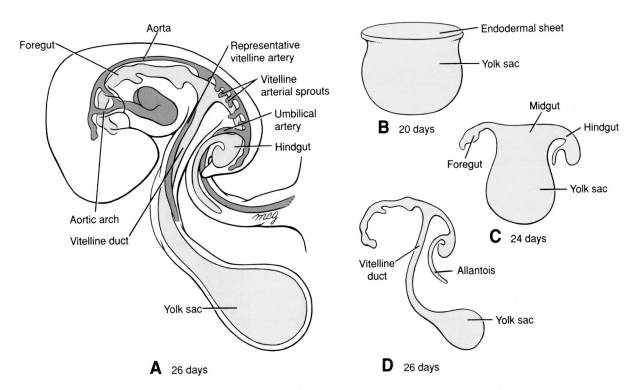

Fig. 9-1. **(A)** The foregut, midgut, and hindgut of the primitive gut tube are formed by the combined action of differential growth and lateral and cephalocaudal folding. The foregut and hindgut are blind-ending tubes that terminate at the buccopharyngeal and cloacal membranes, respectively. The midgut is at first completely open to the cavity of the yolk sac **(B, C).** As folding proceeds, however, this connection is constricted to form the narrow vitelline duct **(D).**

Table 9-1. The Derivatives of the Primitive Gut Tube

REGIONS OF THE DIFFERENTIATED GUT TUBE	ACCESSORY ORGANS DERIVED FROM THE GUT TUBE ENDODERM
Foregut	
Pharynx	Pharyngeal pouch derivatives (see Ch. 12)
Thoracic esophagus	Lungs
Abdominal esophagus	
Stomach	
Superior half of duodenum	Liver parenchyma and hepatic duct epithelium
(superior to the ampulla of Vater)	Gallbladder, cystic duct, and common bile duct
	Dorsal and ventral pancreatic buds (exocrine cells and pancreatic duct epithelium; probably also pancreatic endocrine cells)
Midgut	
Inferior half of duodenum	
Jejunum	
Ileum	
Cecum	
Appendix	
Ascending colon	
Right two-thirds of transverse colon	
Hindgut	
Left one-third of transverse colon	
Descending colon	
Sigmoid colon	
Rectum	Urogenital sinus and derivatives (see Ch. 10)

The primitive abdominal gut is initially a straight tube suspended in the peritoneal cavity by a dorsal mesentery

At the end of the fourth week, almost the entire abdominal gut tube — the portion within the peritoneal cavity, from the abdominal esophagus to the superior end of the developing cloaca — hangs suspended by the dorsal mesentery (see Ch. 6). Except in the region just ventral to the developing stomach, the coelomic cavities in the lateral plate mesoderm on either side of the germ disc coalesce during folding to form a single, continuous peritoneal cavity. In the stomach region the gut tube remains connected to the ventral body wall by the thick septum transversum (see Ch. 6). By the fifth week, the caudal portion of the septum transversum thins to form the **ventral mesentery** connecting the stomach and developing liver to the ventral body wall (Fig. 9-2).

The abdominal foregut gives rise to the stomach, duodenum, liver, pancreas, and gallbladder

The presumptive stomach expands and rotates around two axes

On about day 26, the thoracic foregut begins to elongate rapidly. Over the next 2 days, the presumptive stom-ach, now much farther removed from the lung buds, expands into a *fusiform* (Latin, spindle-shaped) structure that is readily distinguished from the adjacent regions of the gut tube (Fig. 9-3). During the fifth week the dorsal wall of the stomach grows faster than the ventral wall, resulting in the formation of the **greater curvature of the stomach**. Concurrently, deformation of the ventral stomach wall forms the **lesser curvature of the stomach**. Continued differential expansion of the superior part of the greater curvature results in the formation of the **fundus** and **cardiac incisure** by the end of the seventh week.

The stomach rotates during the seventh and eighth weeks. The developing stomach undergoes a 90-degree rotation around a craniocaudal axis so that the greater curvature lies to the left and the lesser curvature lies to the right (Fig. 9-3D). The right and left vagus plexuses, which originally run through the mesoderm on either side of the gut tube, thus rotate to become posterior and anterior vagal trunks in the region of the stomach. The stomach also rotates slightly around a ventrodorsal axis so that the greater curvature faces slightly caudally and the lesser curvature slightly cranially (Fig. 9-3D).

The rotation of the stomach and the secondary fusion of the duodenum to the dorsal body wall create the lesser sac of the peritoneal cavity. The rotations of

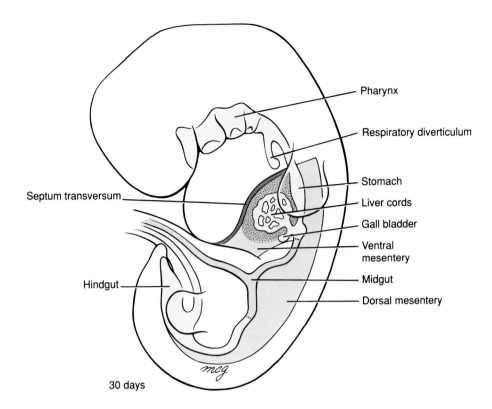

Pharynx

Respiratory diverticulum

Stomach

Liver cords

Gall bladder

Ventral mesentery

Midgut

Dorsal mesentery

Septum transversum

Hindgut

30 days

Fig. 9-2. Structure of the gut tube. The foregut consists of the pharynx, located superior to the respiratory diverticulum, the thoracic esophagus, and the abdominal foregut. The abdominal foregut forms the abdominal esophagus, stomach, and about half of the duodenum and gives rise to the liver, the gallbladder, the pancreas, and their associated ducts. The midgut forms half the duodenum, the jejunum and ileum, the ascending colon, and about two-thirds of the transverse colon. The hindgut forms one-third of the transverse colon, the descending and sigmoid colons, and the upper two-thirds of the anorectal canal. The abdominal esophagus, stomach, and superior part of the duodenum are suspended by dorsal and ventral mesenteries; the abdominal gut tube excluding the rectum is suspended in the abdominal cavity by a dorsal mesentery only.

the stomach bend the presumptive duodenum into a C shape and also displace it to the right until it lies against the dorsal body wall, to which it adheres, thus becoming secondarily retroperitoneal (Fig. 9-4). The rotation of the stomach and fusion of the duodenum create an alcove dorsal to the stomach called the **lesser sac of the peritoneal cavity** (Fig. 9-4). The rest of the peritoneal cavity is now called the **greater sac.**

The lesser sac enlarges as a result of progressive expansion of the dorsal mesogastrium connecting the stom-

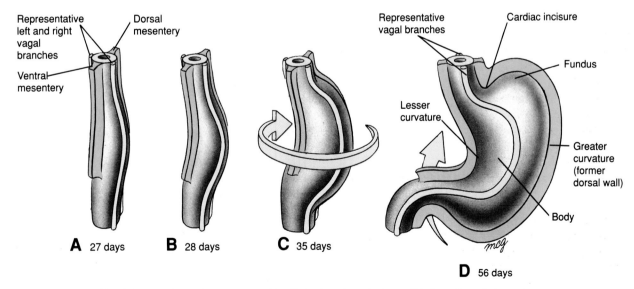

Representative left and right vagal branches

Dorsal mesentery

Ventral mesentery

Representative vagal branches

Cardiac incisure

Fundus

Lesser curvature

Greater curvature (former dorsal wall)

Body

A 27 days   **B** 28 days   **C** 35 days   **D** 56 days

Fig. 9-3. Rotations of the stomach. **(A–C)** Oblique frontal views; **(D)** direct frontal view. The posterior wall of the stomach expands during the fourth and fifth weeks to form the greater curvature. During the seventh week, the stomach rotates clockwise on its longitudinal axis (when viewed from above).

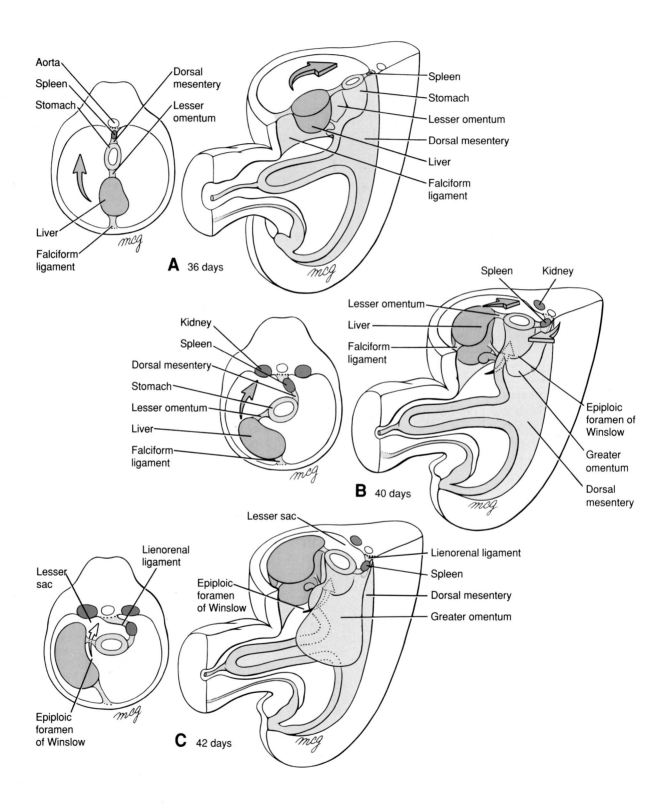

A 36 days

B 40 days

C 42 days

Fig. 9-4. Development of the greater omentum and lesser sac. **(A, B)** The rotation of the stomach and growth of the dorsal mesogastrium create a sac (the greater omentum) that dangles from the greater curvature of the stomach. **(B, C)** When the duodenum swings to the right, it becomes secondarily fused to the body wall, enclosing the space posterior to the stomach and within the expanding cavity of the greater omentum. This space is the lesser sac of the peritoneal cavity. The remainder of the peritoneal cavity is now called the greater sac. The principal passageway between the greater and lesser sacs is the epiploic foramen of Winslow.

ach to the posterior body wall. The resulting large, suspended fold of mesogastrium, called the **greater omentum,** hangs from the dorsal body wall and the greater curvature of the stomach and drapes over more inferior organs of the abdominal cavity (Fig. 9-4C). The portion of the lesser sac directly dorsal to the stomach is now called the **upper recess of the lesser sac,** and the cavity within the greater omentum is called the **lower recess of the lesser sac.** The lower recess, however, is obliterated during fetal life as the anterior and posterior folds of the greater omentum fuse together.

A system of digestive glands develops from endodermal buds of the duodenum

The liver parenchyma, the gallbladder, and their ducts bud from the duodenal endoderm and grow into the septum transversum. On about day 22, a small endodermal thickening, the **hepatic plate,** appears on the ventral side of the duodenum. Over the next few days, cells in this plate proliferate and form a **hepatic diverticulum,** which grows into the inferior region of the septum transversum (Fig. 9-5). The hepatic diverticulum gives

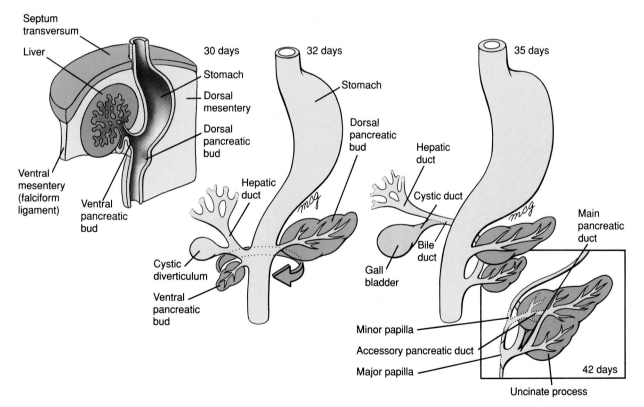

Fig. 9-5. Development of the liver, gallbladder, pancreas, and their duct systems from endodermal diverticulae of the duodenum. The liver bud sprouts during the fourth week and expands in the ventral mesentery. The cystic diverticulum and ventral pancreatic bud also grow into the ventral mesentery, whereas the dorsal pancreatic bud grows into the dorsal mesentery. During the fifth week, the ventral pancreatic bud migrates around the posterior side (former right side) of the duodenum to fuse with the dorsal pancreatic bud. The main duct of the ventral bud ultimately becomes the major pancreatic duct, which drains the entire pancreas.

rise to the ramifying **liver cords,** which become the hepatocytes (parenchyma), to the **bile canaliculi** of the liver, and to the **hepatic ducts.** The mesoblastic **supporting stroma** of the liver, in contrast, develops from splanchnopleuric mesoderm originating near the cardiac region of the stomach.

By day 26, a distinct endodermal thickening appears on the ventral side of the duodenum just caudal to the base of the hepatic diverticulum and buds into the ventral mesentery (Fig. 9-5). This **cystic diverticulum** will form the **gallbladder** and **cystic duct.** As shown in Figure 9-5, no sooner does the cystic diverticulum appear than cells at the junction of the hepatic and cystic ducts proliferate and form the **common bile duct.** As a result, the developing cystic duct is carried away from the duodenum.

The pancreas forms through the fusion of dorsal and ventral pancreatic buds. On day 26, another duodenal bud begins to grow into the dorsal mesentery just opposite the hepatic diverticulum. This endodermal diverticulum is the **dorsal pancreatic bud** (Fig. 9-5). Over the next few days, as the dorsal pancreatic bud elongates into the dorsal mesentery, another endodermal diverticulum, the **ventral pancreatic bud,** sprouts into the ventral mesentery just caudal to the developing gallbladder (Fig. 9-5). By day 32, the main duct of the ventral pancreatic

bud becomes connected to the proximal end of the common bile duct.

During the fifth week, the mouth of the common bile duct and the ventral pancreatic bud migrate posteriorly around the duodenum to the dorsal mesentery (Fig. 9-5). By the early sixth week, the ventral and dorsal pancreatic buds lie adjacent in the plane of the dorsal mesentery, and late in the sixth week the two pancreatic buds fuse to form the definitive pancreas. The dorsal pancreatic bud gives rise to the **head, body,** and **tail** of the pancreas, whereas the ventral pancreatic bud gives rise to the hooklike **uncinate process.** Like the duodenum, the pancreas fuses to the dorsal body wall and becomes secondarily retroperitoneal.

Occasionally, the pancreas forms a complete ring encircling the duodenum, a condition known as **annular pancreas.** As shown in Figure 9-6, this abnormality probably arises when the two lobes of a bilobed ventral pancreatic bud (a normal variation) migrate in opposite directions around the duodenum to fuse with the dorsal pancreatic bud. An annular pancreas compresses the duodenum and may cause gastrointestinal obstruction.

When the ventral and dorsal pancreatic buds fuse, their ductal systems also become interconnected (Fig. 9-5). The duct from the dorsal bud to the duodenum usually degenerates, leaving the ventral pancreatic duct, now called the

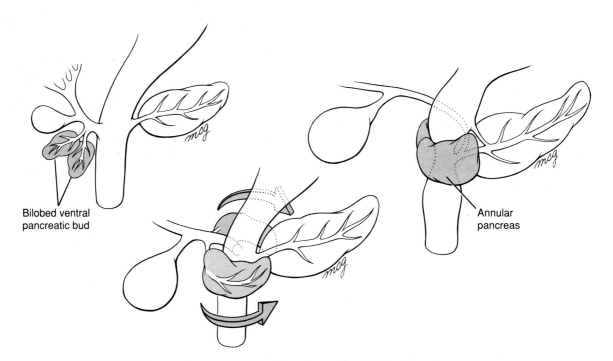

Bilobed ventral pancreatic bud

Annular pancreas

Fig. 9-6. The ventral pancreas may consist of two lobes. If the lobes migrate around the duodenum in opposite directions to fuse with the dorsal pancreatic bud, an annular pancreas is formed.

main pancreatic duct, as the only conduit to the duodenum. The main pancreatic duct and the common bile duct meet and empty their secretions into the duodenum at the **major duodenal papilla** or **ampulla of Vater.** In some individuals, the dorsal pancreatic duct persists as an **accessory pancreatic duct** that empties into the duodenum at a **minor duodenal papilla** (Fig. 9-5).

The **exocrine cells** of the pancreas, which produce digestive enzymes, differentiate from the endoderm of the pancreatic buds. The **pancreatic endocrine cells** in the islets of Langerhans arise from endoderm.

The spleen is derived from the dorsal mesogastrium

As the dorsal mesogastrium of the lesser sac begins its expansive growth at the end of the fourth week, a mesenchymal condensation develops in it near the body wall. This condensation differentiates during the fifth week to form the **spleen,** a vascular lymphatic organ (Fig. 9-4). Smaller splenic condensations called **accessory spleens** may develop near the hilum of the primary spleen. The rotation of the stomach and growth of the dorsal mesogastrium translocate the spleen to the left side of the abdominal cavity. The rotation of the dorsal mesogastrium also establishes a mesenteric connection called the **renalsplenic ligament** between the spleen and the left kidney. The portion of the dorsal mesentery between the spleen and the stomach is called the **gastrosplenic ligament.**

The spleen initially functions as a hematopoietic organ and only later acquires its definitive lymphoid character. During the **preliminary stage** of its development, until 14 weeks, the spleen is strictly hematopoietic. From 15 to 18 weeks (the **transformation stage**) the organ develops its characteristic lobular architecture, and the **stage of lymphoid colonization** then commences as T-lymphocyte precursor cells begin to enter the spleen. Starting at 23 weeks, B-cell precursors arrive and form the **B-cell regions** of the definitive spleen.

The ventral mesentery gives rise to a multitude of structures as it is invaded by the liver

As the liver enlarges, the caudal portion of the septum transversum (the ventral mesentery) is modified to form a number of membranous structures, including the serous coverings of the liver and the membranes that attach the liver to the stomach and to the ventral body wall (Table 9-2). By the sixth week, the enlarging liver splits the two mesothelial layers of the ventral mesentery apart (Fig. 9-7). The serosal membranes of the septum becomes the **visceral peritoneum** that covers almost the entire surface of the liver. At its superior pole, however, the liver tissue makes direct contact with the developing central tendon of the diaphragm and therefore has no peritoneal covering. This zone becomes the **bare area of the liver** (Fig. 9-7). Around the margins of the bare area, the peritoneum covering the inferior surface of the peripheral diaphragm makes a fold or *reflection* onto the surface of the liver. Because this reflection encircles the bare area like a crown, it is called the **coronary ligament.**

The narrow sickle-shaped flap of ventral mesentery that attaches the liver to the ventral body wall differentiates into the membranous **falciform ligament** (Fig. 9-7). The free caudal margin of this membrane carries the umbilical vein from the body wall to the liver. The portion of the ventral mesentery between the liver and the stomach thins out to form the **lesser omentum.** The caudal border of the lesser omentum, connecting the liver to the developing duodenum, is called the **hepatoduodenal ligament** and contains the portal vein, the proper hepatic artery and branches, and the hepatic, cystic, and common bile ducts. The region of the lesser omentum between the liver and the stomach is called the **hepatogastric ligament.**

Table 9-2. Derivatives of the Septum Transversum

REGION OF SEPTUM TRANSVERSUM	DERIVATIVES
Cranial region	Central tendon of the diaphragm Myocytes of the pleuroperitoneal membranes
Central mesenchyme	Hematopoietic cells of liver
Caudal region (ventral mesentery)	Falciform ligament Visceral peritoneum of the liver, including the coronary ligament Visceral peritoneum of the gallbladder Lesser omentum, including the hepatoduodenal and hepatogastric ligaments

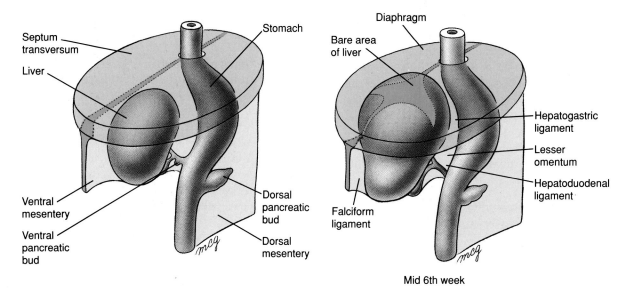

Fig. 9-7. Formation of the liver and associated membranes. As the liver bud grows into the ventral mesentery, its expanding crown makes direct contact with the developing diaphragm. The ventral mesentery that encloses the growing liver bud differentiates into the visceral peritoneum of the liver, which is reflected onto the diaphragm. This zone of reflection, which encircles the area where the liver directly contacts the diaphragm (the bare area), becomes the coronary ligament. The remnant of ventral mesentery connecting the liver with the anterior body wall becomes the falciform ligament, while the ventral mesentery between the liver and lesser curvature of the stomach forms the lesser omentum.

When the stomach rotates to the left and the liver shifts into the right side of the peritoneal cavity, the lesser omentum rotates from a sagittal into a coronal (frontal) plane. This repositioning reduces the communication between the greater and lesser sacs of the peritoneal cavity to a narrow canal lying just posterior to the lesser omentum. This canal is called the **epiploic foramen of Winslow** (Fig. 9-4).

Rotations of the midgut produce the definitive configuration of the small and large intestines

Rapid elongation of the ileum produces a primary intestinal loop that herniates into the umbilicus

By the fifth week, the presumptive ileum, which can be distinguished from the presumptive colon by the presence of a cecal primordium at the junction between the two, begins to elongate rapidly. The growing ileum lengthens much more rapidly than the abdominal cavity itself, and the midgut is therefore thrown into a dorsoventral hairpin fold called the **primary intestinal loop** (Fig. 9-8). The cranial limb of this loop will give rise to most of the ileum, whereas the caudal limb will become the ascend-

ing and transverse colons. At its apex, the primary intestinal loop is attached to the umbilicus by the vitelline duct, and the superior mesenteric artery runs down the long axis of the loop. By the early sixth week, the continuing elongation of the midgut, combined with pressure from the dramatic growth of other abdominal organs (particularly the liver), forces the primary intestinal loop to herniate into the umbilicus (Fig. 9-8B).

The herniated primary intestinal loop undergoes an initial 90-degree counterclockwise rotation

As the primary intestinal loop herniates into the umbilicus, it also rotates around the axis of the superior mesenteric artery (i.e., around a dorsoventral axis) by 90 degrees counterclockwise as viewed from in front, so that the cranial limb moves caudally and to the embryo's right and the caudal limb moves cranially and to the embryo's left (Fig. 9-8B). This rotation is complete by the early eighth week. Meanwhile, the midgut continues to differentiate. The lengthening jejunum and ileum are thrown into a series of folds called the **jejunal-ileal loops,** and the expanding cecum sprouts a wormlike **vermiform appendix** (Fig. 9-8C).

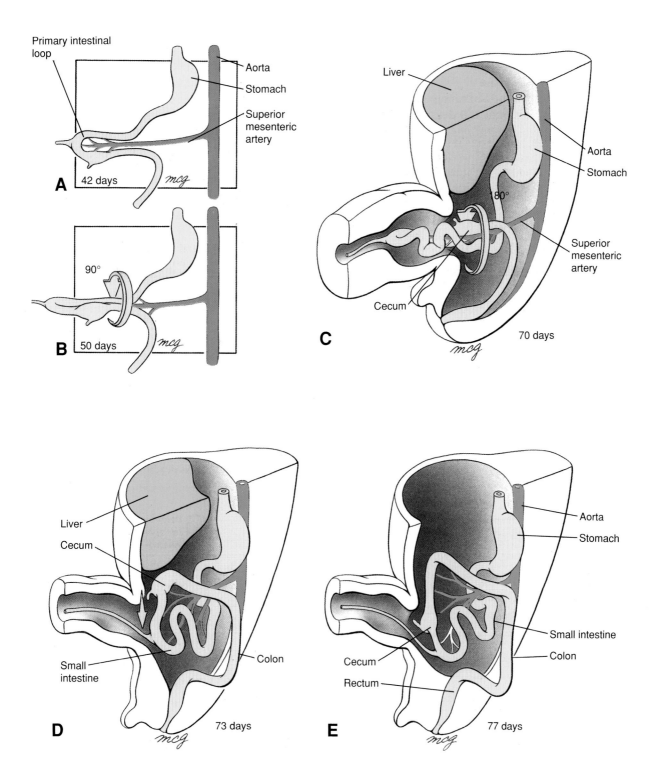

Fig. 9-8. Herniation and rotations of the intestine. **(A, B)** At the end of the sixth week, the primary intestinal loop herniates into the umbilicus, rotating through 90 degrees counterclockwise (in frontal view). **(C)** The small intestine elongates to form jejunal-ileal loops, the cecum and appendix grow, and, at the end of the 10th week, the primary intestinal loop retracts into the abdominal cavity rotating an additional 180 degrees counterclockwise. **(D, E)** During the 11th week, the retracting midgut completes this rotation as the cecum is positioned just inferior to the liver. The cecum is then displaced inferiorly, pulling down the proximal hindgut to form the ascending colon. The descending colon is simultaneously fixed on the left side of the posterior abdominal wall. The jejunum, ileum, and transverse and sigmoid colons remain suspended by mesentery.

During the 10th week, the midgut retracts into the abdomen and rotates an additional 180 degrees

The mechanism responsible for the rapid retraction of the midgut into the abdominal cavity during the 10th week is not understood. As the intestinal loop reenters the abdomen, it rotates counterclockwise through an additional 180 degrees, so that now the retracting colon has traveled a 270-degree circuit relative to the posterior wall of the abdominal cavity (Fig. 9-8C–E). The cecum consequently rotates to a position just inferior to the liver in the region of the right iliac crest. The intestines have completely returned to the abdominal cavity by the 11th week.

The ascending and descending colon become secondarily retroperitoneal

After the large intestine returns to the abdominal cavity, the dorsal mesenteries of the ascending colon and descending colon shorten and fold, bringing these organs into contact with the dorsal body wall, where they adhere and become secondarily retroperitoneal (see Ch. 6). The cecum is suspended from the dorsal body wall by a shortened mesentery shortly after it returns to the abdominal cavity.

In the case of ascending and descending colons, the shortening and folding of the mesenteries is probably related to the relative lengthening of the lumbar region of the dorsal body wall. The transverse colon does not become fixed to the body wall but remains an intraperitoneal organ suspended by mesentery. The most inferior portion of the colon, the sigmoid colon, also remains suspended by mesentery. Figure 9-9 summarizes the final disposition of the gastrointestinal organs with respect to the body wall.

The distal hindgut gives rise to the rectum and the urogenital sinus

The cloaca is partitioned into an anterior primitive urogenital sinus and a posterior rectum

The portion of the primitive gut tube lying just deep to the cloacal membrane forms an expansion called the **cloaca** (Latin, sewer). A slim superoventral diverticulum of the cloaca called the **allantois** extends into the connecting stalk. Between the fourth and sixth weeks, the cloaca is partitioned into a posterior rectum and an anterior **primitive urogenital sinus** by the growth of a coronal partition called the **urorectal septum.** As described in Chapter 10, the uro-

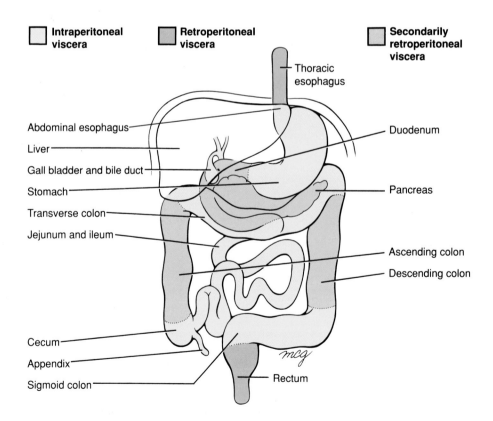

Fig. 9-9. Intraperitoneal, retroperitoneal, and secondarily retroperitoneal organs of the abdominal gastrointestinal tract.

genital sinus gives rise to the bladder, the pelvic urethra, and a lower expansion, the **definitive urogenital sinus.**

The distal edge of the urorectal septum fuses with the cloacal membrane, dividing the membrane into an anterior **urogenital membrane** and a posterior **anal membrane.** The zone of fusion between the urorectal septum and the cloacal membrane becomes the **perineum.**

The urorectal septum is a composite of two mesodermal septal systems

The urorectal septum is a composite structure formed by two integrated mesodermal septal systems: a superior fold called the **Tourneux fold** and a pair of lateral folds called the **Rathke folds** (Fig. 9-10). The Tourneux fold first appears in the fourth week as a crescentic wedge of mesoderm growing inferiorly between the allantois and the cranial end of the cloaca. This coronal partition ceases to grow when it reaches the level of the future pelvic urethra. The Rathke folds arise as a pair of mesodermal bars located on either side of the cloacal cavity near the cloacal membrane and grow toward the midline, where they fuse with each other and with the Tourneux fold to complete the urorectal septum.

The inferior one-third of the anorectal canal forms from an ectodermal pit

The superior two-thirds of the anorectal canal forms from the distal part of the hindgut. The inferior one-third of the anorectal canal, in contrast, is derived from an ectodermal pit called the **anal pit** or **proctodeum** (Fig. 9-11). This pit is created when the mesenchyme around the

anal membrane proliferates to form a raised border. The anal membrane, which thus separates the endodermal and ectodermal portions of the anorectal canal, breaks down in the eighth week. The former location of this membrane is marked in the adult by an irregular folding of mucosa within the anorectal canal, called the **pectinate line.** The vasculature of the anorectal canal is consistent with this dual origin: superior to the pectinate line the canal is supplied by branches of the inferior mesenteric arteries and veins serving the hindgut, whereas inferior to the pectinate line it is supplied by branches of the internal iliac arteries and veins. Anastomoses between tributaries of the superior rectal vein and tributaries of the inferior rectal vein within the mucosa of the anorectal canal may later swell into hemorrhoids if the normal portal blood flow into the inferior vena cava is blocked.

The digestive tube becomes transiently solid and then undergoes recanalization

During the sixth week, the endodermal epithelium of the gut tube proliferates until it completely occludes the gut tube lumen (Fig. 9-13). Over the next 2 weeks, vacuoles develop in this tissue and coalesce until the gut tube is fully **recanalized.** Finally, in the ninth week, the definitive mucosal epithelium differentiates from the endodermal lining of the new gut lumen. *Stenosis* or *duplication* of the digestive tract may result from incomplete recanalization.

The mesodermal coating of the primitive gut tube gives rise to the submucosal connective tissue and smooth muscle layers of the definitive gastrointestinal tract.

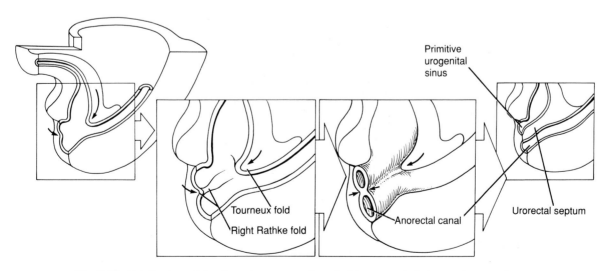

Fig. 9-10. Subdivision of the cloaca into an anterior primitive urogenital sinus and a posterior rectum between 4 and 6 weeks. The urorectal septum that divides the cloaca is composed of three distinct septae. Initially, a superior Tourneaux fold grows inferiorly to the level of the future pelvic uretura. Separation is then completed by left and right Rathke folds that grow in a coronal plane.

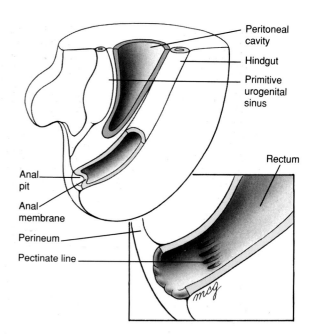

Fig. 9-11. The lower third of the anorectal canal is formed by an ecto-dermal invagination called the anal pit. The border between the superior end of the anal pit and the inferior end of the rectum is demarcated by mucosal folds called the pectinate line in the adult.

APPLICATIONS TO CLINICAL PRACTICE

Segments of the gastrointestinal tract may evaginate through defects of the ventral body wall

If the umbilical ring does not close, midgut/hindgut loops may remain outside the abdominal cavity at birth. This condition, called **omphalocele,** occurs in 2.5 of 10,000 births. The herniated organs may protrude into a membrane-covered sac (Fig. 9-12A). If only amniotic membrane covers the organs, the intestinal loops may have herniated normally during the sixth week but were not retracted. If peritoneum is included in the membrane, the organs may have herniated, retracted normally, and then evaginated secondarily. These defects may result from incomplete lateral folding or from incomplete migration and differentiation of mesoderm that normally forms the muscle and connective tissue in the ventral midline. Defects related to omphalocele involve evagination of the heart **(ectopia cordis;** Fig. 9-12B), **exstrophy of the bladder or cloaca** (Fig. 9-13), and **epispadias** (the right and left halves of the penile tubercle do not completely fuse). Exstrophy of the bladder with epispadias is the most common anomaly in this series (1 in 40,000 births), while exstrophy of the cloaca occurs less frequently (1 in 200,000 births). However, these malformations are about twice as common in males as in females. An unrelated anomaly involving eventration of segments of the gut is called **gastroschisis** (Fig. 9-14). In this condition, how-ever, the abdominal contents herniate through a defect on the right side of the umbilicus that is thought to result from abnormal regression of the right umbilical vein.

Abnormalities of the vitelline duct and the allantois also affect the umbilicus

Normally, the vitelline duct regresses between the fifth and eighth weeks, but in about 2 percent of live-born infants it persists as a remnant of variable length and disposition (Fig. 9-15).

It is about twice as common in males as in females. It typically consists of an intestinal diverticulum 1 to 5 cm long, projecting from the antimesenteric wall of the ileum, about 100 cm from the cecum (Fig. 9-15A). It may remain open to the umbilicus (Fig. 9-15B) or form an enterocyst (Fig. 9-15C) or a fibrous omphalomesenteric ligament (Fig. 9-15D). Collectively these anomalies are called **Meckel's diverticulum.** It is estimated that 15 to 35 percent of individuals with a Meckel's diverticulum develop **intestinal obstruction, gastrointestinal bleeding,** or **bowel sepsis.** Symptoms may closely mimic appendicitis, involving periumbilical pain that later localizes to the lower right quadrant. Mortality in untreated cases is estimated to be 2.5 to 15 percent. In contrast, **incomplete obliteration of the allantois** results in urachal anomalies that may affect the umbilicus (Fig. 9-16). Part or all of the urachus may remain patent, resulting in a

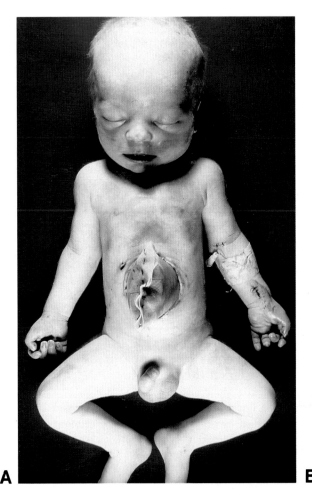
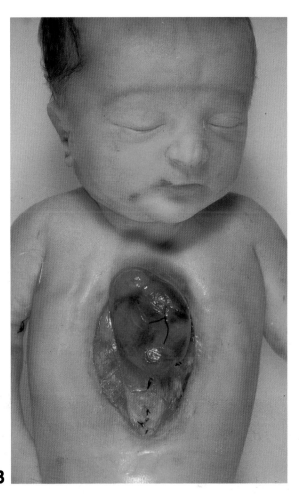

Fig. 9-12. Congenital defects of anterior abdominal wall closure. **(A)** Omphalocele. An omphalocele may be forced back into the abdominal cavity by compressing a Dacron silo. **(B)** Ectopia cordis caused by failure of abdominal wall closure more superiorly. (Photos courtesy of Children's Hospital Medical Center, Cincinnati, OH.)

patent urachus (Fig. 9-16B), a **urachal sinus** (Fig. 9-16C), a **urachal diverticulum** (Fig. 9-16D), or a **urachal cyst** (Fig. 9-16E). Symptoms include leakage of urine from the umbilicus, urinary tract infections and peritonitis resulting from perforation of the urachus, and pain that can be confused with appendicitis. These conditions may be life threatening.

Duplication and stenosis of the gastrointestinal tract

During the sixth week of development, the endodermal epithelium of the gut tube proliferates and completely occludes the lumen. Over the next 2 weeks, however, it vacuolates and is recanalized. **Stenosis** or **duplication** may result from incomplete recanalization, resulting in intestinal obstruction and abdominal pain.

Abnormal rotation and fixation of the primary intestinal loop may result in a variety of malformations

The normal handed asymmetry of the gastrointestinal tract is based on an intricate series of **rotations** and **fixations.** Not surprisingly, errors in one or more of these steps lead to a spectrum of anomalies. In general, these defects can be classified as **nonrotations, reversed rotations,** or **mixed rotations.** In **nonrotations** of the primary intestinal loop, the initial 90-degree counterclockwise rotation occurs but the second 180-degree counterclockwise rotation does not, resulting in a net counterclockwise rotation of only 90 degrees (Fig. 9-17A). This disposes the cranial limb to the right side of the abdominal cavity and the caudal limb to the left side. Since the caudal limb forms most of the colon, this anom-

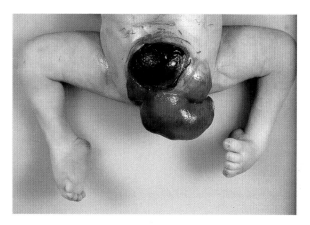

Fig. 9-13. In this case of cloacal exstrophy, the undivided cloaca evaginates from an anterior wall defect at the site of the former cloacal membrane. (Photo courtesy of Children's Hospital Medical Center, Cincinnati, OH.)

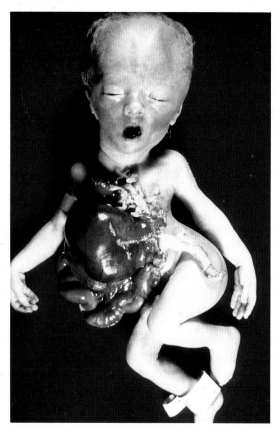

Fig. 9-14. Severe gastroschisis. As is typical, the visceral organs evaginate to the right of the umbilicus. (Photo courtesy of Children's Hospital Medical Center, Cincinnati, OH.)

aly is also called **left-sided colon.** In **reversed rotation** of the primary intestinal loop, the initial 90-degree rotation occurs but the second 180-degree rotation is reversed resulting in a net clockwise rotation of 90 degrees (Fig. 9-17B). This disposes the segments of the small and large intestines in the same pattern as would occur in normal rotation except for one important difference. In reversed rotation, the duodenum lies anterior to the transverse colon. Since this segment of the small intestine fuses to the posterior body wall, the underlying segment of transverse colon may become pinned and obstructed by the duodenum (Fig. 9-17C). In **mixed rotations,** the cranial limb only of the primary intestinal loop rotates 90 degrees, while the caudal limb is the only part of the primary intestinal loop that rotates 180 degrees during retraction in the tenth week. In this case, the cecum becomes fixed at the midline just inferior to the pylorus of the stomach, and the duodenum may become enclosed by a band of thickened peritoneum.

Abnormal midgut rotation or fixation may lead to compression or volvulus of the intestines

Regions of the intestines may be pinned against the body wall as described in reversed rotation, constricted by bands of mesentery as in mixed rotation, or may be suspended from a single point. Such freely suspended coils are prone to torsion or **volvulus,** resulting in obstruction or compromise of the intestinal blood supply and compression of lymphatics (Fig. 9-18). The presence of such rotational abnormalities is usually signaled during childhood by **abdominal pain, bilious vomiting, gastrointestinal bleeding,** and **failure to thrive,** although these anomalies may remain silent until adulthood. Definitive diagnosis often involves barium enema or barium swallow. These defects can be surgically corrected.

The mechanism by which the gastrointestinal tract and other organs develop handed asymmetry is activated long before structural handedness is apparent

In the rare human disorder **situs inversus viscerum** the handedness of all of the viscera is reversed. However, in many other cases, the reversal is incomplete, and subsidiary malformations such as malrotations of the primary intestinal loop may result. Indeed, in most cases, organs exhibit a discordance of sidedness, or **heterotaxia.** For example, folding of the heart may be reversed (**dextrocardia**) while lobulation of the lungs may be normal. The mechanism that underlies the folding and rotations that

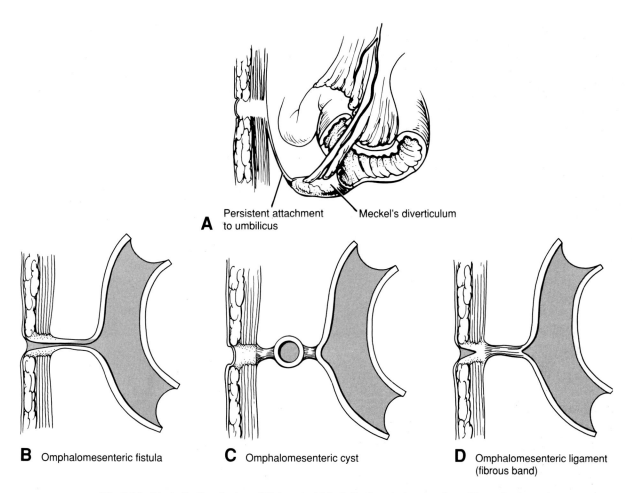

A Persistent attachment to umbilicus   Meckel's diverticulum

B Omphalomesenteric fistula

C Omphalomesenteric cyst

D Omphalomesenteric ligament (fibrous band)

Fig. 9-15. Meckel's diverticulum. **(A)** A typical Meckel's diverticulum is a fingerlike projection of the ileum located about 100 cm proximal to the cecum. A Meckel's diverticulum may form **(B)** a patent fistula connecting the umbilicus with the ileum, **(C)** an isolated cyst suspended by ligaments, or **(D)** a fibrous band connecting the ileum and anterior body wall at the level of the umbilicus. (Photo courtesy of Children's Hospital Medical Center, Cincinnati, OH.)

result in normal handed asymmetry of the human body are partially revealed by two mouse mutants, *iv* and *inv.* Handedness is random in litters of *iv/iv* mice, while handedness is reversed in 100 percent of *inv/inv* mice. One explanation of these differences is that the development of handedness is a two-step process; in the first step, handedness is established in a reverse direction (situs inversus), and in the second step the orientation of the mechanism is reversed, resulting in normal situs. The *iv* mutation could prevent the first step or establishment of the bias mechanism altogether, resulting in random situs. The *inv* mutation could disrupt the switch process, resulting in situs inversus in 100 percent of the offspring.

In situ hybridization experiments suggest that the biasing mechanism is set very early in development and that the protein **sonic hedgehog (Shh)** (see Ch. 3) and members of the **transforming growth factor-β** family may play pivotal roles in the regulation of handed asymmetry in birds and mammals. In chick embryos, Shh is expressed transiently only on the left side of the primitive streak of the gastrulating embryo, while the activin receptor **cAct-R11a** and possibly **activin** are expressed on the right side. Then, somewhat later, the nodal-related gene **cNR-1** is expressed on the left side of the streak. Functional evidence for the role of some of these factors in handedness is demonstrated in experiments where an activin-soaked bead is implanted on the left side of the streak or when chick fibroblast cells transfected with the *Shh* gene are implanted on the right side of the streak. In both cases, the handedness of the embryos is randomized. While *Shh* has not been found to be asymmetrically expressed in normal mouse embryos, as it is in chicks, nor-

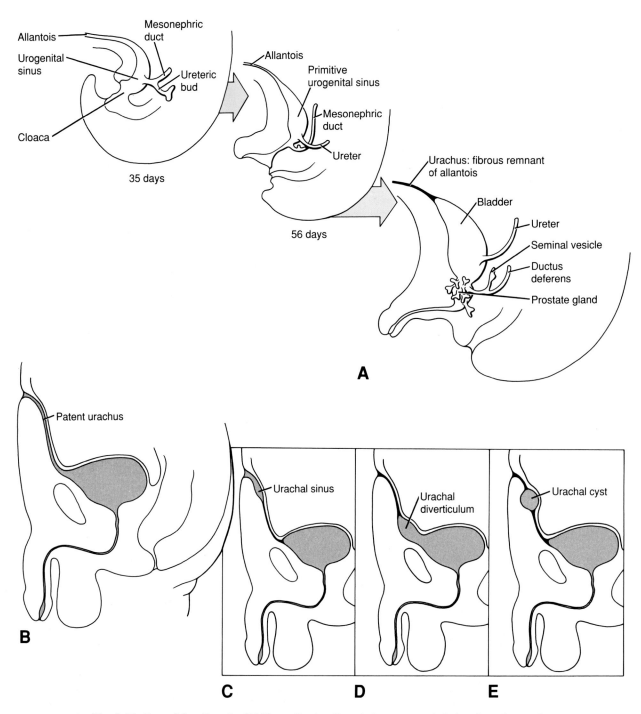

Fig. 9-16. Fate of the allantois. **(A)** Normally, the allantois becomes occluded to form the urachus or median umbilical ligament of the adult. Very rarely, parts of the allantois may remain patent producing **(B)** a urachal fistula, **(C)** a urachal sinus, **(D)** a urachal diverticulum, or **(E)** a urachal cyst.

Fig. 9-17. (A) Nonrotation of the gut (also called left-sided colon). **(B)** Reversed rotation of ▶ the gut. The net rotation is 90 degrees clockwise, so the midgut viscera are brought to their normal locations in the abdominal cavity but the duodenum lies anterior to the transverse colon. **(C)** Mixed rotation of the gut. In this malformation, the cranial and caudal limbs of the primary intestinal loop rotate independently.

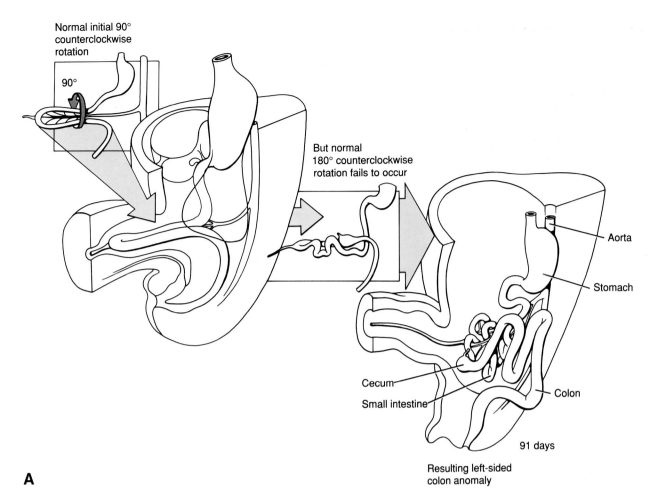

Normal initial 90°
counterclockwise
rotation

90°

But normal
180° counterclockwise
rotation fails to occur

Aorta

Stomach

Cecum

Colon

Small intestine

91 days

Resulting left-sided
colon anomaly

A

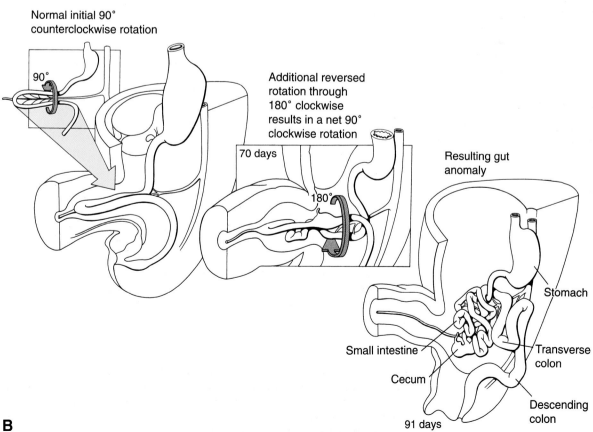

Normal initial 90°
counterclockwise rotation

90°

Additional reversed
rotation through
180° clockwise
results in a net 90°
clockwise rotation

70 days

180°

Resulting gut
anomaly

Stomach

Small intestine

Transverse
colon

Cecum

Descending
colon

91 days

B

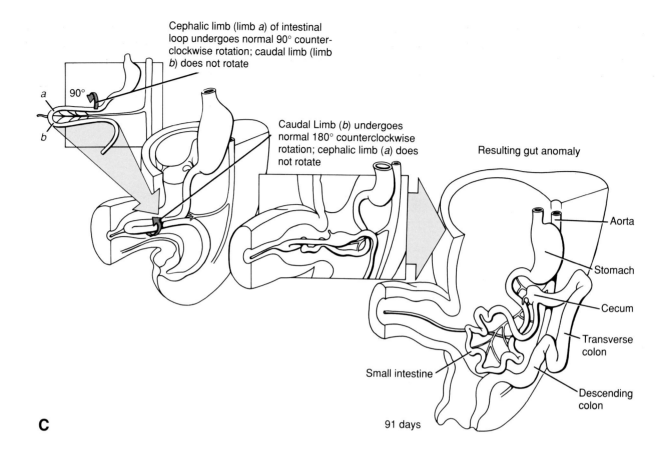

Cephalic limb (limb *a*) of intestinal loop undergoes normal 90° counter-clockwise rotation; caudal limb (limb *b*) does not rotate

Caudal Limb (*b*) undergoes normal 180° counterclockwise rotation; cephalic limb (*a*) does not rotate

Resulting gut anomaly

Aorta

Stomach

Cecum

Transverse colon

Small intestine

Descending colon

91 days

C

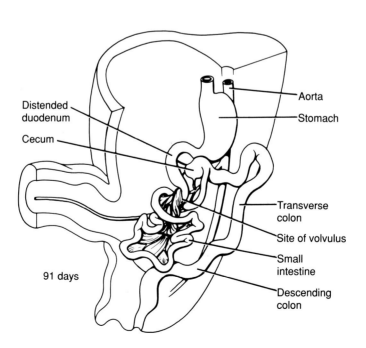

Distended duodenum

Cecum

Aorta

Stomach

Transverse colon

Site of volvulus

Small intestine

Descending colon

91 days

Fig. 9-18. Volvulus. Volvulus may occur as suspended regions of the gut twist around themselves, constricting the intestine and/or compromising its blood supply.

mally the TGF-β family proteins **nodal** and **lefty** are both expressed only on the left side of the mouse primitive streak. Interestingly, in *iv/iv* mutants, where situs is randomized, nodal expression is randomized; it occurs on the right or left side or on both sides or on neither side of the streak. In the *inv/inv* mutant, where situs is reversed, nodal is almost always expressed on the right rather than the left side of the streak.

10

Development of the Urogenital System

Development of the Cervical Nephrotomes, Mesonephric and Metanephric Kidneys, and Urogenital Duct Systems; Development of the Gonads and Genitalia

Development of the **genital system** is closely integrated with that of the **urinary system,** and so they are discussed together in this chapter. Three sequential urinary systems develop from the **intermediate mesoderm:** (1) the **cervical nephrotomes,** which are never functional; (2) a **thoracolumbar mesonephric system,** which functions briefly during embryonic life; and (3) in the fifth week, the intermediate mesoderm forms a **sacral metanephric system,** which ascends to the lumbar region forming the definitive kidneys. This final system develops as each of the **ureteric buds** branch from the mesonephric ducts and grow into a condensation of intermediate mesoderm called the **metanephric blastema.** Reciprocal inductive interactions then result in the differentiation of the **nephrons** within the metanephric blastema, and bifurcation of the ureteric bud forms the collecting system that empties the urine into the bladder. The **bladder** is formed from the superior region of the **primitive urogenital sinus** created by partitioning of the **cloaca** by the **urorectal septum.** The intermediate constricted region of the primitive urogenital sinus gives rise to the prostatic and membranous urethra in males and the membranous urethra in females; the lower expansion, the **definitive urogenital sinus,** forms the **penile urethra** in males and the **vestibule of the vagina** in females. Malformations of the urinary system, such as ectopic ureters or renal agenesis, may result from disturbances of the interaction between the ureteric bud and the metanephric blastema. For example, mutations of regulatory genes that function in this interaction have been implicated in renal congenital diseases like **polycystic kidney disease** and **Wilms' tumor.** Anomalies of the urinary system also result from disruption of the **urorectal septum.**

Migration of the primordial germ cells to the posterior body wall between the fourth and sixth weeks results in induction of the **genital ridges** just medial to the mesonephros on each side of the midline. Enlargement of this ridge is largely a consequence of the proliferation of cells of the coelomic epithelium and the mesonephros that form the **primitive sex cords** that surround the germ cells and of the mesenchyme that forms the gonadal stroma. In males, activation of the sex-determining region on the Y chromosome (SRY) produces a transcription factor, which initiates the **male developmental cascade;** the formation of the testes and the male genital ducts. The absence of SRY in females results in formation of ovaries and female genital ducts. In addition to SRY, genes on the X chromosome and some of the autosomes have been shown to play key roles in male and/or female genital differentiation, and mutations of some of these result in malformations of the genital system or in sex reversals. These include *WT1* (Denys-Drash syndrome, WAGR syndrome), *SOX9* (campomelic dysplasia), and *DAX1* (sex reversal and adrenal hypoplasia). Other anomalies such as pseudohermaphroditism result from abnormal hormone levels or disruptions of hormone receptors.

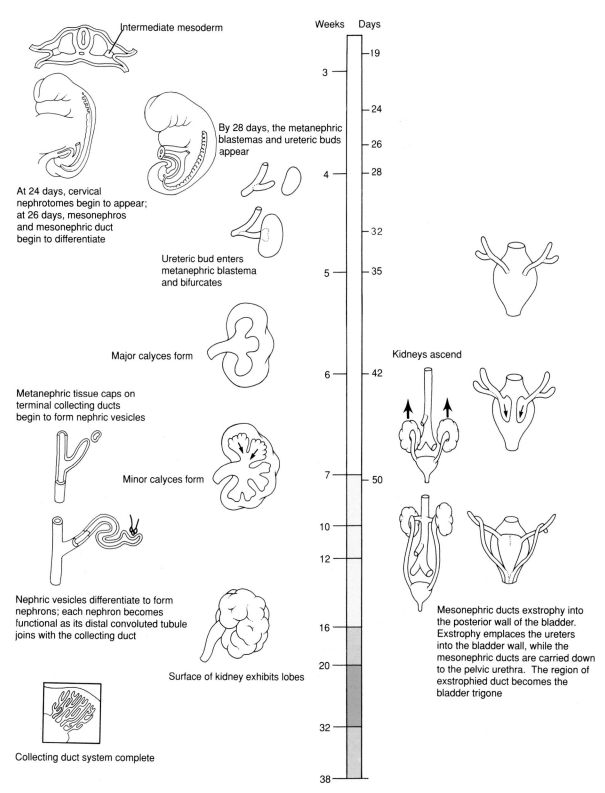

Intermediate mesoderm

At 24 days, cervical nephrotomes begin to appear; at 26 days, mesonephros and mesonephric duct begin to differentiate

By 28 days, the metanephric blastemas and ureteric buds appear

Ureteric bud enters metanephric blastema and bifurcates

Major calyces form

Metanephric tissue caps on terminal collecting ducts begin to form nephric vesicles

Minor calyces form

Nephric vesicles differentiate to form nephrons; each nephron becomes functional as its distal convoluted tubule joins with the collecting duct

Surface of kidney exhibits lobes

Collecting duct system complete

Kidneys ascend

Mesonephric ducts exstrophy into the posterior wall of the bladder. Exstrophy emplaces the ureters into the bladder wall, while the mesonephric ducts are carried down to the pelvic urethra. The region of exstrophied duct becomes the bladder trigone

Weeks   Days

3 — 19

— 24

— 26

4 — 28

— 32

5 — 35

6 — 42

7 — 50

10

12

16

20

32

38

Timeline. Development of the urinary system.

Weeks

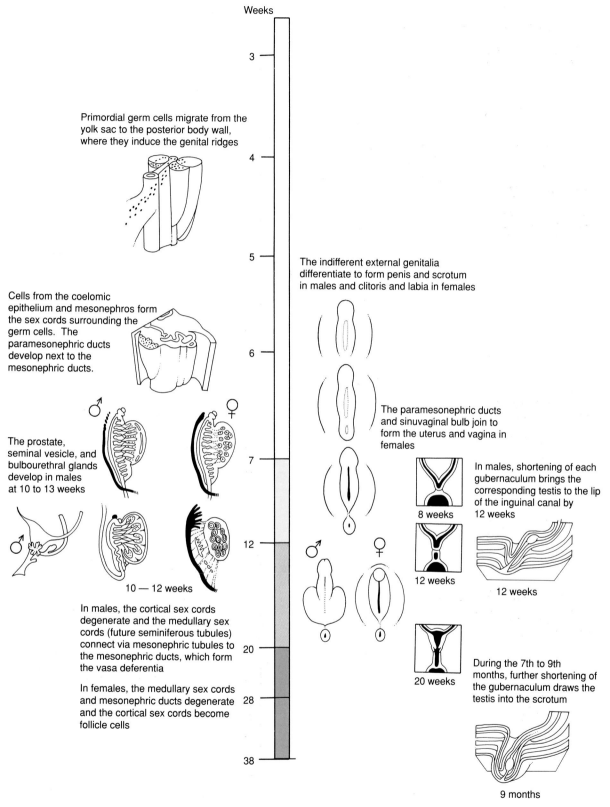

Primordial germ cells migrate from the yolk sac to the posterior body wall, where they induce the genital ridges

Cells from the coelomic epithelium and mesonephros form the sex cords surrounding the germ cells. The paramesonephric ducts develop next to the mesonephric ducts.

The prostate, seminal vesicle, and bulbourethral glands develop in males at 10 to 13 weeks

10 — 12 weeks

In males, the cortical sex cords degenerate and the medullary sex cords (future seminiferous tubules) connect via mesonephric tubules to the mesonephric ducts, which form the vasa deferentia

In females, the medullary sex cords and mesonephric ducts degenerate and the cortical sex cords become follicle cells

The indifferent external genitalia differentiate to form penis and scrotum in males and clitoris and labia in females

The paramesonephric ducts and sinuvaginal bulb join to form the uterus and vagina in females

In males, shortening of each gubernaculum brings the corresponding testis to the lip of the inguinal canal by 12 weeks

8 weeks

12 weeks

12 weeks

During the 7th to 9th months, further shortening of the gubernaculum draws the testis into the scrotum

20 weeks

9 months

Timeline. Development of the genital system.

Three nephric systems develop in craniocaudal sequence

Recall from Chapter 3 that the mesoderm deposited on either side of the midline during gastrulation differentiates into three subdivisions: the paraxial, intermediate, and lateral plate mesoderm (Fig. 10-1). The intermediate mesoderm gives rise to the nephric structures of the embryo, to portions of the gonads, and to the male genital duct system. During embryonic development, three sets of nephric structures develop in craniocaudal succession from the intermediate mesoderm. These are called the **cervical nephrotomes,** the **mesonephroi,** and the **metanephroi** or definitive kidneys.

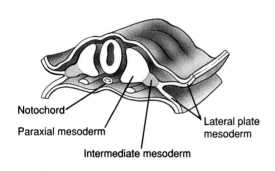

Notochord
Paraxial mesoderm
Intermediate mesoderm
Lateral plate mesoderm

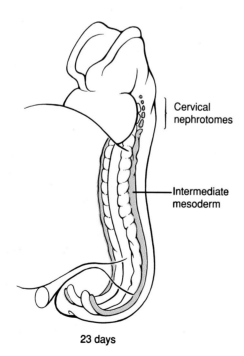

Cervical nephrotomes

Intermediate mesoderm

23 days

Fig. 10-1. The intermediate mesoderm gives rise to paired, segmentally organized nephrotomes from the cervical to the sacral region. Cervical nephrotomes are initially formed early in the fourth week and are sometimes referred to collectively as the pronephros.

The cervical nephrotomes are transient and nonfunctional

Early in the fourth week, each of five to seven paired cervical segments of intermediate mesoderm gives rise to a small, hollow ball of epithelium called a **nephric vesicle** or **nephrotome** (Fig. 10-2A). In humans these units cease developing at the nephrotome stage and therefore seem to be nonfunctional and vestigial. They disappear by day 24 or 25.

The mesonephroi may function as embryonic kidneys and also contribute to the male genital system

The next structures to form in the intermediate mesoderm are the **mesonephroi** (sing., mesonephros) and associated **mesonephric ducts.** Early in the fourth week, **nephric tubules** begin to develop within a pair of elongated swellings of intermediate mesoderm located on either side of the vertebral column from the upper thoracic region to the third lumbar level (Fig. 10-2B–D). These swellings are called the mesonephroi or mesonephric ridges. About 40 mesonephric tubules are produced in craniocaudal succession; thus, several form in each segment. As the more caudal tubules differentiate, however, the more cranial ones regress, so there are never more than about 30 pairs in the mesonephroi. By the end of the fifth week, the cranial regions of the mesonephroi undergo massive regression, leaving only about 20 pairs of tubules occupying the first three lumbar levels.

The mesonephric tubules differentiate into excretory units that resemble an abbreviated version of the adult nephron (Fig. 10-2D). The medial end of the tubule forms a cup-shaped sac, called a **Bowman's capsule,** which wraps around a knot of capillaries called a **glomerulus** to form a **renal corpuscle.** The glomeruli are produced on branches of arteries sprouting from the dorsal aorta. Each renal corpuscle and nephric tubule is collectively called a **mesonephric excretory unit.**

The **mesonephric ducts** first appear at about 24 days as a pair of solid longitudinal rods that condense in the intermediate mesoderm of the thoracic region dorsolateral to the developing mesonephric tubules (Figs. 10-2A and 10-3). These rods grow caudally through the proliferation and migration of the cells at their caudal tips. As the rods grow into the lower lumbar region, they diverge from the intermediate mesoderm and then grow to and fuse with the ventrolateral walls of the cloaca on day 26 (Figs. 10-2 and 10-4; also see Ch. 9 and below). This region of fusion will become a part of the posterior wall of the future bladder. As the rods fuse with the cloaca, they begin to cavitate at their distal ends to form a lumen. This process of canalization progresses cranially, transforming the rods into the mesonephric ducts.

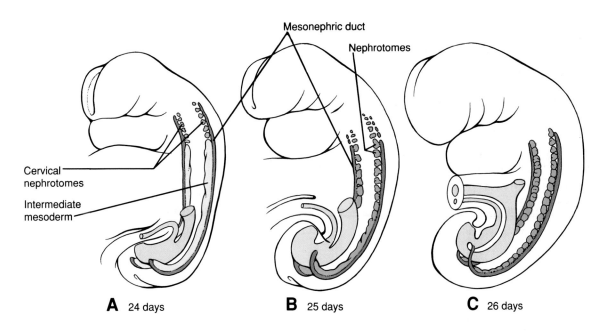

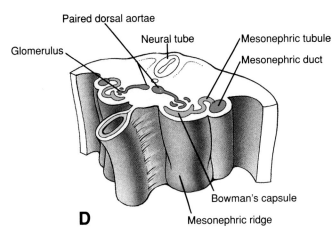

Fig. 10-2. Development of the cervical nephrotomes and mesonephros. (**A**) A pair of cervical nephrotomes forms in each of five to seven cervical segments, but these quickly degenerate during the fourth week. The mesonephric ducts first appear on day 24. (**B, C**) Mesonephric nephrotomes and tubules form in craniocaudal sequence throughout the thoracic and lumbar regions. The more cranial pairs regress as caudal pairs form, and the definitive mesonephroi contain about 20 pairs confined to the first three lumbar segments. (**D**) The mesonephroi contain functional nephric units consisting of glomeruli, Bowman's capsules, mesonephric tubules, and mesonephric ducts.

The lateral tip of each mesonephric tubule fuses with the mesonephric duct, thus opening a passage from the excretory units to the cloaca. The mesonephric excretory units are functional between about 6 and 10 weeks and produce small amounts of urine. After 10 weeks, they cease to function and then regress. As discussed below, the mesonephric ducts also regress in the female. In the male, however, the mesonephric ducts plus a few modified mesonephric tubules persist and form important elements of the male genital duct system.

The definitive metanephroi are induced early in the fifth week by ureteric buds that sprout from the mesonephric ducts

The definitive kidneys or **metanephroi** are induced to form in the intermediate mesoderm of the sacral region by a pair of new structures, the **ureteric buds,** which sprout from the distal portion of the mesonephric ducts on about day 28 (Fig. 10-4A). On about day 32, each ureteric bud penetrates a portion of the sacral intermediate mesoderm called the **metanephric blastema** and begins to bifurcate (Fig. 10-4B). As the ureteric bud branches, each new growing tip (called an **ampulla**) acquires a caplike aggregate of metanephric blastema tissue, giving the metanephros a lobulated appearance. By the middle of the sixth week, the developing metanephros consists of two lobes separated by a sulcus, and, by the end of the 16th week, 14 to 16 lobes have formed (Fig. 10-4C, D). The evidence of these initial branchings of the ureteric bud are eventually obscured as the sulci between the lobes are filled in.

The ureteric bud and metanephric blastema exert reciprocal inductive Effects. The ureters and the col-

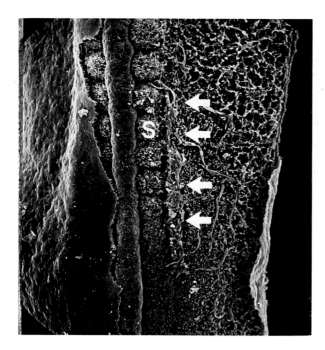

Fig. 10-3. Scanning electron micrograph showing a growing mesonephric duct just adjacent to the somites (S) on one side of an embryo (arrows). The duct is elongating in a craniocaudal direction. (Photo courtesy of Dr. Thomas J. Poole.)

lecting duct system of the kidneys differentiate from the ureteric bud, whereas the **nephrons** (the definitive urine-forming units of the kidneys) differentiate from the metanephric blastema. The differentiation of each of these primordia depends on inductive signals from the other (see Applications to Clinical Practice).

The collecting duct system is produced by sequential bifurcation of the ureteric bud. In the mature kidney, the urine produced by the nephrons flows through a collecting duct system consisting of collecting tubules, minor calyces, major calyces, the renal pelvis, and, finally, the ureter. This system is entirely the product of the ureteric bud. The ureteric bud undergoes an exact sequence of bifurcations (Fig. 10-5), and the expanded major and minor calyces arise through phases of intussusception in which previously formed branches coalesce.

When the ureteric bud first contacts the metanephric blastema, its tip expands to form an initial ampulla that will give rise to the **renal pelvis.** During the sixth week the ureteric bud bifurcates four times, yielding 16 branches. These branches then coalesce to form two to four **major calyces** extending from the renal pelvis. By the seventh week, the next four generations of branches also coalesce, forming the **minor calyces.** By 32 weeks, approximately 11 additional generations of bifurcation have formed one to

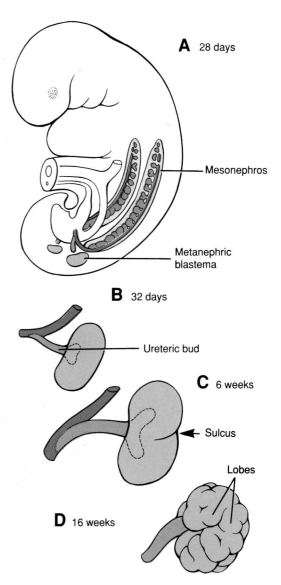

Fig. 10-4. Origin of the metanephric kidneys. **(A)** A metanephric blastema develops from intermediate mesoderm on each side of the body axis early in the fifth week. **(B)** Simultaneously, the metanephric ducts sprout ureteric buds that grow into each metanephric blastema. **(C)** By the sixth week, the ureteric bud bifurcates and the two growing tips (ampullae) induce superior and inferior lobes in the metanephros. **(D)** Additional lobules form during the next 10 weeks in response to further bifurcation of the ureteric buds.

three million branches, which will become the future **collecting tubules (collecting ducts)** of the kidney (Fig. 10-6A). The definitive morphology of the collecting ducts is created by variations in the pattern of branching and by a tendency for distal branches to elongate.

Each nephron originates as a vesicle within the blastemic cap surrounding the ampulla of a collecting duct (Fig. 10-

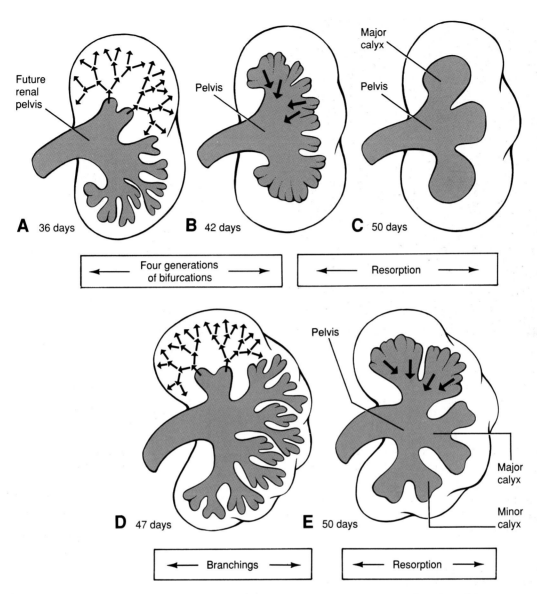

Fig. 10-5. Development of the renal pelvis and calyces. (**A–C**) The first bifurcation of the ureteric bud forms the renal pelvis, and the collapse of the next four generations of bifurcations produces the major calyces. (**D, E**) The next four generations of bifurcation collapse to form the minor calyces of the renal collecting system.

6B). As this vesicle elongates into a tubule, a capillary glomerulus forms near one end of it. The tubule epithelium near the differentiating glomerulus thins and then invaginates to form a Bowman's capsule that surrounds the glomerulus. As in the mesonephros, the unit consisting of Bowman's capsule and the glomerulus is called a **renal corpuscle.** While the renal corpuscle is forming, the lengthening nephric tubule differentiates to form the remaining elements of the nephron: the proximal convoluted tubule, the descending and ascending limbs of the loop of Henle, and the distal convoluted tubule. The de-

finitive nephron with its renal corpuscle is also called a **metanephric excretory unit.**

During the 10th week, the tips of the distal convoluted tubules connect to the collecting ducts, and the metanephroi become functional. Blood plasma from the glomerular capillaries is filtered by the renal corpuscle to produce a dilute glomerular filtrate, which is concentrated and converted to urine by the activities of the convoluted tubules and the loop of Henle. The urine passes down the collecting system into the ureters and thence into the bladder. Even though the fetal kidneys produce urine

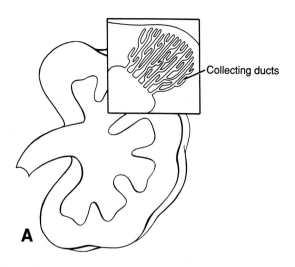

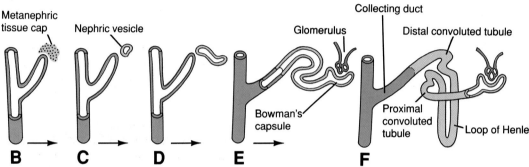

Fig. 10-6. Development of the renal collecting system and nephrons. **(A)** The ureteric buds continue to bifurcate until the 32nd week, producing 1 to 3 million collecting ducts. **(B–F)** The tip of each collecting duct induces the development of a metanephric tissue cap, which differentiates into a renal vesicle. This vesicle ultimately forms a Bowman's capsule and the proximal and distal convoluted tubules and loops of Henle. Functional nephric units (of the type shown in Fig. E) first appear in distal regions of the metanephros at 10 weeks.

throughout the remainder of gestation, their main function is not to clear waste products out of the blood—that task is handled principally by the placenta. Instead, fetal urine is important because it supplements the production of amniotic fluid. Fetuses with bilateral renal agenesis (complete absence of both kidneys) do not make enough amniotic fluid and hence are confined in an abnormally small amniotic space (see Applications to Clinical Practice in Chs. 6 and 15).

The definitive kidney architecture is created between the fifth and 15th weeks. Figure 10-7 shows the structure of the definitive fetal kidney. This architecture reflects the events of the first 10 weeks of renal development, that is, weeks 5 to 15 of development. The kidney is divided into an inner medulla and an outer cortex. The cortical tissue contains the nephrons, whereas the medulla contains collecting ducts and loops of Henle. Each minor calyx

drains a tree of collecting ducts within a **renal pyramid** that converge to form the **renal papilla** (Fig. 10-7). The renal pyramids of the kidney are separated by zones of nephron-containing cortical tissue called **renal columns** or **columns of Bertin.** In the definitive kidney, the cortical tissue thus not only covers the outside of the kidney but also forms piers projecting inward toward the renal pelvis.

The neurons of the kidney, which regulate blood flow and secretory function, arise from neural crest cells that invade the metanephroi early in their development.

The kidneys ascend from their original sacral location to a lumbar site

Between the sixth and ninth weeks, the kidneys ascend to a lumbar site just below the suprarenal glands, (Fig. 10.8).

Several anomalies can arise from variations in this process of ascent. Rarely, a kidney completely fails to as-

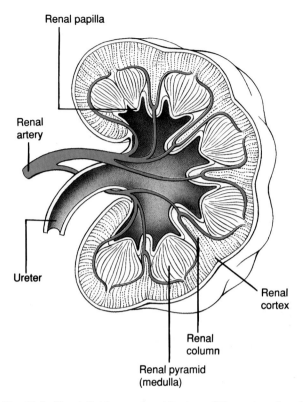

Fig. 10-7. The definitive renal architecture of the metanephros is apparent by the 10th week.

cend, remaining as a **pelvic kidney** (Fig. 10-8C). The inferior poles of the two metanephroi may fuse during the ascent, forming a U-shaped **horseshoe kidney** that crosses over the ventral side of the aorta. During ascent, this kidney becomes caught under the inferior mesenteric artery and therefore does not reach its normal site (Fig. 10-8D). The right kidney usually does not rise as high as the left kidney because of the presence of the liver on the right side, although this is not always the case.

The remainder of the urinary tract differentiates from the hindgut endoderm

Recall from Chapter 9 that the cloacal expansion of the hindgut is partitioned by the urorectal septum into an anterior **primitive urogenital sinus** and a posterior rectum (Fig. 10-9). The primitive urogenital sinus is continuous superiorly with the **allantois** (a hindgut diverticulum that extends into the umbilicus) and is bounded inferiorly by the **urogenital membrane.** It consists of an expanded superior presumptive **bladder,** a narrow neck that becomes the **pelvic urethra,** and an inferior expanded **definitive urogenital sinus.** In males, the pelvic urethra becomes the **membranous** and **prostatic urethra** and the definitive urogenital sinus becomes the **penile urethra.** In females, the pelvic urethra becomes the **membranous ure-**

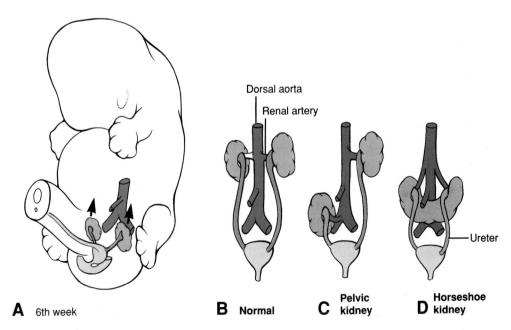

Fig. 10-8. Normal and abnormal ascent of the kidneys. (**A, B**) The metanephroi normally ascend from the sacral region to their definitive lumbar position between the sixth and ninth weeks. (**C**) Infrequently, a kidney may fail to ascend, resulting in a pelvic kidney. (**D**) If the inferior poles of the metanephroi make contact and fuse before ascent, the resulting horseshoe kidney catches under the inferior mesenteric artery.

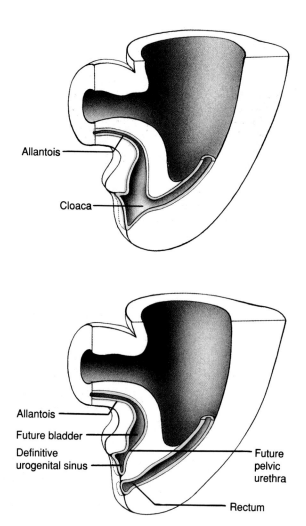

Fig. 10-9. Development of the primitive urogenital sinus. Between weeks 4 and 6, the urorectal septum splits the cloaca into an anterior primitive urogenital sinus and a posterior rectum. The superior part of the primitive urogenital sinus, continuous with the allantois, forms the bladder. The constricted pelvic urethra at the base of the future bladder forms the membranous urethra in females and the membranous and prostatic urethra in males. The distal expansion of the primitive urogenital sinus, the definitive urogenital sinus, forms the vestibule of the vagina in females and the penile urethra in males.

thra, and the definitive urogenital sinus becomes the **vestibule of the vagina.**

While the primitive urogenital sinus is forming, the mesonephric ducts and ureteric buds intercalate into its posterior wall

Concurrently with the septation of the cloaca by the growth of the urorectal septum, the distal portions of the mesonephric ducts and attached ureteric ducts become incorporated into the posterior wall of the presumptive

bladder by a process called **exstrophy** (Fig. 10-10). (*Exstrophy* refers to the eversion of a hollow organ.) Exstrophy begins as the mouths of the mesonephric ducts flare into a pair of trumpet-shaped structures that expand, flatten, and blend into the bladder wall. The superior portion of this trumpet expands and flattens more rapidly than the inferior part, so the mouth of the narrow portion of the mesonephric duct appears to migrate inferiorly along the posterior bladder wall. This process incorporates the distal ureters into the wall of the bladder and causes the mouths of the narrow part of the mesonephric ducts to migrate inferiorly until they open into the pelvic urethra just below the neck of the bladder. The triangular area of exstrophied mesonephric duct wall on the posteroinferior wall of the bladder is called the **trigone** of the bladder. The mesodermal tissue of the trigone is later overgrown by endoderm from the surrounding bladder wall, but the structure remains visible in the adult bladder as a smooth triangular region lying between the openings of the ureters laterally and superiorly and the opening of the pelvic urethra inferiorly. Splanchnopleuric mesoderm associated with the hindgut forms the smooth muscle of the bladder wall in the 12th week.

Several malformations can arise if the ureteric bud sprouts from an incorrect site along the mesonephric duct and therefore is incorrectly emplaced into the posterior wall of the bladder. The consequences of abnormal connection of the ureters is discussed in the Applications to Clinical Practice section of this chapter.

The genital system arises in close conjunction with the urinary system

As discussed in Chapter 1, the gonads are induced to develop by the primordial germ cells that migrate from the yolk sac via the dorsal mesentery to populate the mesenchyme of the posterior body wall in the fifth week (Fig. 10-11A; see also Fig. 1-1). In both sexes, the arrival of the primordial germ cells in the area of the future gonads at about the 10th thoracic level, induces cells in the mesonephros and adjacent coelomic epithelium to proliferate and form a pair of **genital ridges** just medial to the developing mesonephroi (Figs. 10-11B, C, 10-12).

The primitive sex cords develop from cells of the mesonephros and coelomic epithelium

During the sixth week, cells from the mesonephros and coelomic epithelium invade the mesenchyme in the region of the presumptive gonads to form aggregates of supporting cells, the **primitive sex cords,** which completely invest the germ cells (Fig. 10-11B). The genital ridge mesenchyme containing the primitive sex cords is regarded as consisting of **cortical** and **medullary regions.** Both re-

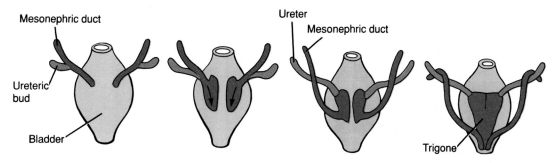

Fig. 10-10. Exstrophy of the mesonephric ducts and ureters into the bladder wall. Between weeks 4 and 6, the root of the mesonephric duct exstrophies into the posterior wall of the developing bladder. This process brings the openings of the ureteric buds into the bladder wall, while the opening of the mesonephric duct is carried inferiorly to the level of the pelvic urethra. The triangular region of exstrophied mesonephric duct incorporated into the posterior bladder wall forms the trigone of the bladder.

gions develop in all normal embryos, but after the sixth week they pursue different fates in the male and female.

The paramesonephric ducts form by invagination of the coelomic epithelium

Also during the sixth week, a new pair of ducts, the **paramesonephric (Müllerian) ducts,** begin to form just lateral to the mesonephric ducts in both male and female embryos (Fig. 10-11B, C). These ducts arise by the craniocaudal invagination of a ribbon of thickened coelomic epithelium extending from the third thoracic segment caudally to the posterior wall of the urogenital sinus. For most of their length, these ducts are enclosed in the basement membrane of the adjacent mesonephric ducts. The caudal tips of the paramesonephric ducts then grow to connect with the pelvic urethra just medial to the openings of the right and left mesonephric ducts. The tips of the two paramesonephric ducts adhere to each other just before they contact the pelvic urethra. The superior ends of the paramesonephric ducts form funnel-shaped openings into the coelom. The further development of the paramesonephric ducts in the female is discussed on pp. 188 and 189.

The male and female genital systems are virtually identical until the end of the sixth week

At the end of the sixth week, the male and female genital systems are indistinguishable in appearance, although subtle cellular differences may already be present. In both sexes, germ cells and sex cords are present in both the cortical and the medullary regions of the presumptive gonads, and complete mesonephric and paramesonephric ducts lie side by side. The **ambisexual** or **indifferent phase** of genital development ends at this point and, from

the seventh week on, the male and female systems pursue diverging pathways.

Male development is instigated by a factor encoded on the Y chromosome; female development occurs in its absence

Key elements of sex differentiation in humans is now well understood (Fig. 10-13). As detailed in Chapter 1, genetic females have two X sex chromosomes, whereas genetic males have an X and a Y sex chromosome. Although the pattern of sex chromosomes determines the choice between male and female developmental path-ways, the subsequent phases of sexual development are controlled not only by sex chromosome genes but also by hormones and other factors, most of which are encoded on the autosomes (see the Applications to Clinical Practice section of this chapter). Recently, a sex-determining factor that controls the choice between the male and female developmental paths has been identified. This sex-determining transcription factor is encoded on the **sex-determining region of the Y chromosome (SRY).** When this factor is synthesized in the sex cord cells of the indifferent presumptive gonad, male development is triggered. If the factor is absent or defective, female development occurs. Thus, femaleness could be seen as the basic developmental path for the human embryo, which is followed unless maleness is actively induced. (The sex-determining protein is discussed further in the Applications to Clinical Practice section at the end of this chapter).

Male genital development begins with the differentiation of Sertoli cells in the medullary sex cords

One of the first events in male genital development is the elaboration of SRY protein within the sex cord cells

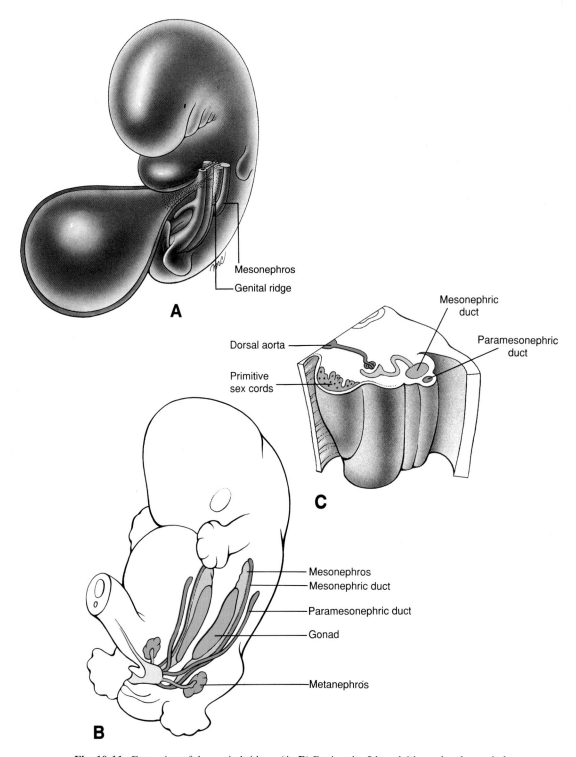

Fig. 10-11. Formation of the genital ridges. **(A, B)** During the 5th and 6th weeks, the genital ridges form in the posterior abdominal wall just medial to the developing mesonephroi in response to colonization by primordial germ cells migrating from the yolk sac. **(C)** The primordial germ cells induce the coelomic epithelium lining the peritoneal cavity as well as cells of the mesonephros to proliferate and form the sex cords.

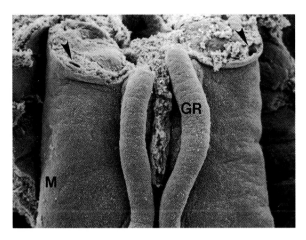

Fig. 10-12. Scanning electron micrographs showing the relationship between the developing genital ridges (GR) and the mesonephroi (M). Arrowheads: Mesonephric ducts. (From Evan AP, Gattone VC II, Blomgren PM. 1984. Application of scanning electron microscopy to kidney development and nephron maturation. Scanning Electron Microsc I:455, with permission.)

(Fig. 10-13). Under the influence of this factor, cells in the *medullary* region of the primitive sex cords begin to differentiate into **Sertoli cells,** while the cells of the *cortical* sex cords degenerate (Fig. 10-14). Sex cord cells will differentiate into Sertoli cells only if they contain the SRY and produce SRY protein; if these are absent, the sex cords differentiate into ovarian follicles.

During the seventh week, the differentiating Sertoli cells organize to form the **testis cords** (Fig. 10-14). At puberty the testis cords associated with the germ cells will become canalized and differentiate into a system of **seminiferous tubules.** The testis cords distal to the presumptive seminiferous tubules also develop lumina and differentiate into a set of thin-walled ducts called the **rete testis** at puberty (see below).

During the seventh week, the testis begins to round up, reducing its area of contact with the mesonephros (Fig. 10-14). This physical isolation of the testis is important since the mesonephros exerts a feminizing influence on the developing gonad. As the testes continue to develop, the degenerating cortical sex cords become separated from the coelomic epithelium by an intervening layer of connective tissue called the **tunica albuginea.**

Contact between the pre-Sertoli cells and the germ cells regulates the development of the male gametes

Although the mechanism has not been elucidated, it is clear that direct cell-to-cell contact between pre-Sertoli cells and primordial germ cells within the medullary sex cords plays a key role in the development of the male gametes. This interaction occurs shortly after the arrival of the primordial germ cells in the region of the presumptive genital ridge. It has the immediate effect of inhibiting further mitosis and also prevents the germ cells from entering meiosis. The remaining phases of male gametogenesis—further germ cell mitosis, differentiation into spermatogonia, meiosis, and spermatogenesis—are thus delayed until puberty (see Ch. 1).

Anti-Müllerian hormone secreted by the pre-Sertoli cells controls several steps in male genital development

As the pre-Sertoli cells begin their morphologic differentiation in response to SRY, they also begin to secrete a glycoprotein hormone called **anti-Müllerian hormone (AMH)** or **Müllerian-inhibiting substance (MIS).** The protein portion of this hormone is a member of the *transforming growth factor-β* family.

AMH causes the paramesonephric ducts to regress in the male. In male embryos, AMH secreted by the pre-Sertoli cells causes the paramesonephric (Müllerian) ducts to regress rapidly between the eighth and tenth weeks (Figs. 10-13, 10-14). Small paramesonephric duct remnants can be detected in the adult male, however, including a small cap of tissue associated with the testis, called the **appendix testis,** and an expansion of the prostatic urethra called the **utriculus prostaticus** (Fig. 10-14).

SRY protein initiates a cascade that induces the differentiation of testosterone-secreting Leydig cells in the testis. In the ninth or tenth week, **Leydig cells** differentiate from mesenchymal cells within the genital ridges, probably in response to the expression of SRY protein by the pre-Sertoli cells (Fig. 10-13). These endocrine cells produce the male sex steroid hormone **testosterone.** At this early stage of development, testosterone secretion is regulated by the peptide hormone **chorionic gonadotropin,** secreted by the placenta, but later in development the pituitary gonadotropins of the male fetus take over control of the masculinizing sex steroids (androgens).

The mesonephric ducts and the accessory glands of the male urethra differentiate in response to testosterone

The mesonephric duct and mesonephric tubules give rise to the vas deferens and ductuli efferentes. Between 8 and 12 weeks, the initial secretion of testosterone stimulates the mesonephric ducts to transform into the spermatic ducts called the **vasa deferentia** (Fig. 10-14). The most

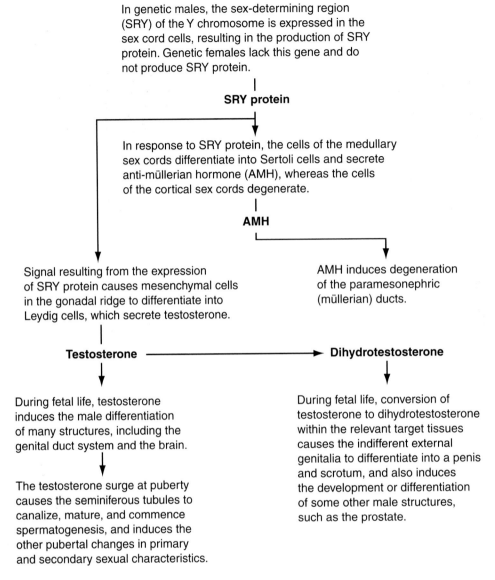

In genetic males, the sex-determining region
(SRY) of the Y chromosome is expressed in the
sex cord cells, resulting in the production of SRY
protein. Genetic females lack this gene and do
not produce SRY protein.

SRY protein

In response to SRY protein, the cells of the medullary
sex cords differentiate into Sertoli cells and secrete
anti-müllerian hormone (AMH), whereas the cells
of the cortical sex cords degenerate.

AMH

Signal resulting from the expression
of SRY protein causes mesenchymal cells
in the gonadal ridge to differentiate into
Leydig cells, which secrete testosterone.

AMH induces degeneration
of the paramesonephric
(müllerian) ducts.

Testosterone ⟶ **Dihydrotestosterone**

During fetal life, testosterone
induces the male differentiation
of many structures, including the
genital duct system and the brain.

During fetal life, conversion of
testosterone to dihydrotestosterone
within the relevant target tissues
causes the indifferent external
genitalia to differentiate into a penis
and scrotum, and also induces
the development or differentiation
of some other male structures,
such as the prostate.

The testosterone surge at puberty
causes the seminiferous tubules to
canalize, mature, and commence
spermatogenesis, and induces the
other pubertal changes in primary
and secondary sexual characteristics.

Fig. 10-13. Differentiation cascade of male genital system development.

cranial end of each mesonephric duct degenerates, leaving a small remnant called the **appendix epididymis,** and the region of the vas deferens adjacent to the presumptive testis differentiates into the convoluted **epididymis.** During the ninth week, 5 to 12 mesonephric ducts in the region of the epididymis make contact with the cords of the future rete testis. It is not until the third month, however, that these **epigenital mesonephric tubules** actually unite with the presumptive rete testis. The epigenital mesonephric tubules are thereafter called the **ductuli efferentes,** and they will provide a pathway from the seminiferous tubules and rete testis tubules to the vas deferens. Meanwhile, the mesonephric tubules at the inferior pole of the developing testis

(called the **paragenital mesonephric tubules**) degenerate, leaving a small remnant called the **paradidymis.**

The seminal vesicle buds form the distal mesonephric duct, whereas the prostate and bulbourethral glands bud form the urethra. The three accessory glands of the male genital system all develop near the junction between the mesonephric ducts and the pelvic urethra (Fig. 10-15). The glandular **seminal vesicles** sprout during the 10th week from the mesonephric ducts near their attachment to the pelvic urethra. The portion of the vas deferens (mesonephric duct) distal to each seminal vesicle is thereafter called the **ejaculatory duct.**

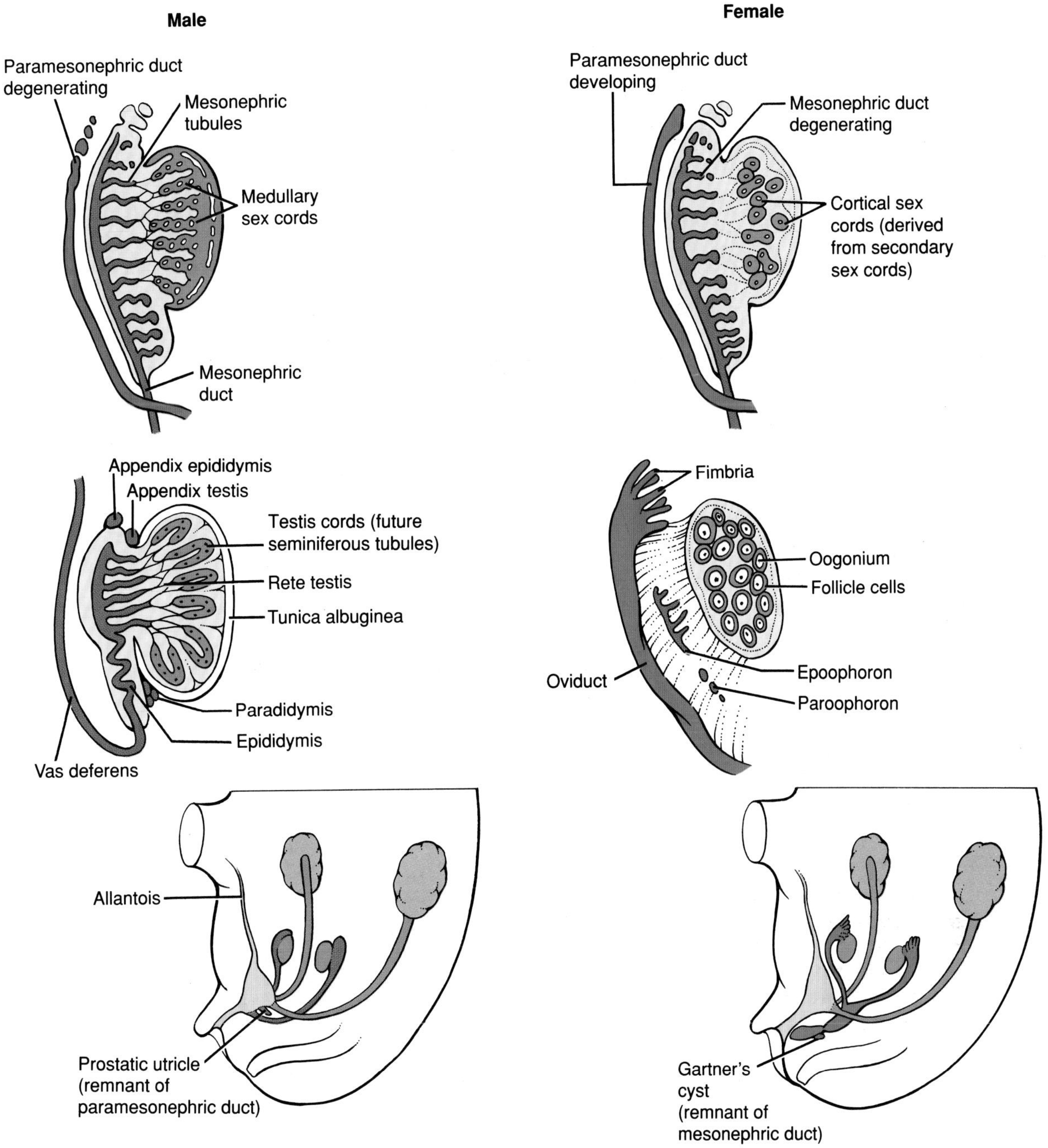

Male

Paramesonephric duct degenerating

Mesonephric tubules

Medullary sex cords

Mesonephric duct

Appendix epididymis
Appendix testis

Testis cords (future seminiferous tubules)

Rete testis

Tunica albuginea

Paradidymis

Epididymis

Vas deferens

Allantois

Prostatic utricle (remnant of paramesonephric duct)

Female

Paramesonephric duct developing

Mesonephric duct degenerating

Cortical sex cords (derived from secondary sex cords)

Fimbria

Oogonium
Follicle cells

Oviduct

Epoophoron
Paroophoron

Gartner's cyst (remnant of mesonephric duct)

Fig. 10-14. Male gonadal development compared with that of the female. The male and female genital systems are virtually identical through the seventh week. In the male, SRY protein produced by the pre-Sertoli cells causes the medullary sex cords to develop into presumptive seminiferous tubules and rete testis tubules and causes the cortical sex cords to regress. Anti-Müllerian hormone produced by the Sertoli cells then causes the paramesonephric ducts to regress and also stimulates the development of Leydig cells, which in turn produce testosterone, the hormone that stimulates development of the male genital duct system, including the vas deferens and the presumptive efferent ductules. In female gonadal development, in the absence of SRY, the medullary sex cords of the female disappear and the cortical sex cords differentiate into follicle cells. The mesonephric ducts and mesonephric tubules disappear except for remnants such as the epoophoron, the paroophoron, and Gartner's cysts. The paramesonephric ducts continue to develop to form the oviducts, the uterus, and the superior part of the vagina.

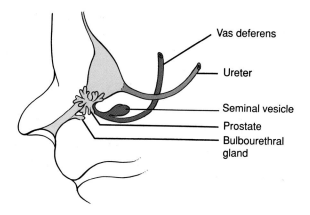

Fig. 10-15. Development of the seminal vesicles, prostate, and bulbourethral glands. These glands are induced by androgens between the 10th and 12th weeks.

The **prostate gland** also begins to develop in the 10th week as a cluster of endodermal evaginations that bud from the pelvic urethra. These presumptive prostatic outgrowths are probably induced by the surrounding mesenchyme, the inductive activity of which probably depends on the conversion of secreted testosterone to another androgenic hormone, **dihydrotestosterone.** The prostatic outgrowths initially form at least five independent groups of solid prostatic cords. By 11 weeks these cords develop a lumen and glandular acini, and by 13 to 15 weeks (just as testosterone concentrations reach a high level) the prostate begins its secretory activity. The mesenchyme surrounding the endoderm-derived glandular portion of the prostate differentiates into the smooth muscle and connective tissue of the prostate.

As the prostate is developing, the paired **bulbourethral glands** sprout from the urethra just inferior to the prostate. As in the prostate, the mesenchyme surrounding the endodermal glandular tissue gives rise to the connective tissue and smooth muscle of this gland.

Eventually, the secretions of the seminal vesicles, prostate, and bulbourethral glands all contribute to the seminal fluid that protects and nourishes the spermatozoa after ejaculation. It should be noted, however, that these secretions are not absolutely necessary for sperm function; spermatozoa removed directly from the epididymis can fertilize oocytes.

In the absence of a Y chromosome, female development occurs

In the female embryo, the somatic sex cord cells do not contain a Y chromosome or SRY region, do not elaborate SRY protein, and therefore do not differentiate into Sertoli cells. In the absence of Sertoli cells and SRY protein,

AMH, Leydig cells, and testosterone are not produced. Male development of the genital ducts and accessory sexual structures therefore is not stimulated, and female development ensues (Fig. 10-14).

In the presumptive ovary, the primitive sex cords degenerate and follicle cells form from secondary cortical sex cords

In genetic females, the primitive sex cords degenerate and the mesothelium of the genital ridge forms secondary cortical sex cords (Fig. 10-14). These secondary sex cords then invest the primordial germ cells to form the follicle cells of the ovary (see Ch. 1).

The female germ cells enter meiosis, but further nuclear development is inhibited by the follicle cells. In the male, the pre-Sertoli cells inhibit germ cell development before meiosis begins. In the female fetus, the germ cells differentiate into oogonia and enter the first meiotic division as primary oocytes before they develop close interactions with the investing follicle cells. The follicle cells then arrest germ cell development until puberty, at which point individual oocytes resume gametogenesis in response to each monthly surge of gonadotropins.

In the absence of AMH, the mesonephric ducts degenerate and the paramesonephric ducts give rise to the fallopian tubes, uterus, and superior vagina

The mesonephric ducts and mesonephric tubules require testosterone for their development. In the female, therefore, they rapidly disappear except for a few vestiges. Two remnants, the **epoophoron** and **paroophoron,** are found in the mesentery of the ovary, and a scattering of tiny remnants called **Gartner's cysts** cluster near the vagina (Figs. 10-14, 10-16C). The paramesonephric ducts, in contrast, develop uninhibited.

Recall that the distal tips of the growing paramesonephric ducts adhere to each other just before they contact the posterior wall of the pelvic urethra. The wall of the pelvic urethra at this point forms a slight thickening called the **sinusal tubercle** (Fig. 10-16A). As soon as the fused tips of the paramesonephric ducts connect with the sinusal tubercle, the paramesonephric ducts begin to fuse from their caudal tips cranially, forming a tube with a single lumen (Fig. 10-16B, C). This tube, called the **genital canal** or **uterovaginal canal,** becomes the superior portion of the vagina and the uterus. The unfused, superior portions of the paramesonephric ducts become the fallopian tubes (oviducts), and the funnel-shaped superior openings of the paramesonephric ducts become the infundibula of the oviducts.

While the uterovaginal canal is forming during the third month, the endodermal tissue of the sinusal tubercle in the posterior urethra continues to thicken, forming a pair of swellings called the **sinuvaginal bulbs** (Fig. 10-16). These structures give rise to the inferior 20 percent of the vagina. The most inferior region of the uterovaginal canal meanwhile becomes occluded by a block of tissue called the **vaginal plate.** The vaginal plate elongates from the third to the fifth month and subsequently becomes canalized by a process of **desquamation** (cell shedding) to form the inferior vaginal lumen.

As the vaginal plate forms, the lower end of the vagina lengthens, and its junction with the urogenital sinus migrates caudally until it comes to rest during the fourth month on the posterior wall of the definitive urogenital sinus (Fig. 10-16C). However, an endodermal membrane temporarily separates the lumen of the vagina from the cavity of the definitive urogenital sinus, which differentiates into the **vestibule of the vagina.** This barrier degenerates partially after the fifth month, but its remnant persists as the vaginal **hymen.** The mucous membrane that lines the vagina and cervix may also be derived from the endodermal epithelium of the definitive urogenital sinus.

The external genitalia develop from the same primordia in both sexes

The early development of the external genitalia is similar in males and females. Early in the fifth week, a pair of swellings called **cloacal folds** develop on either side of the cloacal membrane (Fig. 10-17A). These folds meet just anterior to the cloacal membrane to form a midline swelling called the **genital tubercle.**

The fusion of the urorectal septum with the cloacal membrane in the seventh week creates the **perineum,** which divides the cloacal membrane into an anterior urogenital membrane and a posterior anal membrane. The portion of the cloacal fold flanking the urogenital membrane is now called the **urethral fold** (also the **genital** or **urogenital fold**), and the portion flanking the anal membrane is called the **anal fold.** A new pair of swellings, the

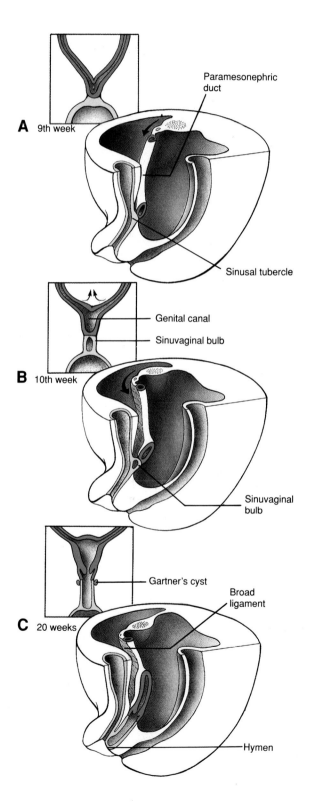

Fig. 10-16. Formation of the uterus and vagina. **(A)** The uterus and superior end of the vagina begin to form as the paramesonephric ducts fuse together near their attachment to the posterior wall of the primitive urogenital sinus. **(B, C)** The ducts then zipper together in a superior direction between the third and fifth months. As the paramesonephric ducts are pulled away from the posterior body wall, they drag a fold of peritoneal membrane with them, forming the broad ligaments of the uterus. **(A–C)** The inferior end of the vagina forms from the sinuvaginal bulbs on the posterior wall of the primitive urogenital sinus.

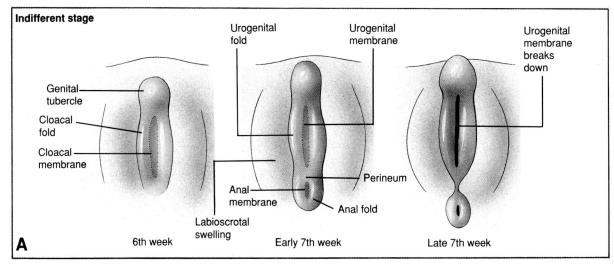

Indifferent stage

Urogenital fold

Urogenital membrane

Urogenital membrane breaks down

Genital tubercle

Cloacal fold

Cloacal membrane

Anal membrane

Perineum

Anal fold

Labioscrotal swelling

A   6th week   Early 7th week   Late 7th week

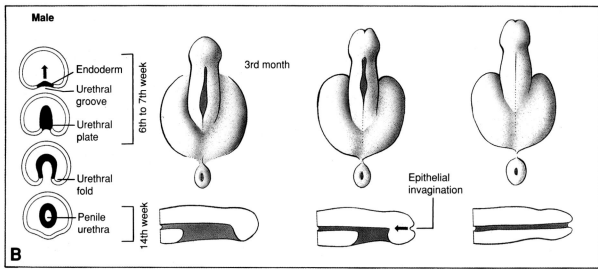

Male

Endoderm

Urethral groove

Urethral plate

6th to 7th week

3rd month

Urethral fold

Penile urethra

14th week

Epithelial invagination

B

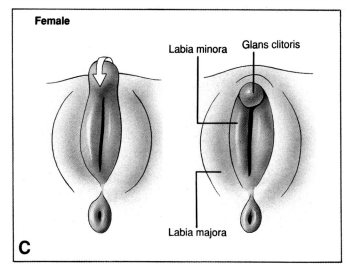

Female

Labia minora

Glans clitoris

Labia majora

C

Fig. 10-17. Formation of the external genitalia in males and females. **(A)** The external genitalia form from a pair of labioscrotal folds, a pair of urogenital folds, and an anterior genital tubercle. Male and female genitalia are morphologically indistinguishable at this stage. **(B)** In males, the urogenital folds fuse, and the genital tubercle elongates to form the shaft and glans of the penis. Fusion of the urogenital folds encloses the definitive urogenital sinus to form most of the penile urethra. A small region of the distal urethra is formed by the invagination of ectoderm covering the glans. The labioscrotal folds give rise to the scrotum. **(C)** In females, the genital tubercle bends inferiorly to form the clitoris, and the urogenital folds remain separated to form the labia minora. The labioscrotal folds form the labia majora.

labioscrotal swellings, then appear on either side of the urethral folds (Fig. 10-17A).

The cavity of the definitive urogenital sinus extends onto the surface of the enlarging genital tubercle in the form of an endoderm-lined **urethral groove** during the sixth week (Fig. 10-17B). This groove becomes temporarily filled by a solid endodermal **urethral plate,** but the urethral plate then recanalizes to form an even deeper groove. In males this groove is relatively long and broad, whereas in females it is shorter and more sharply tapered. In both sexes, an **epithelial tag** is now present at the tip of the genital tubercle. Table 10-1 lists the adult derivatives of the embryonic external genital structures.

The urogenital membrane ruptures in the seventh week, opening the cavity of the urogenital sinus to the amniotic fluid. The genital tubercle elongates to form the **phallus,** and a primordium of the glans clitoris and glans penis is demarcated from the phallic shaft by a **coronary sulcus.**

The appearance of the external genitalia is similar in male and female embryos through the 12th week, and embryos of this age are difficult to sex on the basis of their external appearance.

In the male, the urethral groove becomes the penile urethra and the labioscrotal swellings form the scrotum

Starting in the fourth month, the effects of dihydrotestosterone on the male external genitalia become readily apparent (Fig. 10-17B). The perineal region separating the definitive urogenital sinus from the anus begins to lengthen. The labioscrotal folds fuse at the midline to form the **scrotum,** and the urethral folds also fuse to enclose the **penile urethra.** The penile urethra is completely enclosed by 14 weeks. However, because the urethral groove does not extend onto the glans of the penis, the penile urethra is initially blind ended. The terminal portion of the urethra is created by an ectodermal invagination from the tip of the glans.

It should be noted that the above generally accepted explanation for the closure of the urethral groove has been questioned. An alternative mechanism has been proposed in which the penile urethra is enclosed by an anterior growth of perineal mesoderm, with little or no involvement of the genital folds.

In the female, the perineum does not lengthen and the labioscrotal and urethral folds do not fuse

In the absence of dihydrotestosterone in female embryos, the primitive perineum does not lengthen and the labioscrotal and urethral folds do not fuse across the midline (Fig. 10-17C). The phallus bends inferiorly, becoming the clitoris, and the definitive urogenital sinus becomes the vestibule of the vagina. The urethral folds become the labia minora, and the labioscrotal swellings become the labia majora.

The testes and ovaries both descend under the control of a gubernaculum

During embryonic and fetal life, the testes and the ovaries both descend from their original position at the 10th thoracic level, although the testes ultimately descend much farther. In both sexes, the descent of the gonad depends on a ligamentous cord called the **gubernaculum.** The gubernaculum condenses during the seventh week within the subserous fascia of a longitudinal peritoneal fold on either side of the vertebral column (see Fig. 10-18). The superior end of this cord attaches to the gonad and its expanded inferior end (the **gubernacular bulb**) attaches to the fascia between the developing external and internal oblique muscles in the region of the labioscrotal swellings. At the same time, a slight evagination of the peritoneum, called the **processus vaginalis** or **vaginal process,** develops just adjacent to the inferior root of the gubernaculum.

Inguinal canals develop in both sexes

The **inguinal canal** is a caudal evagination of the abdominal wall that forms when the processus vaginalis grows inferiorly, pushing out a socklike evagination con-

Table 10-1. Development of Male and Female External Genitalia

PRESUMPTIVE ANLAGE	MALE STRUCTURE	FEMALE STRUCTURE
Genital tubercle	Glans and shaft of penis	Glans and shaft of clitoris
Definitive urogenital sinus	Penile urethra	Vestibule of vagina
Urethral fold	Penis surrounding penile urethra	Labia minora
Labioscrotal fold	Scrotum	Labia majora

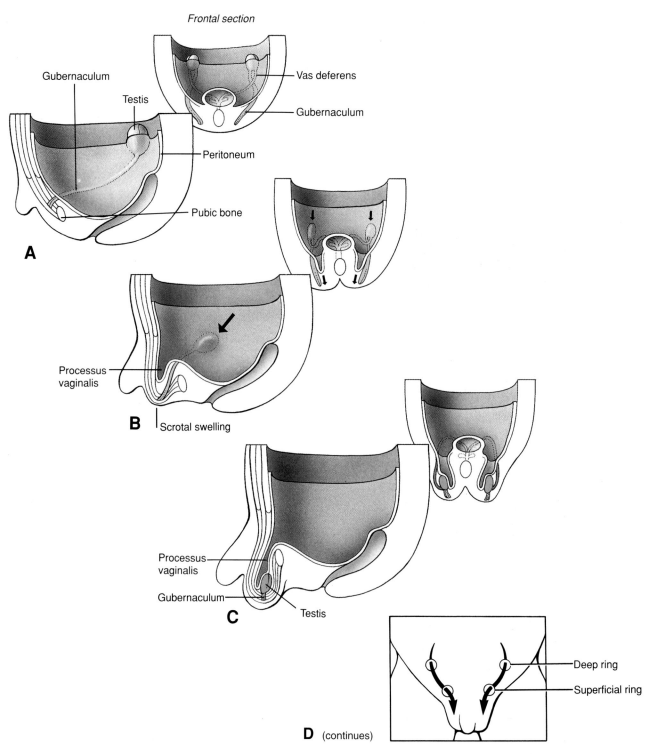

Fig. 10-18. Descent of the testes. **(A–C)** Between the seventh week and birth, shortening of the gubernaculum testis causes the testes to descend from the 10th thoracic level into the scrotum. The testes pass through the inguinal canal in the anterior abdominal wall. **(D)** After the eighth week, a peritoneal evagination called the processus vaginalis forms just anterior to the gubernaculum and pushes out socklike extensions of the transversalis fascia, the internal oblique muscle, and the external oblique muscle, thus forming the inguinal canal. The inguinal canal extends from the base of the everted transversalis fascia (the deep ring) to the base of the everted external oblique muscle (the superficial ring). After the processus vaginalis has evaginated into the scrotum, the gubernaculum shortens and simply pulls the gonads through the canal. The gonads always remain within the plane of the subserous fascia associated with the posterior wall of the processus vaginalis, however.

sisting of the various layers of the abdominal wall (Fig. 10-18). In the male the inguinal canal extends into the scrotum and transmits the descending testes. A complete inguinal canal also forms in females, but plays no role in genital development. The processus vaginalis normally degenerates. Occasionally, however, it remains patent, in which case the inguinal canal may later become the site of an **indirect inguinal hernia** (see Fig. 10-19).

In the male, the inguinal canal conveys the testes to the scrotum and forms the sheath of the spermatic cord. Figure 10-18 illustrates the development of the in-

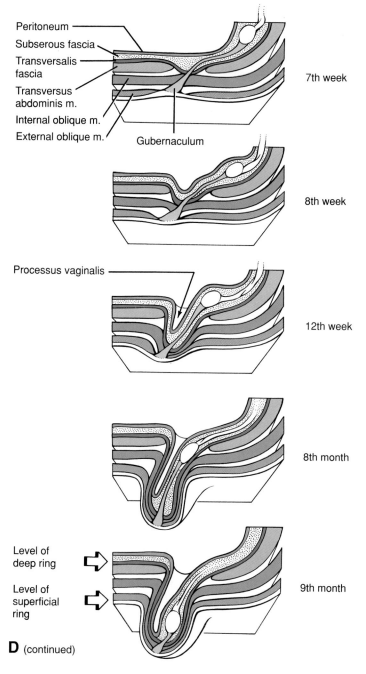

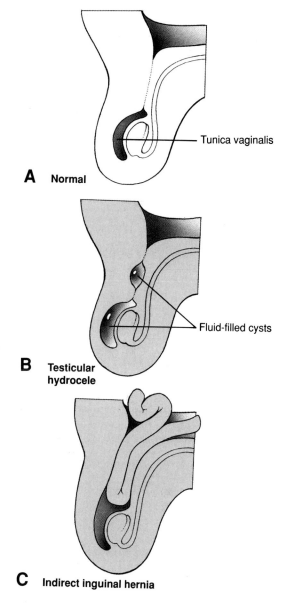

Fig. 10-19. Normal and abnormal development of the processus vaginalis. **(A)** The proximal end of the processus vaginalis normally disintegrates during the first year after birth, leaving a distal remnant called the tunica vaginalis. **(B)** Some proximal remnants may remain, and these and the tunica vaginalis may fill with serous fluid, forming testicular hydroceles in pathologic conditions or subsequent to injury. **(C)** If the proximal end of the processus vaginalis does not disintegrate, abdominal contents may herniate through the processus and inguinal canal into the scrotum. This condition is called congenital inguinal hernia.

guinal canal in the male. During the eighth week, the processus vaginalis begins to elongate caudally, carrying along the bulb of the gubernaculum. The elongating processus successively encounters three layers of the differentiating abdominal wall and pushes them out to form socklike evaginations (Fig. 10-18D). The first layer encountered by the processus is the **transversalis fascia,** lying just deep to the transversus abdominis muscle. This layer will become the **internal spermatic fascia of the spermatic cord.** The processus does not encounter the transversus abdominis muscle itself, since this muscle has a large hiatus in this region. Next, the processus picks up the fibers and fascia of the **internal oblique muscle.** These become the **cremasteric fascia of the spermatic cord.** Finally, the processus picks up a thin layer of **external oblique muscle,** which will become the **external spermatic fascia.**

The inguinal canal can be thought of as a series of weakenings in the layers of the abdominal wall that become stretched out to allow the testes to descend into the scrotum. The superior rim of the canal—the point of weakening and eversion of the transversalis fascia—is called the **deep ring of the inguinal canal** (Fig. 10-18D). The inferomedial rim of the canal formed by the point of eversion of the external oblique muscle is called the **superficial ring of the inguinal canal.**

The testes descend to the deep ring of the inguinal canal by the third month and complete their descent in the seventh to ninth months. Between the 7th and 12th weeks, the extrainguinal portions of the gubernacula shorten and pull the testes down to the vicinity of the deep inguinal ring within the plane of the subserous fascia. The gubernacula shorten mainly by getting fatter at their base; this serves the secondary purpose of enlarging the inguinal canal.

The testes remain in the vicinity of the deep ring from the third to the seventh month, but then enter the inguinal canal in response to renewed shortening of the gubernaculum. The testes remain within the subserous fascia of the processus vaginalis through which they descend toward the scrotum (Fig. 10-18). This second phase of gubernacular shortening is caused by actual reduction and regression of the gubernaculum as a result of the loss of the mucoid extracellular matrix that forms much of its substance. The movement of the testes through the canal is also aided by the increased abdominal pressure created by the growth of the abdominal viscera. By the ninth month, just before normal term delivery, the testes have completely entered the scrotal sac and the gubernaculum is reduced to a small ligamentous band attaching the inferior pole of the testis to the scrotal floor. The actions of testosterone and other **androgens** (male sex steroids) and

the genitofemoral nerve seem to be important for this second phase of testicular descent.

Within the first year after birth, the superior portion of the processus vaginalis is usually obliterated, leaving only a distal remnant sac, the **tunica vaginalis,** which lies anterior to the testis (Figs. 10-19, 10-20). During infancy this sac wraps around most of the testis. Its lumen is normally collapsed, but under pathologic conditions it may fill with serous secretions, forming a testicular hydrocele (Fig. 10-19B).

As mentioned above, it is not rare for the entire processus vaginalis to remain patent, forming a connection between the abdominal cavity and the scrotal sac. During childhood, loops of intestine may herniate into the processus, resulting in an **indirect inguinal hernia** (Fig. 10-19C). Repair of these hernias is the second most common childhood operation.

The ovaries descend and become suspended in the broad ligaments of the uterus. Like the male embryo, the female embryo develops a gubernaculum extending initially from the inferior pole of the gonad to the subcutaneous fascia of the presumptive labioscrotal folds and later penetrating the abdominal wall as part of a fully formed inguinal canal (Fig. 10-21). In the female, the gubernaculum does not shorten, deform, or regress. Nevertheless, it causes the ovaries to descend during the third month and to be swept out into a peritoneal fold called the **broad ligament of the uterus** (Figs. 10-16 and 10-

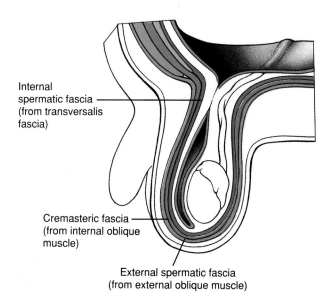

Internal spermatic fascia (from transversalis fascia)

Cremasteric fascia (from internal oblique muscle)

External spermatic fascia (from external oblique muscle)

Fig. 10-20. The three extruded layers of abdominal wall pushed into the scrotum by the evaginating processus vaginalis from three layers of spermatic fascia. These three layers enclose the tunica vaginalis and the testis in a common compartment.

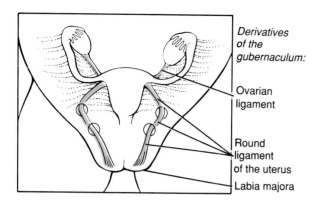

Derivatives
of the
gubernaculum:

Ovarian
ligament

Round
ligament
of the uterus

Labia majora

Fig. 10-21. The ovaries descend to some degree during development and are swept into the broad ligaments while the paramesonephric ducts zipper together to form the uterus. The gubernaculum in the female grows in pace with the body and is attached to the paramesonephric ducts at a crossover point on the posterior body wall. In consequence, the remnant of the female gubernaculum connects the labia majora with the wall of the uterus and is then reflected laterally, attaching to the ovary.

21). This translocation occurs because during the seventh week the gubernaculum becomes attached to the developing paramesonephric ducts where these two structures cross each other on the posterior body wall. As the paramesonephric ducts zipper together from their caudal ends, they sweep out the broad ligaments and simultaneously pull the ovaries into these peritoneal folds.

In the absence of male hormones, the female gubernaculum remains intact and grows in step with the rest of the body. The inferior gubernaculum becomes the **round ligament of the uterus** connecting the fascia of the labia majora to the uterus, and the superior gubernaculum becomes the **ligament of the ovary** connecting the uterus to the ovary.

As in males, the processus vaginalis of the inguinal canal is normally obliterated, but occasionally remains patent and may become the site of an **indirect inguinal hernia.**

APPLICATIONS TO CLINICAL PRACTICE

Renal Anomalies Represent a Significant Percentage of All Congenital Malformations and May Result from Disruption at Many Different Stages of Renal Development

About 10 percent of all newborns have a developmental abnormality of the urinary tract, but most abnormalities do not cause clinical problems. About 45 percent of all cases of **childhood renal failure,** however, arise from anomalous development of the ureteric bud or metanephros, which usually occur together. **Initial specification of the metanephric blastema** requires the expression of the **zinc-finger transcription factor** gene called *WT1*. *WT1* is expressed in the metanephric blastema prior to **formation of the ureteric bud** and is necessary for bud formation based on experiments with transgenic knockout studies in mice. **Mutations of WT1** in humans result in a phenotype that includes anomalies of the kidney and genital development (see below) as well as childhood cancers of the kidney. These **Wilms' tumors,** however, are rare, occurring in only 8 of 1 million individuals. They may be acquired through a dominant or dominant-negative mode of familial inheritance or by sporadic mutation after a second mutation in the normal allele. An unusual mechanism, however, underlies the predisposition of individuals with **Wiedeman-Beckwith syndrome** to develop **renal hyperplasia** and **Wilms' tumor.** These individuals apparently lack the genomic imprinting (see Ch. 2) that normally inactivates the insulin-like growth factor (IGF) gene on the paternal chromosome, and, even though the *WT1* gene is normal, it cannot suppress the activity of the nonimprinted IGF paternal allele. Overexpression of IGF-2 by the paternal gene results in an overabundance of IGF-2 and development of Wilms' tumor. Wilms' tumors are typically diagnosed in the 3- or 4-year-old child and can be treated chemotherapeutically with a cure rate of about 90 percent (refer to discussions of other "developmental regulatory-tumor suppressor" genes such as *DPC4* [a member of the MAD family; Ch. 3], *PTCH* [Chs. 4 and 12], and *DCC* [Ch 13]).

Abnormalities of the ureters also result from anomalies of **induction of the ureteric buds.** For example, an extra ureteric bud may be induced in humans resulting in development of an **ectopic ureter** (Fig. 10-22). As the mesonephric duct undergoes exstrophy into the posterior wall of the bladder, the caudal ureter implants in the normal position, while the root of the originally cranial ureter

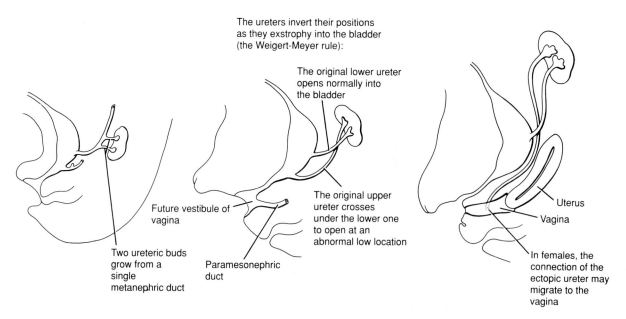

The ureters invert their positions as they exstrophy into the bladder (the Weigert-Meyer rule):

The original lower ureter opens normally into the bladder

Future vestibule of vagina

Two ureteric buds grow from a single metanephric duct

Paramesonephric duct

The original upper ureter crosses under the lower one to open at an abnormal low location

Uterus

Vagina

In females, the connection of the ectopic ureter may migrate to the vagina

Fig. 10-22. Ectopic ureter. An ectopic ureter forms from an anomalous "extra" ureteric bud. The mechanisms of formation of the trigone and placement of the vas deferens and ureters on the posterior wall of the primitive urogenital sinus were largely deduced from the Weigert-Meyer rule.

is carried caudally, forming its final connection to any derivative of the distal mesonephric duct, the pelvic urethra, or the definitive urogenital sinus (Fig. 10-22). The caudal ureteric bud therefore forms a normal or **orthotopic ureter,** while the cranial bud forms an abnormal or **ectopic ureter.** The crossing over of the orthotopic and ectopic ureters is called the **Weigert-Meyer rule** and is part of the evidence from which the mechanism of implantation of the ureters was deduced. In males, an ectopic ureter may drain into the prostatic urethra, the ejaculatory duct, the vas deferens, or the seminal vesicle. These connections thus always open superior to the sphincter urethra muscle and do not result in incontinence, although they may cause painful urination or recurrent infections. In females, ectopic ureters often connect to the vestibule of the vagina or to the uterus, resulting in continuous dribbling of urine unless surgically corrected.

Animal experiments suggest that normal **growth and branching of the ureteric bud** depends on expression of the **proto-oncogene receptor tyrosine kinase c-ret,** as evidenced by the fact that the mouse ureteric bud fails to branch at all in transgenic knockouts of *c-ret.* On the other hand, premature branching of the ureteric bud in humans results in a Y-shaped **bifid ureter** (Fig. 10-23). Most of the kidney is typically drained by the branch attached to its lower pole but contractions of the two branches are asynchronous. Urine may therefore reflux from one branch

into the other, resulting in stagnation of urine, predisposing the individual to infections of the ureter.

The **growth of the metanephric blastema** also requires expression of the **receptor tyrosine kinase c-ret,** since **renal agenesis** is also a characteristic of the mouse *c-ret* knockouts described above. While the causes may be varied and are not understood, both bilateral and unilateral renal ageneses are not uncommon in humans. Human infants born with **bilateral renal agenesis** are stillborn or die within a few days of birth. In addition, complete absence of kidneys results in a reduction of amniotic fluid or **oligohydramnios** (see Ch. 6), and resultant compression of the embryo and fetus by the uterine wall may then result in a spectrum of abnormalities called **Potter syndrome.** This syndrome includes deformed limbs, dry skin, and an abnormal facies (facial appearance) consisting of wide-set eyes, parrot-beak nose, receding chin, and low-set ears. Infants with **unilateral renal agenesis** often live because the remaining kidney undergoes compensatory hypertrophy.

Growth factors and transcription factors play pivotal roles in **differentiation of the metanephric stem cells,** in the **condensation or compaction of the metanephric stem cells,** and in **development of compacted metanephric mesenchyme into tubular renal vesicles (tubulogenesis).**

Animal experiments have also resulted in identification of several factors required for **nephron differentiation and formation of the glomerulus.** These include

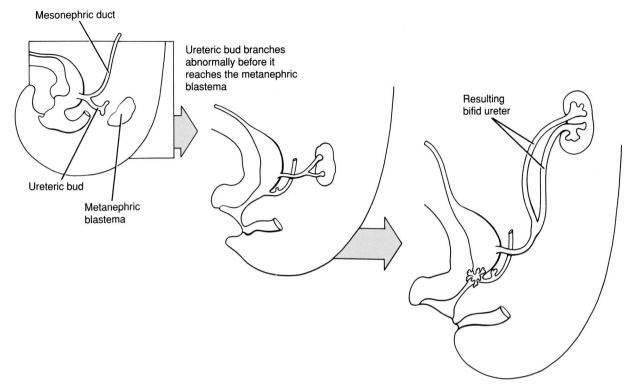

Fig. 10-23. Bifid ureter. A bifid ureter forms when the ureteric bud bifurcates before entering the metanephric blastema.

Mox-1, N-myc, Pax-2, and *Hoxc-9,* to name a few. However, a regulatory gene involved in differentiation of the human nephron has also been mapped to chromosome 16p13.3, and its mutation has been linked to 85 percent of human **autosomal recessive polycystic kidney disease (ARPKD).** While ARPKD is diagnosed in 1 of 10,000 infants, its frequency in stillborn infants suggests that its actual incidence may be 27-fold higher. It is characterized by small multifocal lesions of the proximal tubules and then by cyst formation in the collecting system. The candidate gene product is a protein implicated in cell cycle regulation, and so its disruption may lead to the **epithelial hyperplasia** that underlies this condition.

It is clear that ongoing studies will rapidly expand the list of growth factors and transcription factors that are clinically relevant to the large category of human congenital renal malformations.

Mutation of *WT1* also results in anomalies of genital development

Humans heterozygous for mutation of *WT1* exhibit anomalies of the genital system as well as malformations of the kidneys and Wilms' tumor. In genetic males, these

include **hypospadias** (see below) and **cryptorchidism** (undescended testes); in genetic females, the gonads may consist of **undifferentiated streaks of mesenchyme.** In homozygous knockouts of *Wt-1* in mice, normal thickening of the genital ridge fails to occur, although primordial germ cells enter the presumptive gonadal region. Since *Wt-1* is expressed in the gonadal ridge of normal male mice before expression of SRY, it is thought that its product may directly or indirectly induce SRY expression in the ambisexual gonad of genetic males (Fig. 10-24). **Steroidogenic factor 1 (SF-1)** expression also occurs within the bipotential gonad prior to male–female differentiation and seems to be required for formation of the male and female gonad since its targeted disruption results in their absence. While SF-1 may also play a specific role in development of the testis and in induction of the steroid hydroxylase enzymes, its functional relationships to SRY and the gene encoding **anti-Müllerian substance (AMH)** are not known (Fig. 10-24). Certainly, the targeted disruption of the gene encoding AMH has no effect on the development of the testes in mice. On the other hand, AMH-deficient mice do possess both male and female genital ducts, once again demonstrating AMH's pivotal role in normal regression of the paramesonephric ducts in males.

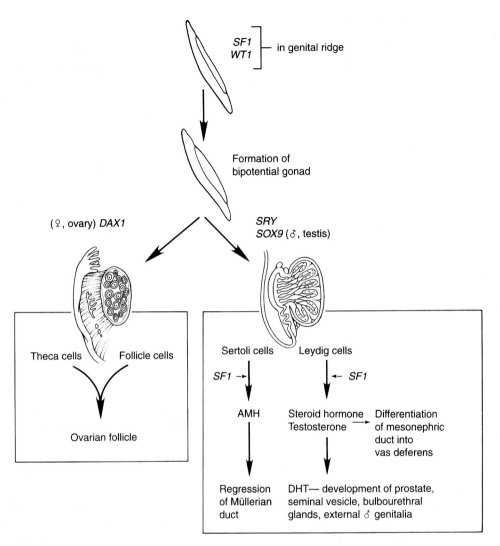

Fig. 10-24. Development cascade of male and female genital development. (Modified from Marx J. 1995. Sharing the genes that divide the sexes for mammals [news.] Science 270:901, with permission.)

Complete sex reversal may occur through disruptions of SRY

It has been known for many years that the Y chromosome instigates development of the testes in humans. The identity of the **sex-determining region** of the Y chromosome and its protein, however, was discovered only recently (Fig. 10-25). Initially, several promising candidates were investigated and rejected, but then a productive strategy arose from the discovery of **human XX males** and **XY females.** The genome of XX males, for example, was found to contain a very small amount of Y chromosome DNA that had been translocated onto the X chromosome, while the XY females were eventually shown to harbor a disruptive mutation of SRY. Analysis of this DNA by using male- and female-specific probes nar-

rowed the location of SRY to region 1 on the short arm. For a brief period, the zinc-finger protein ZFY encoded in the 1A2 interval was considered to be a promising candidate for SRY (Fig. 10-25). However, the 1A1 interval was then cloned and sequenced, and a more suitable SRY candidate was identified. The small protein encoded by this gene is highly conserved throughout nature and shows significant homologies with yeast mating-type protein and with nonhistone nuclear HMG proteins, which are also thought to regulate transcription by binding to DNA.

Sex reversal may be caused by mutation or duplication of genes other than SRY

It has become apparent that only 10 to 15 percent of sex reversals in XY females can be explained by disabling mu-

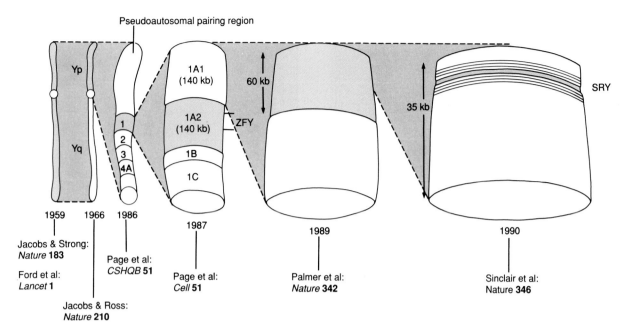

Fig. 10-25. A 31-year history of the search for the sex-determining region of the Y chromosome. (Modified from McLaren A. 1990. What makes a man a man? Nature 346:216, with permission.)

tations of SRY. Indeed, autosomal chromosomal deletions of 9p and 10q and duplications of Xp can lead to a female phenotype in XY individuals with an intact SRY. These individuals possess normal female genital ducts as well as ovaries with normal oocytes. In addition, individuals suffering from the congenital skeletal disease **camptomelic dysplasia** harbor mutations of a gene called *SOX-9* that has been mapped to chromosome 17q24.3–q25.1. These XY individuals also possess a normal SRY but in extreme cases may exhibit completely feminized sex organs. The relationship between skeletal anomalies and the mechanism by which sex reversal in these individuals occurs is unknown. Duplications of xp that result in sex reversal occur in a region that harbors the gene *DAX-1* (**D**osage-dependent sex reversal; **A**drenal hypoplasia congenita; **X** chromosome). Because of the feminization of the genitalia by two copies of *DAX-1* in XY individuals, *DAX-1* may play a role in normal development of the ovary or in suppression of testicular development (Fig. 10-24).

Pseudohermaphroditism is caused by sex hormone anomalies

Genetic males (46,XY) with feminized genitals are called **male pseudohermaphrodites,** and genetic females (46,XX) are called **female pseudohermaphrodites.** Pseudohermaphroditism is always caused by abnormal levels of sex hormones or by abnormalities in sex hormone receptors. Since all male pseudohermaphrodites possess testes that secrete AMH, none possess paramesonephric

duct derivatives. A common manifestation of male pseudohermaphroditism, however, is **hypospadias,** a condition in which the urethra opens onto the ventral surface of the penis. Hypospadias occurs in about 0.5 percent of all live births. In simple cases, a single anomalous opening is located on the underside of the glans or shaft (Fig. 10-26A, B). In more severe cases, the penile urethra has multiple openings or is not enclosed at all. Hypospadias of the glans is probably caused by defective development of the distal ectodermal urethral meatus, whereas openings on the penile shaft represent failures of the urethral folds to fuse. A more severe condition called **penoscrotal hypospadias** occurs when the labioscrotal swellings as well as the urethral folds fail to fuse (Fig. 10-26D, C). This condition is usually accompanied by retarded growth of the phallus so that the genitals appear female at birth. This form of hypospadias may be caused by a deficiency of the enzyme **5α- reductase,** which normally converts testosterone to the derivative androgen **dihydrotestosterone.** While these individuals exhibit penoscrotal hypospadias, they have normal testes within the inguinal canals or labioscrotal swellings and so paramesonephric duct derivatives are absent and the mesonephric ducts differentiate into vasa deferentia. Since pseudohermaphrodites of this type have normal levels of testosterone, their urethral and labioscrotal folds may fuse and the genital tubercle may differentiate into a penis at puberty. These individuals may also be fertile. Male pseudohermaphroditism may also be caused by mutations that affect **enzymes required for the synthesis of testosterone** and its precursors, such as 20,22-desmo-

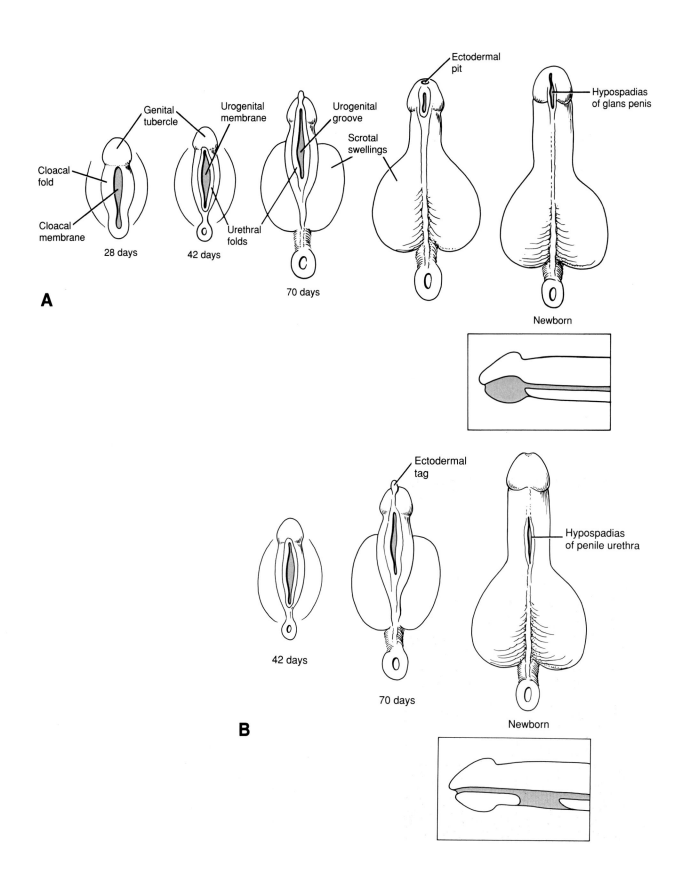

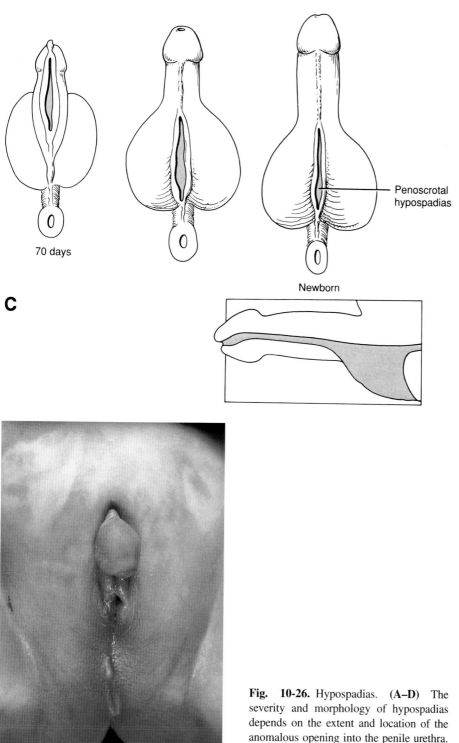

70 days

Newborn

Penoscrotal
hypospadias

C

D

Fig. 10-26. Hypospadias. **(A–D)** The
severity and morphology of hypospadias
depends on the extent and location of the
anomalous opening into the penile urethra.
(D) Infant with penoscrotal hypospadias.
(Fig. D photo courtesy of Children's Hospital Medical Center, Cincinnati, OH.)

lase, 17-hydroxylase, steroid 17,20-desmolase, and 17β-hydroxysteroid dehydrogenase. In these individuals, the mesonephric ducts do not differentiate, the testes do not descend, and the external genitalia appear to be female. However, the testes do produce AMH, and so paramesonephric duct derivatives are absent.

Androgen receptors are abnormal in androgen insensitivity (formerly testicular feminization) syndrome

Male pseudohermaphroditism may also result in cases where mutations have disabled or eliminated the androgen receptors. In these cases, the fetus may exhibit normal or high circulating levels of male steroid hormones, but the target tissues develop as though the androgens were absent. This condition is called **androgen insensitivity syndrome.** As in cases of testosterone deficiency described above, testes are present and AMH is produced so the paramesonephric ducts regress, although a blind-ending vagina may be present. The external genitalia, however, exhibit a female appearance.

Female pseudohermaphroditism is rare

Genetic females may be virilized by exposure to abnormal levels of virilizing sex steroids during fetal development. The source of these androgens may be the hyperplastic adrenal glands. In some cases, progestins used to prevent spontaneous abortion have been suspected. These individuals possess ovaries and female genital ducts such as fallopian tubes, uterus, and vagina, since testes and AMH are absent. The external genitalia, however, exhibit clitoral hypertrophy and fusion of the urethral and labioscrotal folds.

True hermaphrodites have both ovarian and testicular tissue

True hermaphrodites may be chromosomal males (46,XY) or chromosomal females (46,XX) or mosaics (e.g., 45, X/46,XY; 46,XX/47,XXY; or 46,XX/46,XY). In mosaic individuals, ovarian tissue develops from cells without a Y chromosome, whereas testicular tissue develops from cells with a Y chromosome. Hermaphrodites with a 46,XX genotype may actually be mosaics with some cells that are male because of the presence of a fragment of the Y chromosome containing SRY within an X chromosome. 46,XY hermaphrodites are more difficult to explain. The cause may be mosaicism involving mutation of the Y chromosome or ovary-determining regions of the X chromosome. Some of these examples could be caused by duplications or mutations of sex-determining genes on autosomes or X chromosomes. The gonads of true hermaphrodites are usually **ovotestes** containing both seminiferous tubules and follicles. Occasionally, however, an individual has an ovary or ovotestis on one side and a testis on the other. A fallopian tube and single uterine horn may accompany the ovary. A vas deferens always develops in conjunction with the testis. The testis is usually immature, but spermatogenesis is occasionally detectable. A few hermaphroditic individuals have ovulated and conceived, although none has carried a fetus to term. Most hermaphrodites, however, are reared as males, since a phallus is usually present.

Failure to enter puberty may be caused by primary or secondary hypogonadism

When a boy or girl fails to undergo the changes associated with puberty, the cause is usually a deficiency in the amount of sex steroids secreted by the gonads. This pubertal surge is stimulated by increased levels of pituitary gonadotropins, and so the defect may be in the gonads themselves **(primary hypogonadism)** or in the hypothalamus or pituitary **(secondary hypogonadism.)** Most cases of primary hypogonadism are associated with **Klinefelter** or **Turner syndrome.** Klinefelter syndrome occurs in 1 of 500 live male births and is usually caused by an extra X chromosome, acquired during nondisjunction during gametogenesis or early cleavage. The most common karyotype is 47,XXY, although some individuals with Klinefelter syndrome may be mosaics of cells with the normal male karyotype and cells with an abnormal karyotype (e.g., 47,XXY; 48,XXYY; and 45,X) or cells with a normal female karyotype (46,XX) and an abnormal karyotype (47,XXY). In all cases, the Leydig cells fail to produce sufficient male steroids, resulting in small testes and **azoospermia** (lack of spermatogenesis) or **oligospermia** (low sperm count). Many of these individuals also exhibit **gynecomastia** (development of breasts in males) and **eunuchoidism** (elongated extremities). Primary hypogonadism in females is usually associated with **Turner syndrome,** which is much less common than Klinefelter syndrome (1 in 5,000 live female births). The cause is a 45,X karyotype or 45,X/46,XX mosaicism. In addition to failure of normal sexual maturation, these individuals exhibit short stature, webbed neck, coarctation of the aorta, and cervical lymphatic cysts. In **secondary hypogonadism,** individuals have depressed levels of gonadotropins as well as sex steroids, most often because of reduced secretion of gonadotropin-releasing hormone (GnRH) by the hypothalamus (**Kallman syndrome** and **fertile eunuch syndrome** in males). Most of these disorders show autosomal recessive inheritance.

Defective partitioning of the cloaca results in anomalies of urinary, genital, and anorectal structures

In as many as 1 of 5,000 infants, the urorectal septum is incomplete. Depending on the location and size of the defect, a wide range of malformations involving cloacal derivatives and their connections with the ureters and genital ducts may result. For example, **failure of the Rathke folds to develop results in rectourethral fistulas** developing between the primitive urogenital sinus and the rec-

tum (Fig. 10-27). In males, these may take the form of **rectoprostatic urethral fistulas** (Fig. 10-27C) and in females may take the form of a **rectocloacal fistula** (Fig. 10-27D) or a **rectovaginal fistula** (Fig. 10-27E). **Failure of both Tourneux and Rathke folds to form may result**

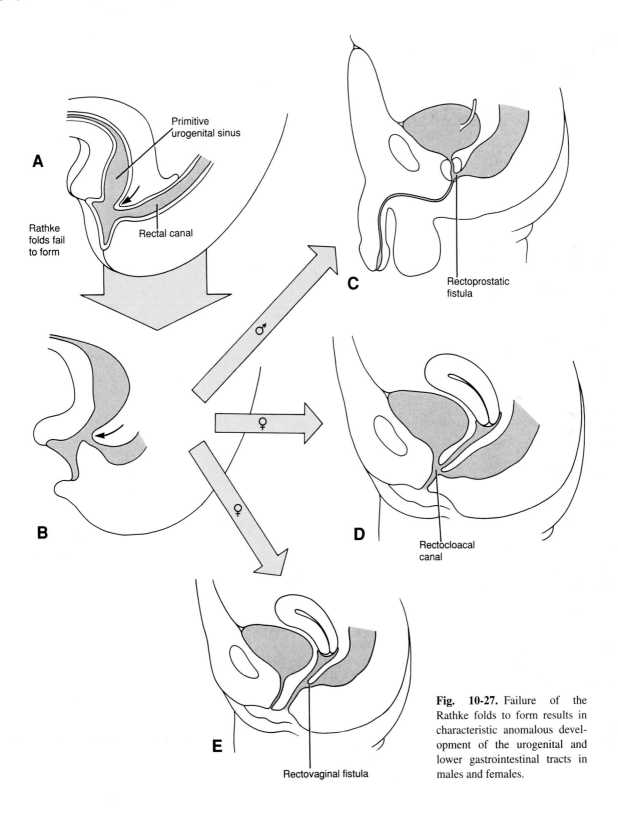

Fig. 10-27. Failure of the Rathke folds to form results in characteristic anomalous development of the urogenital and lower gastrointestinal tracts in males and females.

in a more severe defect called a **rectovesicle fistula** (Fig. 10-28). On the other hand, **malalignment of the Tourneux and Rathke folds** (Fig. 10-29) may result in a **rectourethral fistula** in males (Fig. 10-29B) or a **rectovaginal fistula** in females (Fig. 10-29C, D).

Anal malformations may result from abnormal development of the anal pit, anal membrane, or genital folds

Failure of the anal pit to form results in a blind-ended rectum, a condition called **anal agenesis** (Fig. 10-30A).

In some cases, a thickened anal membrane may fail to rupture or rupture incompletely, conditions respectively called **imperforate anal membrane** or **anal stenosis** (Fig. 10-30B). **Covered anus** may result from excessive fusion of the genital folds, and in some cases a defect in the perineal mesoderm just anterior to the anus results in a malformation called **anocutaneous stenosis** or **anterior anus.**

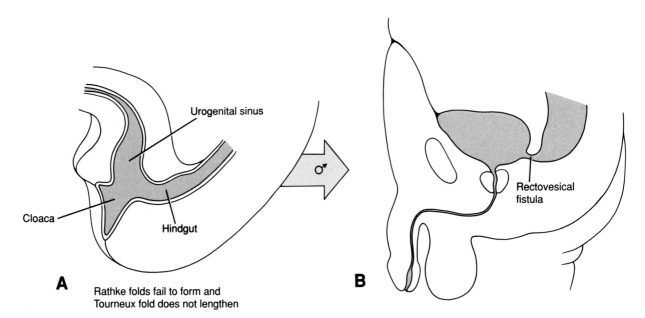

A Rathke folds fail to form and Tourneux fold does not lengthen

B

Fig. 10-28. Failure of the Tourneux and Rathke folds to form may result in the development of a fistula between the rectum and the bladder.

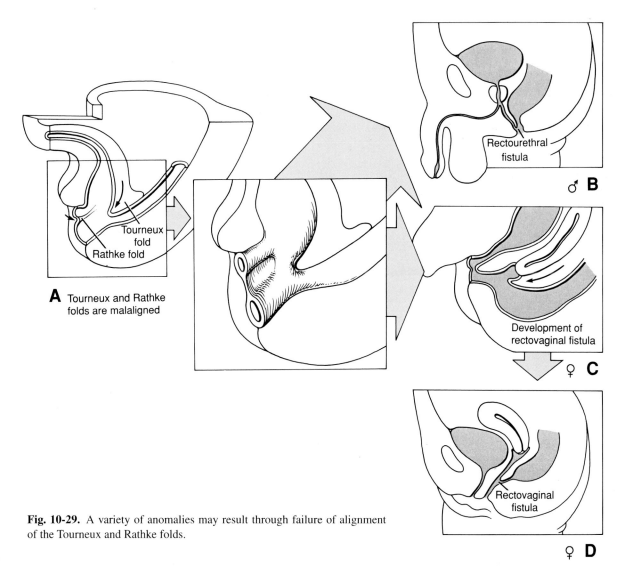

Fig. 10-29. A variety of anomalies may result through failure of alignment of the Tourneux and Rathke folds.

A Tourneux and Rathke folds are malaligned

Tourneux fold

Rathke fold

Rectourethral fistula

♂ **B**

Development of rectovaginal fistula

♀ **C**

Rectovaginal fistula

♀ **D**

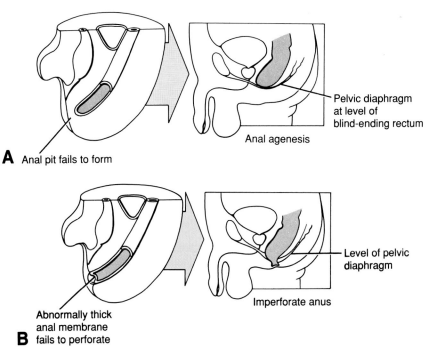

A Anal pit fails to form

Pelvic diaphragm at level of blind-ending rectum

Anal agenesis

B Abnormally thick anal membrane fails to perforate

Level of pelvic diaphragm

Imperforate anus

Fig. 10-30. (A) Anal agenesis resulting from failure of the anal pit to form. **(B)** Imperforate anus may occur in cases where an abnormally thick anal membrane fails to rupture.

11

Development of the Limbs

*Development of the Limb Buds; Functions of
the Apical Ectodermal Ridges and Mesodermal
Core; Formation of the Hand and Foot Plates;
Development of the Appendicular Skeleton
and Musculature*

During the fourth week, the upper **limb buds** are induced by signals from somites in the lower cervical region, while lower limb buds are induced slightly later in the lower lumbar region. The **ectodermal covering** of each limb bud then develops a distal thickening called the **apical ectodermal ridge (AER).** Continued growth of the limb bud is stimulated by several factors, including **fibroblast growth factors (FGFs)** produced within the ridge as well as within its **mesodermal core.** The limb buds also differentiate along three interrelated axes: the proximodistal axis, the craniocaudal axis, and the dorsoventral axis.

Proximodistal differentiation is regulated in part by signals emanating from the AER that induce the expression of growth factors, including the **FGFs, the bone morphogenetic substance (BMP)** family of growth factors, and **HOX** genes. These signals regulate the segment-specific development of limb tissues, including the long bones from **lateral plate mesoderm** within the core and segment-specific muscles from **somite-derived mesoderm.** Indeed, the proximodistal pattern of *HOX* gene expression is directly related to differentiation of each limb segment as shown by transgenic knockouts of *Hox* genes in experimental animals and by the **homeotic transformation** of wrist and ankle bones to hand and foot bones, respectively, in a human family homozygous for a *HOX* gene mutation.

Craniocaudal polarization of the hand or foot plate is controlled by a caudal **zone of polarizing activity (ZPA)** that produces the peptide **sonic hedgehog (Shh).** Not only can **mirror polydactyly** be induced in experimental animals by implantation of an Shh-soaked bead in the cranial edge of the limb bud, but mirror polydactylous mutants ectopically express Shh within a cranial location as well as in the caudal ZPA. Factors expressed in response to Shh signaling include FGFs, BMPs, and *HOX* genes, all of which play downstream roles in digit formation and differentiation. BMP-4, for example, is expressed between the digits and is apparently instrumental in the apoptosis (programmed cell death) that sculpts the digits from the hand and foot plates. Thus, disruptions of homologous factors or *HOX* genes in humans may be responsible for webbing or **syndactyly** (fusion of the digits).

Less is known about the **dorsoventral patterning** of the extremities, but mechanisms similar to those that regulate dorsoventral patterning of the germ disc (Ch. 4) appear to operate here as well. For example, the murine transgenic knockout of *Wnt-7a* results in formation of footpads on both dorsal and ventral sides of the paw. Moreover, as in the germ disc, a *Lim* homeobox gene appears to mediate the effects of *Wnt-7a* on dorsoventral patterning of the limb. While the function of **retinoic acid** in limb development is enigmatic, it clearly plays a role in limb pathogenesis, and, therefore, therapies involving its use during early pregnancy must be avoided. Similarly, application of the spasmolytic **thalidomide** in several new therapies requires physicians to reacquaint themselves with its devastating side effects on development of the limbs and other organs.

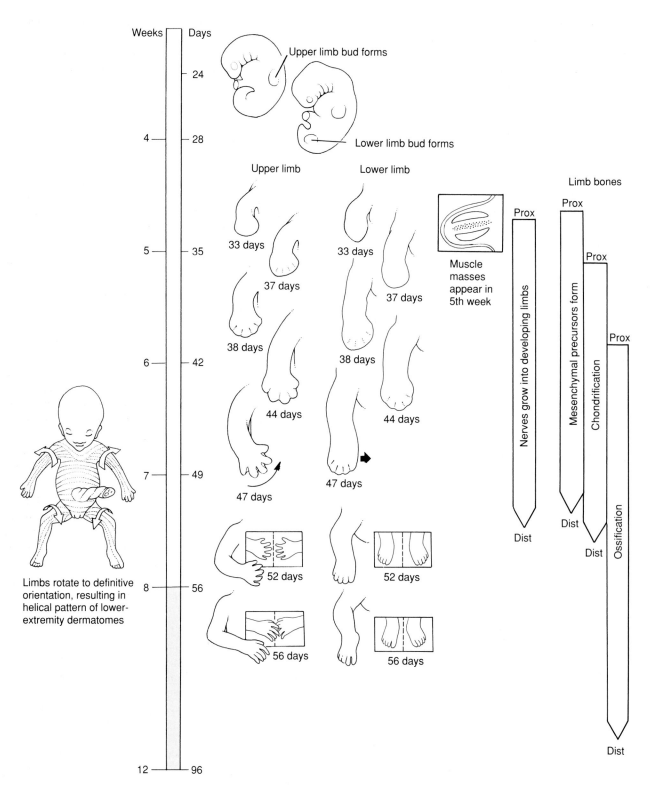

Timeline. Development of the limbs.

The limbs develop through a series of inductive interactions

The formation of limb buds in the lateral plate mesoderm is induced by the adjacent somites

The upper and lower **limb buds** are formed by proliferation of the somatopleuric lateral plate mesoderm in the limb regions of the flank (Fig. 11-1A, B). The upper limb bud appears in the lower cervical region at 24 days, and the lower limb bud appears in the lower lumbar region at 28 days. Each limb bud consists of an outer ectodermal cap and an inner mesodermal core.

The apical ectodermal ridge induces differentiation of the limb buds

As each limb bud forms, the ectoderm along the apex of the bud differentiates into a ridgelike thickening called the **apical ectodermal ridge** (Fig. 11-1C, D). This structure plays an essential role in the differentiation of the limb. Transplantation experiments show that the absence of limbs in these chicks is not due to a defect in the mesodermal core: limb bud mesoderm from this "limbless" mutant is capable of inducing the development of an apical ectodermal ridge and a normal limb if transplanted to the flank of a normal host.

The differentiation of the limb segments is determined by the age of the corresponding portions of core mesoderm

Transplantation experiments in chicks demonstrate that the apical ectodermal ridge induces differentiation throughout the limb bud but does not specify which part of the bud will form which segment of the limb. That "decision" is made by the mesodermal core, apparently on the basis of its age: the late-formed mesenchyme at the tip of the elongating limb bud differentiates into the distal segments of the limb, whereas the early-formed mesenchyme at the base of the bud differentiates into the proximal segments of the limb.

This conclusion is based partly on a series of transplantation experiments carried out on chick wing buds (Fig. 11-2). For example, if a composite artificial wing bud is made by combining the late-formed mesenchyme from the tip of an older bud with the ectodermal cap of a bud of any age, only the distal parts of the wing will form. Conversely, a composite wing bud made by combining an ectodermal cap of any age with the early-formed mesodermal core of a young bud will form an entire limb (see Application to Clinical Practice). On the basis of these and other experiments, it has been suggested that the factor that specifies which limb segment will be formed by a given zone of mesenchyme is the amount of time the mesenchyme has spent under the influence of the apical ridge and that the mesenchymal cells may measure this time by the number of cell divisions they have undergone since the inception of the apical ridge.

Differentiation of the limb buds occurs between the fifth and eighth weeks

Limb development takes place over a 4-week period from the fifth to the eighth weeks. The upper limbs develop slightly in advance of the lower limbs, although by the end of the period of limb development the two limbs are nearly synchronized. Development takes place as follows (Fig. 11-3):

Day 33. In the upper limb, the **hand plate, forearm, arm,** and **shoulder** regions can be distinguished. In the lower limb, a somewhat rounded cranial part can be distinguished from a more tapering caudal part. The distal tip of the tapering caudal part will form the foot.

Day 37. In the hand plate of the upper limb, a central **carpal region** is surrounded by a thickened crescentic flange, the **digital plate,** which will form the fingers. In the lower limb, the **thigh, leg,** and **foot** have become distinct.

Day 38. **Finger rays** (more generally, **digital rays**) are visible as radial thickenings in the digital plate of the upper limb. The tips of the finger rays project slightly, producing a crenulated rim on the digital plate. A process of programmed cell death will gradually sculpt the digital rays out of the digital plate to form the fingers and toes. Programmed cell death takes place in radial **necrotic zones** between the digital rays. The lower limb bud has increased in length and become demarcated from the trunk, and a clearly defined **foot plate** is apparent **on the** caudal side of the distal end of the bud.

Day 44. In the upper limb, the margin of the digital plate is deeply notched and the grooves between the finger rays are deeper. The elbow is obvious. **Toe rays** are visible in the digital plate of the foot, but the rim of the plate is not yet crenulated.

Day 47. The entire upper limb has undergone **horizontal flexion** so that it lies in a parasagittal rather than a coronal plane (Fig. 11-4A). The lower limb has also begun to flex toward a parasagittal plane. The toe rays are more prominent, although the margin of the digital plate is still smooth.

Day 52. The upper limbs are slightly bent at the elbows, and the fingers have developed distal swellings called **tactile pads** (Fig. 11-4B). The hands are slightly flexed at the wrists and meet at the midline in front of the cardiac eminence. The legs are longer, and the feet have begun to approach each other at the midline. The rim of the digital plate is notched.

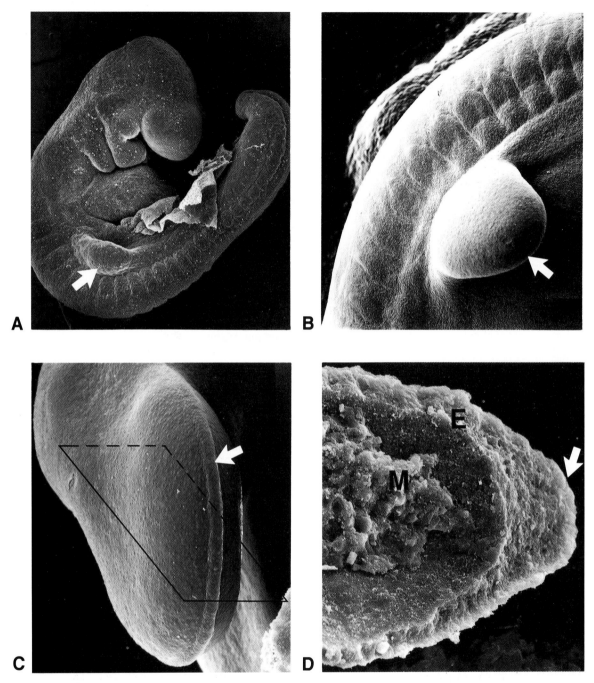

Fig. 11-1. Scanning electron micrographs showing limb buds. The limb buds are formed when somitic mesoderm induces the proliferation of overlying lateral plate mesoderm. **(A)** Embryo with newly formed upper limb bud (arrow). **(B)** By day 29, the upper limb bud (arrow) is flattened and paddle-shaped. **(C)** By day 32, the apical ectodermal ridge (arrow) is visible as a thickened crest of ectoderm at the distal edge of the growing upper limb bud. Rectangle indicates plane of sectioning of Fig. D. **(D)** Limb bud sectioned to show the inner mesenchymal core (M) and the outer ectodermal cap (E). Arrow: apical ectodermal ridge. (Figs. A, C, D from Kelley RO. 1985. Early development of the vertebrate limb: an introduction to morphogenetic tissue interactions using scanning electron microscopy. Scanning Microsc II:827, with permission.)

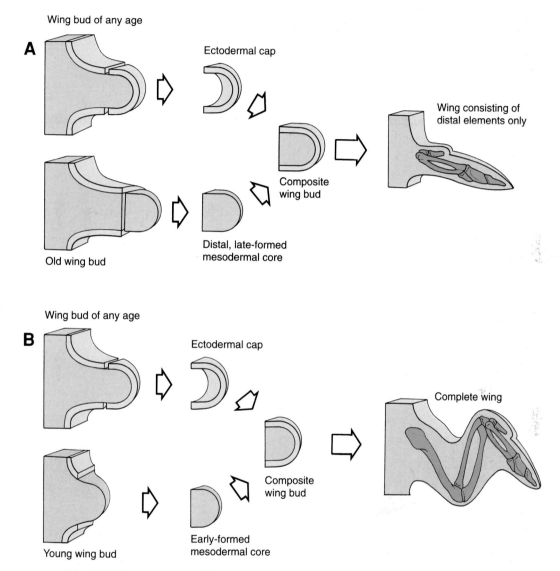

Fig. 11-2. Experiment on chick embryos demonstrating the roles of the apical ectodermal cap and the mesodermal core in limb bud development. **(A)** If an ectodermal cap of any age (even very young) is recombined with the distal end of an old mesenchymal core, the hybrid bud will form only distal elements of the limb. **(B)** If an ectodermal cap from a bud of any age (even very old) is recombined with a complete mesodermal core from a young limb bud, the hybrid bud will form an entire limb. (Modified from Rubin L, Saunders TW. 1972. Ectodermal-mesodermal interactions in the growth of limb buds in the chick embryo: constancy and temporal limits of the ectodermal induction. Dev Biol 28:94, with permission.)

Upper limb

Lower limb

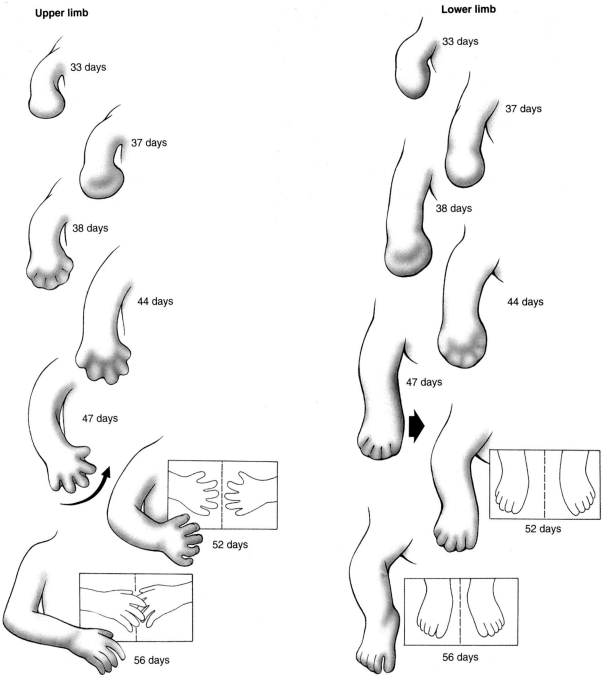

Fig. 11-3. The development of the upper and lower limb buds occurs between the fifth and eighth weeks. Nearly every stage in the development of the lower limb bud takes place several days later than in the upper limb bud.

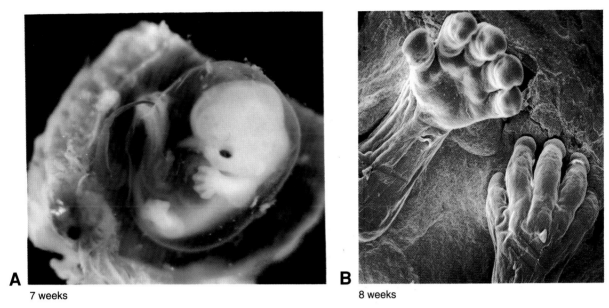

A 7 weeks

B 8 weeks

Fig. 11-4. (A) By 7 weeks, the digits are clearly visible in both upper and lower extremities. **(B)** At 8 weeks, tactile pads are apparent on the distal tips of the fingers. (Fig. A photo courtesy of Dr. Arnold Tamarin.)

Day 56. All regions of the arms and legs are well defined, including the toes. The fingers of the two hands overlap at the midline.

The somites, lateral plate mesoderm, and neural crest contribute to different components within the limb

The quail–chick chimera system has been used to study the cell populations that give rise to the various elements of the limbs. One discovery was that although the lateral plate mesoderm gives rise to the bones, tendons, ligaments, and vasculature of the limbs, the limb *musculature* is derived from somitic mesoderm that migrates into the developing limb bud. A quail–chick chimera experiment demonstrating this point is illustrated in Figure 11-5. If the chick somites at the level of the wing bud are replaced with the corresponding somites from a quail, the wing muscles will be made of quail cells, although the other wing tissues will be made of chick cells.

Other quail–chick experiments involving transplantation of parts of the neural tube have shown that the **melanocytes** and **Schwann cells** of the limb are derived from migrating ectomesenchymal cells of the neural crest.

The limb bones form as mesenchymal condensations that first chondrify and then ossify

With the exception of the clavicle, the bones of the limbs and girdles (constituting the **appendicular skele-**ton) form by ossification of a cartilaginous precursor, a process known as **endochondral ossification.** The clavicle, in contrast, is a **membrane bone:** it forms by direct ossification from mesenchyme in the dermis and lacks a cartilaginous precursor.

The endochondral bones of the limb and their intervening joints form from a rodlike condensation of lateral plate mesenchyme that develops along the long axis of the limb bud (Fig. 11-6). In response to growth factors, **chondrocytes** (cartilage cells) differentiate within this mesenchyme and begin to secrete molecules characteristic of the extracellular matrix of cartilage, such as collagen type II and proteoglycans.

The initial phase of chondrification in the developing limbs results in the deposition of cartilage around the entire axial mesenchymal condensation. This cartilaginous envelope is called the **perichondrium.** Further chondrification is limited to the sites of the future bones, where it creates a cartilaginous model (anlage) of each bone. The mesenchyme in the **interzones**—the sites of the future joints—differentiates into fibrous connective tissue.

After the anlage of each endochondral limb bone has chondrified, the process of **ossification** commences in a region of the bone called the **primary ossification center.** First, mesenchymal cells in the perichondrium differentiate into **osteoblasts** or bone cells. These cells secrete the calcium salt matrix of mineralized bone and form a **primary bone collar** around the circumference of the bone. This primary bone collar thickens as osteoblasts differentiate in progressively more peripheral layers of

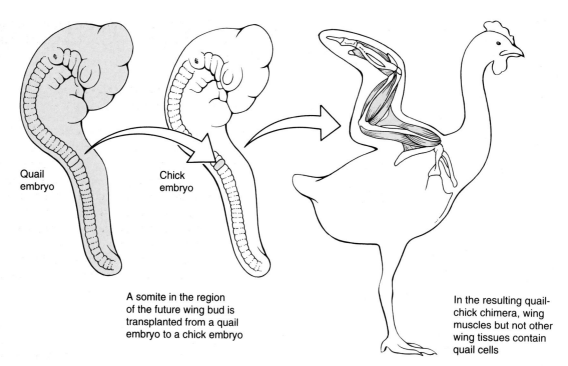

Quail
embryo

Chick
embryo

A somite in the region
of the future wing bud is
transplanted from a quail
embryo to a chick embryo

In the resulting quail-
chick chimera, wing
muscles but not other
wing tissues contain
quail cells

Fig. 11-5. Quail–chick cell tracing experiment demonstrating that the musculature of the limbs forms from somitic mesoderm, whereas the bones form from lateral plate mesoderm. Transplanted somites in the region of limb bud development give rise to limb myocytes. (Modified from Chevallier A, Kieny M, Mauger A. 1977. Limb-somite relationship: origin of the limb musculature. J Embryol Exp Morphol 41:245, with permission.)

the perichondrium. Cells called **osteoclasts,** which break down previously formed bone, also appear and begin to remodel the growing bone. Bone is continually remodeled throughout development and adult life. Ossification also spreads from the primary ossification center toward the ends of the anlage, and the cartilaginous core enclosed by the primary bone collar also begins to ossify to form a loose **trabecular network** of bone.

Shortly after ossification begins, the developing bone is invaded by multiple blood vessels that branch from the limb vasculature (see Ch. 8). One of these vessels eventually becomes dominant and gives rise to the **nutrient artery** that nourishes the bone.

At birth, the **diaphyses** or shafts of the limb bones (consisting of a bone collar and trabecular core) are completely ossified, whereas the ends of the bones, called the **epiphyses,** are still cartilaginous. After birth, **secondary ossification centers** develop in the epiphyses, which gradually ossify. However, a layer of cartilage called the **epiphyseal cartilage plate (growth plate or physis)** persists between the epiphysis and the growing end of the diaphysis (**metaphysis**). Continued proliferation of the chondrocytes in this growth plate allows the diaphysis to lengthen. Finally, when the growth of the body is complete at about 20 years of age, the epiphyses and diaphyses fuse.

Most of the limb bones form between the 5th and 12th weeks

The axial mesenchyme of the limb buds first begins to condense in the fifth week, although at this point the axial condensation is difficult to distinguish from the adjacent somitic mesodermal condensations that will give rise to muscle. In general, the bones of the upper limb form slightly earlier than their counterparts in the lower limb.

By the end of the fifth week, the portion of the axial mesenchymal condensation that will give rise to the proximal limb skeleton (the scapula and humerus in the upper limb; the pelvic bones and femur in the lower limb) is distinct. By the early sixth week, the mesenchymal precursor of the distal limb skeleton is distinct in the upper and lower limbs, and chondrification commences in the humerus, ulna, and radius. By the end of the sixth week, the carpal and metacarpal bones also begin to chondrify. In the lower limb, the femur, the tibia, and, to a lesser extent, the fibula begin to chondrify by the middle of the sixth week, and the tarsals and metatarsals begin to chondrify near the end of the sixth week. By the early seventh week, all the bones of the upper limb except the distal phalanges of the second to fifth digits are

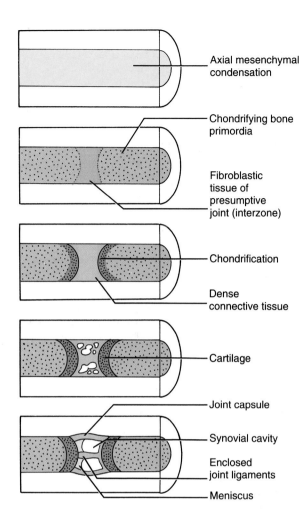

Axial mesenchymal condensation

Chondrifying bone primordia

Fibroblastic tissue of presumptive joint (interzone)

Chondrification

Dense connective tissue

Cartilage

Joint capsule

Synovial cavity

Enclosed joint ligaments

Meniscus

Fig. 11-6. Formation of joints. Cartilage, ligaments, and capsular elements of the joints develop from the interzone regions of the axial mesenchymal condensations that form the long bones of the limbs.

undergoing chondrification. By the end of the seventh week, the distal phalanges of the hand have begun to chondrify, and chondrification is also under way in all the bones of the lower limb except the distal row of phalanges. The distal phalanges of the toes do not chondrify until the eighth week.

The primary ossification centers of most of the limb bones appear in the 7th to 12th weeks. By the early seventh week, ossification has commenced in the clavicle, followed by the humerus, radius, and ulna at the end of the seventh week. Ossification begins in the femur and tibia in the eighth week. During the ninth week the scapula and ilium begin to ossify, followed in the next 3 weeks by the metacarpals, metatarsals, distal phalanges, proximal phalanges, and, finally, the middle phalanges. The ischium and pubis begin to ossify in the 15th and 20th weeks, respectively, while ossification of the calca-

neus finally begins at about 16 weeks. Some of the smaller carpal and tarsal bones do not ossify until early childhood.

The joints of the limbs develop from the mesenchymal interzones

Figure 11-6 illustrates the process by which the **diarthrodial (synovial) joints** connecting the limb bones develop. First, the mesenchyme of the interzones between the chondrifying bone primordia differentiates into **fibroblastic tissue** (undifferentiated connective tissue). This tissue then further differentiates into three layers: a cartilage layer at either end of the future joint, in contact with the adjacent bone primordia, and a central layer of dense connective tissue. The connective tissue of this central layer gives rise to the internal elements of the joint. Proximally and distally, it condenses to form the **synovial tissue** that will line the future joint cavity. Its central zone gives rise to the **menisci** and to **enclosed joint ligaments** such as the cruciate ligaments of the knee. Vacuoles appear within this tissue and coalesce to form the **synovial cavity.** The **joint capsule** arises from the mesenchymal sheath surrounding the entire interzone.

Synchondroidal joints, such as those connecting the bones of the pelvis, also develop from interzones, but the interzone mesenchyme simply differentiates into a single layer of fibrocartilage.

The limb musculature develops from ventral and dorsal condensations of somitic mesoderm

During the fifth week, somitic mesoderm invades the limb bud and forms two large condensations, one dorsal to the axial mesenchymal column and one ventral to it (Fig. 11-7). The cells of the condensations form the anlagen of the limb muscles and differentiate into **myoblasts** (muscle cell precursors). Each muscle increases in mass not only by the growth of myofibrils within each myoblast but also, initially, by continued recruitment of invading somitic mesoderm cells. During this early phase of growth, myoblasts also fuse together to form syncytia. From the fourth month on, however, muscle growth is accomplished primarily by the enlargement of existing muscle fibers.

The dorsal muscle mass gives rise in general to the **extensors** and **supinators** of the upper limb and to the **extensors** and **abductors** of the lower limb, whereas the ventral muscle mass gives rise to the **flexors** and **pronators** of the upper limb and to the **flexors** and **adductors** of the lower limb (Table 11-1). This rule is not absolute, however, some muscles migrate from their site of origin and acquire different functions.

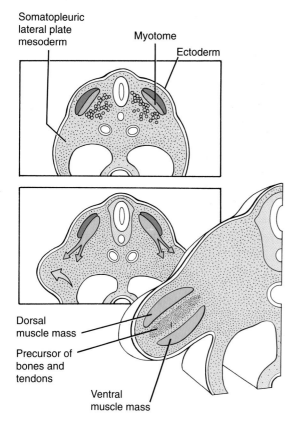

Somatopleuric
lateral plate
mesoderm

Myotome

Ectoderm

Dorsal
muscle mass

Precursor of
bones and
tendons

Ventral
muscle mass

Fig. 11-7. Somitic mesoderm initially forms two major muscle masses in each limb bud. The ventral mass gives rise mainly to flexors, pronators, and adductors, whereas the dorsal muscle mass gives rise mainly to extensors, supinators, and abductors.

Spinal nerve axons innervate specific limb structures by a multistep pathfinding process

As described in Chapter 5, each spinal nerve splits into main branches, the dorsal and ventral primary rami, shortly after it exits the spinal cord. The limb muscles are innervated by branches of the ventral primary rami of spinal nerves C5 through T1 (for the upper limb) and L4 through S3 (for the lower limb). Muscles originating in the dorsal muscle mass are served by *dorsal* branches of these ventral primary rami, whereas muscles originating in the ventral muscle mass are served by *ventral* branches of the ventral primary rami. Thus, the innervation of a muscle shows whether it originated in the dorsal or the ventral muscle mass.

As illustrated in Figure 11-8, the motor axons that innervate the limbs perform an intricate feat of pathfinding to reach their target muscles. The ventral ramus axons destined for the limbs apparently travel to the base of the limb bud by growing along **permissive pathways** (Fig. 11-9A). The growth cones of these axons avoid or are unable to penetrate regions of dense mesenchyme or mesenchyme containing glycosaminoglycans. The axons heading for the lower limb are thus deflected around the developing pelvic anlagen. In both the upper and the lower limb buds, the axons from the nerves cranial to the limb bud grow toward the craniodorsal side of the limb bud, whereas the axons from the nerves caudal to the limb bud grow toward the ventrocaudal side of the limb bud (Fig. 11-9B).

Table 11-1 Muscles Derived from the Ventral and Dorsal Muscle Masses of the Limb Buds

VENTRAL MUSCLE MASS		DORSAL MUSCLE MASS
Upper Limb	**Upper Limb**	**Lower Limb**
Anterior compartment of the arm and forearm	Posterior compartment muscles of the arm and forearm	Anterior compartment muscles of the thigh and leg
All muscles on the palmar surface of hand	Deltoid	Tensor fascia lata
Lower Limb		
Medial compartment muscles of thigh	Lateral compartment muscles of the forearm and hand	Short head of the biceps femoris
Posterior compartment muscles of the thigh except for the short head of the biceps femoris	Latissimus dorsi	Lateral compartment muscles of the leg
Posterior compartment muscles of the leg	Rhomboids	Muscles of the dorsum of the foot
All muscles on the plantar surface of the foot	Levator scapulae	Glutei maximus, medius, and minimus
Obturator internus	Serratus anterior	Piriformis
Gemellus superior and inferior	Teres major and minor	Iliacus
Quadratus femoris	Subscapularis	Psoas
	Supraspinatus (?)	
	Infraspinatus (?)	

Data from Crafts RC. 1985. A Textbook of Human Anatomy. 3rd Ed. Churchill Livingstone, New York.

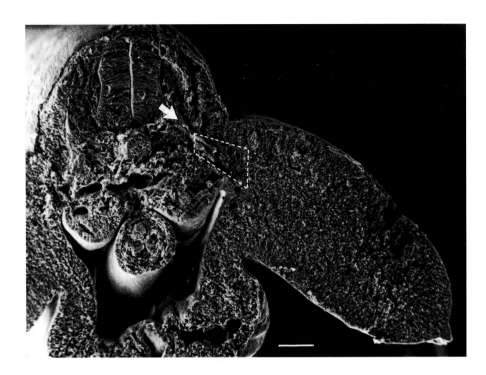

Fig. 11-8. Scanning electron micrograph of a sectioned embryo showing axons entering the limb bud (dotted area). (From Tosney KW, Landmesser LT. 1985. Development of the major pathways for neurite outgrowth in the chick hindlimb. Dev Biol 109:193, with permission.)

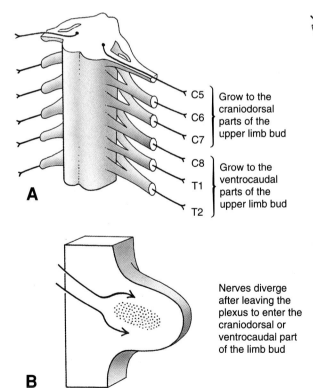

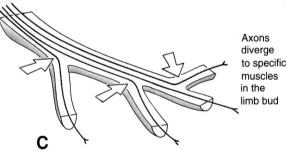

Fig. 11-9. Growth of spinal nerve axons into the limb buds. **(A, B)** Axons grow into the limb buds along permissive pathways. As the axons of the various spinal nerves mingle at the base of the limb buds to form the brachial and lumbosacral plexuses, each axon must "decide" whether to grow into the dorsal or ventral muscle mass. Factors that may play a role in directing axon growth include areas of dense mesenchyme or glycosaminoglycan-containing mesenchyme, which are avoided by outgrowing axons. **(C)** Once the axons grow into the bud, decision points (arrows) under the control of "local factors" may regulate the invasion of specific muscle anlagen by specific axons. (Modified from Tosney K, Landmesser LT. 1984. Pattern and specificity of axonal outgrowth following varying degrees of chick limb bud ablation. J Neurosci 4:2518, with permission.)

Once the motor axons arrive at the base of the limb bud, they mix in a specific pattern to form the **brachial plexus** of the upper limb and the **lumbosacral plexus** of the lower limb. This zone thus constitutes a **decision-making region** for the axons.

Once the axons have sorted out in the plexus, the growth cones continue into the limb bud, presumably traveling along permissive pathways that lead in the general direction of the appropriate muscle compartment. Axons from the dorsal divisions of the plexuses tend to grow into the dorsal side of the limb bud and thus innervate mainly extensors, supinators, and abductors; axons from the ventral divisions of the plexus grow into the ventral side of the limb bud and thus innervate mainly flexors, pronators, and adductors. Over the last part of an axon's path, from the point where it leaves its major nerve trunk to the point where it innervates a specific muscle axonal pathfinding is probably regulated by cues produced by the muscle itself (Fig. 11-9C).

Once the motor axons have found their targets, sensory fibers innervate the sensory end organs in the limbs. The sensory axons apparently grow along the motor axons to the vicinity of the appropriate sensory end or-gans, and then local cues direct them to their respective end organs.

The segmental pattern of limb innervation is complicated by limb bud rotation

As described above, the upper and lower limb buds rotate from their original coronal orientation into a roughly parasagittal orientation. Subsequently (between the sixth and eighth weeks), they also rotate around their long axis. The upper limb rotates slightly laterally so that the elbow points caudally and the original ventral surface of the limb bud becomes the cranial surface of the limb. The lower limb rotates medially so that the knee points cranially and the original ventral surface of the limb bud becomes the caudal surface of the limb. As shown in Figure 11-10, this rotation causes the originally straight segmental pattern of lower limb innervation to twist into a spiral. The rotation of the upper limb is less extreme than that of the lower limb and is accomplished partly through the caudal migration of the shoulder girdle. Moreover, some of the dermatomes in the upper limb bud exhibit overgrowth and come to dominate the limb surface.

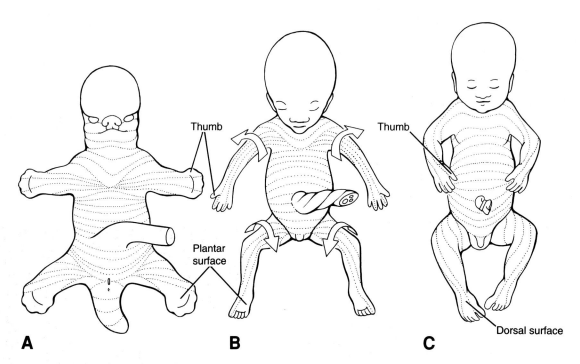

Fig. 11-10. Rotation of the limbs. The dramatic medial rotation of the lower limbs during the sixth to eighth weeks causes the mature dermatomes to spiral down the limb. The configuration of the upper limb dermatomes is partially modified by more limited lateral rotation of the upper limb during the same period.

APPLICATIONS TO CLINICAL PRACTICE

Humans exhibit a wide range of limb defects

Major categories of human limb defects include (1) **reduction defects,** in which part of a limb (**meromelia;** Fig. 11-11A) or an entire limb (**amelia;** Fig. 11-11B) is missing; (2) **duplication defects,** in which supernumerary limb elements are present (**polydactyly** or the presence of extra digits is the most common example; Fig. 11-11C); and (3) **dysplasia,** which includes **syndactyly** or fusion of the digits (Fig. 11-12) and **gigantism,** or excessive growth of parts of the limb. Historically, the nomenclature of limb defects has been somewhat imprecise (Table 11-2), although most limb defects can be attributed to specific causes, including (1) arrest of development; (2) failure of differentiation of component primordia; (3) **homeotic transformations** and duplication of components; (4) hyperplasia; (5) hypoplasia; (6) focal defects such as amniotic band syndrome; and (7) general skeletal abnormalities that incidentally affect the limbs such as **osteogenesis imperfecta.** Limb abnormalities can also be characterized with respect to the part of the limb affected (e.g., limb **segment** [thigh or forearm] or compartment [extensor vs. flexor]). Most human limb defects appear to have a multifactorial basis. In a few cases, familial associations or teratogens are involved. Yet others arise from indirect causes.

Familial associations indicate a genetic basis for some limb abnormalities

Polydactyly and **ectrodactyly** tend to run in families with an autosomal dominant, autosomal recessive, or X-linked pattern of inheritance. Other limb anomalies known to be transmitted as autosomal dominant traits include **partial tibia, general micromelia, triphalangeal thumbs, lobster claw hand and foot** (Fig. 11-3), and the **Adams-Oliver syndrome.** An autosomal recessive disease characterized by the fusion of digits (**syndactyly)**

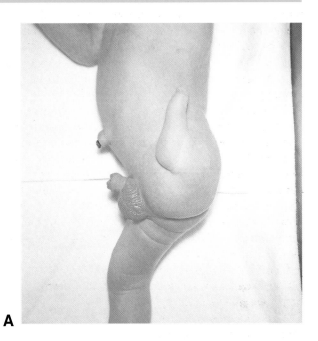

A

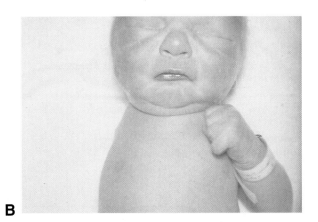

B

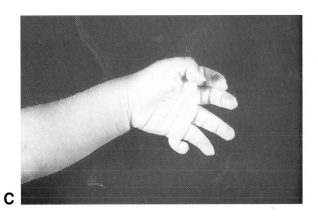

C

Fig. 11-11. (A) Meromelia. In this example, the distal end of a lower limb has not completely formed. (Photo courtesy of Children's Hospital Medical Center, Cincinnati, OH.) **(B)** Amelia. In this example, an entire upper limb failed to form. (Photo courtesy of Children's Hospital Medical Center, Cincinnati, OH.) **(C)** Polydactyly. One of the hands has six digits. (Photo courtesy of Children's Hospital Medical Center, Cincinnati, OH.)

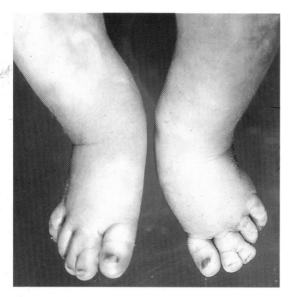

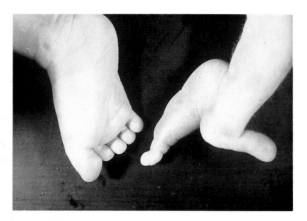

Fig. 11-13. Some limb anomalies, such as lobster claw hand or foot, are sometimes inherited as autosomal dominant traits. (Photo courtesy of Children's Hospital Medical Center, Cincinnati, OH.)

Fig. 11-12. Syndactyly. In this severe case, even the bony elements of digits 2 and 3 are fused together. Less severe cases may exhibit only a web of skin between the digits. (Photo courtesy of Children's Hospital Medical Center, Cincinnati, OH.)

and the **homeotic transformation** of metacarpal and metatarsal segments to carpals and tarsals, respectively, results from mutation of the *HOX* gene *HOXD*13 (Fig. 11-14). Some chromosomal anomalies, such as trisomy 18, cause limb defects.

Environmental teratogens cause limb defects

A variety of drugs, **metabolic poisons,** and other **environmental teratogens** cause limb defects in experimental animals. These include 5′-fluoro-2-deoxyuridine, an inhibitor of thymidylate synthase; acetazolimide, a carbonic

anhydrase inhibitor; and triethyl melamine, an alkylating agent. Cadmium, which inhibits a range of metalloenzymes including carbonic anhydrase, is also known to induce limb deformities in mice and rats. **Hyperthermia,** resulting from febric (fever-causing) disease may also produce limb defects in nonhuman primates. Of particular importance to physicians, however, are the teratogenic effects of therapeutic drugs. Four such drugs known to cause limb defects in animals or humans are **aspirin, dimethadione, retinoic acid,** and **thalidomide.**

The thalidomide incident is a tragic example of drug teratogenicity

The drug **thalidomide** was first marketed as a spasmolytic under the trade name Contergan and was thought to be virtually free of side effects. However, a baby of a man who worked for the manufacturer in West Germany and who had been given free samples for his pregnant wife was born without ears on December 25, 1956. Within a year an epidemic of limb embryopathy began throughout West Germany, and hindsight shows that the incidence of thalidomide-induced embryopathy paralleled thalidomide sales during the next 6 to 7 years, with a lag of about 7 to 8 months (Fig. 11-15). This relationship was apparent in about 20 countries. Malformations included major defects such as amelia and phocomelia (Fig. 11-16) and minor deformities such as hypoplasia of the thumb. Limb malformations were often accompanied by defects such as anotia, duodenal stenosis, and cardiac defects. It is estimated that about 5,850 individuals were affected. About 40 percent of these "thalidomide babies" died soon after birth, leaving 3,900 survivors. Thalido-

Table 11-2.   Some Common Terms for Limb Malformations

TERM	DEFINITION
Meromelia	Absence of part of a limb
Amelia, ectromelia	Absence of one or more limbs
Phocomelia	Short, ill-formed upper or lower limbs—named for their resemblance to the flippers of a seal
Hemimelia	Stunting of distal limb segments
Acrodolichomelia	Disproportionately large hands or feet
Ectrodactyly	Absence of any number of fingers or toes
Polydactyly	Presence of extra digits or parts of digits
Syndactyly	Fusion of digits
Adactyly	Absence of all the digits on a limb

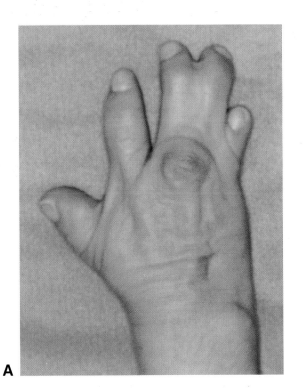

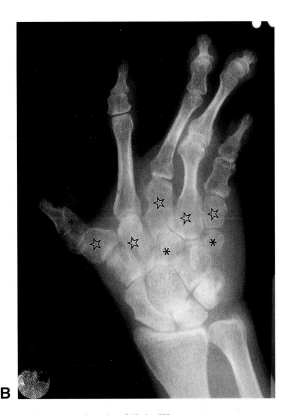

Fig. 11-14. (A) Hand and **(B)** X-ray of homozygous individual. Note syndactyly of digits III, IV, and V, their single knuckle, the transformation of metacarpals I, II, III, and V to short carpal-like bones (stars), two additional carpal bones (asterisks), and short second phalanges. The radius ulna and proximal carpal bones appear normal. (From Muragaki Y, Mundlos S, Upton J et al. 1996. Altered growth and branching patterns in synpolydactyly caused by mutations in *HOXD13*. Science 272:548, with permission.)

mide apparently resulted in limb embryopathies when taken during the sensitive period of limb morphogenesis (4 to 8 weeks).

While realization of thalidomide's teratogenicity in the early 1960s led to prohibitions of its use, limited research has provided insights into its mechanism of action. It is now thought that thalidomide may disrupt cell adhesion in the limb by downregulating cell surface adhesion receptors or by inhibiting angiogenesis. Recent studies have also demonstrated that thalidomide may have many beneficial uses. For example, it has now been utilized in the treatment of autoimmune and inflammatory conditions in humans, including symptoms of **AIDS, lupus erythematosis, leprosy, Jessner-Kanof lymphocytic infiltration of the skin, cutaneous** and **pulmonary sarcoidosis, chronic graft-vs.-host disease).** In Brazil, where leprosy is more common, thalidomide has been used for several years. As a consequence, at least 46 new cases of thalidomide embryopathy have occurred. It is, therefore, most important that physicians be aware of thalidomide's teratogenic potency when treating women of reproductive age.

Limb malformations may result from indirect causes

Occasionally, a band of tissue detaches from the amnion and wraps around part of the embryo, constricting its growth and causing malformations. These **amniotic bands** may amputate or constrict a developing limb or may induce facial dysplasia (Fig. 11-17). It has been argued that related defects may arise by local disruption of vasculature. In other cases, reduction defects may arise because of a constricted uterine environment resulting from oligohydramnios, a bicornate uterus (the consequence of incomplete fusion of the paramesonephric ducts; see Ch. 10), or large benign tumors of the uterine myometrium.

Modern research has also revealed several steps of limb development susceptible to disruption and pathogenesis

The limb bud differentiates with respect to three axes: its own proximodistal axis and the craniocaudal and

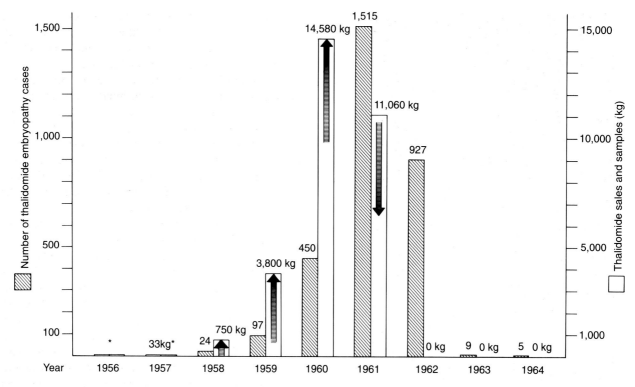

Fig. 11-15. The frequency of limb embryopathy in Germany between 1956 and 1967 compared with the sales of thalidomide. The correlation of thalidomide sales with limb embryopathies strongly indicated the teratogenic role of the drug. *Premarketing samples (low volume of samples in 1956).

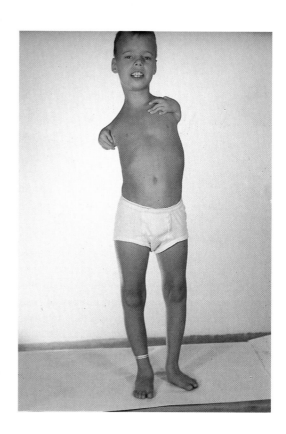

Fig. 11-16. Phocomelia. While phocomelia may be inherited, it was also a common limb defect in offspring of pregnant women who ingested thalidomide. (Photo courtesy of Children's Hospital Medical Center, Cincinnati, OH.)

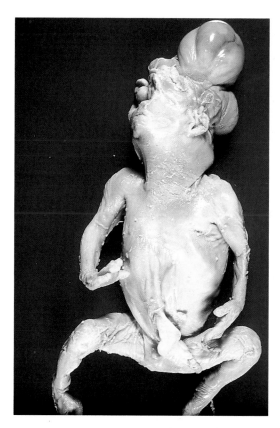

Fig. 11-17. Amniotic band syndrome. Generalized limb defects as well as craniofacial and trunk anomalies may arise when bands of amniotic membrane detach from the chorion and wrap around growing body structures. (Photo courtesy of Children's Hospital Medical Center, Cincinnati, OH.)

dorsoventral axes of the organism (Fig. 11-18). The proximodistal axis defines the sequence of limb segments (shoulder girdle–arm–forearm–wrist–hand/pelvis–thigh–leg–ankle–foot); the craniocaudal axis defines the differ-

entiation of the first digit to the fifth digit; and the dorsoventral axis defines the differentiation of extensor from flexor compartments. Cells in the limb must "know" where they are with respect to all three axes.

For example, **positional signaling** in the **proximodistal axis** is at first dependent on induction of the lateral plate mesoderm within the mesodermal core of the limb by intrinsic signals from adjacent somites and from midline structures, possibly **insulin** and **IGF-I.** Then limb bud outgrowth is maintained by factors produced within the ectoderm of the apical ectodermal ridge (AER) and the mesodermal core itself, especially by members of the **fibroblast growth factor family.**

Amazingly, a bead soaked in fibroblast growth factor-1 (FGF-1), FGF-2, FGF-4, or FGF-8 is able to stimulate development of an entire supernumerary limb within the flank between the orthotopic limbs (Fig. 11-19). Factors diffusing from the AER may also be instrumental in induction of *MSX1* (a homeobox gene), several ***HOX* genes,** and genes encoding the transforming-β superfamily members, bone morphogenetic protein-2 (BMP-2) and BMP-7. BMP-2 and other BMP family members have been implicated in processes of mesenchymal condensation, **chondrogenesis,** and **osteogenesis** in limb bud skeletal elements. Morover, most 5′ members of the *HOXA* and *HOXD* clusters (9 to 13) are expressed in a distal to proximal transcriptional cascade within the growing limb bud and their expression can be correlated with development of specific skeletal elements of upper and lower limb segments (Fig. 11-20). A test of the developmental role of *HOX* gene expression in proximodistal differentiation of the limb is a double knockout of *Hoxa-11* and *Hoxd-11* genes in mice. While disruption of one or the other of these genes has subtle effects on skeletal morphology, the double null mutation of *Hoxa-11* and *Hoxd-11* results in complete absence of the ulna and radius. The relevance of these findings to human

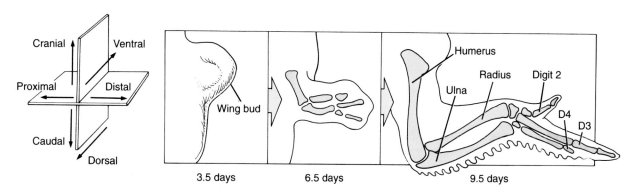

Fig. 11-18. The limb buds of birds and other vertebrates grow with respect to three axes of symmetry: craniocaudal, dorsoventral, and proximodistal. (Modified from Alberts B, Bray D, Lewis J et al. 1983. Molecular Biology of the Cell. Garland, New York, with permission.)

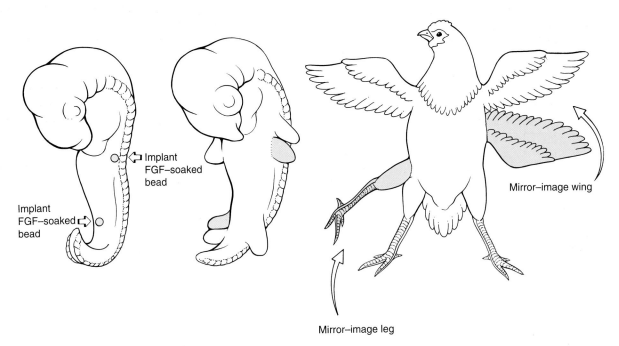

Fig. 11-19. FGF-soaked bead produces supernumerary limb.

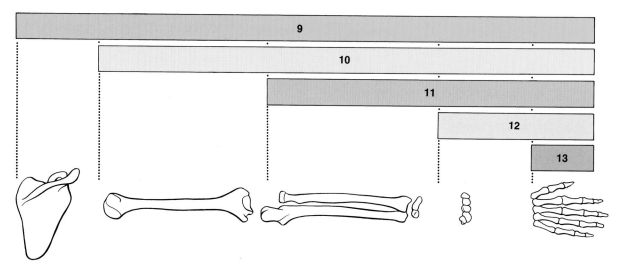

Fig. 11-20. *Hoxd* gene expression patterns in relation to definitive segments of the upper extremity. (Modified from Davis AP, Witte DP, Hsieh-Li HM et al. 1995. Absence of radius and ulna in mice lacking *Hoxa-11* and *Hoxd-11*. Nature. 375:791, with permission.)

clinical practice is illustrated by the spontaneous human mutation of *HOXD13* that results in the **homeotic transformation** described above (see Fig. 11-14).

Craniocaudal differentiation of the limb may require the asymmetric expression of sonic hedgehog

The classic series of experiments on craniocaudal limb differentiation was performed in the 1960s with chick wing buds. When a small piece of tissue was transplanted from the caudal edge of a donor wing bud to the cranial edge of a host wing bud, the cranial half of the wing bud formed extra digits that were the mirror image of the normal digits on the caudal half of the wing bud (Fig. 11-21). It was proposed that the transplanted tissue fragment produced a morphogenetic substance or **morphogen** that diffused to form a gradient across the wing bud and determined which digit would be produced in which position: a high morphogen gradient would induce digit 4, while

progressively lower concentrations would induce digits 3 and 2 (digits 1 and 5 do not form in chicken wings).

The caudal tissue region responsible for this digit-determining activity was called the **zone of polarizing activity (ZPA;** Fig. 11-21). The search for the polarizing signal molecule expressed specifically within the ZPA at first led to **retinoic acid,** since a retinoic acid-soaked bead implanted in the cranial edge of the limb bud was able to induce **mirror polydactyly** (Fig. 11-22; and see below). However, a more definitive candidate for the polarizing function of the ZPA is the protein **sonic hedgehog (Shh),** a factor identified in avian and mammalian embryos and mapped to human chromosome 7q (see Chs. 3, 4, and 9). Indeed, in chicks and mice, limb bud Shh is normally expressed only within the limb bud within the caudal region of the limb bud mesenchyme, in the region of the ZPA. Moreover, Shh is expressed at the cranial edge of the inverted limb buds ectopically induced with an FGF-4-soaked bead (Fig. 11-23A). Shh is also expressed at both caudal and cranial edges of limb buds in

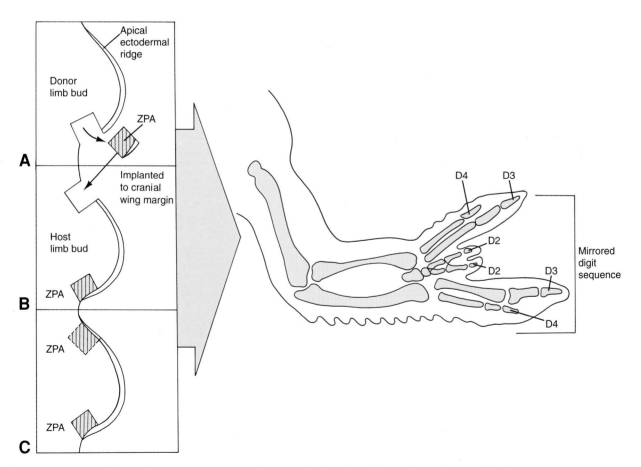

Fig. 11-21. Transplantation of the zone of polarizing activity (ZPA) of one limb bud to the cranial edge of another will induce mirror polydactyly. (Modified from Alberts B, Bray D, Lewis J et al. 1983. Molecular Biology of the Cell. Garland, New York, with permission.)

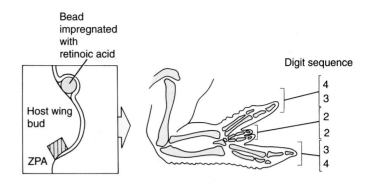

Bead impregnated with retinoic acid

Host wing bud

ZPA

Digit sequence

4
3
2
2
3
4

Fig. 11-22. Transplantation of a retinoic-acid-soaked bead to the cranial edge of a chick wing bud induces mirror polydactyly. (Modified from Eichele G, Tickle C, Alberts BM. 1984. Micro-controlled release of biologically active compounds in chick embryos: beads of 200 μm diameter for the local release of retinoids. Anal Biochem 142:542, with permission.)

Luxoid mouse mutants, a mouse characterized by **mirror-image polydactyly** (Fig. 11-23B). Results of experiments involving implantation of the FGF-4-soaked beads, just described, support the idea that FGF-4 from the AER induces Shh expression in the mesenchyme of the ZPA.

As in regulation of proximodistal patterning, the mechanism by which Shh then mediates the development of the normal **craniocaudal patterning** of the limb, especially with respect to **differentiation of the digits,** may also involve BMP and *Hox* gene expression. For example, the

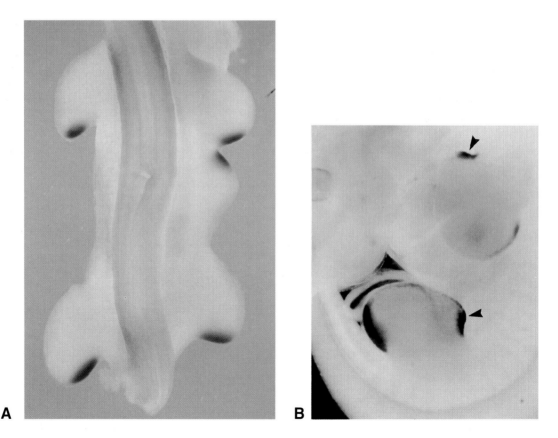

A

B

Fig. 11-23. (A) Whole mount in situ hybridization (shh mRNA) shows Shh expression in a chick embryo 48 hours after application of an FGF-2 bead similar to that in Figure 2 in Cohn et al (1995). Cell 80:739. (With permission from Martin J. Cohn.) **(B)** In situ hybridization showing both Shh and FGF-4 mRNA in normal caudal ZPA at ectopic location (arrow heads). (From Chan DC, Laufer E, Tabin C, Leder P. 1995. Polydactylous limbs in Strong's Luxoid mice result from ectopic polarizing activity. Development 121:1971.)

expression of specific *Hox* genes in chick limbs is also correlated with development of individual digits within the developing wing and leg (Fig. 11-24). In addition, Shh is able to activate these *Hox* genes. The possible clinical relevance of these findings is illustrated by the **disruptions of digit formation** that occur in humans harboring a mutation of *Hoxd-13* (Fig. 11-14).

While a role for BMP-4 has not been well-defined in craniocaudal patterning, this member of the BMP family and its receptor apparently play a pivotal role in **separating the digits.** The developing digits are first revealed as radial thickenings within the hand and foot plates. The separation of the differentiating digits from one another is facilitated by programmed cell death (apoptosis) within necrotic zones between the digital rays. This localized apoptosis may be under the control of bone BMPs. For example, when the function of BMP receptors is disrupted, apoptosis fails to occur, and the chick foot remains webbed like that of a duck (Fig. 11-25A, B). The possibility that BMPs may be disrupted in **syndactyly** in humans has not been directly demonstrated but is suggested by these findings.

The dorsoventral differentiation of the limb bud is regulated by Wnt-7a

Function of the cell surface- and extracellular matrix-associated Wnt family member Wnt-7a in dorsoventral differentiation of the limbs is implied by its restricted expression within the dorsal limb bud ectoderm. Moreover, if the ectodermal covering of the limb bud is surgically

reversed, dorsoventral polarity of the skeletal elements is reversed. Consistent with this observation, striking dorsal-to-ventral transformations of the paw are exhibited in null mutants of mice in which the gene expressing Wnt-7a is disrupted. While ventral structures remain relatively normal, the dorsal side of the paw assumes ventral characteristics. Apparently, the dorsoventral signaling mechanism must involve factors other than Wnt-7a, however, since only the paw is affected in this knockout. Indeed, Wnt-7a has been shown to induce the expression of *Lmx-1*, a *Lim* homeobox gene, and thus to dorsalize the limb bud in a manner similar to dorsalization of the embryo as a whole (see Ch. 3). Moreover, ectopic expression of *Lmx-1* is able to dorsalize the limb, showing that this homeobox gene mediates the dorsalizing signal expressed by Wnt-7a within the dorsal ectoderm.

While the role of retinoic acid in patterning of the limb is controversial, its actions are clinically significant

Vitamin A-induced limb defects were first described decades ago, and in the early 1970s the teratogenic effects of excess retinoic acid became apparent and have been verified many times throughout the intervening years. It seems likely that vitamin A and many of its biologically active analogs behave as teratogens. Indeed, as noted, the finding that implicated vitamin A in ZPA activity supported the possibility that it even acted as an endogenous morphogen in limb development (see Fig. 11-21). However, careful measurements of concentrations of several

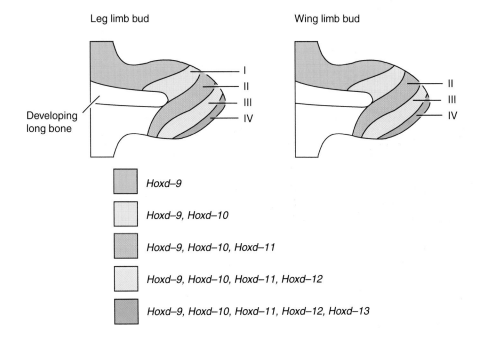

Fig. 11-24. *Hoxd* gene expression patterns in foot plate and "hand" plate of chick leg and wing buds, respectively. Note how territories of *Hoxd* gene expressions define the territories of future digits I, II, III, and IV in the foot plate and II, III, and IV in the "hand" plate. (Modified from Morgan BA, Tabin C. 1994. *Hox* genes and growth: early and late roles in limb bud morphogenesis. Development (suppl) 181, with permission.)

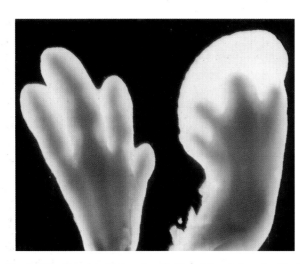

Fig. 11-25. Normal chicken foot (left) and foot infected with the mutant *BMPR-1B* gene at stage 14. (From Zou H, Niswander L. 1996. Requirement for BMP signaling in interdigital apoptosis and scale formation. Science 272:738, with permission.)

bioactive forms of vitamin A and cytoplasmic retinoic acid binding proteins in chickens and mice have produced equivocal results. Moreover, transgenic knockouts of many of these factors have produced such inconsistent results that presently a functional relationship between free vitamin A concentrations and craniocaudal patterning of the limb is enigmatic. However, it must be emphasized that, as controversial as the role of vitamin A may be in normal limb development, the evidence strongly implicates this factor in congenital pathogenetic malformation of the limbs and many other organs. As a consequence, vitamin A intake by pregnant mothers should not be deficient or excessive. Moreover, physicians must carefully consider the teratogenicity of retinoic acid and related compounds when treating women of reproductive age with medications containing these substances.

12

Development of the Head, the Neck, and the Eyes and Ears

Formation of the Skull; Differentiation of the Pharyngeal Arch Cartilages, Muscles, and Nerves; Development of the Tongue and Pharyngeal Pouch Derivatives; Morphogenesis of the Face; Development of the Eyes; Development of the Ears

The human skull is composed of three major skeletal elements; (1) a **chondrocranium** or **neurocranium** with **sensory capsules,** (2) the **cranial vault,** and (3) the **facial skeleton.** The chondrocranium is homologous to the primitive brain housing of the jawless fishes; the facial skeleton develops within the **pharyngeal arches,** which descend from the gill (branchial) arches of the jawed fishes; and the cranial vault is modified from the secondary skeletal armor of a line of bony fishes. The chondrocranium is formed from paraxial mesoderm while the cranial vault and facial skeleton are derived from neural crest.

Many craniofacial abnormalities involve these skeletal elements. For example, the sutures between the membrane bones of the skull may fuse prematurely **(craniosynostosis),** resulting in deformation of the skull and compression of the cerebrum. Other craniofacial malformations result from anomalous development of the five pairs of pharyngeal arches that form in humans. Arch-related abnormalities may be heritable or induced by teratogens, such as retinoic acid or its bioactive analogs. The disruption of neural crest cell migration directly affects the development of facial skeletal elements. However, abnormal migration of neural crest indirectly influences development of arch-specific aortic arch arteries and striated muscles derived from somitomeres and occipital somites. Abnormal development of the cranial nerves that characterize each arch as well as glandular derivatives of the **pharyngeal pouches** and the thyroid gland, which forms from the endodermal mucosa of the tongue, may also occur. Effects of retinoic acid are mediated by disruptions of the combinatorial *HOX* gene codes that specify the unique development of each arch.

The face develops from five swellings, including the paired **maxillary** and **mandibular swellings** of the first pharyngeal arch. The fifth component is the large **frontonasal prominence.** Normally these swellings, or processes derived from them, fuse together during development of the face. Anomalies of the fusion process result in abnormal **facial clefts,** including **cleft lip** and **cleft palate.** The most common facial abnormality, however, is the **holoprosencephalic** spectrum of anomalies that includes **fetal alcohol syndrome (FAS).** FAS is thought to be the single most common cause of mental retardation in the Western world and apparently results from disturbances in development of the forebrain, predominantly by alcohol, in the third week. The holoprosencephalic spectrum of anomalies also affects midfacial development, resulting in microcephaly or lack of the philtrum, a single nostril, and hypotelorism (close-set eyes) or cyclopia. While holoprosencephalic anomalies are most often caused by alcohol, they may also be heritable, as in **Meckel syndrome.**

Many of the craniofacial anomalies described in this chapter can be induced by therapeutic drugs such as isotretinoin (used for treatment of acne), by the anticonvulsant phenytoin (dilantin), or from alcohol consumption. They are, therefore, readily preventable.

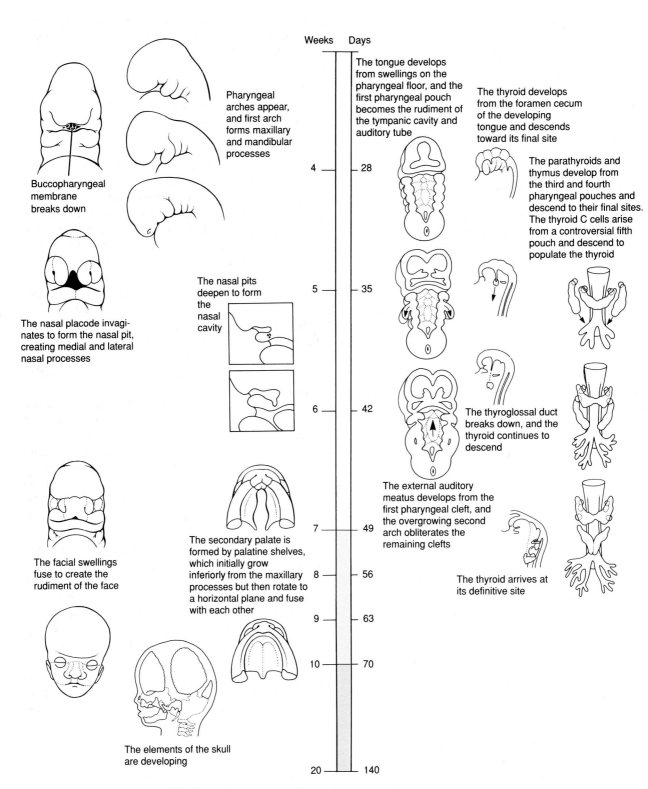

Weeks   Days

Buccopharyngeal membrane breaks down

Pharyngeal arches appear, and first arch forms maxillary and mandibular processes

The nasal placode invaginates to form the nasal pit, creating medial and lateral nasal processes

The nasal pits deepen to form the nasal cavity

The facial swellings fuse to create the rudiment of the face

The secondary palate is formed by palatine shelves, which initially grow inferiorly from the maxillary processes but then rotate to a horizontal plane and fuse with each other

The elements of the skull are developing

The tongue develops from swellings on the pharyngeal floor, and the first pharyngeal pouch becomes the rudiment of the tympanic cavity and auditory tube

The thyroid develops from the foramen cecum of the developing tongue and descends toward its final site

The parathyroids and thymus develop from the third and fourth pharyngeal pouches and descend to their final sites. The thyroid C cells arise from a controversial fifth pouch and descend to populate the thyroid

The thyroglossal duct breaks down, and the thyroid continues to descend

The external auditory meatus develops from the first pharyngeal cleft, and the overgrowing second arch obliterates the remaining clefts

The thyroid arrives at its definitive site

4 — 28
5 — 35
6 — 42
7 — 49
8 — 56
9 — 63
10 — 70
20 — 140

Timeline. Development of the head, neck, and pharyngeal structure.

Development of the Head and Neck

A head and neck specialized for active predation arose during early vertebrate evolution: our progenitors had small and simple heads

The vertebrates arose from a group of simple, filter-feeding aquatic organisms called **protochordates.** A prominent structure of living protochordates is the expanded **pharyngeal chamber** used in filter feeding. This chamber is supported by a cartilaginous **branchial basket.** Water and suspended food particles are drawn into the pharynx through the mouth; the water is expelled through **gill pores** or **gill slits** located on either side of the pharynx; and the edible particles proceed down the gut tube.

Some other characteristic vertebrate features—particularly the presence of a notochord, segmented axial musculature, and a head—probably developed in response to the active life of larval protochordates.

The most primitive vertebrates, the **jawless fishes (agnathans),** do not have a movable jaw. Most extinct forms appear to have been filter feeders or detritus feeders (Fig. 12-1A), although the living forms, the lamprey and hagfishes, pursue specialized blood-sucking and scavenging modes of life. The brain of agnathans (which is large compared with that of protochordates) is cradled in a bony or cartilaginous **chondrocranium,** which is connected to the persistent notochord as well as to the newly developed spinal column (Fig. 12-1A). The branchial skeleton supports the **branchial bars (gill bars)** between the gill slits or gill pores and is also anchored to the chondrocranium. The gill bars bear gills in which the blood is oxygenated, and each is therefore served by a **branchial arch artery** (see below and Ch. 8).

In an extinct line of fishes, the first gill bar became hinged and eventually was transformed into a pair of upper and lower jaws (Fig. 12-1B). This innovation made possible the pursuit and capture of living prey. The improvements to the sensory and propulsive apparatus necessitated by this new mode of life made additional demands on the brain, which progressively enlarged. All these developments together laid the foundations for the evolution of the familiar human head and neck.

The human skull is composed of distinct groups of bones derived from discrete evolutionary precursors

The cranial skeleton of fishes is composed of (1) the **chondrocranium,** which encloses the brain and helps to form the **sensory capsules** that support the olfactory organs, eyes, and inner ears; (2) an external armor of **membrane (dermal) bones;** and (3) the **visceral skeleton** or **viscerocranium** that supports the gill bars and jaws. These components can still be distinguished in the genesis of the human skull (Fig. 12-1C, D).

The brain is cradled in the chondrocranium and roofed by the membrane bones of the skull vault

The chondrocranium of primitive fishes is the forerunner of the human **skull base.** In humans, as in fishes, the chondrocranium develops from three pairs of cartilaginous precursors—the **prechordal cartilages (trabeculae cranii),** the **hypophyseal cartilages,** and the **parachordal cartilages**—which are arranged in series and underlie the brain from the interorbitonasal region to the cranial end of the vertebral column (Fig. 12-2A). The caudalmost pair of elements, the parachordal cartilages, are derived from the occipital sclerotomes plus the first cervical sclerotome and thus represent modified vertebral elements (see Ch. 4). The cranial two pairs of elements appear to be derived mostly from neural crest. The bones of the chondrocranium (as the name indicates) are preformed in cartilage and ossify by the process of **endochondral ossification** (see Ch. 11).

The membrane-bone armor that covers the skull of our piscene ancestors (bony fishes) is represented in humans by the membrane bones of the skull, comprising the flat bones of the **cranial vault** or **calvaria,** as well as many bones of the face (Fig. 12-1C, D). These bones grow by the direct ossification of mesenchyme in the presumptive dermis and therefore are not preformed in cartilage. The mesenchyme from which they develop is derived from neural crest.

The bones of the cranial vault do not complete their growth during fetal life. The soft, fibrous sutures that join them at birth permit the skull vault to deform as it passes through the birth canal and also allow it to continue growing throughout infancy and childhood. Six large, membrane-covered **fontanelles** occupy the areas between the corners of cranial vault bones at birth (Fig. 12-3). The posterior fontanelle closes by 3 months after birth, but the anterior fontanelle normally remains open until 1.5 years of age. Palpation of this fontanelle can be used to detect elevated intracranial pressure or premature closure of the skull sutures.

The special sense organs are protected by sensory capsules

As the simple sense organs of the protochordates gave way to the more sophisticated olfactory, ocular, and auditory/vestibular systems of the vertebrates, three pairs of skeletal capsules evolved to house and protect these organs. In humans these capsules are formed from por-

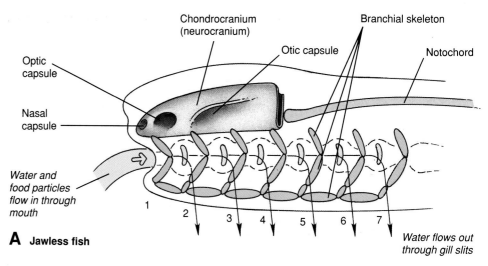

A Jawless fish

Fig. 12-1. The evolutionary origin of the human skull from the pharyngeal arch skeleton, braincase, and dermal bones of primitive vertebrates. (**A, B**) The pharyngeal arches of humans are modified from the gill apparatus (branchial arches) of primitive vertebrates. The skeletal elements of the gill bars formed the foundation for the development of the human jaw and neck skeleton. (**C, D**) The expanding brain in the line of fishes leading to humans was housed in a cranium formed partly by the chondrocranium and partly by membrane bones derived from the dermis. Membrane bones also form a large part of the highly modified facial skeleton of humans.

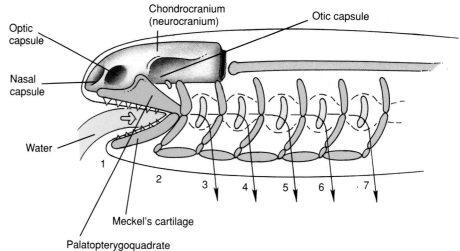

B Primitive jawed fish

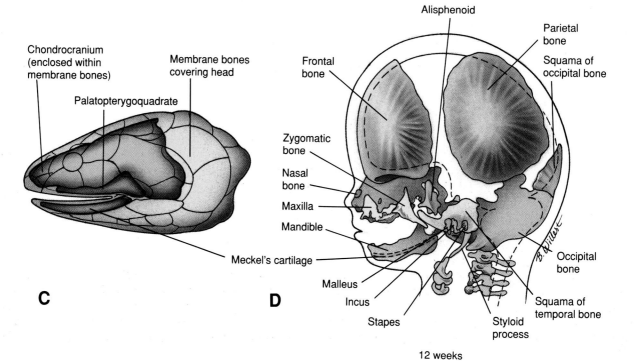

C

D

12 weeks

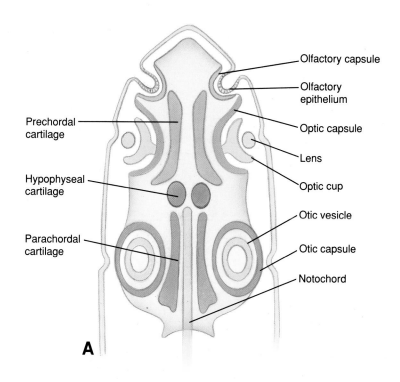

Olfactory capsule

Olfactory epithelium

Optic capsule

Lens

Optic cup

Otic vesicle

Otic capsule

Notochord

Prechordal cartilage

Hypophyseal cartilage

Parachordal cartilage

A

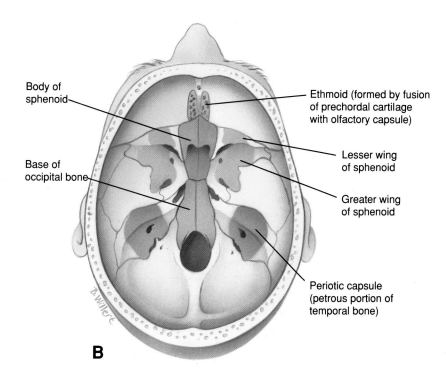

Body of sphenoid

Base of occipital bone

Ethmoid (formed by fusion of prechordal cartilage with olfactory capsule)

Lesser wing of sphenoid

Greater wing of sphenoid

Periotic capsule (petrous portion of temporal bone)

B

Fig. 12-2. The base of the skull in humans is derived from three pairs of cartilaginous plates formed in early ancestors: the prechordal, hypophyseal, and parachordal cartilages. Sensory capsules became increasingly complex throughout evolutionary history.

tions of the prechordal and hypophyseal cartilages and from bones derived from elements of the primitive capsules of evolutionary ancestors (Fig. 12-2). The nasal capsules of humans include the **ethmoid** bone, derived from the prechordal cartilages, and the **nasal** and **turbinate** bones. The human orbit includes the body of the sphenoid bone, which is derived from the hypophyseal cartilages, and the greater and lesser wings of the sphenoids. The otic capsules of humans are descendants of primitive otic capsule ossification centers, which fuse

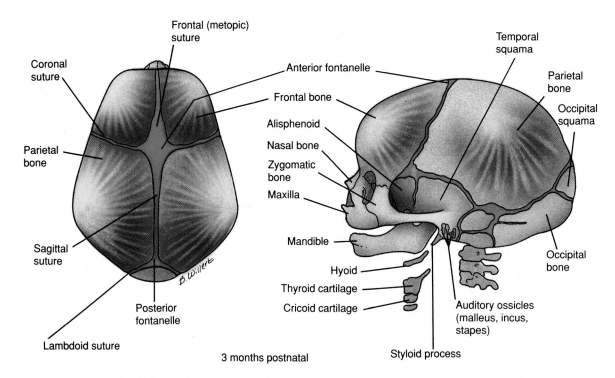

Fig. 12-3. The brain in humans is mostly enclosed by the dermal bones of the cranial vault. These bones do not fuse together until early childhood. The unfused sutures allow the cranium to deform during birth and to expand during childhood as the brain grows.

together into a single mass called the **periotic** or **petromastoid bone.**

The sensory capsules arise from cranial somitomeres, occipital somites and neural crest.

Much of the human face and neck is derived from the ancient gill apparatus

The jawless fishes improved the respiratory and filter-feeding systems of the protochordates by transforming the rigid branchial basket into a series of movable gill bars on either side of the pharynx. These arches still develop embryonically in all vertebrates. In jawed vertebrates, the first arch gives rise to the upper and lower jaws. The remaining arches form the gills in fishes and many structures of the face and neck in humans.

Each embryonic arch (branchial or pharyngeal) consists of a mesodermal core lined on the outside with ectoderm and on the inside with endoderm (Fig. 12-4D). Each contains a central cartilaginous skeletal element, striated muscle anlagen innervated by an arch-specific cranial nerve, and an aortic arch artery. In fishes, the blood pumped out of the single ventricle is distributed to the arch arteries and thence to the capillary beds of the gills. The blood is oxygenated in the gills by the water flowing through the gill slits and then reenters the dorsal portion of the arch artery for distribution to the body via the dorsal aortae (see Fig. 8-2).

In jawed fishes, forcible expansion of the pharyngeal cavity is often used to suck prey into the mouth. Thus, the branchial arches of jawed fishes, like those of filter-feeding jawless fishes, may function in feeding as well as respiration. The pharyngeal arches of humans also participate in both these functions: they give rise, for example, to the jaws and the muscles of chewing and swallowing. Other human pharyngeal arch derivatives have been adapted to the new function of communication: the second arch contributes to the muscles of facial expression, and the fourth and sixth arches contribute to the tongue and larynx, which are used in vocalization.

The five human pharyngeal arches form in craniocaudal sequence. The pharyngeal arches of human embryos initially resemble the gill arches of fish except that the gill slits never become perforated. Instead, the external **pharyngeal clefts** between the arches remain separated from the apposed, internal **pharyngeal pouches** by thin **pharyngeal membranes.** These membranes are three layered, consisting of ectoderm, mesoderm, and endoderm.

Although the number of branchial arches is somewhat variable among the fishes, the five pharyngeal arches that develop in human embryos correspond to numbers 1, 2, 3, 4, and 6 of the primitive complement in the evolutionary line leading to land vertebrates. Arch 5 either never forms in humans or forms as a short-lived rudiment and promptly regresses. The pharyngeal arches form in craniocaudal succession (Fig. 12-4A–C): the first arch appears on day 22; the second and third arches appear sequentially on day 24; and the fourth and sixth arches appear sequentially on day 29. Table 12-1 summarizes the origin and fate of the skeletal element,

artery, muscles, and cranial nerve of each of the pharyngeal arches.

The skeletal elements of the pharyngeal arches are derived from midbrain and hindbrain neural crest or from lateral plate mesoderm. Most of the cartilages that form within the pharyngeal arches develop from the neural crest of the midbrain and hindbrain regions, although the cartilages of arches 4 and 6 apparently develop

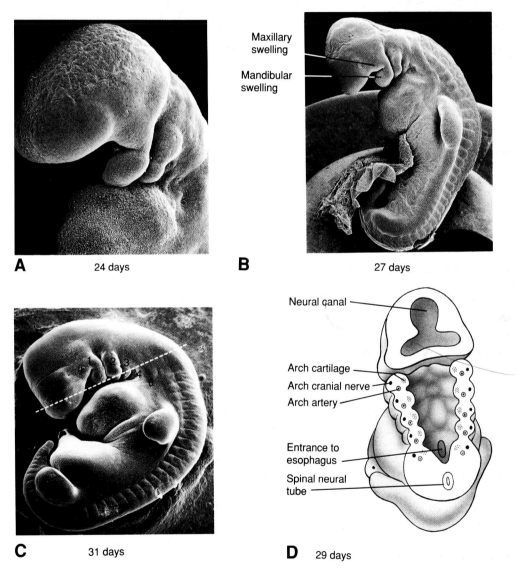

A   24 days

Maxillary swelling
Mandibular swelling

B   27 days

C   31 days

Neural canal

Arch cartilage
Arch cranial nerve
Arch artery

Entrance to esophagus
Spinal neural tube

D   29 days

Fig. 12-4. Formation of the pharyngeal arches. The pharyngeal arches form in craniocaudal sequence during the fourth and fifth weeks. (**A**) By day 24, the first two arches have formed. (**B**) By day 27, the first three arches have formed, and the left first arch is visibly divided into maxillary and mandibular swellings. (**C**) By the early fifth week, all five arches have formed. The dashed line indicates the plane of the section shown (at a slightly earlier stage) in Fig. D. (**D**) Schematic cross section through the pharyngeal arches, showing the cartilage, artery, and cranial nerve in each arch. (Figs. A and B photos courtesy of Dr. Arnold Tamarin.)

Table 12-1. The Derivatives of the Pharyngeal Arches and Their Tissues of Origin

PHARYNGEAL ARCH	ARCH ARTERY[a]	SKELETAL ELEMENTS	MUSCLES	CRANIAL NERVE[b]
1	Terminal branch of maxillary artery	Derived from arch cartilages (originating from neural crest): From maxillary cartilage: alisphenoid, incus From mandibular (Meckel's) cartilage: malleus Derived by direct ossification from arch dermal mesenchyme: maxilla, zygomatic, squamous portion of temporal bone, mandible	Muscles of mastication (temporalis, masseter, and pterygoids), myelohyoid, anterior belly of the digastric, tensor tympani, tensor veli palatini (originate from cranial somitomere 4)	Maxillary and mandibular division of trigeminal nerve (V)
2	Stapedial artery (embryonic), corticotympanic artery (adult)	Stapes, styloid process, stylohyoid ligament, lesser horns and upper rim of hyoid (derived from the second-arch [Reichert's] cartilage; originate from neural crest)	Muscles of facial expression (orbicularis oculi, orbicularis oris, risorius, platysma, auricularis, fronto-occipitalis, and buccinator), posterior belly of the digastric, stylohyoid, stapedius (originate from cranial somitomere 6)	Facial nerve (VII)
3	Common carotid artery, root of internal carotid	Lower rim and greater horns of hyoid (derived from the third-arch cartilage; originate from neural crest)	Stylopharyngeus (originate from cranial somitomere 7)	Glossopharyngeal nerve (IX)
4	Arch of aorta, right subclavian artery; original sprouts of pulmonary arteries	Laryngeal cartilages (derived from the fourth-arch cartilage; originate from lateral plate mesoderm)	Constrictors of pharynx, cricothyroid, levator veli palatini (originates from occipital somites 2 to 4)	Superior laryngeal branch of vagus nerve (X)
6	Ductus arteriosus; roots of definitive pulmonary arteries	Laryngeal cartilages (derived from the sixth-arch cartilage; originate from lateral plate mesoderm)	Intrinsic muscles of larynx (originate from occipital somites 1 and 2)	Recurrent laryngeal branch of vagus nerve (X)

[a]See Chapter 8 for a thorough discussion of aortic arch artery development.

[b]See Chapter 13 for a thorough discussion of the cranial nerves.

from lateral plate mesoderm. As discussed in Chapter 5, the neural crest in the trunk region migrates mainly by the active movement of the neural crest cells. The neural crest of the cranial region also tends to migrate passively along with the displacement of the surrounding tissue.

Figure 12-5 shows the skeletal elements derived from each arch. All the bones that develop from the pharyngeal arch cartilages themselves are endochondral. Some of these cartilages in humans, however, become completely encased within membrane bones that form by the direct ossification of dermal mesenchyme (also of neural crest origin).

In mammals, the first arch gives rise to the incus and malleus of the middle ear and to the endochon-

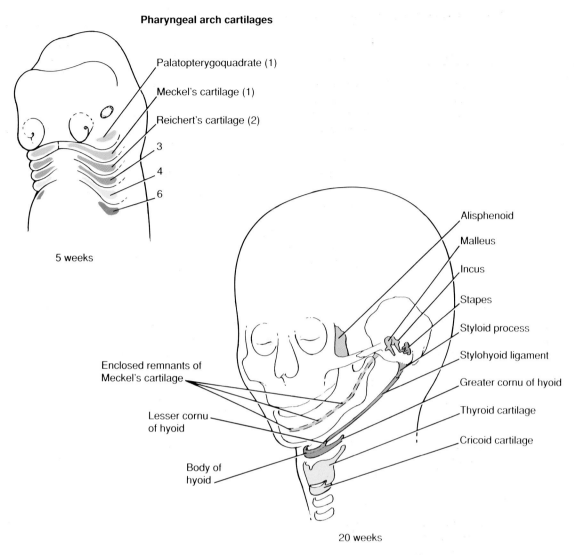

Pharyngeal arch cartilages

Palatopterygoquadrate (1)

Meckel's cartilage (1)

Reichert's cartilage (2)

3

4

6

5 weeks

Alisphenoid

Malleus

Incus

Stapes

Styloid process

Stylohyoid ligament

Greater cornu of hyoid

Thyroid cartilage

Cricoid cartilage

Enclosed remnants of
Meckel's cartilage

Lesser cornu
of hyoid

Body of
hyoid

20 weeks

Fig. 12-5. Fate of the pharyngeal arch cartilages. These cartilages give rise to a small bone of the orbit, to elements of the jaw skeleton, to the three auditory ossicles, and to the hyoid and laryngeal skeleton.

dral and dermal bones of the upper and lower jaw. As the first pharyngeal arch develops, it is remodeled to form a cranial **maxillary swelling** and a caudal **mandibular swelling** (Fig. 12-4A–C). These processes give rise to the upper and lower jaws, respectively. Each process contains a central cartilaginous element. The central cartilages are produced by neural crest cells arising in the region of the embryonic midbrain (mesencephalon) and cranial portion of the hindbrain (metencephalon). The central cartilages of the maxillary swellings are called **palatopterygoquadrate bars,** and the central cartilages of the mandibular swellings are called **Meckel's cartilages.**

In humans and other mammals, the jaws consist almost entirely of membrane bones that ensheathe some of the cartilages of the first arch and therefore receive little con-

tribution from the viscerocranium (Fig. 12-1D). Instead, the first-arch cartilages of mammals give rise mainly to two ossicles of the middle ear: the maxillary cartilage forms the **incus,** and the mandibular cartilage forms the **malleus.** The maxillary cartilage also gives rise to a small bone called the **alisphenoid** located in the orbital wall, which represents a remnant of the old endochondral upper jaw. A small remnant of Meckel's cartilage can be distinguished in the core of the mandible. The maxilla, zygomatic, temporal squamosa, and most of the mandible are all membrane bones.

The temporomandibular joint is a mammalian invention. There is a curious reason why the incus and malleus bones of the mammalian middle ear form from the first-arch cartilage. In all jawed vertebrates except mammals, the jaw joint is formed by endochondral bones developing from the maxillary and mandibular cartilages, even though other portions of the jaw may be made of membrane bones. Among the immediate ancestors of mammals, however, a second, novel jaw articulation developed between two membrane bones: the mandible and the temporal squamosa. As this new **temporomandibular joint** became dominant, the bones of the ancient endochondral jaw articulation shifted into the adjacent middle ear and joined with the preexisting stapes to form the unique three-ossicle auditory mechanism of mammals.

There is some dispute as to how the temporomandibular joint develops in the embryo. Some researchers believe that the joint forms within a single mesenchymal condensation that differentiates into temporal and mandibular portions in response to a morphogenetic field. Other workers report that the joint forms from two mesenchymal condensations—a **temporal** or **glenoid blastema** associated with the temporal bone and a **condylar blastema** associated with the mandible—which slowly grow to meet each other. The joint forms between the 7th and 11th weeks, and it is thought that temporomandibular joint malformations may be caused by teratogens acting during this sensitive period.

The second-arch cartilage has evolved to support the jaw, tongue, and larynx and also gives rise to the stapes. After the jaws evolved, the second-arch cartilage was recruited as a bracing element to help support them. This function is still detectable in humans. The human second-arch cartilage, called **Reichert's cartilage,** undergoes endochondral ossification to form the **stapes** of the middle ear, the **styloid process** of the temporal bone, the fibrous **stylohyoid ligament,** and the **lesser horns (cornua)** and upper rim of the **hyoid** bone (Fig. 12-5). The hyoid bone is stabilized by muscle attachments to the styloid process and mandible and, through its muscular attachments to the larynx and the tongue, serves in both swallowing and vocalization. Reichert's cartilage is formed from neural crest cells derived from the cranial end of the myelencephalon (the caudal subdivision of the rhombencephalon).

The third pharyngeal arch also contributes to the hyoid. The cartilage of the third arch develops from neural crest cells that originate in the midregion of the myelencephalon. It ossifies endochondrally to form the **greater horns** (cornua) and **lower rim** of the **hyoid** bone (Fig. 12-5).

The fourth and sixth arches contribute to the larynx. The mesoderm of the fourth and sixth arches together gives rise to the larynx, consisting of the **thyroid,** **cuneiform, corniculate, arytenoid,** and **cricoid** cartilages (Fig. 12-5). These cartilages are formed from lateral plate mesoderm rather than from neural crest. The development of the larynx begins in the fifth week as a pair of mesodermal condensations called the **arytenoid swellings** form in the region of the sixth arch. These condensations begin to chondrify in the early seventh week to form the arytenoid cartilages. The chondrification of the thyroid and cricoid cartilages begins at about the same time, and late in the seventh week the cuneiform and corniculate cartilages begin to form.

The epiglottis develops at the location of the fourth arch but may not form from pharyngeal arch mesoderm. The **epiglottal cartilages** do not appear until the fifth month, long after the other pharyngeal arch cartilages have formed. This fact supports the view that the epiglottal cartilages develop from mesenchyme that immigrates into the fourth-arch area long after the arch itself has differentiated. Other studies, however, have detected mesodermal condensations within an epiglottal swelling of the fourth arch as early as the sixth week, raising the possibility that the chondrification of this cartilage is merely greatly delayed relative to the other arch cartilages.

The third aortic arch arteries give rise to vessels that supply the head and neck

In human embryos, as in fishes, the arch artery system initially takes the form of a basketlike arrangement of five pairs of arteries, which arise from the expansion at the end of the truncus arteriosus called the **aortic sac** and pass through the pharyngeal arches to empty into the paired dorsal aortae (Fig. 12-6).

Arterial blood reaches the head via paired vertebral arteries that form from intersegmental artery anastomoses and via the **common carotid** arteries. The common carotid arteries branch to form the **internal** and **external carotid arteries.** The common carotids and the roots of the internal carotids are derived from the third-arch arteries, whereas the distal portions of the internal carotids are derived from the cranial extensions of the paired dorsal aortae (see also Fig. 8-3). The external carotid arteries sprout de novo from the common carotids. The endothelium of the head vasculature and aortic arch arteries is derived from paraxial mesoderm.

The paraxial mesoderm of each pharyngeal arch gives rise to functionally related muscles

The musculature of the pharyngeal arches is derived from the paraxial mesoderm of the somitomeres and oc-

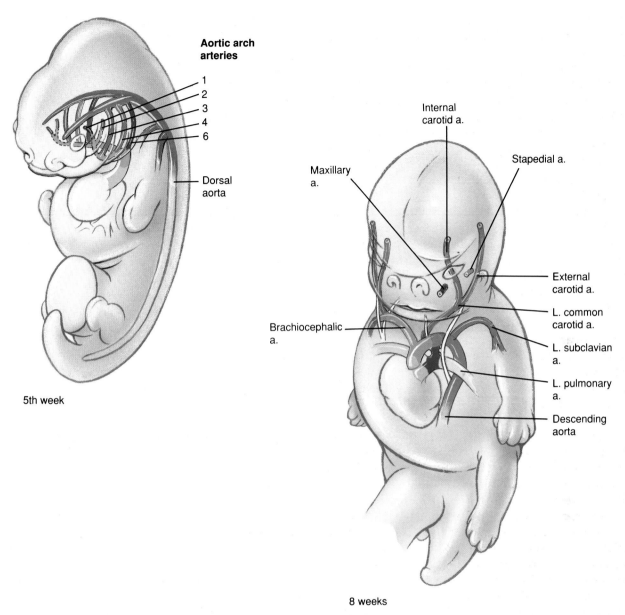

Aortic arch arteries

1
2
3
4
6

Dorsal aorta

5th week

Internal carotid a.

Maxillary a.

Stapedial a.

External carotid a.

L. common carotid a.

Brachiocephalic a.

L. subclavian a.

L. pulmonary a.

Descending aorta

8 weeks

Fig. 12-6. Fate of the pharyngeal arch arteries. These arteries are modified to form definitive arteries of the upper thorax, neck, and head (see Ch. 8).

cipital somites. The muscles that form in each arch are innervated by a cranial nerve branch specific to that arch, and each muscle drags its nerve behind it as it migrates. Thus, even though the pharyngeal arch muscles intermingle as they move to their final locations on the face and neck, the origin of each muscle can be determined from its innervation. Figure 12-7 shows the muscles derived from the pharyngeal arches.

In the first arch, paraxial mesoderm derived from the fourth cranial somitomere gives rise to the **muscles of mastication** (the **temporalis, masseter,** and **medial** and **lateral pterygoids),** as well as to the **myelohyoid, ante-**

rior belly of the digastric, tensor tympani, and **tensor veli palatini** muscles (Fig. 12-7).

In the second arch, paraxial mesoderm from the sixth cranial somitomere gives rise to the **muscles of facial expression,** including the **orbicularis oculi, orbicularis oris, risorius, platysma, auricularis, fronto-occipitalis,** and **buccinator** muscles, as well as to the **posterior belly of the digastric,** the **stylohyoid,** and the **stapedius** muscles.

In the third arch, paraxial mesoderm from the seventh somitomere gives rise to a single muscle: the long, slender **stylopharyngeus,** which originates on the styloid process and inserts into the wall of the pharynx.

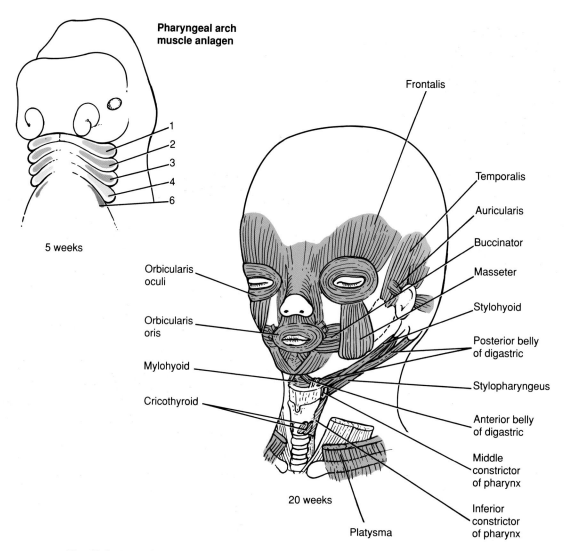

Pharyngeal arch muscle anlagen

1
2
3
4
6

5 weeks

Frontalis

Temporalis

Auricularis

Buccinator

Masseter

Stylohyoid

Posterior belly of digastric

Stylopharyngeus

Anterior belly of digastric

Middle constrictor of pharynx

Inferior constrictor of pharynx

Orbicularis oculi

Orbicularis oris

Mylohyoid

Cricothyroid

20 weeks

Platysma

Fig. 12-7. Fate of the pharyngeal arch musculature. The pharyngeal arch muscles develop from paraxial mesoderm derived mainly from cranial somitomeres and occipital somites. The myoblasts of the sixth arch become the intrinsic laryngeal muscles (not shown).

This muscle raises the pharynx during vocalization and swallowing.

Muscles originating in the fourth arch are the **superior, middle,** and **inferior constrictors** of the pharynx, the **cricothyroid,** and the **levator veli palatini,** which function in vocalization and deglutition. The mesoderm giving rise to these muscles is derived from the second to fourth occipital somites and the first cervical somite.

Paraxial mesoderm derived from the first and second occipital somites becomes associated with the sixth pharyngeal arch to form **intrinsic musculature of the larynx** (Figs. 12-5 and 12-7). The lateral **cricoarytenoids, thyroarytenoids,** and **vocalis** muscles are thus primarily devoted to the function of vocalization.

A cranial nerve innervates each pharyngeal arch

Four cranial nerves arising in the hindbrain supply branches to the pharyngeal arches and their derivatives (Fig. 12-8). (See Ch. 13 for a complete discussion of the 12 cranial nerves.) The maxillary and mandibular swellings of the first arch are innervated, respectively, by the **maxillary** and **mandibular branches** of the **trigeminal** nerve (cranial nerve V). The second arch is innervated by the **facial** nerve (nerve VII); the third arch, by the **glossopharyngeal** nerve (nerve IX); and the fourth and sixth arches, respectively, by the **superior laryngeal** and **recurrent laryngeal** branches of the **vagus** nerve (nerve X).

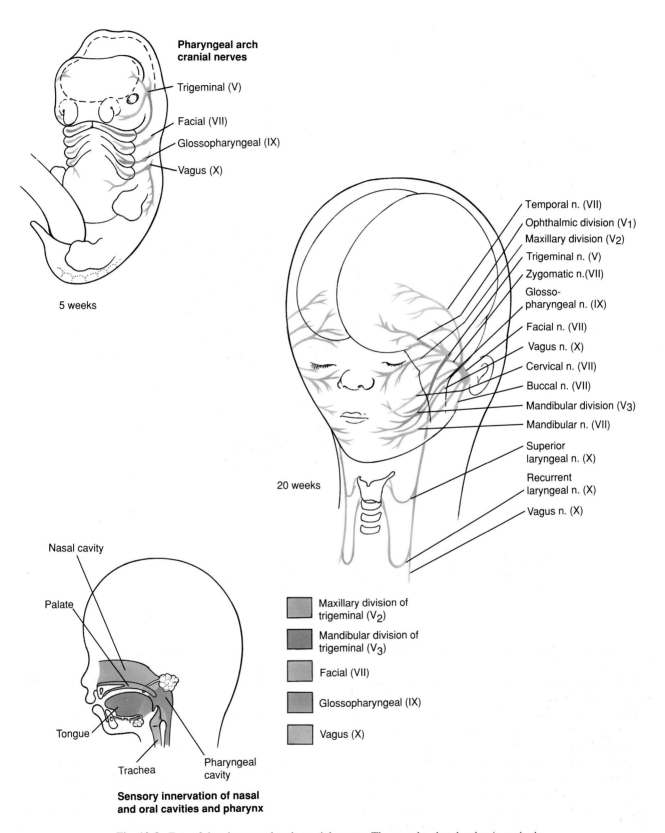

Pharyngeal arch cranial nerves

Trigeminal (V)

Facial (VII)

Glossopharyngeal (IX)

Vagus (X)

5 weeks

Temporal n. (VII)
Ophthalmic division (V₁)
Maxillary division (V₂)
Trigeminal n. (V)
Zygomatic n.(VII)
Glosso-pharyngeal n. (IX)
Facial n. (VII)
Vagus n. (X)
Cervical n. (VII)
Buccal n. (VII)
Mandibular division (V₃)
Mandibular n. (VII)
Superior laryngeal n. (X)
Recurrent laryngeal n. (X)
Vagus n. (X)

20 weeks

Nasal cavity

Palate

Tongue

Trachea

Pharyngeal cavity

Sensory innervation of nasal and oral cavities and pharynx

Maxillary division of trigeminal (V₂)

Mandibular division of trigeminal (V₃)

Facial (VII)

Glossopharyngeal (IX)

Vagus (X)

Fig. 12-8. Fate of the pharyngeal arch cranial nerves. The muscles that develop in each pharyngeal arch are served by the cranial nerve that originally innervates that arch.

As discussed in Chapter 13, the various cranial nerves carry different combinations of somatic motor, autonomic, and sensory fibers. In all cases, however, the somatic motor neurons develop in the basal (ventral) columns of the brain, whereas the sensory neurons are located in cranial nerve ganglia. Unlike the sensory neurons of the dorsal ganglia of the spinal cord, which all arise from neural crest cells, some cranial nerve sensory neurons arise from special areas of ectoderm known as **neurogenic ectodermal placodes.** These placodes are discussed in detail in Chapter 13. The remaining cranial nerve sensory cells arise from rhombencephalic neural crest.

The sensory innervation of the ventral side of the face is supplied by the ophthalmic, maxillary, and mandibular divisions of the trigeminal nerve, as would be expected from the fact that the dermis in this region develops from neural crest cells that migrate into the first pharyngeal arch and frontonasal prominence of the face (see below). The sensory innervation of the dorsal side of the head and neck is supplied by the second and third cervical spinal nerves. The sensory innervation to the endodermal derivatives of the pharynx is supplied by cranial nerves V, VII, IX, and X, as described in Figure 12-8.

The face develops from five facial swellings

The basic morphology of the face is created between the 4th and 10th weeks by the development and fusion of five prominences: an unpaired **frontonasal process** plus the two **maxillary swellings** and two **mandibular**

swellings of the first pharyngeal arches (Fig. 12-9). The spectrum of congenital facial defects known as **facial clefts**—including cleft lip and cleft palate—result from the failure of some of these facial processes to fuse correctly. These relatively common congenital anomalies are discussed in the Applications to Clinical Practice section of this chapter.

All five facial swellings appear by the end of the fourth week. During the fifth week, the paired maxillary swellings enlarge and grow ventrally and medially. Simultaneously, a pair of ectodermal thickenings called the **nasal placodes (nasal discs, nasal plates)** appear on the frontonasal process and begin to enlarge (Figs. 12-9 and 12-10). In the sixth week, the ectoderm at the center of each nasal placode invaginates to form an oval **nasal pit,** thus dividing the raised rim of the placode into **lateral** and **medial nasal processes** (Fig. 12-10A). The groove between the lateral nasal process and the adjacent maxillary swelling is called the **nasolacrimal groove.** During the seventh week, the ectoderm at the floor of this groove invaginates into the underlying mesenchyme to form a tube called the **nasolacrimal duct.** This duct is invested by bone during the ossification of the maxilla. After birth, it functions to drain excess tears from the conjunctiva of the eye into the nasal cavity.

During the sixth week, the medial nasal processes migrate toward each other and fuse to form the primordium of the bridge and septum of the nose (Fig. 12-10A, B). By the end of the seventh week, the inferior tips of the medial nasal processes expand laterally and inferiorly and fuse to form the **intermaxillary process** (Fig. 12-10C, D). The

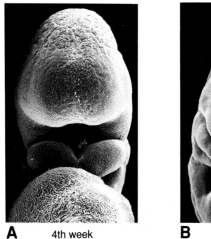

A   4th week

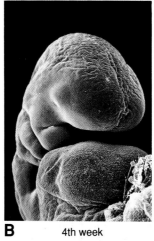

B   4th week

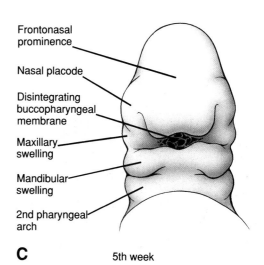

C   5th week

Frontonasal prominence

Nasal placode

Disintegrating buccopharyngeal membrane

Maxillary swelling

Mandibular swelling

2nd pharyngeal arch

Fig. 12-9. Origin of the human face and mouth. The face develops from five primordia that appear in the fourth week: the frontonasal prominence, the two maxillary swellings, and the two mandibular swellings. The buccopharyngeal membrane breaks down to form the opening to the oral cavity. (Figs. A and B photos courtesy of Dr. Arnold Tamarin.)

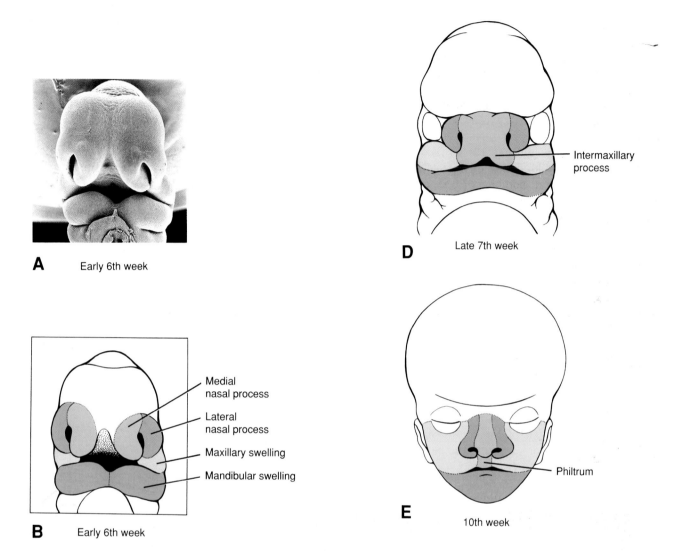

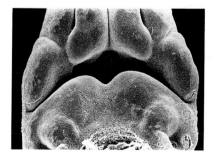

A   Early 6th week

Medial nasal process

Lateral nasal process

Maxillary swelling

Mandibular swelling

B   Early 6th week

D   Late 7th week

Intermaxillary process

E   10th week

Philtrum

C   Early 7th week

Fig. 12-10. Development of the face. (**A, B**) In the sixth week, the nasal placodes of the frontonasal prominence invaginate to form the nasal pits and the lateral and medial nasal processes. (**C, D**) In the seventh week, the medial nasal processes fuse at the midline to form the intermaxillary process. (**E**) By the 10th week, the inter-maxillary process forms the philtrum of the upper lip. The dotted lines in Figs. B, D, and E represent regions of fusion of facial primordia. (Figs. A and C photos courtesy of Dr. Arnold Tamarin.)

tips of the maxillary swellings grow to meet the intermaxillary process and fuse with it. On the upper lip, the intermaxillary process gives rise to the **philtrum** (Fig. 12-10E).

Although the two mandibular swellings appear to be separated by a fissure midventrally (Fig. 12-9A), they actually form in continuity with each other like the rest of the pharyngeal arches. The transient intermandibular depression is filled in during the fourth and fifth weeks by proliferation of mesenchyme, creating the primordium of the lower lip (Fig. 12-9C). Meanwhile, on day 24, the buccopharyngeal membrane ruptures to form a broad, slitlike embryonic mouth (Fig. 12-9C). The mouth is reduced to its final width during the second month as the fusion of the lateral portions of the maxillary and mandibular swellings creates the cheeks (Fig. 12-10D, E).

The nasal passages are formed by the deepening of the nasal pits

Figure 12-11 illustrates the process by which the nasal pits give rise to the nasal passages. At the end of the sixth week, the deepening nasal pits fuse to form a single ectodermal nasal sac. From the end of the sixth week to the beginning of the seventh week, the floor and posterior wall of the nasal sac form a thickened, plate-like fin of ectoderm, called the **nasal fin.** Vacuoles develop in the nasal fin, thinning it to a membrane called the **oronasal membrane.** This membrane ruptures during the seventh week to form an opening called the **primitive choana.** The floor of the nasal cavity is formed by a posterior extension of the intermaxillary process called the **primary palate.**

The secondary palate enlarges the nasal cavity, and the nasal septum divides it into two nasal passages

During the eighth and ninth weeks, the medial walls of the maxillary processes produce a pair of thin medial extensions called the **palatine shelves** (Fig. 12-12A, B). At first these shelves grow downward parallel to the lateral surfaces of the tongue. At the end of the ninth week, however, they rotate rapidly upward into a horizontal position and then fuse with each other and with the primary palate

Fig. 12-11. Formation of the nasal cavity and primitive choana. (**A, B**) The nasal pits invaginate to form a single nasal cavity separated from the oral cavity by a thick partition called the nasal fin. (**C–E**) The nasal fin thins to form the oronasal membrane, which breaks down completely to form the primitive choana. The posterior extension of the intermaxillary process forms the primary palate. (Fig. D photo courtesy of Dr. Arnold Tamarin.)

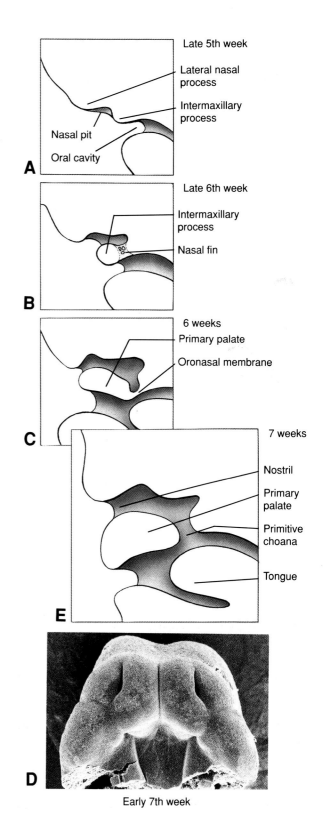

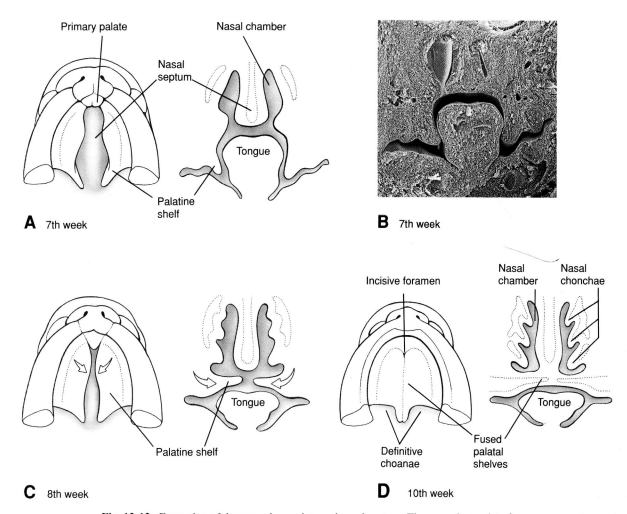

Fig. 12-12. Formation of the secondary palate and nasal septum. The secondary palate forms from palatine shelves that grow medially from the maxillary swellings. During the same period, growth of the nasal septum separates the left and right nasal passages. The palatine shelves at first grow inferiorly on either side of the tongue (**A, B**), but then rapidly rotate upward to meet in the midline (**C**), where they fuse with each other and with the inferior edge of the nasal septum (**D**). (Fig. B photo courtesy of Dr. Arnold Tamarin.)

to form the **secondary palate** (Fig. 12-12C, D). Fusion occurs first at the ventral end of the palatine shelves and proceeds dorsally.

Mesenchymal condensations in the ventral portion of the secondary palate undergo endochondral ossification to form the bony **hard palate.** In the dorsal portion of the secondary palate, myogenic mesenchyme condenses to give rise to the musculature of the soft palate.

While the secondary palate is forming, ectoderm and mesoderm of the frontonasal process and the medial nasal processes proliferate to form a midline **nasal septum** that grows down from the roof of the nasal cavity to fuse with the upper surface of the primary and secondary palates along the midline (Fig. 12-12). The nasal cavity is now divided into two **nasal passages,** which open into the

pharynx behind the secondary palate through an opening called the **definitive choana.**

The postnatal development of the air sinuses significantly alters the relative sizes of the face and cranial vault

At birth, the ratio of the volume of the facial skeleton to the volume of the cranial vault is about 1:7. During infancy and childhood this ratio steadily decreases, mainly as a result of the development of teeth (see Ch. 14) and the growth of the four pairs of **paranasal sinuses: the maxillary, ethmoid, sphenoid,** and **frontal sinuses.** These sinuses develop from invaginations of the nasal cavity that extend into the bones.

The *maxillary sinuses* appear during the third fetal month as invaginations of the nasal sac that slowly expand within the maxillary bones. The resulting cavities are small at birth but expand throughout childhood.

The *ethmoid sinuses* appear during the fifth fetal month as invaginations of the middle meatus of the nasal passages (the space underlying the middle nasal concha) and grow into the ethmoid bone. These sinuses do not complete their growth until puberty.

The *sphenoid sinuses* represent extensions of the ethmoid sinuses into the sphenoid bones. These extensions first appear in the fifth postnatal month and continue to enlarge throughout infancy and childhood.

The *frontal sinuses* do not appear until the fifth or sixth postnatal year and expand throughout adolescence. Each frontal sinus consists of two independent spaces that develop from different sources. One forms by the expansion of the ethmoid sinus into the frontal bone, and the other develops from an independent invagination of the middle meatus of the nasal passage. Because these cavities never coalesce, they drain independently.

The first pharyngeal cleft becomes the external acoustic meatus, and the remaining three clefts disappear

As described earlier, the pharyngeal arches are separated by pharyngeal clefts externally and by pharyngeal pouches internally (Figs. 12-4 and 12-13). The first pharyngeal cleft and pouch, located between the first and second pharyngeal arches, participate in the formation of the ear: the first cleft becomes the **external acoustic meatus,** and the first pouch expands to form a cavity called the **tubotympanic recess,** which differentiates to become the **tympanic cavity** of the middle ear and the **auditory (eustachian) tube** (Fig. 12-13).

The remaining three pharyngeal clefts are normally obliterated during development. During the fourth and fifth weeks, the rapidly expanding second pharyngeal arch overgrows these clefts and fuses caudally with the cardiac eminence, enclosing the clefts in a transient, ectoderm-lined **lateral cervical sinus** (Fig. 12-13B, C). This space normally disappears rapidly and completely.

The first pharyngeal cleft and the lateral cervical sinus may form anomalous cysts or fistulae

Infrequently, duplication of the first pharyngeal cleft results in the formation of an ectoderm-lined **first-cleft sinus** or **cervical aural fistula** located in the tissues inferior or ventral to the external acoustic meatus (Fig. 12-14C). A fully enclosed first-cleft sinus may become apparent as a swelling just inferior or ventral to the auricle or external ear. Alternatively, it may drain to the exterior through a cervical aural fistula, which usually opens into the external auditory canal. Depending on its position, a first-cleft cyst or fistula may threaten the facial nerve if it becomes infected and may require resection.

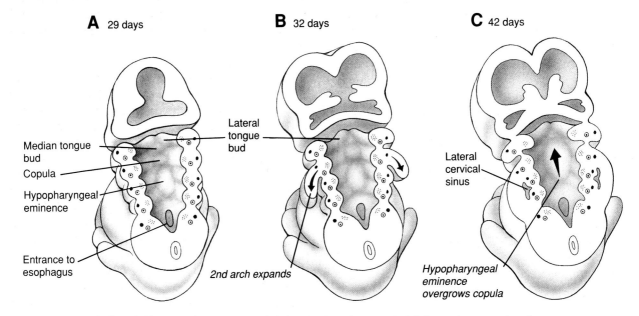

A 29 days   **B** 32 days   **C** 42 days

Median tongue bud

Copula

Hypopharyngeal eminence

Entrance to esophagus

Lateral tongue bud

2nd arch expands

Lateral cervical sinus

Hypopharyngeal eminence overgrows copula

Fig. 12-13. Fate of the pharyngeal clefts. The first pharyngeal cleft forms the external auditory meatus. The second pharyngeal arch expands and fuses with the cardiac eminence to cover the remaining pharyngeal clefts, which form the transient lateral cervical sinus.

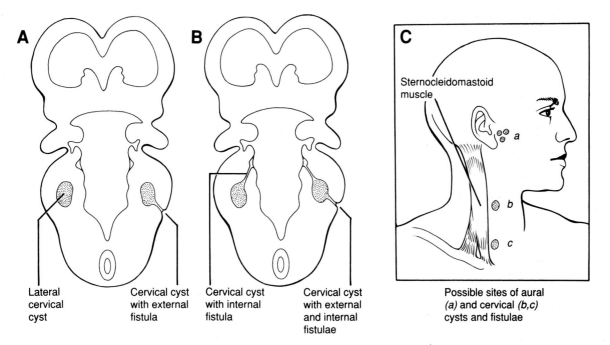

A Lateral cervical cyst · Cervical cyst with external fistula

B Cervical cyst with internal fistula · Cervical cyst with external and internal fistulae

C Sternocleidomastoid muscle · Possible sites of aural (a) and cervical (b,c) cysts and fistulae

Fig. 12-14. Abnormal cysts produced by the lateral cervical sinus or first pharyngeal cleft. The lateral cervical sinus occasionally persists in the form of an abnormal lateral cervical cyst. (**A, B**) Such cysts may be isolated or may connect to the skin of the neck by an external cervical fistula or to the pharynx by an internal fistula, or both. (**C**) Lateral cervical cysts are located just medial to the anterior border of the sternocleidomastoid muscle. Anomalous derivatives of the first pharyngeal cleft known as aural cysts may form anterior to the ear.

The lateral cervical sinus occasionally persists on one or both sides in the form of a **cervical cyst** located just ventral to the ventral border of the sternocleidomastoid muscle (Fig. 12-14). A completely enclosed cyst may expand to form a palpable lump as its epithelial lining desquamates or if it becomes infected. Occasionally, the cyst communicates either with the skin via an **external cervical fistula** or with the pharynx via an **internal cervical fistula.** Internal cervical fistulae most commonly open into the embryonic derivative of the second pouch, the palatine tonsil. Less often, they communicate with derivatives of the third pouch (see below). Rarely, a cervical cyst has both internal and external fistulae. Cysts of this type may be diagnosed by the drainage of mucus through the small opening of the external fistula on the neck just medial to the ventral border of the sternocleidomastoid. Cervical cysts are usually of minor clinical importance but may require resection if they become seriously infected.

The tongue and thyroid develop from pharyngeal arch tissue

The tongue develops from pharyngeal arches 1, 3, and 4 and from occipital somite mesoderm

At the end of the fourth week, the floor of the pharynx consists of the five pharyngeal arches and the intervening pharyngeal pouches. The development of the tongue begins late in the fourth week when the first arch forms a median swelling called the **median tongue bud** or **tuberculum impar** (Fig. 12-15A). An additional pair of lateral swellings, the **distal tongue buds** or **lateral lingual swellings,** develop on the first arch early in the fifth week and rapidly expand to overgrow the median tongue bud. These swellings continue to grow throughout embryonic and fetal life and form the anterior two-thirds of the tongue (Fig. 12-15B–D).

Late in the fourth week, the second arch develops a midline swelling called the **copula** (Fig. 12-15A). This swelling is rapidly overgrown during the fifth and sixth weeks by a midline swelling of the third and fourth arches called the **hypopharyngeal eminence,** which gives rise to the posterior one-third of the tongue. The hypopharyngeal eminence expands mainly by the growth of third-arch endoderm, whereas the fourth arch contributes only a small region on the most posterior aspect of the tongue (Fig. 12-15C, D). Thus, the bulk of the tongue mucosa is formed by the first and third arches. Table 12-2 summarizes the developmental origins of the parts of the tongue.

The surface features of the definitive tongue reflect its embryonic origins. The boundary between the first-arch and third-arch contributions—roughly, the boundary between the anterior two-thirds and posterior one-third of the tongue—is marked by a transverse groove called the **terminal sulcus** (Fig. 12-15D). The line of fusion be-

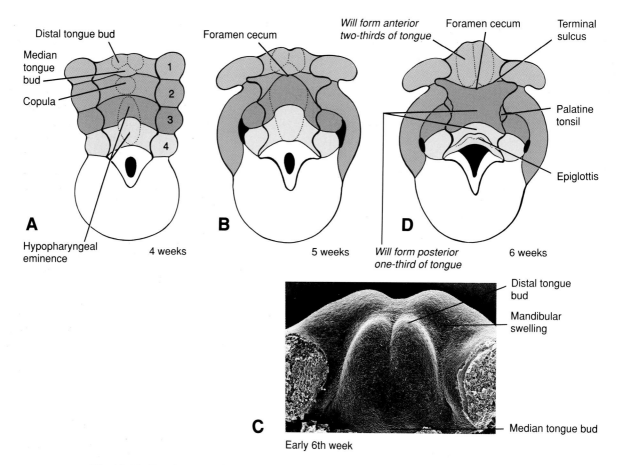

Fig. 12-15. Development of the tongue mucosa from the endoderm of the pharyngeal floor. The mucosa of the anterior two-thirds of the tongue develops primarily from the distal tongue buds (lateral lingual swellings) of the first pharyngeal arch, whereas the mucosal lining of the posterior one-third of the tongue is formed by overgrowth of the copula of the second arch by the hypopharyngeal eminence of the third and fourth arches. (Photo courtesy of Dr. Arnold Tamarin.)

Table 12-2. Development of the Tongue from Pharyngeal Arches 1 through 4 and the Occipital Somites

EMBRYONIC PRECURSOR	INTERMEDIATE STRUCTURE	ADULT STRUCTURE	INNERVATION
Pharyngeal arch 1	Median tongue bud	Overgrown by lateral lingual swellings	Lingual branch (sensory) of mandibular division of trigeminal nerve (V)
	Lateral lingual swellings	Mucosa of anterior two-thirds of tongue	Chorda tympani from facial nerve (VII; innervating arch 2) (innervates all taste buds except vallate papillae)
Pharyngeal arch 2	Copula	Overgrown by other structures	
Pharyngeal arch 3	Large, ventral part of hypopharyngeal eminence	Mucosa of most of posterior one-third of tongue	Sensory branch of glossopharyngeal nerve (IX) (also supplies vallate papillae)
Pharyngeal arch 4	Small, dorsal part of hypopharyngeal eminence	Mucosa of small, dorsal region of tongue	Sensory fibers of superior laryngeal branch of vagus nerve (X)
Occipital somites	Myoblasts	Intrinsic muscles of tongue	Hypoglossal nerve (XII)
		Palatoglossus muscle	Pharyngeal plexus of vagus nerve (X)

tween the right and left distal tongue buds is marked by a midline groove, the **median sulcus,** on the anterior two-thirds of the tongue. A depression called the **foramen cecum** is visible where the median sulcus intersects the terminal sulcus. As discussed below, this depression is the site of origin of the thyroid gland.

All the muscles of the tongue except the palatoglossus are formed by mesoderm derived from the myotomes of the occipital somites, and the proliferation of this mesoderm is responsible for most of the growth of the tongue primordia. The innervation of the tongue muscles is consonant with their origin: all the muscles except the palatoglossus are innervated by the **hypoglossal nerve** (cranial nerve XII), which is the cranial nerve associated with the occipital somites, whereas the palatoglossus is innervated by the **pharyngeal plexus of the vagus** (nerve X).

The mucosal covering of the tongue is derived from pharyngeal arch endoderm and is innervated by sensory branches of the corresponding four cranial nerves (Table 12-2). The general sensory receptors on the anterior two-thirds of the tongue are supplied by a branch of the mandibular nerve (cranial nerve V_3) called the **lingual nerve.** The taste buds of the anterior two-thirds of the tongue are supplied by a special branch of the facial nerve (cranial nerve VII) called the **chorda tympani.** In contrast, the vallate papillae (a row of large taste buds flanking the terminal sulcus) and the general sensory endings over most of the posterior one-third of the tongue are supplied by the **glossopharyngeal nerve.** The small area on the most posterior aspect of the tongue that is derived from the fourth pharyngeal arch receives sensory innervation from the **superior laryngeal** branch of the vagus nerve.

The thyroid gland develops from an invagination of the tongue endoderm and migrates to a ventrocaudal location

Figure 12-16 illustrates the embryogenesis of the thyroid gland. The gland primordium first appears in the late fourth week as a small, solid mass of endoderm proliferating at the apex of the foramen cecum on the developing

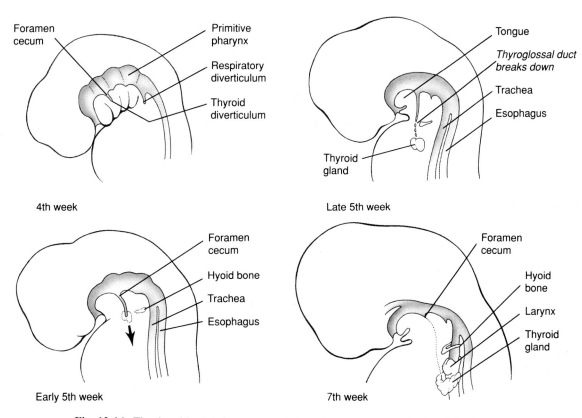

Fig. 12-16. The thyroid originates as an endodermal proliferation at the tip of the foramen cecum of the developing tongue and migrates inferiorly to its final site anterior and inferior to the larynx. Until the fifth week, the thyroid remains connected to the foramen cecum by the thyroglossal duct. The gland reaches its final site in the seventh week.

tongue. The thyroid primordium descends through the tissues of the neck at the end of a slender **thyroglossal duct.** The thyroglossal duct breaks down by the end of the fifth week, and the isolated thyroid, now consisting of lateral lobes connected by a well-defined isthmus, continues to descend, reaching its final position just inferior to the cricoid cartilage by the seventh week. The thyroid gland begins to function as early as the 10th to the 12th week in human embryos.

Normally, the only remnant of the thyroglossal duct is the foramen cecum itself. Occasionally, however, a portion of the duct persists either as an enclosed **thyroglossal cyst** or as a **thyroglossal sinus** communicating with the surface of the neck. Rarely, a fragment of the thyroid becomes detached during the descent of the gland and forms a patch of ectopic thyroid tissue, which may be located anywhere along the route of descent.

Pharyngeal pouches 2 to 5 give rise to tissues of the immune system and endocrine glands

The second pharyngeal pouch gives rise to the palatine tonsils

The palatine tonsils arise from the endoderm lining the second pharyngeal pouch (located between the second and third arches) and from the mesoderm of the second pharyngeal membrane and adjacent regions of the first and second arch (Fig. 12-17). Development of these tonsils begins early in the third month as the epithelium of the second pouch proliferates to form solid endodermal buds or ledges growing into the underlying mesoderm, which will give rise to the tonsillar stroma. The central cells of the buds later die and slough, converting the solid

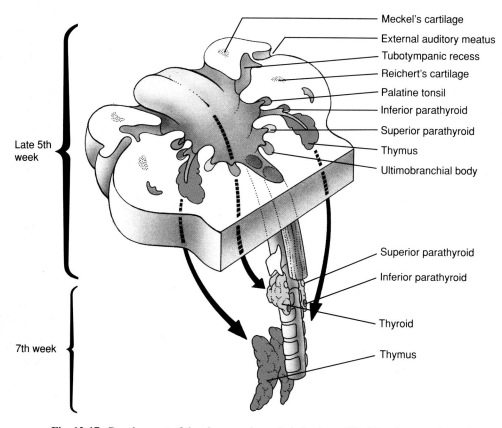

Fig. 12-17. Development of the pharyngeal pouch derivatives. All of the pharyngeal pouches give rise to adult structures. These are the tubotympanic recess (pouch 1), the palatine tonsils (pouch 2), the inferior parathyroid glands and thymus (pouch 3), the superior parathyroid glands (pouch 4), and the ultimobranchial (telopharyngeal) body (inferior part of pouch 4 or, possibly, a hypothetical pouch 5). The parathyroids, thymus primordia, and ultimobranchial bodies separate from the lining of the pharynx and migrate to their definitive locations within the neck and thorax.

buds into hollow **tonsillar crypts,** which are rapidly infiltrated by lymphoid tissue. The definitive lymph follicles of the tonsil do not form until the last three months of prenatal life, however.

Similar lymphatic tonsils, called **pharyngeal tonsils,** develop in association with mucous glands of the pharynx. The major pharyngeal tonsils are the **adenoids,** the **tubal tonsils** (associated with the auditory tubes), and the **lingual tonsils** (associated with the posterior regions of the tongue). Minor intervening patches of lymphoid tissue also form.

The thymus arises from the third pharyngeal pouch and migrates to a position just dorsal to the sternum

The two thymic primordia arise at the end of the fourth week in the form of endodermal proliferations at the end of ventral elongations of the third pharyngeal pouches (Figs. 12-17 and 12-18). These endodermal proliferations form hollow tubes that invade the underlying mesoderm and later transform into solid, branching cords. These cords are the primordia of the polyhedral **thymic lobules.** The underlying mesoderm is derived from neural crest.

Between the fourth and seventh weeks, the thymus glands lose their connections with the pharynx and migrate to their definitive location inferior and ventral to the developing thyroid and just dorsal to the sternum. There they fuse to form a single, bilobate thymus gland. By 12 weeks, each thymic lobule is 0.5 to 2 mm in diameter and has a well-defined cortex and medulla. The whorl-like **Hassall's corpuscles** within the medulla apparently arise from the ectodermal cells of the third pharyngeal cleft, whereas the loosely organized **epithelial reticulum** of the thymus is of endodermal origin. The lobules are supported by mesenchymal septa. Shortly after the thymus forms it is infiltrated by lymphocytes derived from stem cells in the yolk sac, omentum, and liver. These lymphocytes presumably home on the thymus by a chemotactic mechanism.

The thymus is highly active during the perinatal period and continues to grow throughout childhood, reaching its maximum size at puberty. After puberty the gland involutes rapidly and is represented only by insignificant fatty vestiges in the adult.

The parathyroids arise from pharyngeal pouches 3 and 4

The rudiments of the **inferior parathyroid glands (parathyroids III)** form in the dorsal portion of the third pouch early in the fifth week (Figs. 12-17 and 12-18). They detach from the pharyngeal wall and migrate inferi-

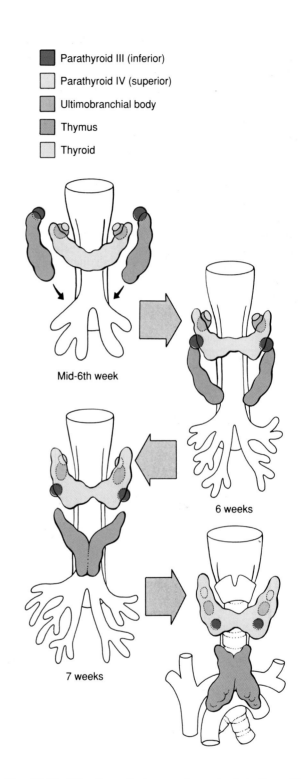

Fig. 12-18. Migration of pharyngeal pouch derivatives. The parathyroid glands and the ultimobranchial bodies migrate inferiorly to become embedded in the posterior wall of the thyroid gland. The two parathyroids exchange position as they migrate: parathyroid III becomes the inferior parathyroid, whereas parathyroid IV becomes the superior parathyroid.

orly and medially, coming to rest by the seventh week on the dorsal side of the inferior end of the thyroid lobes.

Early in the fifth week, the rudiments of the **superior parathyroid glands (parathyroids IV)** form in the fourth pouch. They detach from the pharynx and migrate inferiorly and medially, coming to rest by the seventh week in a position slightly superior to the inferior parathyroid glands.

The ultimobranchial (telopharyngeal) bodies arise from a controversial fifth pharyngeal pouch

During the fifth week, a minor invagination appears just caudal to the fourth pharyngeal pouch (Fig. 12-17). This invagination has been described by many embryologists as a **fifth pharyngeal pouch.** Almost immediately after they appear, these invaginations become populated by epithelial cells, which form the rudiments of the paired **ultimobranchial bodies** (Fig. 12-18). These rudiments immediately detach from the pharyngeal wall and migrate medially and caudally to implant in the dorsal wall of the thyroid gland, where they differentiate into the calcitonin-producing **C cells (parafollicular cells)** of the thyroid.

The salivary glands arise from ectoderm and endoderm in the pharyngeal region

Three pairs of salivary glands develop in humans: the **parotid, submandibular,** and **sublingual** glands. The parotid gland develops from a groovelike invagination of ectoderm that forms in the crease between the maxillary and mandibular swellings. This groove differentiates into a tubular duct that sinks into the underlying mesenchyme but maintains a ventral opening at the angle of the primitive mouth. As the cheek portions of the maxillary and mandibular swellings fuse, this opening is transferred to the inner surface of the cheek. The blind dorsal end of the tube differentiates to form the parotid gland, whereas the stem of the tube becomes the parotid duct. Similar invaginations of the endoderm in the floor of the oral cavity and in the paralingual sulci on either side of the tongue give rise to the submandibular and sublingual salivary glands, respectively.

Development of the Eyes

The eyes begin their development as diverticulae of the forebrain early in the fourth week

The first morphologic evidence of the eyes is the formation of an **optic primordium** and **optic sulcus** in the future diencephalic region of the prosencephalic (fore-brain) neural folds at 22 days (Fig. 12-19A, B). These structures are induced and supported in their initial growth by interactions with the adjacent pharyngeal endoderm and head mesoderm.

By the time the cranial neuropore close on day 24, the optic primordia have developed into lateral evaginations of the neural tube called **optic vesicles** (Fig. 12-19C, D). The walls of the optic vesicles are continuous with the neurectoderm of the future brain, and the cavity or **ventricle** within the optic vesicles is continuous with the neural canal. As the optic vesicle forms, it is surrounded by a sheath of mesenchyme that consists partly of neural crest cells that detach from the optic vesicle itself. This sheath begins to form on day 24 and completely envelops the optic vesicle on day 26 (Fig. 12-19C).

By day 28, the distal face of the optic vesicle (called the **retinal disc**) reaches the surface ectoderm, from which it is separated only by a few mesenchymal cells. On about day 32, the retinal disc invaginates into the expanded tip of the optic vesicle to form a goblet-shaped **optic cup** (Fig. 12-20D–F). Simultaneously, the stem of the otpic vesicle narrows to form the hollow **optic stalk.** The lumen of the optic cup remains continuous with the ventricle of the forebrain through the optic stalk. Blood vessels gain access to the interior of the optic cup through a longitudinal groove, the **choroidal (retinal) fissure,** that develops on the ventral surface of the optic stalk (see Fig. 12-22).

The lens develops from an ectodermal placode that forms adjacent to the optic cup

As soon as the optic cup reaches the surface ectoderm, the ectoderm apposed to it thickens to form a **lens placode** (Fig. 12-20).

Lens induction apparently begins when definitive endoderm first arrives next to the prospective lens ectoderm early in gastrulation. Later in gastrulation, the neural plate may pass inductive signals to the presumptive lens through the plane of the nurectoderm. During embryonic folding, the heart mesoderm also exerts a significant inductive effect when it comes into proximity with the prospective lens.

Immediately after the lens placode appears on day 32, it invaginates to form a **lens pit** (Fig. 12-20A, B, D). By day 33, the placode pinches off from the surface ectoderm, becoming a hollow **lens vesicle.** This event coincides with the invagination of the retinal disc, and the newly formed lens vesicle sits within the optic cup. A gelatinous matrix called the **primary vitreous body** is subsequently secreted into the **lentiretinal space** between the lens vesicle and the inner wall of the expanding optic cup (Fig. 12-12E). The lens vesicle becomes surrounded by a mesenchymal capsule as it forms.

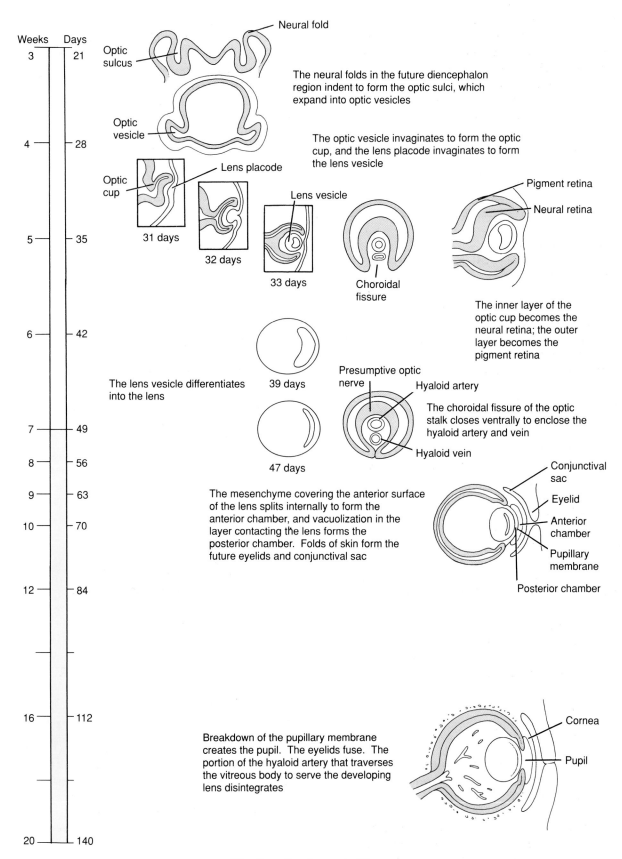

Neural fold

Optic sulcus

The neural folds in the future diencephalon region indent to form the optic sulci, which expand into optic vesicles

Optic vesicle

The optic vesicle invaginates to form the optic cup, and the lens placode invaginates to form the lens vesicle

Optic cup

Lens placode

Lens vesicle

Pigment retina

Neural retina

31 days

32 days

33 days

Choroidal fissure

The inner layer of the optic cup becomes the neural retina; the outer layer becomes the pigment retina

The lens vesicle differentiates into the lens

39 days

Presumptive optic nerve

Hyaloid artery

The choroidal fissure of the optic stalk closes ventrally to enclose the hyaloid artery and vein

47 days

Hyaloid vein

The mesenchyme covering the anterior surface of the lens splits internally to form the anterior chamber, and vacuolization in the layer contacting the lens forms the posterior chamber. Folds of skin form the future eyelids and conjunctival sac

Conjunctival sac

Eyelid

Anterior chamber

Pupillary membrane

Posterior chamber

Breakdown of the pupillary membrane creates the pupil. The eyelids fuse. The portion of the hyaloid artery that traverses the vitreous body to serve the developing lens disintegrates

Cornea

Pupil

Weeks Days
3   21
4   28
5   35
6   42
7   49
8   56
9   63
10   70
12   84
16   112
20   140

Timeline. Development of the eyes.

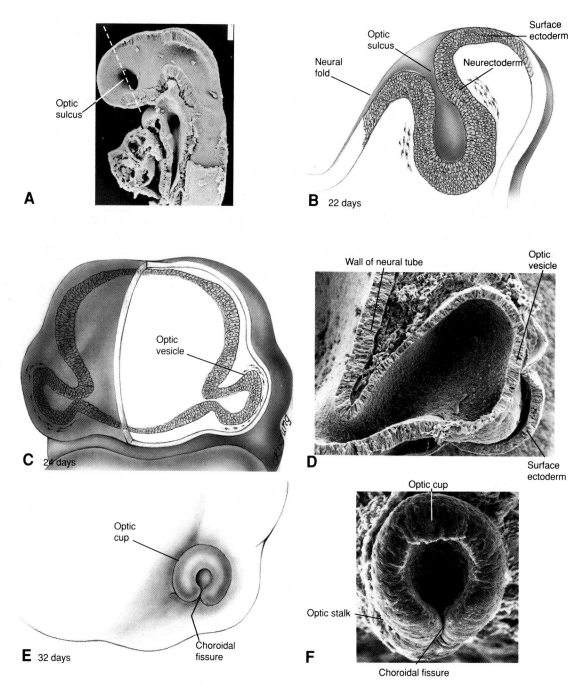

Fig. 12-19. Formation of the optic vesicle and optic cup. (**A, B**) The optic vesicle begins to form as an evagination of the diencephalic neural folds on day 22, before the cranial neuropore has closed. (**C, D**) By day 24, the optic vesicles lie adjacent to the surface ectoderm. (**E, F**) During the fifth week, the optic vesicle invaginates to become the optic cup, and the choroidal fissure forms on the inferior surface of the optic cup and stalk. (Fig. A from Morriss-Kay G. 1981. Growth and development of pattern in the cranial neural epithelium of rat embryos during neurulation. J Embryol Exp Morphol 65:225, with permission. Fig. D from Garcia-Porrero JA, Colvee E, Ojeda JL. 1987. Retinal cell death occurs in the absence of retinal disc invagination. Anat Rec 217:395, with permission. Fig. F from Morse D, Mc-Cann PS. 1984. Neurectoderm of the early embryonic rat eye. Invest Ophthalmol Vis Sci 25:899, with permission.)

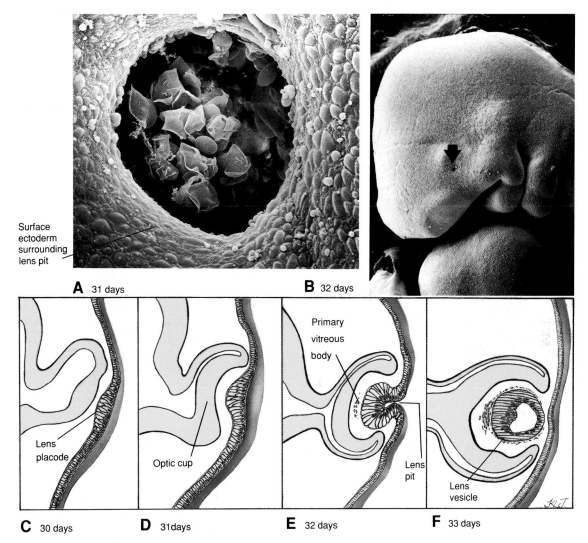

Surface
ectoderm
surrounding
lens pit

A 31 days

B 32 days

Primary
vitreous
body

Lens
placode

Optic cup

Lens
pit

Lens
vesicle

C 30 days   **D** 31days   **E** 32 days   **F** 33 days

Fig. 12-20. Formation of the lens placode and lens vesicle. Contact with the optic cup is necessary for the maintenance and development of the lens placode, although other influences are apparently more important in its induction. (**A–E**) During the fifth week, the lens placode begins to invaginate to form the lens pit (arrow in Fig. B). (**E, F**) The invaginating lens placode pinches off to form a lens vesicle enclosed in the optic cup. (Fig. A photo courtesy of Dr. Arnold Tamarin.)

Beginning on day 33, the cells of the posterior (deep) wall of the lens vesicle differentiate to form long, slender, anteroposteriorly oriented **primary lens fibers** (Figs. 12-20F and 12-21). The elongation of these cells transforms the deep wall of the lens vesicle into a rounded **lens body,** obliterating the cavity of the lens vesicle by the late seventh week. After the eighth week, the primary lens fibers are augmented by a new population of **secondary lens fibers** that arise from the simple epithelium that differentiates from cells of the anterior wall of the lens vesicle.

The lens and retina are vascularized by the hyaloid branch of the ophthalmic artery

As soon as the lens vesicle forms on day 32, it becomes vascularized by a branch of the ophthalmic artery called the **hyaloid artery,** which also vascularizes the developing retina (Fig. 12-22A). This artery gains access to the lentiretinal space via the choroidal fissure on the ventral surface of the optic stalk. The lips of the choroidal fissure fuse by day 37, enclosing the hyaloid artery and its accompanying vein in a canal within the ventral wall of the

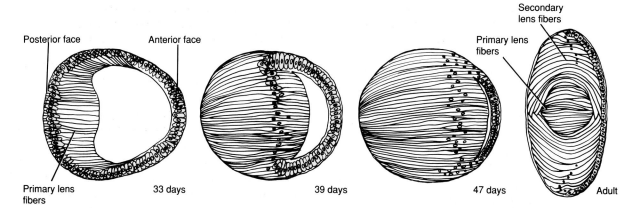

Fig. 12-21. Differentiation of the lens. The lens develops rapidly in the fifth to seventh weeks as the cells of its posterior wall elongate and differentiate to form the primary lens fibers. Secondary lens fibers begin to form in the third month.

optic stalk (Fig. 12-22B–D). When the lens matures during fetal life and ceases to need a blood supply, the portion of the hyaloid artery that crosses the vitreous body degenerates. Even in the adult, however, the course of this former artery is marked by a conduit through the vitreous body called the **hyaloid canal.** The proximal portion of the hyaloid artery becomes the **central artery of the retina,** which supplies blood to the retina.

The outer and inner walls of the optic cup differentiate into the pigment and neural retinas, respectively

The two walls of the optic cup give rise to the two layers of the retina: the thick inner wall of the cup (the former retinal disc) becomes the **neural retina,** which contains the light-receptive **rods** and **cones** plus associated

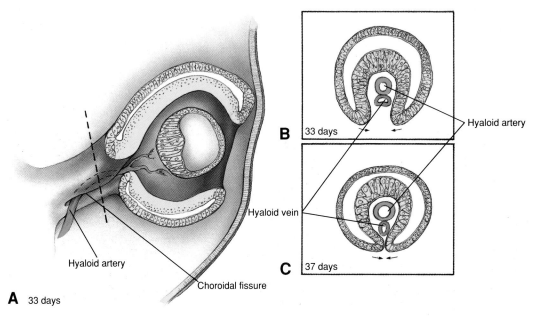

Fig. 12-22. Vascularization of the lens and retina. (**A**) As the lens vesicle detaches from the surface ectoderm, it becomes vascularized by the hyaloid vessels, which gain access to the lens through the choroidal fissure. (**B, C**) During the seventh week the edges of the choroidal fissure fuse together, enclosing the hyaloid artery and vein in the hyaloid canal. When the lens matures, the vessels serving it degenerate, and the hyaloid artery and vein become the central artery and vein of the retina.

neural processes, and the thin outer wall of the cup becomes the melanin-containing **pigment retina** (Fig. 12-23). These two walls are initially separated by a narrow **intraretinal space.**

Melanin first appears in the cells of the developing pigment retina on day 33. Differentiation of the neural retina begins at the end of the sixth week as the layer of cells adjacent to the intraretinal space (which is homologous to the proliferative neuroepithelium lining the neural tube; see Ch. 4) begins to produce waves of cells that migrate inward toward the vitreous body. By the sixth week, these cells form two cellular embryonic retinal layers: an **outer neuroblastic layer** and an **inner neuroblastic layer.**

By the ninth week, two additional membranes develop to cover the two surfaces of the neural retina. An **external limiting membrane** is interposed between the pigment retina and the proliferative zone of the neural retina, and the inner surface of the retina is sealed off by an **inner limiting membrane** (Fig. 12-23B).

The definitive cell layers of the mature neural retina arise from the inner and outer neuroblastic layers. The rods and cones, which form the outermost layer of the mature neural retina, are derived from the outer neuroblastic layer. The inner neuroblastic layer gives rise to the **ganglion cells** and **supporting cells** of the retina. In the sixth week, the ganglion cells sprout axons that emerge onto the inner surface of the retina and grow across it toward the optic stalk. These axons form the definitive **fiber layer** that lines the inner surface of the retina. All the cell layers of the definitive retina are apparent by the eighth month.

Nerve fibers from the retina grow to the brain through the optic stalk, transforming it into the optic nerve

The nerve fibers that emerge from the retinal ganglion cells in the sixth week travel through the optic stalk to reach the brain. The stalk lumen is gradually obliterated by the growth of these fibers, and by the eighth week the hollow optic stalk is transformed into the solid **optic nerve** (cranial nerve II). Just before the two optic nerves enter the brain, they join to form an X-shaped structure called the **optic chiasm.** Within the chiasm, about half the fibers from each optic nerve cross over to the contralateral (opposite) side of the brain. The resulting combined bundle of ipsilateral and contralateral fibers on each side then grows back to the lateral geniculate body of the thalamus (see Ch. 13), where the fibers synapse starting in the eighth week. Over 1 million nerve fibers grow from each retina to the brain.

The intraretinal space between the neural and pigment retinas disappears by the seventh week. The two layers of the retina never fuse firmly, however, and various types of trauma—even a simple blow to the head—can cause **retinal detachment** between them.

The mesenchymal capsule of the optic vesicle gives rise to the choroid, the sclera, and the anterior chamber

During weeks 6 and 7, the mesenchymal capsule that surrounds the optic cup differentiates into two layers: an inner, pigmented, vascular layer called the **choroid** and

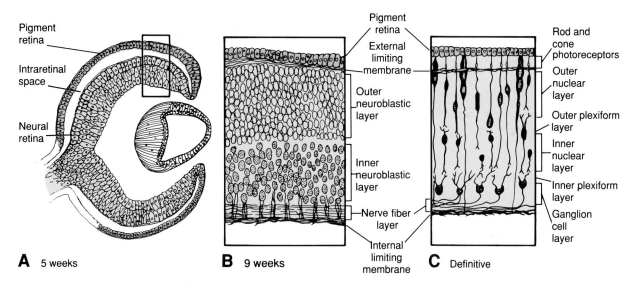

Fig. 12-23. Differentiation of the inner layer of the optic cup to form the neural retina. The definitive layers of the neural retina do not develop until late fetal life.

an outer, fibrous layer called the **sclera** (Fig. 12-24). The choroid layer is homologous in origin with the pia mater and arachnoid membranes investing the brain (the leptomeninges), and the sclera is homologous with the dura mater. The tough sclera supports and protects the delicate inner structures of the optic globe.

Late in the sixth week, the mesenchyme surrounding the optic cup invades the region between the lens and the surface ectoderm, thus forming a complete mesenchymal jacket around the developing globe. During the seventh week, the mesenchyme overlying the lens splits into two layers that enclose a new cavity called the **anterior chamber of the eye** (Fig. 12-24C). The anterior (superficial) wall of this chamber is continuous with the sclera of the optic globe, and the posterior (deep) wall is continuous with the choroid.

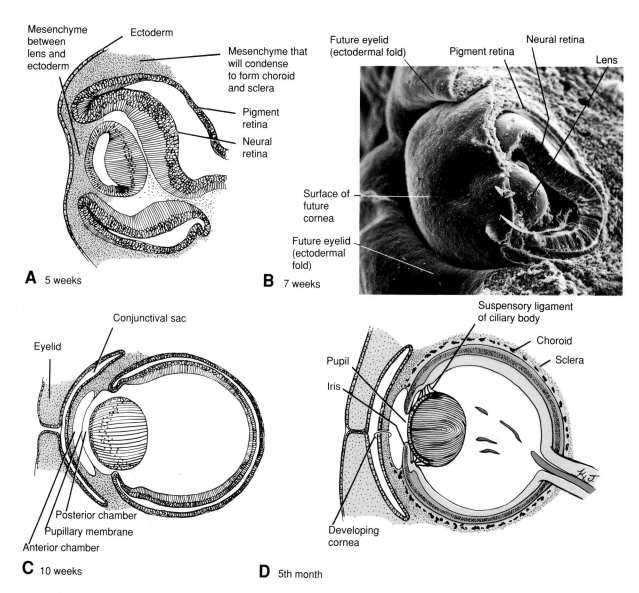

Fig. 12-24. Development of the anterior and posterior chambers, the eyelids, and the coverings of the optic globe. (**A, B**) Mesenchyme surrounds the developing eyeball (optic globe) between the fifth and seventh weeks to form the choroid and sclera. (**C, D**) Vacuolization within this mesenchyme in the seventh week forms the anterior chamber. Shortly thereafter, vacuolization in the layer of mesenchyme immediately anterior to the lens forms the posterior chamber. The pupillary membrane, which initially separates the anterior and posterior chambers, breaks down in early fetal life. The upper and lower eyelids form as folds of surface ectoderm. They fuse together by the end of the eighth week and separate again between the fifth and seventh months.

The two inner layers of the cornea form from the superficial wall of the anterior chamber, and the third (outer) layer forms from the overlying ectoderm. By the eighth week, the superficial wall of the anterior chamber differentiates into two layers: a thin inner epithelium lining the anterior chamber (called the **mesothelium of the anterior chamber**) and, external to it, an **acellular postepithelial layer.** Mesenchymal cells rapidly invade the latter and convert it to a cellular **stromal layer (substantia propria).** The anterior chamber mesothelium and the substantia propria constitute the two deep layers of the cornea, which thus are of mesodermal origin. In contrast, the outer layer of the cornea, called the **anterior epithelium,** is derived from the overlying surface ectoderm.

The inner wall of the anterior chamber forms the pupillary membrane. When the anterior chamber forms, its thick posterior wall rests directly against the lens. The deep layers of this wall subsequently break down by a process of vacuolization to create a new space, the **posterior chamber,** between the lens and the thin remaining layer of the wall (Fig. 12-24C). This thin remaining layer, called the **pupillary membrane,** breaks down early in the fetal period to form the opening called the **pupil** through which the anterior and posterior chambers communicate. On rare occasions, the pupillary membrane fails to break down completely, leaving strands that traverse the pupil. The posterior chamber eventually expands to underlie the iris and part of the ciliary body (see below), as well as the pupil.

The rim of the optic cup and the overlying choroidal mesenchyme form the iris and ciliary body

At the end of the third month, the anterior rim of the optic cup and its overlying choroidal mesenchyme expand to form a thin ring that projects between the anterior and posterior chambers and overlaps the lens (Fig. 12-24B). This ring differentiates into the **iris** of the eye. The inner surface of the iris is lined by a thin epithelium that represents the two fused layers of the optic cup; the remainder of the iris differentiates from choroidal mesoderm. The circumferentially arranged smooth muscle bundles of the **pupillary muscles** in the iris form from neural crest-derived ectomesenchymal cells in the choroid. These muscles act as a diaphragm, controlling the diameter of the pupil and thus the amount of light that enters the eye.

Just posterior to the developing iris, the optic cup and overlying choroid differentiate to form the **ciliary body.** The lens is suspended from the ciliary body by a radial network of elastic fibers called the **suspensory ligament** of the lens. Around the insertions of these fibers, the optic cup epithelia of the ciliary body proliferate to form a ring of highly vascularized, feathery elaborations that are specialized to secrete the fluid that fills the optic globe. Ectomesenchymal cells in the choroid of the ciliary body differentiate to form the smooth muscle bundles of the **ciliary muscle,** which controls the shape and hence the focusing power (accommodation) of the lens.

The extrinsic ocular muscles develop from mesenchyme adjacent to the optic cup

The first of the extraocular muscles to appear are the **lateral** and **superior rectus** muscles, which begin to condense adjacent to the mesenchymal sheath of the optic vesicle as early as day 28. Within a few days, the insertions of these muscles on the globe also begin to condense. By the early sixth week, the **superior oblique** muscle appears, followed by the **medial rectus** and the common primordium of the **inferior rectus** and **inferior oblique.** The **trochlea**—the ligamentous pulley for the superior oblique muscle—does not appear until early in the eighth week, at about the same time that the muscle of the upper eyelid, the **levator palpebrae superioris,** is formed by delamination from the superior rectus muscle. The connective tissue associated with the extrinsic ocular muscles is derived from neural crest.

The extrinsic ocular muscles are innervated by three cranial nerves: the **oculomotor nerve** (cranial nerve III), the **trochlear nerve** (cranial nerve IV), and the **abducent nerve** (cranial nerve VI). The oculomotor nerve reaches the vicinity of the developing eye early in the fifth week and innervates the levator palpebrae superioris; the superior, inferior, and medial recti; and the inferior oblique. The trochlear and abducent nerves appear at the end of the fifth week and innervate the superior oblique and the lateral rectus, respectively.

The eyelids form from folds in the surface ectoderm and associated mesenchyme

By the sixth week, small folds of ectoderm with a mesenchymal core appear just cranial and caudal to the developing cornea (Fig. 12-24). These upper and lower eyelid primordia rapidly grow toward each other, meeting and fusing by the eighth week. The space between the fused eyelids and the cornea, which is lined with ectoderm-derived epithelium, is called the **conjunctival sac.** The eyelids separate again between the fifth and seventh months.

The **lacrimal glands** form from invaginations of the ectoderm at the superolateral angles of the conjunctival sacs but do not mature until about 6 weeks after birth. The tear fluid produced by the glands is excreted into the conjunctival sac, where it lubricates the cornea.

Development of the Ears

The inner ear forms by invagination of an otic placode in the surface ectoderm of the head

Late in the third week, a thickening of the surface ectoderm called the **otic placode** or **otic disc** appears next to the rhombencephalic (hindbrain) region of each neural fold (Fig. 12-25). This placode is the primordium of the membranous labyrinth of the inner ear, including the sensory receptors for hearing and balance, and of the **statoacoustic ganglion** of the **vestibulocochlear nerve** (cranial nerve VIII), which innervates these receptors. The growth of the head causes the otic placode to be translocated caudally to the level of the second pharyngeal arch. During the fourth week, the otic placode gradually invaginates to form first an **otic pit** and then a closed, hollow **otic vesicle** (Fig. 12-25). A stem of ectoderm briefly connects the otic vesicle to the surface but disintegrates at the end of the fourth week.

The otic vesicle differentiates into a dorsal endolymphatic sac, an intermediate utricle, and a ventral saccule

By day 26 of the fourth week, the dorsomedial region of the otic vesicle begins to elongate, forming an **endolymphatic appendage** (Fig. 12-26A, B). Simultaneously, the rest of the otic vesicle differentiates into an expanded **utricle** and a tapered, ventral **saccule.** The endolymphatic appendage elongates over the following week, and its distal portion expands to form an **endolymphatic sac,** which is connected to the utricle by a slender **endolymphatic duct** (Fig. 12-26C).

During the fifth week, the ventral tip of the saccule begins to elongate and coil, forming a **cochlear duct,** which is the primordium of the cochlea (Fig. 12-26D, E). The connection between the developing cochlea and the saccule constricts to form the **ductus reuniens.** During the seventh week, cells of the cochlear duct differentiate to form the **spiral organ of Corti** (the structure that bears the hair cell receptors responsible for transducing sound vibrations into electrical impulses). The organ of Corti is innervated by the sensory neurons of the **spiral ganglion (cochlear ganglion)** tucked into the coil of the cochlea. The fibers from the spiral ganglion form the **cochlear branch** of the vestibulocochlear nerve, and they synapse in the medial geniculate bodies of the brain (see Ch. 13).

During the seventh week, three flattened diverticulae grow from the utricular portion of the otic vesicle and differentiate sequentially to form the **anterior, posterior,** and **lateral semicircular ducts** (Fig. 12-26D, E); timeline). A small expansion called the **ampulla** forms at one end of each semicircular duct. The hair cell sensory structures in the ampullae and the utriculus, which are responsible for detecting the accelerations and orientation of the head, are innervated by the **vestibular ganglion** of the vestibulocochlear nerve. The fibers of this ganglion form the **vestibular branch** of the vestibulocochlear nerve.

Beginning in the ninth week, the mesenchyme surrounding the membranous labyrinth chondrifies to form a cartilage called the **otic capsule.** During the third to fifth months, the layer of cartilage immediately surrounding the membranous labyrinth undergoes vacuolization to form a cavity somewhat larger than the membranous labyrinth. The membranous labyrinth is suspended in this cavity in a fluid called **perilymph,** and the space between the membranous labyrinth and the walls of the otic capsule is called the **perilymphatic space.** The otic capsule ossifies between 16 and 23 weeks to form the **petrous portion** of the **temporal bone** (Fig. 12-27). Continued ossification later produces the mastoid portion of the temporal bone. The bony enclosure that houses the membranous labyrinth and the perilymph is called the **bony labyrinth.**

The middle ear cavity and auditory tube are derived from the first pharyngeal pouch and are lined by endoderm

As mentioned earlier in this chapter, the first pharyngeal pouch elongates to form a **tubotympanic recess,** which subsequently differentiates to form the expanded **tympanic cavity** of the middle ear and the slender **auditory (eustachian) tube,** which connects the tympanic cavity to the pharynx. During the seventh week, the cartilaginous precursors of the three **auditory ossicles** condense in the mesenchyme of the first and second arches near the tympanic cavity (Fig. 12-26). As described earlier in this chapter, the cartilage of the mandibular process gives rise to the malleus, the cartilage of the maxillary process to the incus, and the cartilage of the second arch to the stapes. The developing ossicles remain embedded in the mesenchyme adjacent to the tympanic cavity through the eighth month of gestation. Their associated middle ear muscles—the **tensor tympani** and the **stapedius**—form in the ninth week from first- and second-arch mesenchyme.

During the ninth month of development, the mesenchyme surrounding the auditory ossicles and associated muscles disperses, and the tympanic cavity expands to enclose them (Figs. 12-26E and 12-27). The endoderm that lines the tympanic cavity therefore jackets the ossicles and also forms transient endodermal mesenteries that suspend the ossicles in the cavity until their definitive supporting ligaments develop.

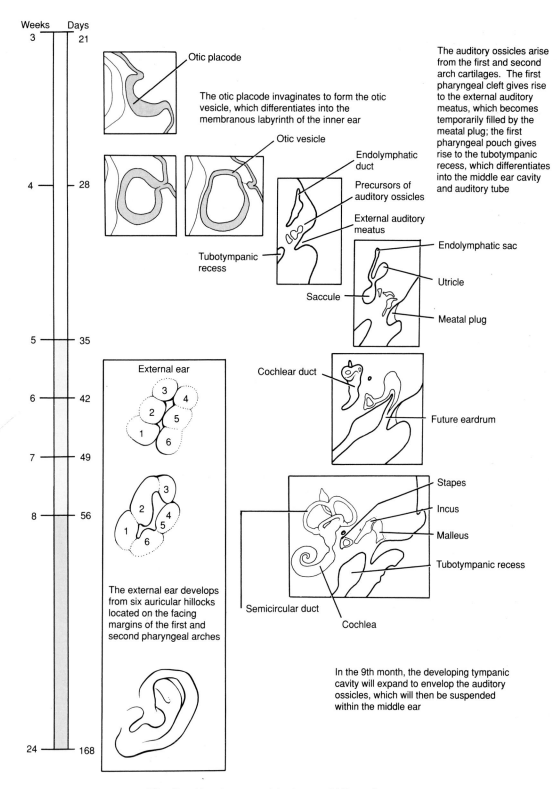

Timeline. Development of the inner, middle, and outer ears.

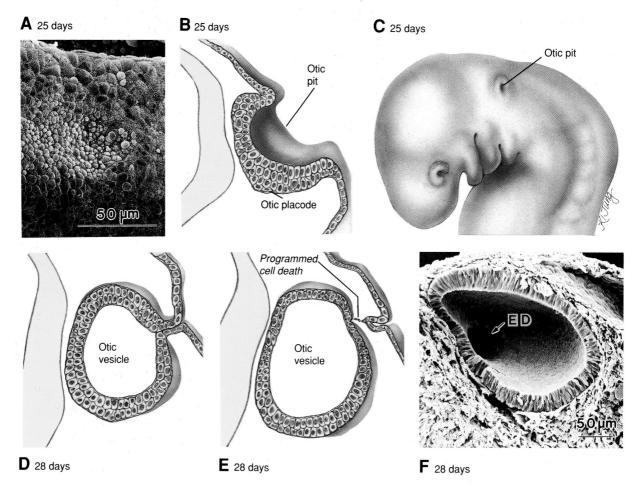

A 25 days

B 25 days

Otic
pit

Otic placode

C 25 days

Otic pit

D 28 days

Otic
vesicle

E 28 days

Programmed
cell death

Otic
vesicle

F 28 days

ED

Fig. 12-25. Formation of the otic vesicle. (**A**) The otic placode appears in the surface ecto-derm adjacent to the rhombencephalon late in the third week. (**B, C**) By day 25, the placode invaginates to form the otic pit. (**D–F**) By the end of the fourth week, continued invagination forms the otic vesicle, which quickly detaches from the surface ectoderm (ED, endolym-phatic duct). (Figs. A and F from Kikuchi T, Tonosaki A, Takasaka T. 1988. Development of apical-surface structures of mouse otic placode. Acta Otolaryngol 106:200, with permission.)

Meanwhile, the pharyngeal membrane separating the tympanic cavity from the external auditory meatus (de-rived from the first pharyngeal cleft) develops into the **tympanic membrane** or **eardrum** (Fig. 12-26E). The tympanic membrane is composed of an outer lining of ectoderm, an inner lining of endoderm, and an interven-ing mesodermal layer called the **fibrous stratum.** As described below, the definitive ectodermal layer of the tympanic membrane is formed during the process of re-canalization that created the definitive external auditory meatus.

During the ninth month, the tympanic cavity expands into the mastoid part of the temporal bone to form the **mastoid antrum.** The **mastoid air cells** in the mastoid portion of the temporal bone do not form until about 2

years of age, when the action of the sternocleidomastoid muscle on the mastoid part of the temporal bone induces the mastoid process to form.

The external ear is derived from the first pharyngeal cleft and the first and second pharyngeal arches

The external ear consists of the funnel-shaped **external auditory meatus** and the **auricle (pinna).** The precursor of the external auditory meatus develops by deepening of the first pharyngeal cleft during the sixth week. However, the ectodermal lining of the deep portion of this tube later proliferates, producing a solid core of tissue called the **meatal plug** that completely fills the medial end of the

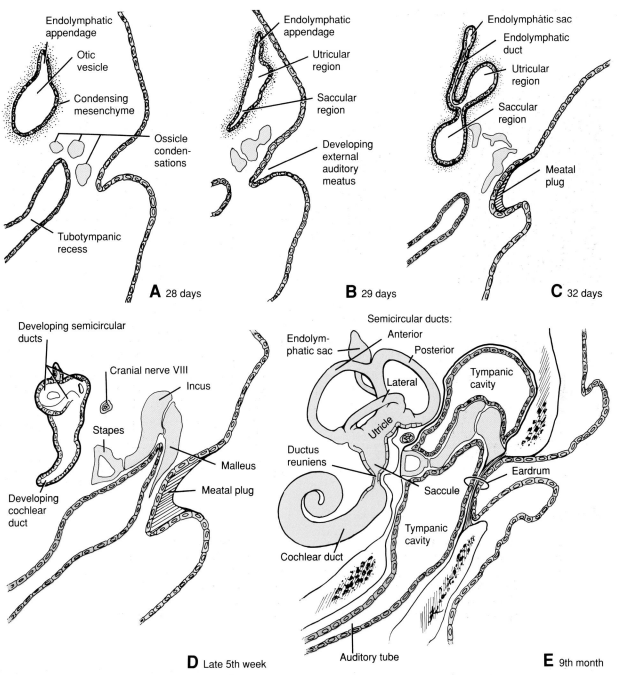

Fig. 12-26. Development of the ear. The components of the inner, middle, and outer ears arise in coordination from several embryonic structures. The otic vesicle gives rise to the membranous labyrinth of the inner ear and to the eighth nerve ganglia. (**A, B**) The superior end of the otic vesicle forms an endolymphatic appendage, and the body of the vesicle then differentiates into utricular and saccular regions. (**C, D**) The endolymphatic appendage elongates to form the endolymphatic sac and duct; the utricle gives rise to the three semicircular ducts; and the inferior end of the saccule elongates and coils to form the cochlear duct. Simultaneously, the three auditory ossicles arise from mesenchymal condensations formed by the first and second pharyngeal arches; the first pharyngeal pouch enlarges to form the tubotympanic recess (the future middle ear cavity), and the first pharyngeal cleft (the future external auditory meatus) becomes filled with a transient meatal plug of ectodermal cells. (**E**) Finally, in the ninth month, the tubotympanic cavity expands to enclose the auditory ossicles, forming the functional middle ear cavity. The definitive eardrum represents the first pharyngeal membrane and is thus a three-layered structure comprising ectoderm, mesoderm, and endoderm.

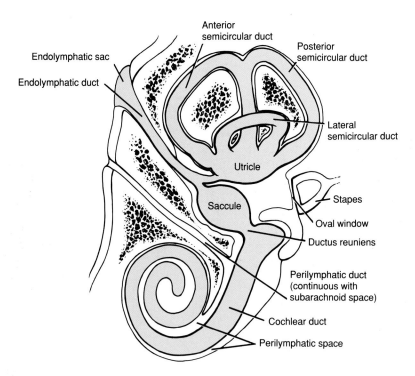

Fig. 12-27. The definitive membranous labyrinth is suspended in the fluid-filled perilymphatic space within the bony labyrinth of the petrous portion of the temporal bone. The perilymphatic space is connected to the subarachnoid space by the perilymphatic duct. The membranous labyrinth itself is filled with endolymph.

external auditory meatus by week 26. Canalization of this plug begins almost immediately and produces the medial two-thirds of the definitive meatus. The meatus does not achieve its final length until the age of 9 or 10 years.

The auricle develops from three pairs of **auricular hillocks** that arise during the fifth week on the facing edges of the first and second arches (Fig. 12-28). From ventral to dorsal, the hillocks on the first arch are called the **tragus, helix,** and **cymba concha,** and the hillocks on the second arch are called the **antitragus, antihelix,** and **concha.** During the seventh week the auricular

hillocks begin to enlarge, differentiate, and fuse to produce the definitive form of the auricle. As the face develops, the auricle is gradually translocated from its original location low on the side of the neck to a more lateral and cranial site.

The absence or abnormal development of one or more of the auricular hillocks may result in malformations of the auricle. A defect that suppresses the growth of all the hillocks results in **microtia** (small auricle) or **anotia** (absence of the auricle). Accessory hillocks may also form, producing ectopic **auricular tags.**

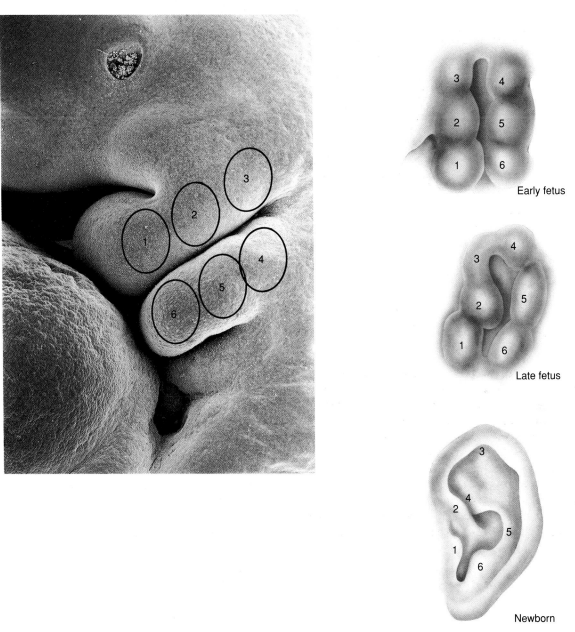

Fig. 12-28. Differentiation of the auricle. The auricle develops from six auricular hillocks, which arise on the apposed surfaces of the first and second pharyngeal arches. (Fig. A photo courtesy of Dr. Arnold Tamarin.)

APPLICATIONS TO CLINICAL PRACTICE

Craniofacial defects represent a large proportion of all human congenital malformations

It is estimated that the **craniofacial anomalies**—including malformations of the cranial vault, clefting defects, malformations of the forebrain and midface process, and anomalies of the pharyngeal arches—account for approximately one-third of all congenital defects. Most arise through multifactorial effects, but some have a genetic basis and others are caused by teratogens such as alcohol, retinoic acid analogs, phenytoin, toluene, cigarette smoking, ionizing radiation, and hyperthermia.

Premature calvarial synostosis results in malformations of the skull

A familial condition called **craniofrontonasal dysplasia syndrome** is characterized by a tall narrow skull called **acrocephaly (tower skull),** which arises through the premature closure or synostosis of the coronal suture. This syndrome may also include **hypertelorism** and **clefting** of the nose and upper lip. On the other hand, premature closure of the suture between the frontal bones results in a triangular skull shape called **trigonocephaly** and may occur in response to alcohol during early embryonic development (see below). Other craniofacial syndromes involving premature synostosis of cranial sutures include **Crouzen** and **Apert syndromes** (Fig. 12-29).

Alcohol consumed in early pregnancy may produce devastating effects on brain and midface development

Disturbances in the early induction of the forebrain (prosencephalon) can result in a spectrum of abnormalities known as **holoprosencephaly.** The forebrain anomalies characteristic of holoprosencephaly result from defective development of the ventromedial forebrain and include deficiencies of the olfactory nerves, olfactory bulbs, olfactory tracts, basal olfactory cortex, and associated structures like the limbic lobe, hippocampus, and mammillary bodies. The corpus callosum is sometimes affected, but the hindbrain is usually normal. Disturbances of forebrain development also affect development of midfacial structures resulting in a short upturned nose, a long upper lip with deficient philtrum, a highly arched palate, **retrognathia** (short retracted lower jaw), and **microcephaly** (small skull). In severe cases, derivatives of the nasal placode are affected; the medial nasal processes

and intermaxillary process may fail to form (Fig. 12-30A), and the nasal septum and ethmoid bones may be deficient. The nose may have only a single nostril (**cebocephaly;** Fig. 12-30B), and the eyes may be close set (**hypotelorism;** Fig. 12-30C). Sometimes only a single eye is present (**cyclopia;** Fig. 12-30D).

The majority of cases of holoprosencephaly are caused by consumption of alcohol during the period when events responsible for forebrain induction are taking place. The same effects have been produced by administration of alcohol to mice during the appropriate sensitive period. Alcohol-related holoprosencephaly is thought to be the major cause of **mental retardation** in the Western World. This condition, called **fetal alcohol syndrome (FAS),** may affect as many as 2 in 1,000 live-born infants and as many as 1 in 6 in some subpopulations. It must be recognized that

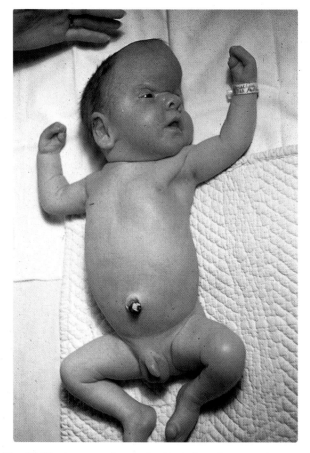

Fig. 12-29. Apert syndrome. In this infant, the coronal sutures have fused prematurely, and the cranium has therefore been forced to adopt a "tower skull" (acrocephalic) shape to accommodate the growing brain. (Photo courtesy of Dr. David Billmire.)

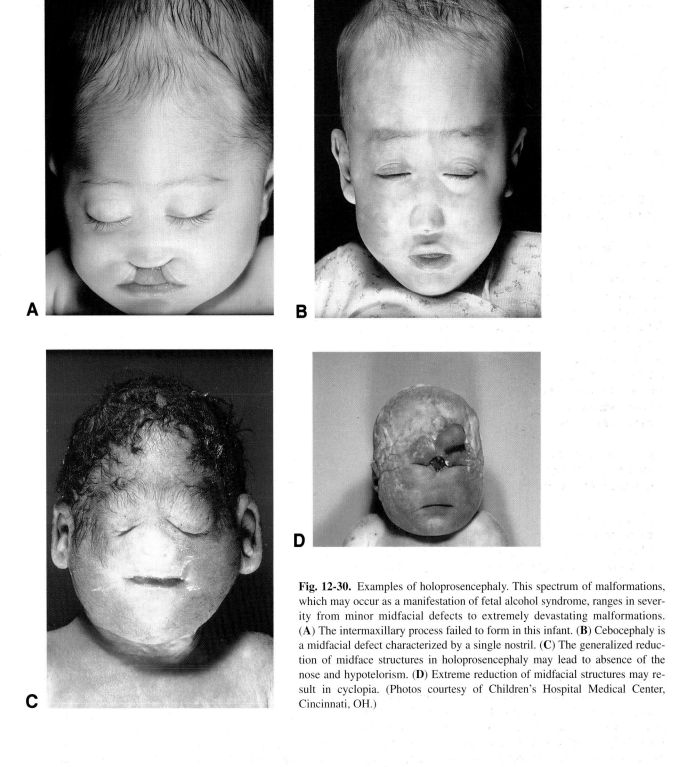

Fig. 12-30. Examples of holoprosencephaly. This spectrum of malformations, which may occur as a manifestation of fetal alcohol syndrome, ranges in severity from minor midfacial defects to extremely devastating malformations. (**A**) The intermaxillary process failed to form in this infant. (**B**) Cebocephaly is a midfacial defect characterized by a single nostril. (**C**) The generalized reduction of midface structures in holoprosencephaly may lead to absence of the nose and hypotelorism. (**D**) Extreme reduction of midfacial structures may result in cyclopia. (Photos courtesy of Children's Hospital Medical Center, Cincinnati, OH.)

the most severe effects of alcohol occur in the first month of pregnancy, typically when a woman does not know she is pregnant. While avoidance of alcohol throughout pregnancy is recommended, it is of the utmost importance that **couples who are planning a pregnancy** must be advised of these devastating effects. Other teratogens like toluene may also result in holoprosencephaly, and offspring of diabetic mothers appear to be at increased risk. Holoprosencephaly may also occur in trisomies 13, 18, and 21. Some cases of holoprosencephaly may be caused by mutation as in the autosomal recessive **Meckel syndrome** (Fig. 12-31).

The expression of Sonic hedgehog by prechordal plate mesoderm is required for normal forebrain and midface development

The knockout of the signaling molecule Sonic hedgehog (Shh) in a transgenic mouse is extraordinarily in-

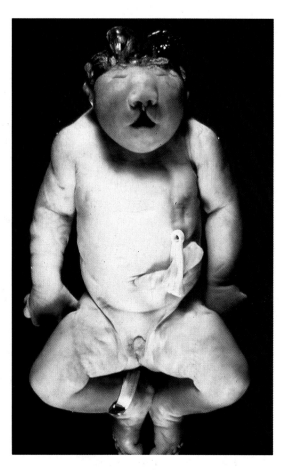

Fig. 12-31. Meckel syndrome. Holoprosencephalic defects of the midface, including absence of the olfactory bulbs, are common manifestations of this autosomal recessive syndrome. (Photo courtesy of Children's Hospital Medical Center, Cincinnati, OH.)

structive. First, with respect to this chapter, the abnormalities of craniofacial development exhibited by these null mutants provide evidence that Shh expression is required for normal forebrain and midfacial development since these animals exhibit cyclopia, the most severe form of the holoprosencephalic spectrum of anomalies. As in the case of the interaction between the notochord and ventral spinal cord, Shh expression in the prechordal mesoderm appears to play a key role in the induction of ventral midline structures in the forebrain. As might be expected, development of ventral midline structures in the presumptive spinal cord, such as the floor plate and motor columns, are also disrupted. While the notochord forms in these animals, it rapidly degenerates, supporting the possibility that normal expression of Shh is required for maintenance of the notochord.

This interesting knockout also sheds light on possible reasons for some common associations of craniofacial, limb, and axial abnormalities in humans. These animals also exhibit distal limb disruptions and axial skeletal anomalies including the disruption of vertebral and rib development. Recall from Chapter 4 that Shh expressed by the notochord induces the medial region of the somite to form the sclerotome. Recall from Chapter 11 that Shh plays a key role in craniocaudal differentiation of the limb buds. The reductions of distal limb structures in this knockout also suggests that Shh may play some role in proximodistal differentiation of the limb buds as well.

Holoprosencephaly may result from disturbances of cholesterol metabolism

It is now clear that normal Shh signaling depends on an autoprocessing step that cleaves the molecule into C- and N-terminal fragments. During this process, the C fragment functions as a **cholesterol transferase** that covalently links cholesterol to the amino fragment as a lipophilic adduct converting the amino fragment to an active Shh signaling factor. Thus it should not be surprising that holoprosencephalic malformations occur in pups born to rats treated with inhibitors of cholesterol biosynthesis. Similarly, this relationship between cholesterol and Shh signaling may also explain the occurrence of holoprosencephalic and limb abnormalities in humans suffering from the autosomal recessive disorder **Smith-Lemli-Opitz syndrome (SLOS).** It is estimated that this autosomal recessive disease, which is characterized by elimination of activity of the last enzyme in the cholesterol pathway, affects about 1 in 9,000 births (alive and stillborn). The mechanism by which alcohol may disrupt the Shh signaling process is not understood.

Facial clefts arise from teratogenic or genetic causes

Complete or partial failure of fusion between any of the facial swellings is called a **facial cleft,** which can be unilateral or bilateral. The most common types are **cleft lip** (Figs. 12-32 and 12-33) and **cleft palate** (Fig. 12-33). Although cleft lip and cleft palate often occur together, the defects differ in their distribution with respect to sex, familial association, race, and geography and therefore probably have different etiologies. For example, **cleft lip** has been ascribed to underdevelopment of mesenchyme in the maxillary swellings that results in inadequate contact of the maxillary swelling with the medial nasal process and intermaxillary process. The defect may occur because of inadequate migration of neural crest or excessive cell death during modeling of the nasal placode and maxillary swelling. The cleft may be a minor notch in the vermilion border of the lip to a cleft that completely sepa-

rates the lateral lip from the philtrum and nasal cavity. Some clefts involve the soft tissue only, while others may separate the bony premaxilla and primary palate from the maxillary bone. Cleft lip may be induced by several common drugs including the anticonvulsant phenytoin (dilantin), vitamin A, and some vitamin A analogs, particularly the oral anti-acne drug isotretinoin (Accutane). In contrast, **cleft palate** results from failure of the palatine shelves to fuse during the 7th to 10th weeks and may result from a variety of errors. These include inadequate growth of the palatine shelves, failure of the shelves to elevate at the proper time, an excessively wide head, failure of the shelves to fuse, and secondary rupture after fusion. Cleft palate may, therefore, result from a wide range of congenital insults and genetic errors. Most cases are multifactorial in etiology, although an X-linked cleft palate syndrome has been described. Teratogens such as phenytoin, vitamin A and its analogs, and some corticosteroid anti-inflammatory drugs may also cause cleft palate.

Pharyngeal arch defects may be caused by vascular disruptions

Not surprisingly, errors in the development of the numerous pharyngeal arch and pouch elements that contribute to the human head and face can cause varied malformations. After cleft lip and cleft palate, the most common group of facial malformations are defects caused by underdevelopment of the first and second arches, collectively known as **craniofacial microsomia** (*microsomia* is from the Greek word for *small body*). The most common of these defects is a lateral cleft, in which incomplete fusion of the maxillary and mandibular processes in the cheek region results in a cleft extending from the corner of the mouth to as far as the tragus of the auricle. In contrast to the facial clefts described above, this malformation may arise from secondary ischemic necrosis caused by an expanding hematoma arising from the stapedial artery system. The group of deformities known as **hemifacial microsomia** are also thought to arise in many cases by the same vascular mechanism. In these deformities, the lateral cleft of the face is usually not large, but the posterior portion of the mandible, the temporomandibular joint, the muscles of mastication, and the outer and middle ear may all be underdeveloped. Figure 12-34 illustrates **Goldenhar syndrome,** a particularly severe member of this group.

Pharyngeal arch defects may result from direct disturbances of neural crest cell migration

The syndromes classified as **mandibulofacial dysostosis** may resemble the above vascular-related deformities

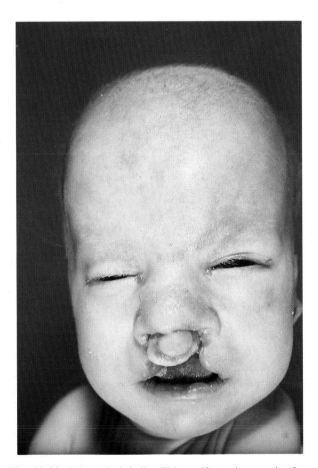

Fig. 12-32. Bilateral cleft lip. This malformation results from failure of the medial nasal processes to fuse with the maxillary swellings. (Photo courtesy of Children's Hospital Medical Center, Cincinnati, OH.)

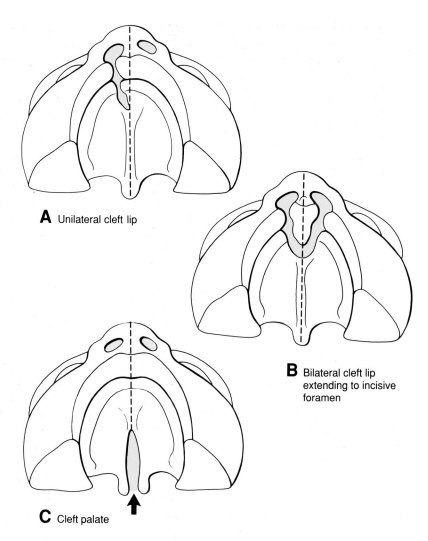

Fig. 12-33. Cleft lip and cleft palate. (**A, B**) Cleft lip. The cleft may involve the lip only or extend posteriorly along one or both edges of the primary palate. (**C**) Cleft palate results from failure of the palantine shelves to properly fuse during development of the secondary palate. Cleft lip and cleft palate appear to represent distinct errors of development.

but arise by very different mechanisms. In these disorders, underdevelopment of the lower face and mandible and associated abnormalities of the palate and external ears result from a deficit of mesenchyme in the **first** and **second pharyngeal arches.** This deficit may result from defective migration or proliferation of neural crest cells or, alternatively, from excessive cell death. Two genetic syndromes involving mandibulofacial dysostosis are **Treacher-Collins syndrome** and **Hallerman-Streif syndrome.** It is thought that the former may be an autosomal dominant form and the latter an autosomal recessive form of the same genetic syndrome. Other cases of mandibulofacial dysostosis apparently arise through diverse etiologies. The oral anti-acne drug isotretinoin can cause similar abnormalities in humans if administered during the first month and in experimental animals if administered during the comparable period of development.

A related complex of congenital malformations known as **DiGeorge syndrome** mainly affects the **third** and **fourth pharyngeal arches.** It is characterized by three groups of malformations: (1) minor craniofacial defects, including micrognathia (small jaw), low-set ears, auricular abnormalities, cleft palate, and hypertelorism; (2) total or partial agenesis of the derivatives of the third and fourth pharyngeal pouches (the thymus and parathyroid glands); and (3) cardiovascular anomalies, including persistent truncus arteriosus and interrupted aortic arch. This syndrome may be caused by abnormalities of neural crest migration and proliferation occurring during the formation of the third and fourth arches, that is, slightly later in development than for the cases of mandibulofacial dysostosis described above. The inclusion of cardiac abnormalities is explained by the migration of neural crest cells through the third to the sixth pharyngeal arches to form the aorticopulmonary septum (see Ch. 7). Although some cases of DiGeorge syndrome are associated with partial monosomy of chromosome 22, the syndrome also occurs among offspring of alcoholic women. Experiments have shown that

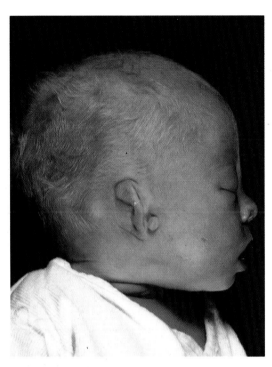

Fig. 12-34. An infant with Goldenhar syndrome, exhibiting characteristic hemifacial microsomia anomalies of the ear. These defects apparently are caused by an expanding hematoma of the stapedial artery system. (Photo courtesy of Children's Hospital Medical Center, Cincinnati, OH.)

acute administration of alcohol to animals during the period of third and fourth arch development can result in a spectrum of anomalies similar to DiGeorge syndrome.

Some pharyngeal arch anomalies may result from disruption of the segmental development of the brain and the pharyngeal arches

The cranial paraxial mesoderm and the brain of vertebrate embryos are transiently segmented. As described in Chapter 3, the paraxial mesoderm initially differentiates into whorl-like structures called **somitomeres**. Most somitomeres proceed to form somites. The first seven cranial somitomeres, however, never form somites. The four somitomeres that develop next to the caudal half of the hindbrain, however, differentiate to form the four occipital somites. The neural tube also displays segmentation early in its development (see Ch. 13). This segmentation is clearest in the hindbrain (rhombencephalon), which is transiently divided into a series of small swellings called neuromeres or, more specifically, **rhombomeres**. Nine rhombomeres form in rats, fishes, and humans; eight have been detected in the chick. In this case, the rhombomeres

are spatially related to the first three pharyngeal arches and their cranial nerves; the first three pharyngeal arches are each aligned with two pairs of rhombomeres (Fig. 12-35).

Segmentation of the pharyngeal arches is regulated by combinatorial *HOX* gene codes

It is now apparent that each rhombomere is specified by a **combinatorial code of *HOX* gene expression** similar to that described for the paraxial mesoderm and somites in the trunk (see Ch. 4). In fact, the cranial expression boundaries of several *Hox* genes coincide exactly with rhombomere boundaries, providing a basis for the unique developmental function of each rhombomere (Fig. 12-35). Moreover, the hypothesis that the *Hox* gene code specifies development of the pharyngeal arches has been tested in several transgenic knockouts.

For example, knockout of *Hoxa-1* results in severe alteration of rhombomeres 4 and 5. Rhombomere 4 is significantly reduced, and rhombomere 5 is almost absent. The parts of these rhombomeres that remain fuse with rhombomere 6 to form a single "fourth" rhombomere. As a consequence, the motor nuclei of facial and abducens nerves that normally develop within rhombomeres 4, 5, and 6 (Fig. 12-35) are not formed. Alternatively, the targeted disruption of *Hoxa-3* results in failure of development of the thymus, an organ derived from the third pharyngeal pouch, which lies within the normal expression territory of this switch gene. Development of the thyroid gland, which develops from the foramen cecum between the first and second arch, is also reduced. Targeted disruption of *Hoxa-2*, however, produces a truly dramatic effect. Indeed, the effect can be described as a **homeotic transformation of pharyngeal arch 2 to pharyngeal arch 1.** The resulting mice exhibit duplication of first arch structures. One explanation for this result is that a *Hox*-independent ground pattern drives development of the first pharyngeal arch and underlies development of the second pharyngeal arch. Knockout of the *Hoxa-2* gene in arch 2 thus transforms the overriding *Hoxa-2*-driven developmental program of the second arch to the basic ground pattern-driven program of the first arch. All of these results taken together as well as evidence from many other studies support the hypothesis that the specific development of each pharyngeal arch depends on interactions of unique constellations of elements within each rhombomere.

The unique specification of each neural crest subpopulation occurs prior to migration into respective pharyngeal arches

Even when rhombencephalic neural crest cells and dorsal regions of the rhombencephalon are ablated, the

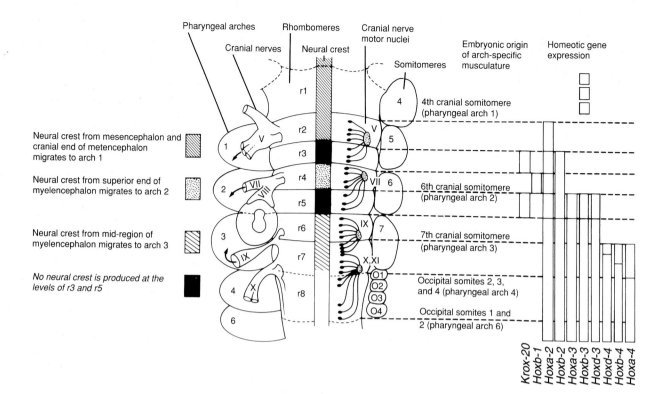

Fig. 12-35. Stylized depiction of the brain stem showing the spatial relationships of the pharyngeal arches, neuromeres, cranial nerves, cranial nerve motor nuclei, neural crest domains, somitomeres and somites, and *Hox, Eux-1, Pax-2,* and *Krox-20* gene expression. (*Krox-20, Eux-1,* and *Pax-2,* like the *Hox* genes, have been implicated in transcription regulation.) (Data from Lumsden A, Keynes R. 1989. Segmental patterns of neuronal development in the chick hindbrain. Nature [London] 337:424; Wilkinson DG, Bhatt S, Cook M et al. 1989. Segmental expression of *Hox-2* homeobox-containing genes in the developing mouse hindbrain. Nature [London] 341:405; Jacobson AG. 1992. Somitomeres: mesodermal segments of the head and trunk. In Hanken J, Hall BH [eds]: The Vertebrate Skull. University of Chicago Press, Chicago; and Krumlauf R. 1993. *Hox* genes and pattern formation in the branchial region of the vertebrate head. TIG 9:106.)

neural crest cells regenerating from the cut edge of the hindbrain (see above) continue to express *Hox* genes unique to their regions of origin. This result and other transplantation experiments support the likelihood that the rhombomere-specific identity of these cells is determined by unique patterns of *Hox* gene expression within these specific segments of the neural tube, prior to neural crest cell detachment and migration. In addition, it seems likely from transplantation experiments that the neural crest cells of a given arch direct the arch-specific development of the striated muscles of that arch.

Retinoic acid may play a role in normal development of the head and neck

While it is clear that **retinoic acid** is a potent craniofacial teratogen, especially affecting arches 1 and 2, this presumptive morphogen has also been implicated in nor-

mal differentiation of head and neck structures. Ectopic application of retinoic acid to developing chick embryos, for example, transforms rhombomeres 2/3 to rhombomeres 4/5. Recall from Chapter 4 that excess retinoic acid results in a caudalization of axial structures in the trunk. In addition, the application of excess retinoic acid inhibits neural crest migration, resulting in hypoplasia of the first three arches.

More direct evidence of the role of retinoic acid in normal development of the head and neck, however, is provided by the results of double RAR receptor knockout experiments. These knockouts result in arch-related craniofacial abnormalities. Finally, the mediation of retinoic acid effects by *Hox* genes is supported by the discovery of **retinoic acid response elements** in **enhancers** of *Hoxa-1* and *Hoxa-2.* In addition, knockouts of these elements abolish the normal expression of *Hoxa-1* and *Hoxa-2* in the neural epithelium caudal to the fourth rhombomere.

CHAPTER

13

Development of the Brain and Cranial Nerves

Development of the Regions of the Brain;
Organization of the Cranial Nerves and Their
Nuclei and Ganglia; Cytodifferentiation in the
Brain; Development of the Ventricular System

SUMMARY

The primordia of the **three primary brain vesicles** are first visible as broadenings in the neural plate. Following neurulation in the fifth week, the **prosencephalon** then subdivides into a **telencephalon** and a **diencephalon,** and the **rhombencephalon** subdivides into a **metencephalon** and a **myelencephalon,** thus creating **five secondary brain vesicles,** along with the **mesencephalon.** The brain is also transiently divided into smaller segments called **neuromeres** and undergoes flexion at three points.

Cytodifferentiation of the neural tube begins in the **rhombencephalon** at the end of the fourth week. At first, the neuroepithelium produces the neuroblasts and then the glioblasts and ependyma. The neuroblasts form the gray matter, and the growing neuronal fibers establish the white matter. The brain stem is then organized into a pair of basal columns and a pair of alar columns. Laterally these columns are separated by a groove called the **sulcus limitans;** dorsally and ventrally they are separated by the **roof plate** and **floor plate.** The 12 pairs of **cranial nerve motor nuclei** develop from the brain stem basal plates, and the **cranial nerve associational nuclei** develop from alar plates. All of these are organized into seven columns, which correspond to the types of function they serve. The peripheral neurons of the sensory and parasympathetic cranial nerve pathways reside in peripheral ganglia and are partly derived from neural crest and partly from ectodermal placodes.

The **myelencephalon** gives rise to the **medulla oblongata,** which is the portion of the brain most similar to the spinal cord. The **metencephalon** gives rise to the **pons** and to the **cerebellum.** Congenital anomalies of the cerebellum and their causes are described in the Applications to Clinical Practice section of this chapter. The **mesencephalon** contains nuclei of three cranial nerves as well as various other structures. In particular, the alar plates give rise to the superior and inferior colliculi. The **forebrain** has no basal plates.

The alar plates of the **diencephalon** are divided into a dorsal portion and a ventral portion. The ventral **hypothalamus** controls visceral activities such as heart rate and pituitary secretion, while the dorsal thalamus serves as a relay center. The most dorsal epithalamus gives rise to the pineal gland. A ventral outpouching of the diencephalon called the **infundibulum** and a matching diverticulum of the stomodeal roof called **Rathke's pouch** form the **pituitary gland.** Diencephalic outpouchings also form the eyes. The two **cerebral hemispheres** arise as lateral outpouchings of the **telencephalon** and grow rapidly to cover the diencephalon and mesencephalon. The hemispheres are joined by fiber tracts called **commissures.** The olfactory bulbs and olfactory tracts arise from the telencephalon and synapse with the primary olfactory neurosensory cells that differentiate in the nasal placodes. The neural canal within the secondary brain vesicles gives rise to the ventricular system of the brain. The cerebrospinal fluid that fills the ventricle system is produced mainly by secretory choroid plexuses.

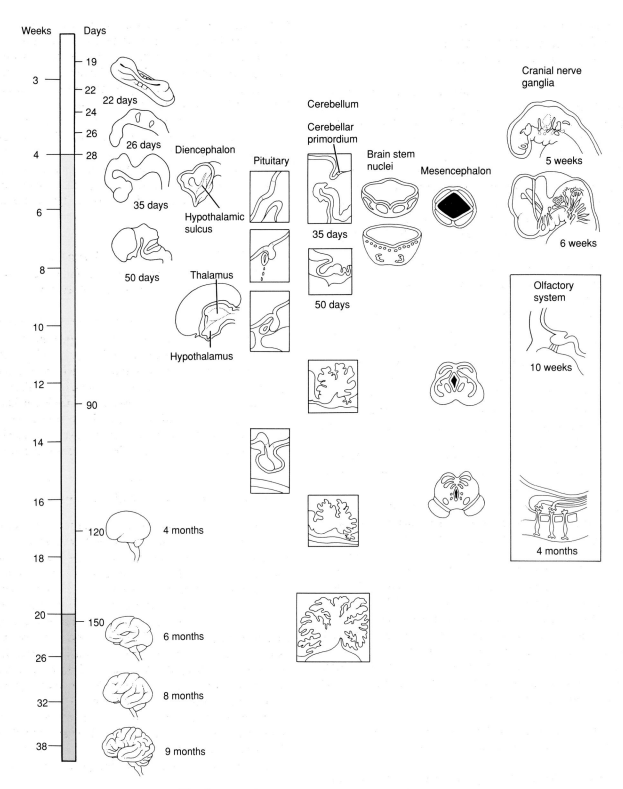

Weeks   Days

3   19
         22 days
         22
         24
         26
         26 days

4   28   Diencephalon   Pituitary   Cerebellum
                                                               Cerebellar
                     35 days   primordium   Brain stem
6   nuclei   Mesencephalon
                     Hypothalamic
                     sulcus   35 days
8
         50 days   50 days
                     Thalamus
10
                     Hypothalamus

12

         90

14

16

         120   4 months

18

20
         150   6 months

26

32   8 months

38   9 months

Cranial nerve ganglia

5 weeks

6 weeks

Olfactory system

10 weeks

4 months

Timeline. Development of the brain and cranial nerves.

The three primary brain vesicles subdivide to form five secondary brain vesicles

Chapters 3 and 4 describe how the central nervous system (CNS) arises as a neural plate from the ectoderm of the germ disc and folds to form the neural tube. The presumptive brain is visible as the broad cranial portion of the neural plate. Even on day 19, before neurulation begins, the three major divisions of the brain—the **prosencephalon (forebrain), mesencephalon (midbrain),** and **rhombencephalon (hindbrain)**—are demarcated by indentations in the neural folds. The future eyes appear as outpouchings from the forebrain neural folds by day 22 (see Ch. 12). Neurulation begins on day 22, and the cranial neuropore closes on day 24. The three brain divisions are then marked by expansions of the neural tube called **primary brain vesicles** (Fig. 13-1A, B).

By day 21, an additional series of narrow swellings called **neuromeres** becomes apparent in the future brain (Fig. 13-1B). At least six neuromeres may form in the presumptive prosencephalon (P1 to P6), one (M1) in the presumptive mesencephalon, and nine in the presumptive rhombencephalon. The nine hindbrain segments consist of a single **isthmic segment,** occupying the constricted isthmic region of the rhombencephalon, and eight **rhombomeres,** numbered r1 through r8. The neuromeres are transient structures and become indistinguishable by the early sixth week. Their possible relation with the segmentation of the paraxial mesoderm and pharyngeal arches is discussed in the Applications to Clinical Practice section of Chapter 12.

During the fifth week, the prosencephalon and rhombencephalon each subdivide into two portions, thus converting the three primary brain vesicles into five **secondary brain vesicles** (Fig. 13-1C). The prosencephalon divides into a cranial **telencephalon** ("end-brain") and a caudal **diencephalon** ("between-brain"). The rhombencephalon divides into a cranial **metencephalon** ("behind-brain") and a caudal **myelencephalon** ("medulla-brain"). Within each of the brain vesicles, the neural canal is expanded into a cavity called a **primitive ventricle.** These primitive ventricles will become the definitive ventricles of the mature brain (see Fig. 13-15).

The brain folds at the mesencephalic, cervical, and pontine flexures

Between the fourth and eighth weeks, the brain tube folds sharply at three locations (Fig. 13-1). The first of these folds to develop is the **mesencephalic flexure (cranial flexure)** in the midbrain region (see Ch. 6). The prosencephalon rotates ventrally and then posteriorly around this hinge during the fourth and fifth weeks until it is folded back under the mesencephalon. Ventral flexion begins during the fifth week at the **cervical flexure** between the myelencephalon and the spinal cord and continues through the eighth week. The development of the cranial and cervical flexures is closely related to the craniocaudal folding of the embryonic disc (see Ch. 6).

During the fifth week, reverse, dorsal flexion begins at the location of the developing pons. By the eighth week, the deepening of this **pontine flexure** has folded the metencephalon (including the developing cerebellum) back onto the myelencephalon. The pontine flexure may form as a result of differential growth in the ventral part of the metencephalon.

The fundamental organization of the brain stem and cranial nerves is similar to that of the spinal cord and spinal nerves

For purposes of description, the brain can be divided into two parts: the **brain stem,** which represents the cranial continuation of the spinal cord and is similar to it in organization, and the **higher centers,** which are extremely specialized and retain little trace of a spinal cord-like organization. The brain stem consists of the myelencephalon, the metencephalon derivative called the **pons,** and the mesencephalon. The higher centers consist of the cerebellum (derived from the metencephalon) and the forebrain.

The brain stem is initially organized into basal and alar columns

As described in Chapter 4, the neurons of the developing spinal cord aggregate to form four plates or cell columns: two **basal (ventral) columns** and two **alar (dorsal) columns.** The basal columns contain the somatic and visceral motor neurons, and the alar columns contain the association neurons that synapse with *afferent* (incoming) fibers from the sensory neurons of the dorsal root ganglia. The axon of an association neuron may synapse with motor neurons on the same (ipsilateral) or opposite (contralateral) side of the cord, forming a reflex arc, or may ascend to the brain. The outgoing (*efferent*) motor neuron fibers exit via the ventral roots.

The primitive pattern is much less easy to detect in the forebrain. Basal plates are entirely lacking in the forebrain. The diencephalon has alar plates, but it is not clear whether the gray matter of the telencephalon represents alar plates.

The early differentiation of the brain stem is similar to that of the spinal cord

In the brain stem, as in the spinal cord, all the cell types of the CNS except the microglia are produced by the neu-

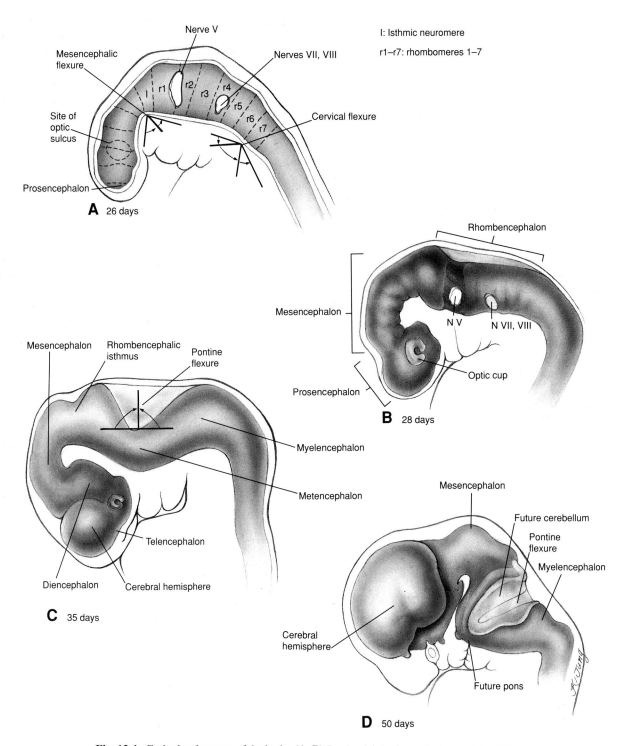

Fig. 13-1. Early development of the brain. **(A, B)** By day 26 the future brain consists of three primary brain vesicles (the prosencephalon, mesencephalon, and to begin bending at the mesencephalic and cervical flexures. **(C, D)** Further subdivision of the brain vesicles creates five secondary vesicles: the rhombencephalon divides into the metencephalon and myelencephalon, and the prosencephalon divides into the diencephalon and telencephalon. The cerebral hemispheres appear and expand rapidly. The pontine flexure folds the metencephalon back against the myelencephalon.

roepithelium lining the neural canal (see Ch. 4). An initial wave of proliferation produces the neuroblasts, which migrate peripherally. As neuroblast production tapers off, a second wave produces the glioblasts, which also migrate peripherally and differentiate to form astrocytes and oligodendrocytes. The layer of neuroepithelium lining the neural canal then differentiates to form the ependyma (see Fig. 4-16).

The neuroblasts aggregate to form a **mantle zone** surrounding the proliferating neuroepithelium, which is then called the **ventricular zone.** Neuronal fibers produced by the mantle neurons form a **marginal zone** external to the mantle layer. The mantle layer gives rise to the **gray matter** of the CNS, whereas the marginal layer gives rise to the **white matter,** so called because of the whitish color imparted by the fatty myelin sheaths that wrap around many of the nerve fibers. In the CNS, these sheaths are formed by oligodendrocytes rather than by Schwann cells. The marginal layer contains the nerve fibers entering and leaving the CNS as well as the fiber tracts coursing to higher or lower levels in the CNS.

The differentiation of the neural tube begins in the region of the rhombencephalon. Because this portion of the brain stem contains most of the cranial nerve nuclei, its morphogenesis will now be described.

The walls of the rhombencephalon splay apart to form a troughlike fourth ventricle with a thin roof plate

The roof and floor plates of the spinal cord are narrow and lie at the bottom of deep grooves. In the rhombencephalon, in contrast, the walls of the neural tube splay open dorsally so that the roof plate is stretched and widened and the alar and basal plates lie nearly parallel to each other in an oblique plane (Fig. 13-2). The rhombencephalic neural canal (future fourth ventricle) is diamond shaped in dorsal view, with the widest point located at the pontine flexure. The dorsal margin of the alar plate, from which the roof plate arises, is called the **rhombic lip.** Cranial to the pontine flexure, the rhombic lip is thickened and laps over onto the roof of the neural canal. This metencephalic portion of the rhombic lip will give rise to the cerebellum.

The thin rhombencephalic roof plate consists mainly of a layer of ependyma and is covered by a well-vascularized layer of pia mater called the **tela choroidea.** On either side of the midline, the pia and ependyma form a zone of minute, fingerlike structures projecting into the fourth ventricle. This zone, called a **choroid plexus,** is specialized to secrete cerebrospinal fluid. Similar choroid plexuses develop in the ventricles of the forebrain. Cerebrospinal fluid circulates constantly through the central canal of the spinal cord and ventricles of the brain and also through the subarachnoid space surrounding the CNS, from which it is reabsorbed into the blood. The fluid gains access to the subarachnoid space via three holes that open in the roof plate of the fourth ventricle: a single **median aperture (foramen of Magendie)** and two **lateral apertures (foramina of Luschka).**

The cranial nerve nuclei appear in the brain stem during the fifth week

All of the 12 cranial nerves except the first (olfactory) and second (optic) arise from nuclei located in the brain stem. These nuclei are among the earliest structures to develop in the brain. The basal plates of the rhombencephalon are the first neuronal aggregations in the CNS. By day 28, all the brain stem cranial nerve motor nuclei are distinguishable. As in the spinal cord, the alar plates of the brain stem form somewhat later than the basal plates, appearing in the middle of the fifth week. The cranial nerve associational nuclei are all distinguishable by the end of the fifth week. Figure 13-5 (see below) illustrates the development of the cranial nerves.

The cranial nerves are motor, sensory, or mixed

Although the cranial nerves show homologies to spinal nerves, they are much less uniform in composition. Three cranial nerves are exclusively sensory (I, II, and VIII); four are exclusively motor (IV, VI, XI, and XII); one is mixed sensory and motor (V); one is motor and parasympathetic (III); and three include sensory, motor, and parasympathetic fibers (VII, IX, and X). The motor and sensory fibers of the cranial nerves nevertheless bear the same basic relation to the cell columns of the brain that the ventral and dorsal roots bear to the cell columns of the spinal cord. Table 13-1 summarizes the relations of the cranial nerves to the subdivisions of the brain.

The cranial nerve nuclei of the brain stem are organized into seven columns on the basis of function

In the same way that the basal plates of the spinal cord are organized into somatic motor and autonomic motor columns (see Ch. 4), the basal and alar cranial nerve nuclei of the brain stem are organized into seven columns that subserve particular functions. Although seven columns form, some textbooks describe only six functions, three motor and three sensory. Figure 13-3 shows the arrangement of the seven columns of basal and alar cranial nerve nuclei in the brain stem. In the rhombencephalon, the columns are initially laid out in a rough plane from ventro-

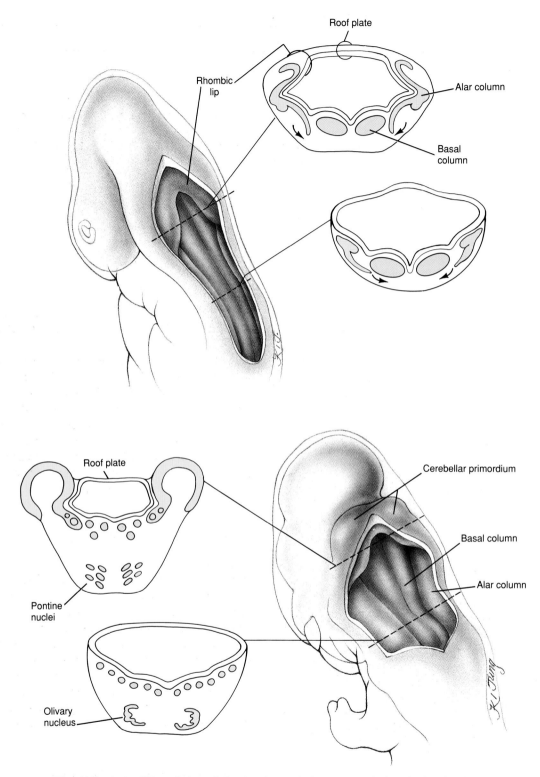

Fig. 13-2. Early differentiation of the rhombencephalon. The roof plate in the rhomben-cephalic region forms a wide, transparent membrane over the fourth ventricle. The basal and alar columns give rise to the motor and associational nuclei, respectively, of most of the cra-nial nerves, as well as to other structures. Extensions of the alar columns also migrate ven-trally to form pontine and olivary nuclei.

Table 13-1.   Location of the Cranial Nerve Nuclei

BRAIN REGION	ASSOCIATED CRANIAL NERVES
Telencephalon	Olfactory (I)
Diencephalon	Optic (II)
Mesencephalon	Oculomotor (III)
Metencephalon	Trochlear (IV) (Arises in the metencephalon but is later displaced into the mesencephalon)
	Trigeminal (V) (The trigeminal sensory nuclei arise in the metencephalon and myelencephalon but are later displaced partly into the mesencephalon. The trigeminal motor nucleus arises in the metencephalon and remains there.)
	Abducens (VI)
	Facial (VII)
	Vestibulocochlear (VIII)
Myelencephalon	Glossopharyngeal (IX)
	Vagus (X)
	Accessory (XI)
	Hypoglossal (XII)

medial to dorsolateral. Only two of the columns penetrate into the mesencephalon. Starting with the most ventromedial, the three basal (motor) columns are as follows:

1. The *somatic efferent* column consists of the nucleus of the hypoglossal nerve (XII) in the caudal rhombencephalon, the nucleus of nerve VI more cranially in the rhombencephalon, and the nuclei of nerves IV and III in the mesencephalon. The latter three cranial nerves innervate extrinsic ocular muscles.

2. The *branchial efferent* (sometimes called *special visceral efferent*) column contains three nuclei serving nerves V, VII, X, IX, and XI and is confined to the rhombencephalon. The branchial efferent nuclei serving nerves V and VII are located cranially in the rhombencephalon; caudally, the elongated **nucleus ambiguus** supplies branchial efferent fibers for nerves IX, X, and XI. These nerves innervate muscles of the pharyngeal arches (V, VII, IX, and X) and the trapezius and sternocleidomastoid muscles (XI).

3. The *visceral efferent* (sometimes called *general visceral efferent)* column includes two nuclei located in the rhombencephalon. The **salivatory nuclei** innervate the salivary and lacrimal glands via nerves VII and IX. Just caudal to this nucleus is the **dorsal nucleus of the vagus,** which contains preganglionic parasympathetic neurons innervating the viscera. The Edinger-Westphal nucleus (III) is located in the mesencephalon. This nerve innervates the sphincter pupillae and ciliary muscles of the eye.

From ventromedial to dorsolateral, the four alar (associational) columns are as follows:

1. The general *visceral afferent* column consists of the nucleus that receives interoceptive information via the glossopharyngeal (IX) and vagus nerve (X).

2. The first *special afferent* column (sometimes called the *special visceral afferent* column) consists of the **nu-cleus of the tractus solitarius,** which receives taste impulses via the facial (VII), glossopharyngeal (IX), and vagus (X) nerves.

3. The *general afferent* column consists of the neurons that receive impulses of general sensation (touch, temperature, pain, etc.) from areas of the face served by the trigeminal (V) and facial (VII) nerves and from the oral, nasal, and pharyngeal and laryngeal cavities (V, IX, and X).

4. The second *special afferent* column (sometimes called the *special somatic afferent* column) consists of the **cochlear** and **vestibular nuclei,** which subserve the special senses of balance and hearing.

Some brain stem nuclei migrate after they form

Not all of the nuclei that develop within the basal and alar columns remain where they form. The branchial efferent nucleus of the facial nerve, for example, travels first dorsocaudally and then ventrally to arrive at a location deeper than would be expected on the basis of its function. The nucleus ambiguus also migrates, as do some of the non-cranial nerve nuclei of the rhombencephalon, such as the **olivary** and **pontine nuclei,** which arise from the alar plate but migrate to a ventral position (Fig. 13-2). As CNS neurons migrate, their axons elongate; thus, the path of a nucleus can be reconstructed by tracing its axons.

Parasympathetic and sensory ganglia develop in association with some cranial nerves

As in the rest of the body, the peripheral neurons of the cranial nerve sensory and parasympathetic pathways are

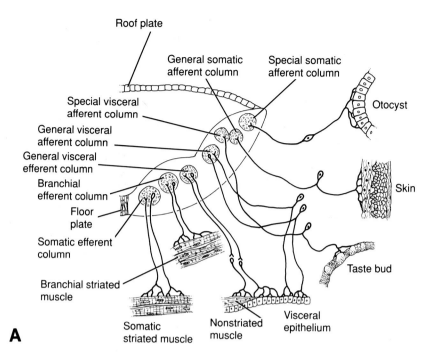

Fig. 13-3. Organization of the brain stem cranial nerve nuclei. The basal columns give rise to motor (efferent) cranial nerve nuclei and the alar columns to associational (afferent) cranial nerve nuclei. These nuclei can be grouped into seven discontinuous columns, each subserving a specific type of function. **(A)** Idealized organization of the brain stem cranial nerve nuclei into seven columns. **(B)** View of the brain stem showing the locations of the cranial nerve nuclei making up the seven columns. The efferent nuclei are shown on the left and the afferent nuclei on the right. (Fig. A modified from Williams PL, Warwick R, Dyson M, Bannister LH. 1989. Gray's Anatomy. Churchill Livingstone, Edinburgh, with permission.)

housed in ganglia that lie outside the CNS. Like the rest of the autonomic system, the cranial parasympathetic system consists of two neuron pathways: the central neuron of each pathway resides in a CNS nucleus, and the peripheral neuron resides in a ganglion. The cranial sensory and parasympathetic ganglia appear during the end of the fourth week and beginning of the fifth week (Table 13-2, and see Fig. 13-5). The cranial nerve sensory ganglia are comparable to the dorsal root ganglia of the spinal cord. The cranial nerve parasympathetic ganglia can be divided into two groups: the ganglia associated with the vagus nerve, which are located in the walls of the visceral organs (gut, heart, lungs, pelvic organs, etc.; see Ch. 5), and the parasympathetic ganglia of cranial nerves III, VII, and IX, which innervate structures in the head. The head receives sympathetic innervation via nerves from the cervical chain ganglia (see Ch. 5).

Cranial nerve parasympathetic ganglia arise from the neural crest of the brain

The origin of the neural crest cells giving rise to the various cranial nerve parasympathetic ganglia has been

determined by using quail–chick chimera experiments. Each ganglion arises from neural crest located at roughly the same level as the corresponding brain stem nucleus (Figs. 13-4 and 13-5A; see also Fig. 12-8). Thus, the **ciliary ganglion** of the oculomotor nerve (III) is formed by neural crest arising in the caudal part of the diencephalon and cranial part of the mesencephalon; the **sphenopalatine** and **submandibular ganglia** of the facial nerve (VII) are formed by neural crest cells that migrate from the cranial end of the rhombencephalon; and the **otic ganglion** of the glossopharyngeal nerve (IX), as well as the enteric ganglia served by the vagus nerve, are derived from neural crest originating in the caudal portion of the rhombencephalon (see Ch. 5).

Cranial nerve sensory ganglia are derived partly from neural crest and partly from ectodermal placodes

Quail–chick chimera experiments have shown that the cranial nerve sensory ganglia have a dual origin (Fig. 13-5A–C). Some are formed from neural crest in the same way as the dorsal root ganglia of the spinal nerves, but

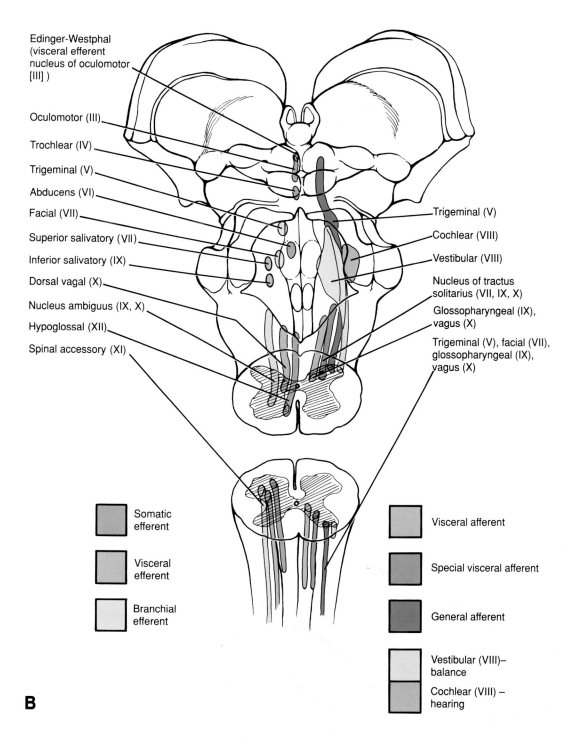

Edinger-Westphal (visceral efferent nucleus of oculomotor [III])

Oculomotor (III)

Trochlear (IV)

Trigeminal (V)

Abducens (VI)

Facial (VII)

Superior salivatory (VII)

Inferior salivatory (IX)

Dorsal vagal (X)

Nucleus ambiguus (IX, X)

Hypoglossal (XII)

Spinal accessory (XI)

Trigeminal (V)

Cochlear (VIII)

Vestibular (VIII)

Nucleus of tractus solitarius (VII, IX, X)

Glossopharyngeal (IX), vagus (X)

Trigeminal (V), facial (VII), glossopharyngeal (IX), vagus (X)

Somatic efferent

Visceral efferent

Branchial efferent

Visceral afferent

Special visceral afferent

General afferent

Vestibular (VIII)– balance

Cochlear (VIII) – hearing

B

others are derived partially or exclusively from **ectodermal placodes.** Three of these placodes—the nasal, lens, and otic placodes—were discussed in Chapter 12. In addition, a series of four **epibranchial placodes** develop as ectodermal thickenings just dorsal to the four pharyngeal clefts, and a more diffuse **trigeminal placode** develops in the area between the epibranchial placodes and the otic placode.

As discussed later in this chapter, the nasal placodes give rise to the primary neurosensory cells of the olfactory epithelium, and the axons of these cells form the olfactory nerve (I). With some exceptions, the remaining cranial nerve sensory ganglia show a regular stratification with respect to their origin: the ganglia (or portions of ganglia) that lie closest to the brain are derived from neural crest, whereas the neurons of ganglia (or portions

Table 13-2.   Origins of the Neurons in the Cranial Nerve Ganglia

CRANIAL NERVE	GANGLION AND TYPE	ORIGIN OF NEURONS
Olfactory (I)	Olfactory epithelium (primary neurons of the olfactory pathway) (special afferent)	Nasal placode
Oculomotor (III)	Ciliary ganglion (visceral efferent)	Neural crest of the caudal diencephalon and cranial mesencephalon
Trigeminal (V)	Trigeminal ganglion (general afferent)	Neural crest of the caudal diencephalon and cranial mesencephalon; trigeminal placode
Facial (VII)	Superior ganglion of nerve VII (general and special afferent)	Rhombencephalic neural crest; 1st epibranchial placode
	Inferior (geniculate) ganglion of nerve VII (general and special afferent)	1st epibranchial placode
	Sphenopalatine ganglion (visceral efferent)	Rhombencephalic neural crest
	Submandibular ganglion (visceral efferent)	Rhombencephalic neural crest
Vestibulocochlear (VIII)	Acoustic (cochlear) ganglion (special afferent)	Otic placode
	Vestibular ganglion (special afferent)	Otic placode plus some contribution from neural crest
Glossopharyngeal (IX)	Superior ganglion (general and special afferent)	Rhombencephalic neural crest
	Inferior (petrosal) ganglion (general and special afferent)	2nd epibranchial placodes
	Otic ganglion (visceral efferent)	Rhombencephalic neural crest
Vagus (X)	Superior ganglion (general afferent)	Rhombencephalic neural crest
	Inferior (nodose) ganglion (general and special afferent)	3rd and 4th epibranchial placodes
	Vagal parasympathetic (enteric) ganglia (visceral efferent)	Rhombencephalic neural crest

thereof) lying farther from the brain are formed by placode cells. The supporting cells of all cranial nerve sensory ganglia, however, are derived from neural crest.

The **trigeminal (semilunar) ganglion** of cranial nerve V has a mixed origin: the proximal portion arises mainly from diencephalic and mesencephalic neural crest, whereas the neurons of the distal portion arise mainly from the diffuse trigeminal placode. The sensory ganglia associated with the second, third, fourth, and sixth pharyngeal arches are derived from the corresponding epibranchial placodes and from neural crest. Each of these nerves has both a proximal and a distal sensory ganglion. The combined **superior ganglion** of nerves IX and X is formed by rhombencephalic neural crest, whereas the neurons of the **inferior (petrosal) ganglion** of nerve IX are derived from the second epibranchial placode and those of

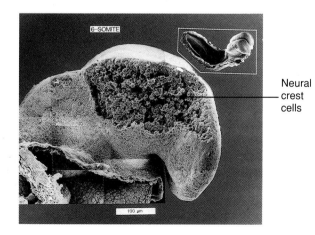

Neural crest cells

Fig. 13-4. Scanning electron micrograph showing neural crest cells migrating over the surface of the neural fold in the region of the future brain. In the brain region, the crest cells detach and begin to migrate while the neural folds are still broadly open. In the spinal cord region, in contrast, the neural crest detaches as the folds fuse together along the midline. (From Tan SS, Morriss-Kay G. 1985. The development and distribution of the cranial neural crest in the rat embryo. Cell Tissue Res 240:403, with permission.)

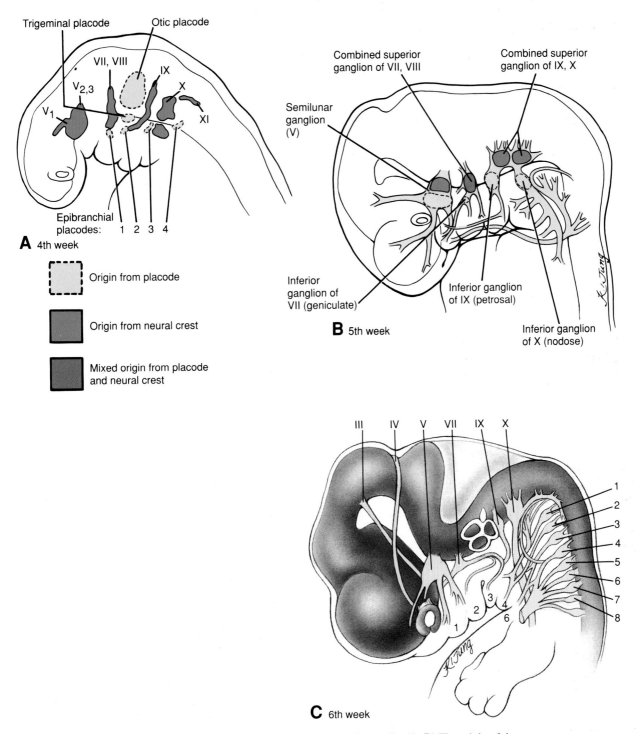

Fig. 13-5. Development of the cranial nerves and their ganglia. (**A, B**) The origin of the cranial nerve ganglia from neural crest and from ectodermal placodes. The cranial nerve parasympathetic ganglia arise solely from neural crest, whereas the neurons in the cranial nerve sensory ganglia arise from neural crest, from placode cells, or from a mixture of both. The glia in all cranial nerve ganglia are derived from neural crest. (**C**) The definitive arrangement of cranial nerves is apparent by the sixth week.

the **inferior (nodose) ganglion** of nerve X are derived from the third and fourth epibranchial placodes. The **superior combined ganglion** of nerves VII and VIII is derived from both the first epibranchial placode and the rhombencephalic neural crest, but the neurons of the **inferior (geniculate) ganglion** of nerve VII are derived exclusively from the first epibranchial placode. As mentioned in Chapter 12, the distal ganglia of cranial nerve VIII—the **vestibular ganglion** and the **cochlear ganglion**—differentiate from the otic placode.

The rhombencephalon gives rise to the medulla oblongata, the pons, and the cerebellum

The medulla oblongata serves mainly as a relay center between the spinal cord and the rest of the brain

The myelencephalon differentiates to form the **medulla oblongata,** which is the portion of the brain most similar to the spinal cord. In addition to housing most of the cranial nerve nuclei, the medulla serves as a relay center between the spinal cord and the higher brain centers and also contains centers and nerve networks that regulate respiration, the heartbeat, reflex movements, and a number of other functions.

The pons is composed largely of white matter tracts that serve the cerebellum

The metencephalon gives rise to two structures: the **pons,** which functions mainly to relay signals between the spinal cord and the cerebral and cerebellar cortices, and the **cerebellum,** which is a center for balance and postural control. The pons (named after the Latin word for bridge) consists mainly of massive fiber tracts that relay information between the cerebrum, the cerebellum, and the spinal cord (Fig. 13-6). These tracts arise primarily from the marginal layer of the basal columns of the metencephalon. In addition, ventrally located **pontine nuclei** relay input from the cerebrum to the cerebellum (Fig. 13-2).

The cerebellum is a specialization of the metencephalic alar plates

The cerebellum is derived largely from the rhombic lips of the metencephalon. It begins to develop at the end of the sixth week and continues to grow after birth, although its gross morphology is similar in the newborn and the adult.

The metencephalic rhombic lips thicken at the end of the sixth week to produce a pair of **cerebellar plates**

(cerebellar primordia) (Fig. 13-7; see also Fig. 13-2). By the second month, the cranial portions of the growing rhombic lips meet across the midline, forming a single primordium that covers the fourth ventricle. This primordium initially bulges only into the fourth ventricle and does not protrude dorsally. By the middle of the third month, however, the growing cerebellum begins to bulge dorsally, forming a dumbbell-shaped swelling at the cranial end of the rhombencephalon.

At this stage, the developing cerebellum is separated into cranial and caudal portions by a transverse groove called the **posterolateral fissure.** The caudal portion, consisting of a pair of **flocculonodular lobes,** represents the most primitive part of the cerebellum. The larger cranial portion consists of a narrow median swelling called the **vermis** connecting a pair of broad **cerebellar hemispheres.** This cranial portion grows much faster than the flocculonodular lobes and becomes the dominant component of the mature cerebellum.

The cerebellar vermis and hemispheres undergo an intricate process of transverse folding as they develop. The major **primary fissure** deepens by the end of the third month and divides the vermis and hemispheres into a cranial **anterior lobe** and a caudal **middle lobe** (Fig. 13-7C, D). These lobes are further divided into a number of **lobules** by the development of additional transverse fissures (starting with the **secondary** and **prepyramidal fissures),** and the surface of the lobules is thrown into closely packed, leaflike transverse gyri called **folia.** These processes of fissuration and foliation continue throughout embryonic and fetal life and have the result of vastly increasing the surface area of the cerebellar cortex (Fig. 13-7E, F).

The gray matter of the cerebellar nuclei and cortex is produced by two proliferative zones

The cerebellum has two types of gray matter: a group of internal **deep cerebellar nuclei** and an external **cerebellar cortex.** Four deep nuclei form on each side: the **dentate, globose, emboliform,** and **fastigial nuclei.** All the input to the cerebellar cortex is relayed through these nuclei. The cerebellar cortex has an extremely regular cytoarchitecture that is similar over the entire cerebellum. The cell types of the cortex are arranged in layers.

The deep nuclei and cortex of the cerebellum are produced by a complex process of differentiation (Fig. 13-8). As elsewhere in the neural tube, the neuroepithelium of the metencephalic rhombic lips undergoes an initial proliferation to produce ventricular, mantle, and marginal layers (Fig. 13-8A). However, in the third month a second layer of proliferating cells appears in the most superficial layer of the marginal zone. The ventricular proliferating layer is now called the **inner germinal layer,** and the

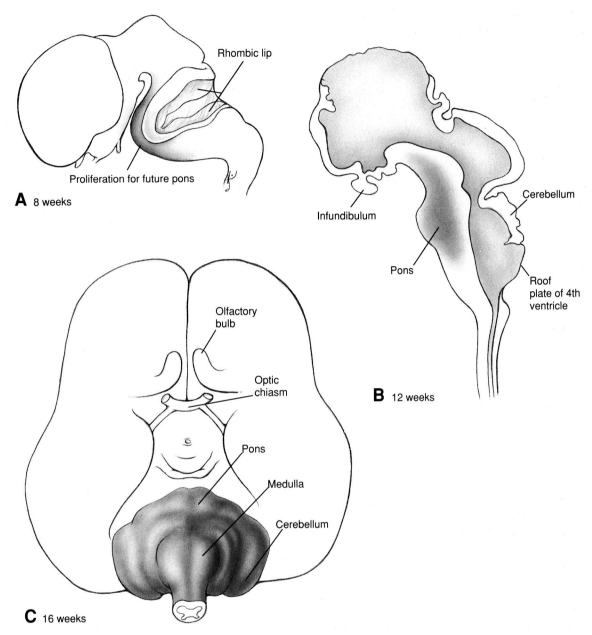

Fig. 13-6. **(A–C)** Development of the pons. The pons is formed by proliferation of cells and fiber tracts on the ventral side of the metencephalon.

new layer is called the **external germinal layer** (or, sometimes, the **external granular layer**) (Fig. 13-8B).

Starting in the fourth month, the internal and external germinal layers undergo highly regulated cell divisions that produce the various populations of cerebellar neuroblasts. The internal germinal layer gives rise to the **primitive nuclear neuroblasts,** which migrate to form the cerebellar nuclei (Fig. 13-8C). In addition, this layer produces two types of neuroblasts that migrate to the cortex: the **primitive Purkinje neuroblasts,** which differentiate to

form the Purkinje cells, and the **Golgi neuroblasts,** which differentiate to form the Golgi cells. As each primitive Purkinje neuroblast migrates toward the cortex, it reels out an axon that maintains synaptic contact with neuroblasts in the developing cerebellar nuclei. These axons will constitute the only efferents of the mature cerebellar cortex. The Purkinje cells form a distinct **Purkinje cell layer** just underlying the external germinal layer.

The external germinal layer undergoes three waves of proliferation to produce, in succession, the three re-

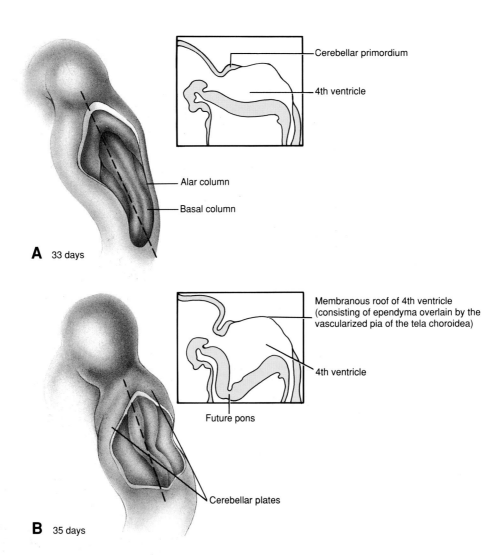

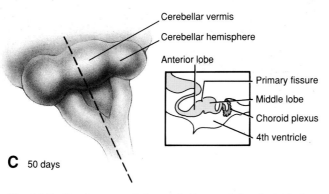

Fig. 13-7. Development of the cerebellum and the choroid plexus of the fourth ventricle. **(A, B)** Proliferation of cells in the rhombic lips of the metencephalon forms the cerebellar plates. **(C)** Further growth creates two lateral cerebellar hemispheres and a central vermis. The primary fissure appears and divides the cerebellum into anterior and middle lobes. A choroid plexus develops in the roof plate of the fourth ventricle. *(Figure continues.)*

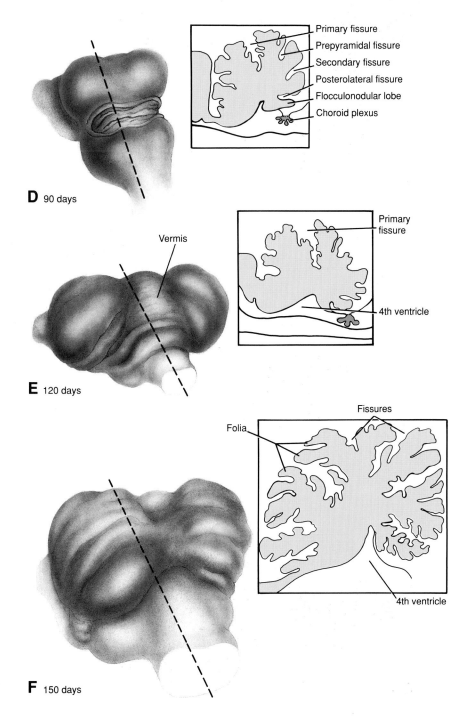

Fig. 13-7. *(Continued)* **(D–F)** Continued fissuration subdivides the expanding cerebellum into further lobes and then, starting in the third month, into lobules and folia. This process greatly increases the area of the cerebellar cortex.

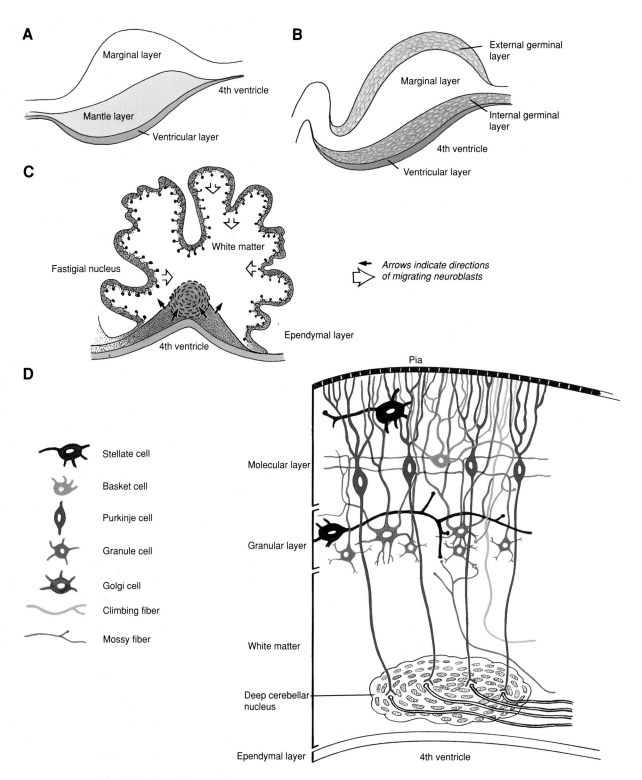

Fig. 13-8. Cytodifferentiation of the cerebellum. **(A)** During the second month, the cranial regions of the rhombic lips form typical ventricular, mantle, and marginal zones. **(B)** During the third month, neuroblasts are produced by proliferation both in an internal germinal layer adjacent to the ventricular zone and in a novel external germinal layer that forms in the most peripheral region of the marginal layer. **(C, D)** Neuroblasts produced by the external germinal layer migrate inward or remain in place to form basket neuroblasts, granule neuroblasts, and stellate neuroblasts. Neuroblasts produced by the internal germinal layer include the Purkinje neuroblasts, which migrate outward, and the nuclear neuroblasts, which form the deep cerebellar nuclei. (Modified from Williams PL, Warwick R, Dyson M, Bannister LH. 1989. Gray's Anatomy. Churchill Livingstone, Edinburgh, with permission.)

maining neuroblast populations of the cerebellar cortex: the **basket neuroblasts,** the **granule neuroblasts,** and the **stellate neuroblasts** (Fig. 13-8D). The granule neuroblasts and some of the basket and stellate neuroblasts are displaced to a location deep to the Purkinje cells, where they form the **granular layer** of the definitive cortex. The remaining basket and stellate cells remain superficial to or closely associated with the Purkinje cells and form the **molecular layer** of the definitive cortex.

As the waves of neurogenesis subside, the germinal layers produce the glioblasts of the cerebellum, which differentiate into astrocytes (including the specialized cerebellar Bergmann cells) and oligodendrocytes.

The mesencephalon is primarily a relay center but also contains cranial nerve nuclei, visual and auditory centers, and other structures

Much of the mesencephalon is composed of white matter, principally the massive tracts that connect the forebrain with the hindbrain and spinal cord. The midbrain also contains a number of important neuronal centers, including four cranial nerve nuclei.

The midbrain contains nuclei of three cranial nerves, but only the oculomotor nuclei originate in the midbrain

As mentioned earlier, the motor nuclei of the oculomotor (III) and trochlear (IV) nuclei are located in the mesencephalon, as is a portion of the sensory nucleus of the trigeminal nerve (V) called the **mesencephalic trigeminal nucleus** (Fig. 13-9). Of these nuclei, however, only the two serving the oculomotor nerve arise from mesencephalic neuroblasts; the trochlear and mesencephalic trigeminal nuclei originate in the metencephalon and are secondarily displaced into the mesencephalon. The two nuclei of the oculomotor nerve are the somatic motor **oculomotor nucleus,** which controls the movements of all but the superior oblique and lateral rectus extrinsic ocular muscles, and the general visceral efferent **Edinger-Westphal nucleus,** which supplies parasympathetic pathways to the pupillary constrictor and the ciliary muscles of the globe.

The superior and inferior colliculi develop from alar plate neuroblasts that migrate into the mesencephalic roof plate

The **superior** and **inferior colliculi** are visible as four prominent swellings on the dorsal surface of the mid-

brain. The superior colliculi receive fibers from the retinas and mediate ocular reflexes. The inferior colliculi, in contrast, form part of the perceptual pathway by which information from the cochlea is relayed to the auditory areas of the cerebral hemispheres. The colliculi are formed by mesencephalic alar plate cells that proliferate and migrate medially into the roof plate (Fig. 13-9). The roof plate thickening produced by these cells is subsequently divided by a midline groove into a pair of lateral **corpora bigemina,** which are later subdivided into inferior and superior colliculi by a transverse groove. The synapses in the superior colliculi form precise spatial maps of the corresponding sensory fields.

The midbrain neural canal forms the narrow cerebral aqueduct

During development, the primitive ventricle of the mesencephalon becomes the narrow **cerebral aqueduct** (Fig. 13-9). The cerebrospinal fluid produced by the choroid plexuses of the forebrain normally flows through the cerebral aqueduct to reach the fourth ventricle. However, various conditions can cause the aqueduct to become blocked during fetal life. Obstruction of the flow of cerebrospinal fluid through the aqueduct results in the congenital condition called **hydrocephalus,** in which the third and lateral ventricles are swollen with fluid, the cerebral cortex is abnormally thin, and the sutures of the skull are forced apart (Fig. 13-10).

The most evolutionarily advanced and complex structures of the brain arise from the prosencephalon

The prosencephalon consists of two secondary brain vesicles, the diencephalon and the telencephalon. The walls of the diencephalon differentiate to form a number of neuronal centers and tracts, described below. In addition, the roof plate, floor plate, and ependyma of the diencephalon give rise to several specialized structures through mechanisms that are relatively unique. These structures include the **choroid plexus** and **circumventricular organs,** the **posterior lobe of the pituitary gland (neurohypophysis),** and the **optic vesicles.** The origin of the optic cups from the diencephalic neural folds was described in Chapter 12.

The telencephalon gives rise to the **cerebral hemispheres** and to the commissures and other structures that join them. It also forms the **olfactory bulbs** and **olfactory tracts,** which, along with the olfactory centers and tracts of the cerebral hemispheres, collectively constitute the **rhinencephalon** ("nose-brain").

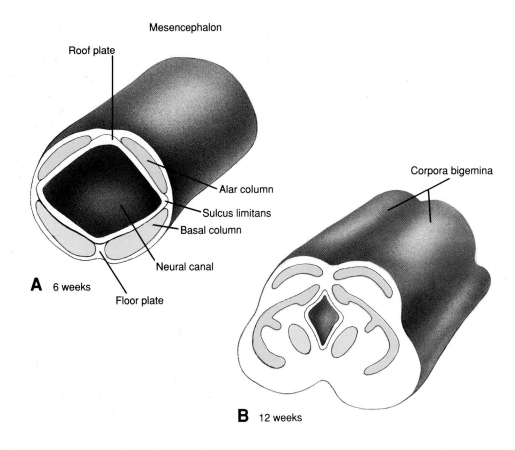

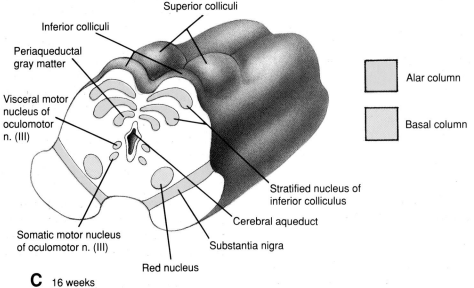

Fig. 13-9. Development of the mesencephalon. (**A, B**) A shallow longitudinal groove develops on the dorsal surface of the mesencephalon between weeks 6 and 12, creating the corpora bigemina. (**C**) Over the next month, a transverse groove subdivides these swellings to produce the superior and inferior colliculi. The mesencephalic alar columns form the stratified nuclear layers of the colliculi, the periaqueductal gray matter, and the substantia nigra. The mesencephalic basal columns form the red nuclei.

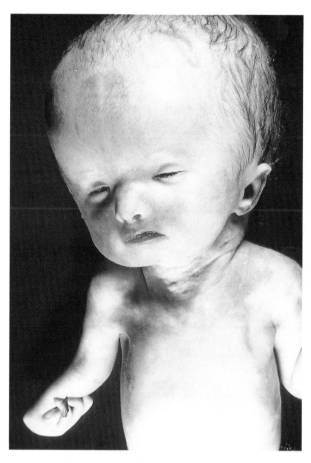

Fig. 13-10. Hydrocephaly. Obstruction of the cerebral aqueduct causes the developing forebrain ventricles to become swollen with cerebrospinal fluid. Infants born with this condition may be retarded. However, incipient hydrocephaly can now be detected in utero using ultrasound and can be corrected by inserting a pressure valve that allows the excess cerebrospinal fluid to vent into the amniotic cavity. (Photo courtesy of Children's Hospital Medical Center, Cincinnati, OH.)

The diencephalic alar plate forms the thalamus, hypothalamus, and epithalamus

As mentioned above, the walls of the diencephalon are formed by alar plates; basal plates are lacking. These plates form three embryonic swellings, the **thalamus, hypothalamus,** and **epithalamus** (Fig. 13-11). The thalamus and hypothalamus differentiate to form complexes of nuclei that serve a diverse range of functions. The thalamus acts primarily as the relay center for the cerebral cortex: it receives all the information (sensory and other) projecting to the cortex from subcortical structures, processes it as necessary, and relays it to the appropriate cortical area(s). Within the thalamus, the sense of sight is handled by the **lateral geniculate body** and the sense of hearing by the **medial geniculate body.** The hypothalamus regulates the endocrine activity of the pituitary as well as many autonomic responses. It participates in the limbic system, which controls emotion, and coordinates emotional state with the appropriate visceral responses. The hypothalamus also controls the level of arousal of the brain (sleep and waking). The small epithalamus gives rise to a few miscellaneous structures, described below.

At the end of the fifth week, the thalamus and hypothalamus are visible as swellings on the inner surface of the diencephalic neural canal, separated by a deep groove called the **hypothalamic sulcus** (Fig. 13-11A). The thalamus grows disproportionately after the seventh week and becomes the largest element of the diencephalon. The two thalami usually meet and fuse across the third ventricle at one or more points called **interthalamic adhesions** (Fig. 13-12).

By the end of the sixth week, a shallow groove called the **sulcus dorsalis** separates the thalamus from the epithalamic swelling, which forms in the dorsal rim of the diencephalic wall and the adjoining roof plate (Fig. 13-11B, C). The epithalamic roof plate evaginates to form a midline diverticulum that differentiates into the endocrine **pineal gland.** The epithalamus also forms a neural structure called the **trigonium habenulae** (including the **nucleus habenulae**) and two small commissures, the **posterior** and **habenular commissures.** The growth of the thalamus eventually obliterates the sulcus dorsalis and displaces the epithalamic structures dorsally.

Retinal fibers from the optic cup project to the lateral geniculate bodies. As described in Chapter 12, the nerve fibers from the retina grow back through the optic nerve to the diencephalon. Just before they enter the brain, nerve fibers growing from both eyes meet to form the **optic chiasm,** a joint structure in which some of the fibers from each side cross over to the other side (decussate). The resulting bundles of ipsilateral and contralateral fibers then project back to the lateral geniculate bodies, where they synapse to form a map of the visual field. Not all retinal fibers project to the lateral geniculate bodies; as mentioned above, some of them terminate in the superior colliculus, where they mediate ocular reflex control.

The diencephalic roof plate and ependyma form the choroid plexus and circumventricular organs of the third ventricle

Cranial to the epithalamus, the diencephalic roof plate remains epithelial in character. This portion of the roof plate differentiates along with the overlying pia to form the paired choroid plexuses of the third ventricle. Else-

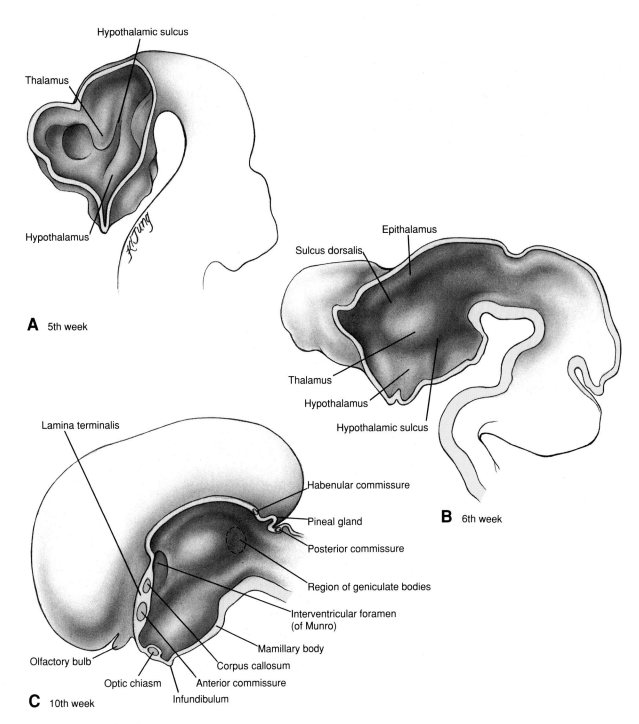

Fig. 13-11. Development of the diencephalon. **(A)** The thalamus and hypothalamus become demarcated by a hypothalamic sulcus during the fifth week. **(B)** By the end of the sixth week, the thalamus is clearly differentiated from the more dorsal epithalamus by a shallow groove called the sulcus dorsalis. **(C)** By 10 weeks, additional specializations of the diencephalon are apparent, including the mamillary body, the pineal gland, and the posterior lobe of the pituitary. The optic sulci, the posterior and habenular commissures, and the geniculate bodies are also specializations of the diencephalon.

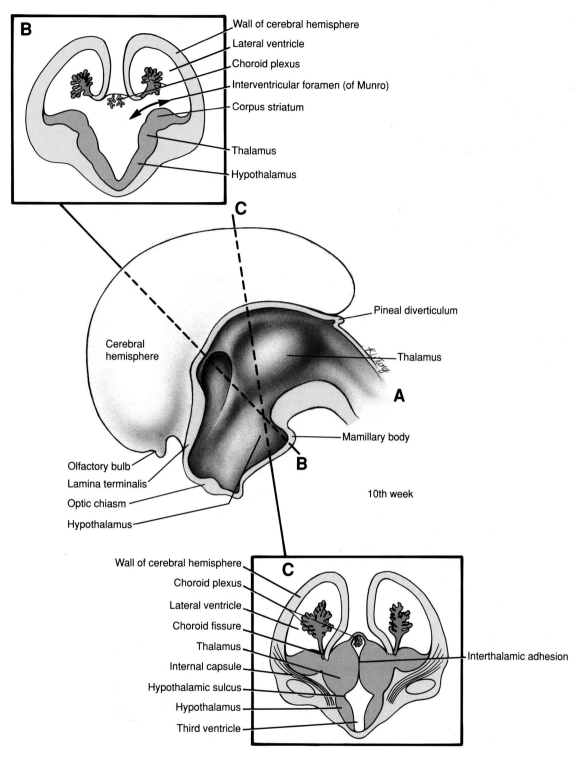

Fig. 13-12. Development of the cerebral hemispheres and lateral ventricles. The lateral ventricle in each hemisphere communicates with the third ventricle through an interventricular foramen (of Münro). The choroid fissure running the length of each lateral ventricle contains a choroid plexus, which produces cerebrospinal fluid. The fibers growing to and from the cerebral cortex form the massive fiber bundle called the internal capsule. The thalami function primarily as relay centers that process information destined for the cerebral hemispheres. The growing thalami meet across the third ventricle, forming the interthalamic adhesion.

where in the third ventricle, the ependyma forms a number of unique secretory structures that add specific metabolites and neuropeptides to the cerebrospinal fluid. These structures, collectively known as the **circumventricular organs,** include the **subfornical organ,** the **organum vasculosum of the lamina terminalis,** and the **subcommissural organ.**

The pituitary is formed by the diencephalon and by Rathke's pouch

During the third week, a diverticulum called the **infundibulum** develops in the floor of the third ventricle and grows ventrally toward the stomodeum (Figs. 13-11C and 13-13). Simultaneously, an ectodermal placode appears in the roof of the stomodeum and invaginates to form a diverticulum called **Rathke's pouch,** which grows dorsally toward the infundibulum. Rathke's pouch eventually loses its connection with the stomodeum and forms a discrete sac that is appressed to the cranial surface of the infundibulum. This sac differentiates to form the **adenohypophysis** of the pituitary. The cells of its anterior surface give rise to the **anterior lobe** proper of the pituitary, and a small group of cells on the posterior surface of the pouch form the functionally distinct **pars intermedia.** Meanwhile, the distal portion of the infundibulum differentiates to form the **posterior pituitary (neurohypophysis).** The lumen of the infundibulum is obliterated by this process, but a small proximal pit, the **infundibular recess,** persists in the floor of the third ventricle.

The telencephalon forms the cerebral hemispheres, their connecting commissures, and the olfactory bulbs and tracts

The cerebral hemispheres arise as lateral diverticulae of the telencephalon

The cerebral hemispheres first appear on day 32 as a pair of bubblelike outgrowths of the telencephalon. By 16 weeks, the rapidly growing hemispheres are oval and have expanded back to cover the diencephalon. The thin roof and lateral walls of each hemisphere represent the future **cerebral cortex** (Fig. 13-14A). The floor is thicker and contains a neuronal aggregation called the **corpus striatum,** which will give rise to two of the three **basal nuclei** of the cerebral hemispheres (the third is contributed by the diencephalon) (Fig. 13-12B). As the growing hemispheres press against the walls of the diencephalon, the meningeal layers that originally separate the two structures disappear, so that the neural tissue of the thalami becomes continuous with that of the floor of the cerebral hemispheres. This former border is eventu-

ally crossed by a massive fiber bundle called the **internal capsule,** which passes through the corpus striatum and carries fibers from the thalamus to the cerebral cortex as well as from the cerebral cortex to lower regions of the brain and spinal cord (Fig. 13-12C).

The cerebral hemispheres are initially smooth-walled. Like the cerebellar cortex, however, the cerebral cortex folds into an increasingly complex pattern of lobes and gyri as the hemispheres grow. This process begins in the fourth month with the appearance of a small indentation called the **lateral cerebral fossa** in the lateral wall of the hemisphere (Fig. 13-14A, B). The caudal end of the lengthening hemisphere curves ventrally and then grows forward across this fossa, creating the **temporal lobe** of the cerebral hemisphere and converting the fossa into a deep cleft called the **lateral cerebral sulcus.** The portion of the cerebral cortex that originally forms the medial floor of the fossa is covered by the temporal lobe and is called the **insula.**

By the sixth month, several other cerebral sulci have appeared. These include the **central sulcus,** which separates the frontal and parietal lobes, and the **occipital sulcus,** which demarcates the occipital lobe. The detailed pattern of gyri that ultimately forms on the cerebral hemispheres varies somewhat from individual to individual.

A choroid plexus forms in the choroid fissure of the lateral ventricles

Each cerebral hemisphere contains a diverticulum of the telencephalic primitive ventricle called the **lateral ventricle.** The lateral ventricle initially occupies most of the volume of the hemisphere but is progressively constricted by the thickening of the cortex. However, along the line between the floor and the medial wall of the hemisphere, the cerebral wall does not thicken but instead remains thin and epithelial. This zone forms a longitudinal groove in the ventricle; this groove is called the **choroid fissure** (Fig. 13-12C). A choroid plexus develops along the choroid fissure. As shown in Figure 13-15, the lateral ventricle extends the whole length of the hemisphere, reaching anteriorly into the frontal lobe and, at its posterior end, curving around to occupy the temporal lobe.

The opening between each lateral ventricle and the third ventricle persists as the **interventricular foramen (foramen of Monro).**

The cytodifferentiation of the cerebral cortex is complex

The neuroepithelium of the cerebral hemispheres is initially much like that of other parts of the neural tube. Studies on cerebral histogenesis have shown, however, that the process of proliferation, migration, and differ-

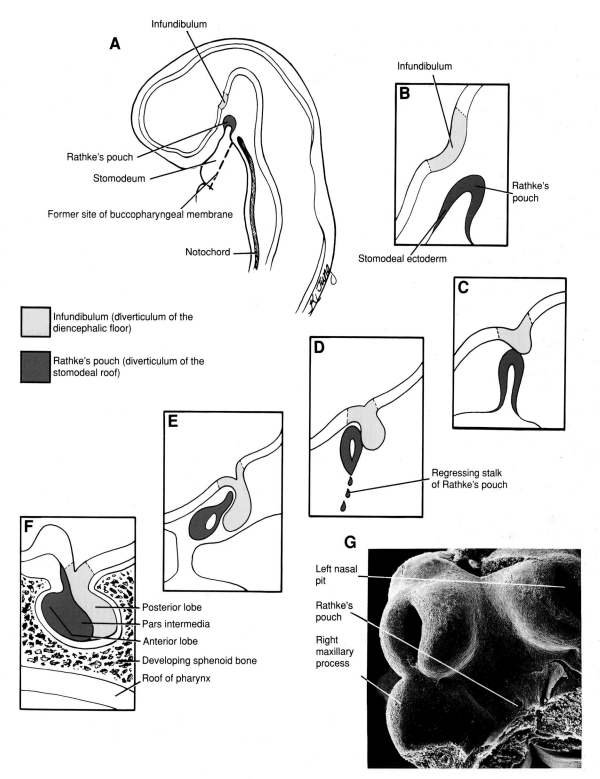

Fig. 13-13. (A–G) Development of the pituitary. The pituitary gland is a compound structure. The posterior lobe forms from a diverticulum of the diencephalic floor called the infundibulum, whereas the anterior lobe and pars intermedia form from an evagination of the ectodermal roof of the stomodeum called Rathke's pouch. Rathke's pouch detaches from the stomodeum and becomes associated with the developing posterior pituitary. **(G)** Scanning electron micrograph of the roof of the embryonic oral cavity, showing the opening to Rathke's pouch. (Fig. G photo courtesy of Dr. Arnold Tamarin.)

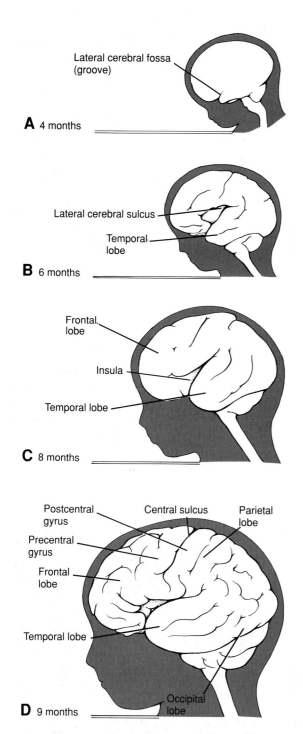

Lateral cerebral fossa
(groove)

A 4 months

Lateral cerebral sulcus

Temporal
lobe

B 6 months

Frontal
lobe

Insula

Temporal lobe

C 8 months

Postcentral   Central sulcus   Parietal
gyrus   lobe

Precentral
gyrus

Frontal
lobe

Temporal lobe

Occipital
lobe

D 9 months

Fig. 13-14. Growth and folding of the cerebral hemispheres during fetal life. Growth of the cerebral hemispheres is continuous throughout embryonic and fetal development and continues after birth. **(A, B)** In the fourth month, the formation of the narrow lateral cerebral fossa delineates the temporal lobe of the cerebral hemisphere. By the sixth month, additional clefts delineate the frontal, parietal, and occipital lobes. **(C, D)** Additional sulci and gyri form throughout the remainder of fetal life.

entiation by which the mature cortex is produced is unique (Fig. 13-16). Moreover, the details of this process vary from place to place in the cortex and are not fully understood.

The first neuroblasts produced in the ventricular layer form neuronal fibers, which grow out of the ventricular layer to form a thin, superficial **marginal zone.** This thin fiber layer immediately underlies the developing pia and remains the most superficial layer of the cortex. Many of these neuroblasts then migrate outward to form an **intermediate zone,** which is intercalated between the ventricular layer and the marginal zone. Some of the cells from the intermediate zone, plus new neuroblasts produced in the ventricular layer, then migrate outward to form a transient lamina called the **cortical plate** between the intermediate zone and the marginal zone. At this point the ventricular zone gradually ceases to produce neuroblasts, and neuroblast production is taken over by a layer of proliferating cells between the ventricular and intermediate layers, called the **subventricular zone.** Neuroblasts from the subventricular zone migrate peripherally through the intermediate zone to establish a **subplate** layer just deep to the cortical plate. Some of these neurons then migrate through the earlier generations of neuroblasts in the cortical plate to establish outer laminae within the cortical plate. Together, the cortical plate and subplate give rise to the cerebral cortex. The cerebral cortex is made up of several cell layers, which vary in number from three in the phylogenetically oldest parts to about six in the dominant **neocortex.** The intermediate layer, meanwhile, has become relatively devoid of neuroblast cell bodies and differentiates into the **white matter** of the cerebral hemispheres. It must be made clear that the sequence and timing of these events vary considerably in different regions of the hemispheres.

The olfactory bulbs and olfactory tracts are derived from the cranial telencephalon

As described in Chapter 12, the nasal placodes appear at the end of the fourth week. Very early, some cells in the nasal placode differentiate to form the **primary neurosensory cells** of the future olfactory epithelium. At the end of the fifth week, these cells sprout axons that cross the short distance to penetrate the most cranial end of the telencephalon (Fig. 13-17A). The subsequent ossification of the ethmoid bone around these axons creates the perforated cribriform plates.

In the sixth week, as the nasal pits differentiate to form the epithelium of the nasal passages, the area at the tip of each cerebral hemisphere where the axons of the primary neurosensory cells synapse begins to form an outgrowth called the **olfactory bulb** (Figs. 13-17 and 13-18). The cells in the olfactory bulb that synapse with the axons of

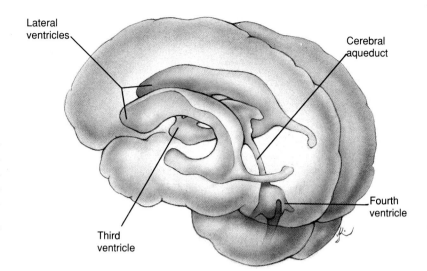

Fig. 13-15. The cerebral ventricles. The expansions of the neural canal in the primary and secondary brain vesicles and cerebral hemispheres give rise to the cerebral ventricles. The ventricle system consists of the lateral ventricles in the cerebral hemispheres, the third ventricle in the diencephalon, the narrow cerebral aqueduct (of Sylvius) in the mesencephalon, and the fourth ventricle in the rhombencephalon.

the primary sensory neurons differentiate to become the secondary sensory neurons of the olfactory pathways. The axons of these cells synapse in the olfactory centers of the cerebral hemispheres. As the changing proportions of the face and brain lengthen the distance between the olfactory bulbs and their point of origin on the hemispheres, the axons of the secondary olfactory neurons lengthen to form stalklike CNS **olfactory tracts.** Traditionally, the olfactory tract and bulb together are referred to as the **olfactory nerve.**

The telencephalon produces the commissures that connect the cerebral hemispheres

The commissures that connect the right and left cerebral hemispheres form from a thickening at the cranial end of the telencephalon, which represents the zone of final neuropore closure. This area can be divided into a dorsal **commissural plate** and a ventral **lamina terminalis.**

The first fiber tract to develop in the commissural plate is the **anterior commissure,** which forms during the sev-

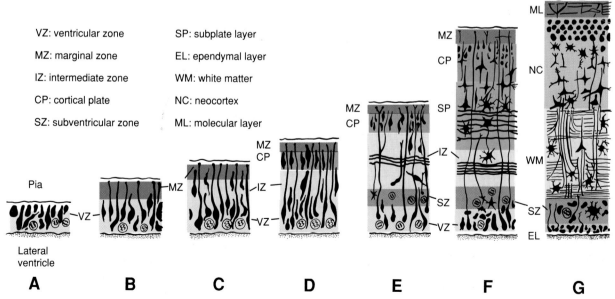

Fig. 13-16. (A–G) Cytodifferentiation of the cerebral neocortex. Although the timing of neuroblast formation varies widely in different regions of the cerebral hemispheres, the general scheme illustrated here is typical for all regions. See text for explanation.

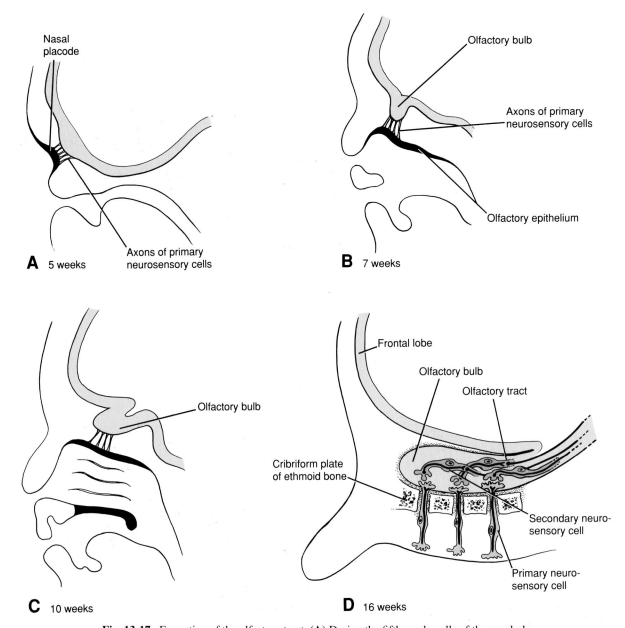

Fig. 13-17. Formation of the olfactory tract. **(A)** During the fifth week, cells of the nasal placode differentiate into the primary neurosensory cells of the olfactory tract and produce axons that grow into the presumptive olfactory bulb of the adjacent telencephalon and synapse there with secondary neurons. **(B–D)** As development continues, the elongating axons of the secondary olfactory neurons in the olfactory bulb produce the olfactory tract.

enth week and interconnects the olfactory bulbs and olfacatory centers of the two hemispheres (Fig. 13-18). During the ninth week, the **hippocampal** or **fornix commissure** forms between the right and left hippocampi (a phylogenetically old portion of the cerebral hemisphere that is located adjacent to the choroid fissure). A few days later, the massive, arched **corpus callosum** begins to form, linking together the right and left neocortices along their entire length. The most anterior part of the corpus

callosum appears first, and its posterior extension (the **splenium**) forms later in fetal life.

Most of the growth of the brain takes place after birth

At birth the brain is about 25 percent of its adult volume. Some of the postnatal growth of the brain is due to increase in the size of neuronal cell bodies and to the pro-

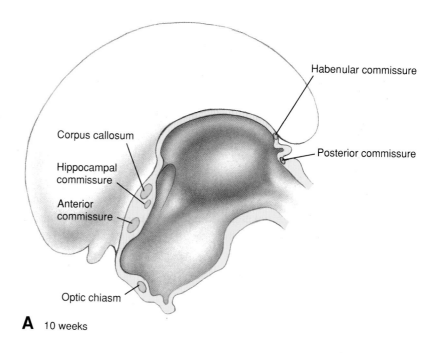

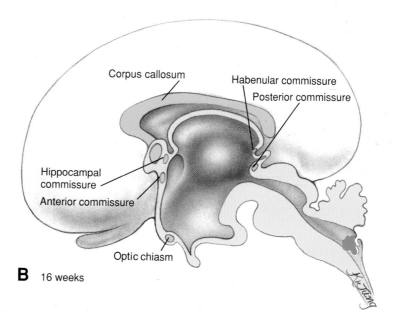

Fig. 13-18. (A & B) Formation of the commissures. The telencephalon gives rise to commissural tracts that integrate the activities of the left and right cerebral hemispheres. These include the anterior and hippocampal commissures and the corpus callosum. The small posterior and habenular commissures arise from the epithalamus.

liferation of neuronal processes. Most of this growth, however, results from the myelination of nerve fibers.

Neuronal histogenesis is regulated by neurotrophic factors, neuron-glia interactions, extracellular matrix molecules, and sex steroids

The manner in which the 10 billion to 1 trillion neurons of the human brain become organized and interconnected is a problem of daunting complexity. Not only do the neu-

rons themselves proliferate, migrate, and differentiate according to a precise pattern, but also their cell processes display awesome pathfinding abilities. The cellular and molecular mechanisms that control these processes have become the subject of intense scientific interest. Because the neuronal architecture of the cerebellar cortex is extremely regular and well understood, the cerebellum is a favored object for research on neuronal differentiation.

Research has also focused on the mechanisms by which specific chemical **neurotrophic factors** control the survival and growth of various types of neuron. Interest in these substances is particularly high because they may lead to an understanding not only of congenital defects of nervous system development but also of the involutional changes that occur with aging and because they may eventually be used in devising therapies for CNS injuries and diseases. The first neurotrophic factor to be identified was **nerve growth factor,** which supports the growth of sympathetic, parasympathetic, and sensory nerve fibers in the periphery. An intensive search was then carried out for agents that would have more specific effects. **Brain-derived growth factor** (mentioned in Ch. 4 in the context of neural crest migration) seems to prevent the death of cells in the nodose ganglion and in dorsal root ganglia. **Purpurin,** a protein present in the retina, has been shown to enhance the adhesion of retinal neurons in vitro; **apolipoprotein E** apparently abets the incorporation of lipids into the membrane of regenerating neurites; and **S100b,** a factor found in the brain, can stimulate the elongation of telencephalic neurons in cell culture.

Some of the widespread effects of members of the growth factor family of molecules have been mentioned in previous chapters. Several growth factors, including **epidermal growth factor, basic** and **acidic fibroblast growth factors, insulinlike growth factors,** and **insulin** all promote neuronal survival and neurite outgrowth. Some of these effects are exerted directly; others are mediated by glial cells. One important way in which glial cells regulate neurite growth is by secreting extracellular matrix substances that guide and control neurite growth. Such an activity has been demonstrated for astrocytes and Schwann cell tumors. Extracellular matrix components that have been shown to affect neurite growth include **laminin, heparan sulfate proteoglycan, fibronectin,** and **collagen.**

Sex steroids are also known to influence both the organization and the functioning of the brain. It has been demonstrated, for example, that the number of neurons in a nucleus of the medial preoptic area of the rat brain is determined partly by the level of circulating male sex steroids.

APPLICATIONS TO CLINICAL PRACTICE

Cellular and molecular basis of human cerebellar malformations

The human cerebellum is subject to a variety of developmental disorders, including **hypoplasias** (underdevelopment), **dysplasias** (abnormal tissue development), and **heterotopias** (abnormal location of gray matter). Many of these disorders cause abnormalities of lobular and foliar architecture distinctive enough that a diagnosis can be made from a gross specimen or by magnetic resonance imaging (MRI), computed tomography (CT), or ultrasonography. A number of these disorders also cause characteristic **cerebellar ataxias** (disruptions of coordination).

Mercury poisoning may result in focal damage to the granular layer of the cerebellum and ataxia in humans. Many cerebellar anomalies are caused by chromosomal anomalies and single-gene mutations. Trisomy 13, for example, is typified by gross brain abnormalities that affect the cerebellum and cerebrum. In the cerebellum, the vermis is hypoplastic and neurons are heterotopically located in the white matter. Cerebellar dysplasia, usually of the vermis, is also characteristic of trisomy 18 and Down syndrome (trisomy 21) and may involve abnormalities of the Purkinje and granule cell layers. A variety of chromosome deletion syndromes, including 5p⁻ (**cri du chat**), 13q⁻, and 4p⁻, also may cause cerebellar anomalies.

Many cerebellar ataxias are acquired through autosomal recessive inheritance. One of the most common human ataxia syndromes is **Friedreich's ataxia,** which affects the dorsal root ganglia, spinal cord, and cerebel-

lum. It is characterized by clumsy gait, ataxia of the upper limbs, and dysarthria (disturbed speech articulation). Other autosomal recessive cerebellar ataxia syndromes are **Joubert syndrome, Gillespie syndrome, Marinesco-Sjögren syndrome,** and **Dandy-Walker syndrome. Paine syndrome** is a cerebellar ataxia that is inherited as an X-linked recessive trait. Two forms of autosomal dominant cerebellar ataxia syndromes have been mapped to human chromosomes 6p and 12q. Many of these heritable recessive syndromes also cause such dramatic cerebellar malformations that they can be diagnosed by CT, MRI, or ultrasonography.

The mutations that cause some of the recessive heritable cerebellar ataxias are known to affect the metabolism of mucopolysaccharides, lipids, and amino acids. In the cerebellum, these mutations cause effects such as a deficiency of Purkinje cells (mucopolysaccharidosis III), abnormal accumulation of lipid (juvenile ganglioidosis), and reduced myelin formation (phenylketonuria). The disorder called **olivopontocerebellar atrophy** seems in some cases to be caused by a deficiency in the excitatory neurotransmitter glutamate, resulting in turn from a deficiency in the enzyme glutamate dehydrogenase.

Insight into the cause of cerebellar defects has been gained by studying mouse mutants with cerebellar ataxias

A more detailed understanding of the cellular and molecular mechanisms that cause various cerebellar anomalies has been gained by research on an intriguing series of mouse mutants that display a spectrum of cerebellar ataxias. Many of these strains were created in the late 19th and early 20th centuries by amateur zoologists who bred them for their strange gaits. When it was later realized that these unusual behaviors were caused by specific errors in cerebellar development, many of the strains were revived and bred for scientific research.

The strange gaits of many of the ataxic mouse mutants can be correlated with defects in the cerebellar cytoarchitecture. For example, the high-stepping, broad-based gait of the mutant **"stumbler"** is apparently caused by defects in the Purkinje cells. The mutant **"meander tail"** also has abnormal Purkinje cells, but in this case the abnormality is limited to the anterior lobe of the cerebellum. Interestingly, the *Wnt-3* proto-oncogene (see below), while expressed normally in the posterior lobe of meander tail mutants, is not expressed in the anterior cerebellar lobe of this strain. The **"vibrator"** displays a rapid postural tremor that is caused by progressive degeneration of cerebellar neurons, whereas defects in myelination account for the unstable locomotion, tremor, and seizures of the mutant **"shiverer."** The poor myelination in these mice appears to be caused by a primary deficit of myelin basic proteins throughout the nervous system. **"Tottering"** mice exhibit ataxia and intermittent movement disorders that are correlated with reductions in the thickness of the molecular layer of the cerebellar paramedian lobule.

In vitro studies have revealed a basis for cerebellar pathogenesis in the "Weaver" mutant

Normally, the granule cell neuroblasts that arise in the external germinal layer of the developing cerebellum produce bipolar processes and then migrate inward to populate the granule layer, reeling out an axon behind them as they travel. In the homozygous recessive **"weaver"** mutant *(wv/wv),* the granule cells fail to produce processes, fail to migrate, and then die prematurely. Evidence from in vitro studies on explants of developing cerebellum indicates that granule cells make a special "migration junction" with astrocyte processes that is essential for normal migration and synapse formation. These junctions are easy to see in explants of normal cerebellum but do not form in explants of "weaver" mutant cerebellum. A series of experiments was carried out in which wild-type and weaver astrocytes and neurons were mixed in vitro. It was found that wild-type neurons interact normally with "weaver" astrocytes but that weaver granule cells do not form junctions with wild-type astrocytes and do not migrate along astrocyte processes. Thus, the "weaver" mutation apparently affects the granule cell and not the astrocytes.

Studies of "staggerer"–wild-type chimeras suggest a mechanism for the numerical matching of Purkinje and granule cells

In the normal cerebellum, the number of granule cells is precisely matched to the number of Purkinje cells. This matching is accomplished by a process of **histogenetic cell death,** by which the great overabundance of granule cell neuroblasts initially produced by the external germinal layer is reduced to the correct number. Various experiments have indicated that this process is automatically controlled by the number of Purkinje cells: apparently, granule cells die unless they make contact with the dentritic arbor of a Purkinje cell. This model was tested by using "staggerer" –wild-type chimeras made by aggregating eight-cell "staggerer" embryos with wild-type embryos and then reinserting them into the uterus of a pseudopregnant mother. This technique results in the birth of animals with widely different numbers of normal and wild-type Purkinje cells. Examination revealed a linear relationship between the number of granule cells and the number of wild-type Purkinje cells, confirming the hypothesis that granule cell survival depends on the presence of appropriate Purkinje cell targets.

In situ hybridization and gene targeting implicate the proto-oncogene *Wnt* family in cerebellar development

A proto-oncogene is a normal gene that can become a tumor-promoting oncogene if it mutates or if its expression is disturbed. The clinical interest of these genes is obvious. Moreover, many proto-oncogenes have proved to be important regulators of cell proliferation and differentiation.

By using the technique of in situ hybridization, the proto-oncogene *Wnt-1 (int-1)* has been shown to be expressed in the developing central nervous system. In the neural plate, messenger RNA for this gene is localized predominantly in the presumptive mesencephalon and metencephalon. Later in development, the expression of the gene extends caudally to include the myelencephalon and spinal cord. The gene is also expressed to a minor degree in adult mouse spermatids. Interestingly, mice homozygous for the recessive mutation "swaying" *(sw)* have been shown to harbor a deletion of a single base pair within the *Wnt-1* locus. These mice also exhibit malformation of the anterior cerebellum and are characterized by ataxia and hypertonia (extreme muscle tension). To investigate the role of this gene, mutants in which the gene was nonfunctional were produced by using gene-targeting technology. Embryos homozygous for this nonfunctional "null allele" usually die in utero or shortly after birth, and those that survive are severely ataxic. Examination of animals that died in utero or soon after birth showed that the mesencephalon and cerebellum were completely absent. One animal that survived to adulthood did have the caudal part of the cerebellum, suggesting that differences in the penetrance of the null allele may be regulated by a craniocaudal gradient. Significant midbrain or cerebellar defects are exhibited by transgenic mice homozygous for a targeted deletion of the engrailed-1 or engrailed-2 homeobox gene, respectively, providing evidence for the functional interaction between engrailed and *Wnt*. In other studies, however, the expression of *Wnt-3* does not seem to be affected by the deletion of the engrailed-2 homeobox gene.

The cerebellar ataxias displayed by the various strains of mice described in this chapter resemble some human cerebellar ataxias, although direct comparisons are not currently justified. Nevertheless, it is clear that the investigation of such mutants will lead to new insights into the regulation of neuronal proliferation, pathfinding, and synaptogenesis in the human cerebellum.

14

Development of the Integumentary System

Development of the Skin, Hair, Epidermal Glands, Nails, and Teeth

S U M M A R Y

The **integument** consists of two layers: the **epidermis** and the **dermis.** The epidermis is formed primarily by embryonic surface ectoderm, although it is also colonized by melanocytes from neural crest, Langerhans cells (immune cells of bone marrow origin), and pressure-sensing Merkel cells. The dermis is derived from the somatopleuric lateral plate mesoderm and dermatomes.

The single layered ectoderm begins to proliferate just after neurulation to produce an outer layer of simple squamous epithelium called the **periderm.** At this time the inner proliferating layer of cells is called the **basal layer.** In the 11th week, the basal layer produces a new intermediate layer between itself and the periderm. The basal layer is now called the **stratum germinativum,** which produces epidermal cells throughout life. By the 21st week, the intermediate layer is replaced by the definitive three layers of the outer epidermis. The layers of the epidermis represent a maturation series: keratinocytes produced by the stratum germinativum differentiate as they pass outward, forming the intermediate layers and the flattened, dead cells of the horny layer, which are finally sloughed from the surface of the skin. As the epidermis develops, the overlying periderm is shed into the amniotic fluid. Several disorders of epidermal proliferation occur in humans, including **psoriasis.** Disorders of keritinization include **lamellar ichthyosis** and **harlequin fetus.** The latter condition usually results in death just after birth.

The **dermis** contains blood vessels, nerves, muscle bundles, and sensory structures. The superficial layer of the dermis develops **dermal papillae,** which interdigitate with downward projections of the epidermis called **epidermal ridges.**

The skin forms several specialized structures, including hair, nails, ectodermal placodes, and epidermal glands. **Hair follicles** grow down from the stratum germinativum into the dermis. The epidermal glands, including **sebaceous glands, apocrine glands, sweat glands,** and **mammary glands,** also arise as diverticulae of the epidermis. **Supernumerary nipples** or **breasts** may form anywhere along the lines of the **mammary ridges** that form the breasts (from thigh to axilla). The primordia of the **fingernails** and **toenails** arise on the palmar and plantar surface of the digits and then migrate around to the dorsal side.

The first sign of **tooth development** is the formation of a U-shaped epidermal ridge called the **dental lamina** along the crest of the upper and lower jaws. Twenty downgrowths from the dental lamina combine with underlying concentrations of **neural crest-derived mesenchyme** to form the tooth buds of the **primary (deciduous) teeth.** The **secondary, permanent teeth** are formed by secondary tooth buds that sprout from these primary buds. The inner cells of the dental papilla give rise to the tooth pulp, and nerves and blood vessels gain access to the pulp through the tips of the tooth roots.

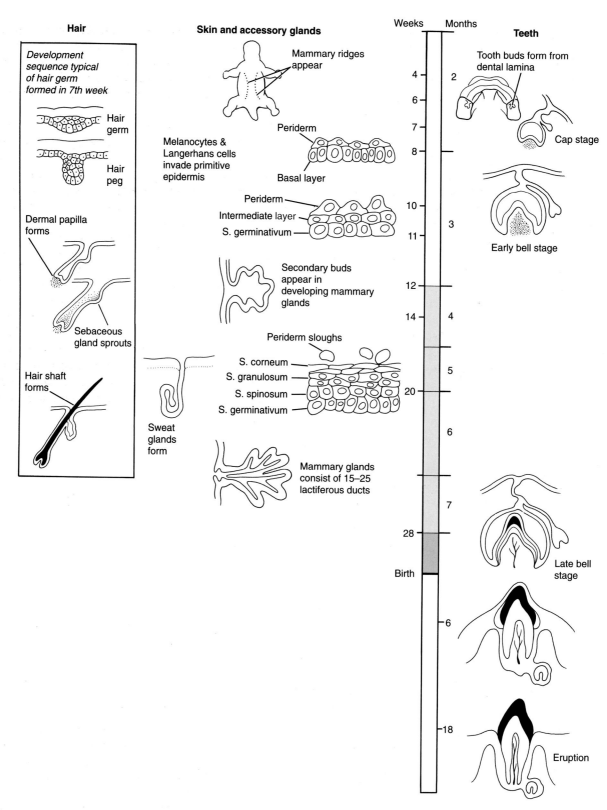

Hair

Development sequence typical of hair germ formed in 7th week

Hair germ

Hair peg

Dermal papilla forms

Sebaceous gland sprouts

Hair shaft forms

Skin and accessory glands

Mammary ridges appear

Melanocytes & Langerhans cells invade primitive epidermis

Periderm

Basal layer

Periderm

Intermediate layer

S. germinativum

Secondary buds appear in developing mammary glands

Periderm sloughs

S. corneum

S. granulosum

S. spinosum

S. germinativum

Sweat glands form

Mammary glands consist of 15–25 lactiferous ducts

Weeks   Months

4   2

6

7

8

10

11   3

12

14   4

5

20

6

7

28

Birth

6

18

Teeth

Tooth buds form from dental lamina

Cap stage

Early bell stage

Late bell stage

Eruption

Timeline. Development of the integument and integumentary derivatives.

The surface ectoderm gives rise to most cells of the epidermis, and mesoderm gives rise to the dermis

The ectoderm first produces an external layer of periderm and then differentiates into the definitive four-layered epidermis

The ectoderm covering of the embryo is initially a single cell thick. Just after neurulation, in the fourth week, the surface ectoderm proliferates to form a new outer layer of simple squamous epithelium called the **periderm** (Fig. 14-1A). The underlying layer of proliferating cells is now called the **basal layer.** The cells of the periderm are gradually sloughed into the amniotic fluid. The periderm is normally shed completely by the 21st week, but in some fetuses it persists until birth, forming a "shell" or "cocoon" around the new-born infant, which is removed by the physician or shed spontaneously during the first weeks of life. These babies are called **collodion babies.**

In the 11th week, proliferation of the basal layer produces a new **intermediate layer** just deep to the periderm (Fig. 14-1B). This layer is the forerunner of the outer layers of the mature epidermis, and the basal layer, now

called the **germinative layer** or **stratum germinativum,** constitutes the layer of stem cells that will continue to replenish the epidermis throughout life. The cells of the intermediate layer contain the **keratin** proteins characteristic of differentiated epidermis and therefore are called **keratinocytes.**

During the early part of the fifth month, at about the time the periderm is shed, the intermediate layer is replaced by the three definitive layers of keratinocytes: the inner **stratum spinosum,** the middle **stratum granulosum,** and the outer **stratum corneum** or **horny layer** (Fig. 14-2). This transformation, which involves **apoptosis** or **programmed cell death,** begins at the cranial end of the fetus and proceeds caudally. The layers of the epidermis represent a maturational series: presumptive keratinocytes are constantly produced by the stratum germinativum, differentiate as they pass outward to the stratum corneum, and finally are sloughed from the surface of the skin.

The stem cells of the stratum germinativum are the only dividing cells of the epidermis. They contain a dispersed network of keratin filaments and are connected by cell-to-cell membrane junctions called **desmosomes.** As cells produced in the stratum germinativum move into the overlying, four-to-eight-cell-thick stratum spinosum, they

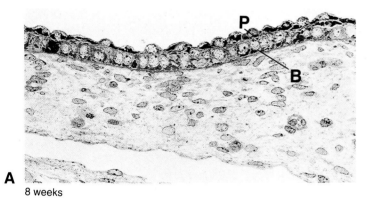

A 8 weeks

B 11 weeks

Fig. 14-1. Differentiation of the ectoderm into the primitive epidermis. (**A**) At 8 to 9 weeks, the surface ectoderm has begun to proliferate to form a periderm layer (P). The proliferating layer is now called the basal layer (B). (**B**) By week 11, the basal layer (B) produces an intermediate layer (I), while a complete but irregular outer layer of periderm (P) is still apparent. (From Holbrook KA, Dale BA, Smith LT et al. 1987. Markers of adult skin expressed in the skin of the first trimester fetus. Curr Probl Dermatol 16:94, with permission.)

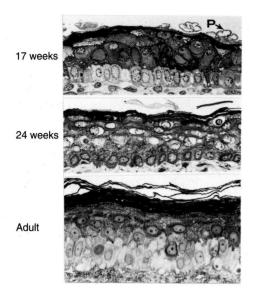

Fig. 14-2. Differentiation of the mature epidermis. The periderm (P) is sloughed during the fourth month and normally is absent by week 21. The definitive epidermal layers, including the stratum spinosum, stratum granulosum, and stratum corneum, begin to develop during the fifth month. (From Foster C, Bertram JF, Holbrook KA. 1988. Morphometric and statistical analyses describing the in utero growth of human epidermis. Anat Rec 222:201, with permission.)

begin to manufacture large amounts of two keratin proteins and also of **envelope proteins** that cover the inner surface of the plasma membrane. Production of keratins and envelope proteins ceases as the cells move into the stratum granulosum, but a protein called **filagrin** is produced that helps to bundle the keratin filaments within the cell. In addition, the enzyme **transglutaminase** cross-links the envelope proteins. Finally, lytic enzymes are released within the cell, metabolic activity ceases, and the resulting flattened, scalelike, terminally differentiated keratinocytes enter the stratum corneum.

Many factors regulate the production and differentiation of epidermal cells

The "decision" of a cell in the stratum germinativum to remain in the pool of proliferating cells or to move into the stratum spinosum and begin differentiating is regulated by a number of interacting agents, including several growth factors. Epidermal growth factor, transforming growth factor-α, transforming growth factor-β, keratin growth factor, calcium, retinoic acid, BIG, a ligand for ECK (a member of the EPH receptor tyrosine kinase family) and the interleukin cytokines IL-1α and Il-6 all appear to play essential and distinct roles in maintaining the balance between proliferation and differentiation in the stratum germinativum. Some of these factors have been

mentioned in previous chapters in connection with other roles they play in development. Transcriptional factors, which regulate the expression of specific genes, also play a role in the regulation of keratinocyte differentiation.

Not surprisingly, imbalances in this complex dynamic control system can result in disorders of skin proliferation. For example, excessive levels of transforming growth factor-α, which appears to be an autoregulator of epidermal proliferation since it is produced by keratinocytes themselves, can result in **psoriasis** and other hyperproliferative skin diseases. It has been hypothesized that overproduction of this substance can also lead to cancer. Transforming growth factor-β may be involved in arresting proliferation once a cell has begun to differentiate into a mature keratinocyte. CD8+ T cells may act as effectors in pathology of psoriatic lesions.

A number of heritable disorders result in excessive keratinization of the skin. For example, infants suffering from **lamellar ichthyosis** have skin that scales off in flakes, sometimes over the whole body. These infants require special care but are usually viable. **Harlequin fetuses,** in contrast, have rigid, deeply cracked skin and usually die shortly after birth. These babies suffer from a defect in the mechanism that bundles keratin fibers in the cells of the stratum granulosum. As a consequence, the keratinocytes do not mature properly and cannot be sloughed from the surface of the stratum corneum.

Gorlin syndrome (nevoid basal cell carcinoma syndrome; NBCCS) is an autosomal dominant disorder occurring in about 1:50,000–100,000 individuals. NBCCS maps to chromosome 9q22.3 and in addition to developmental anomalies consistent with disruption of the sonic hedgehog signaling pathway, the syndrome is also characterized by predisposition to several cancers including **basal cell carcinoma (BCC).** This latter finding supports the view that PTCH is a **tumor suppressor gene.** Nonneoplastic disorders of epidermal derivatives also characterize NBCCS including **odontogenic keratocysts** and **pathognomonic dyskeratotic pitting** of the hands and feet. The odontogenic keratocysts, or jaw cysts, arise from the **dental lamina** (see below). Both **sporadic** and **hereditary** forms of BCCs occur in humans, but this phenotype is variable (age of onset and frequency), suggesting that other modifier genes or environmental factors such as exposure to sunlight may play a role in their pathogenesis.

Melanocytes, Langerhans cells, and Merkel cells appear in the fetal epidermis

In addition to keratinocytes, the epidermis contains a few types of less abundant cells, including melanocytes, Langerhans cells, and Merkel cells. As mentioned in Chapter 4, the pigment cells or **melanocytes** of the skin differentiate from neural crest cells that detach from the neural tube in the sixth week and migrate to the developing epidermis. Although morphologic and histochemical studies do not detect melanocytes in the human epidermis until the 10th to 11th week, studies using monoclonal antibodies directed against antigens characteristic of melanocyte precursors have identified these cells in the epidermis as early as the sixth to seventh weeks (Fig. 14-3A). Thus, it may take neural crest cells only a few days to a week to migrate to the epidermis. Melanocytes are also found in the dermis during fetal life, but at least the vast majority of these are probably in transit to the epidermis. Recall from the Applications to Clinical Practice section of Chapter 5 that c-kit ligand and c-kit receptor play a pivotal role in migration of melanocytes to the skin.

The density of melanocytes increases during fetal life, reaching a peak of about 2,300 cells/mm³ at the end of the third month, after which it drops to the final value of about 800 cells/mm³. Melanocytes represent between 5 and 10 percent of the cells of the epidermis in the adult. In the 10th week many melanocytes become associated with the developing hair follicles (see below), where they function to donate pigment to the hairs.

Melanocytes function as a sunscreen, protecting the deeper layers of the skin from solar radiation, which can cause not only sunburn but also, in the long run, cancer. Unfortunately, melanocytes themselves are relatively likely to produce tumors. Most of these remain benign, but sometimes they give rise to the highly malignant type of cancer called **melanoma.**

The **Langerhans cells** are the macrophage immune cells of the skin, functioning both in contact sensitivity (allergic skin reactions) and in immune surveillance against invading microorganisms. They arise in the bone marrow and first appear in the epidermis by the seventh week (Fig. 14-3B). Langerhans cells continue to migrate into the epidermis throughout life.

Merkel cells are pressure-detecting mechanoreceptors. In humans, they are found only in the thick skin of the palmar or plantar (foot sole) regions. They lie at the base of the epidermis and are associated with underlying nerve endings in the dermis. Although the origin of these cells is not clear, they contain keratin and form desmosomes with adjacent keratinocytes; therefore, they may represent a modified type of keratinocyte. They appear in the fourth to sixth months.

The dermis is derived from both the dermatomes and the somatopleuric mesoderm

The dermis or **corium**—the layer of skin that underlies the epidermis and contains blood vessels, hair follicles, nerve endings, sensory receptors, etc.—is a mesodermal tissue with a dual embryonic origin. Most of it is derived from the somatopleuric layer of the lateral plate mesoderm, but part of it is derived from the dermatomal divisions of the somites. During the third month, the outer layer of the developing dermis proliferates to form ridge-like **dermal papillae** that protrude into the overlying epi-

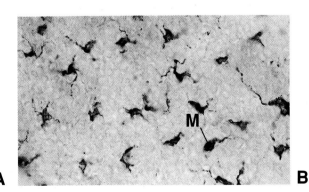
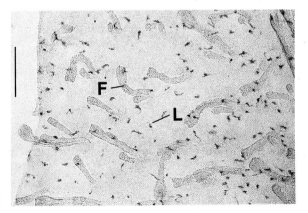

Fig. 14-3. Specialized cells of the epidermis. (**A**) Melanocytes (M) first appear in the embryonic epidermis during the sixth and seventh week. (**B**) Langerhans cells (L) migrate into the epidermis from the bone marrow starting in the seventh week. F, hair follicle. (Fig. A from Holbrook KA. 1988. Structural abnormalities of the epidermally derived appendages in skin from patients with ectodermal dysplasia: insight into developmental errors. Birth Defects Orig Artic Ser 24:15, with permission. Fig. B from Foster C, Holbrook KA. 1989. Ontogeny of Langerhans cells in human embryonic and fetal skin: cell densities and phenotypic expression relative to epidermal growth. Am J Anat 1984:157, with permission.)

dermis (Fig. 14-4). The intervening protrusions of the epidermis into the dermis are called **epidermal ridges.** This superficial region of the dermis is called the **papillary layer,** whereas the thick underlying layer of dense, irregular connective tissue is called the **reticular layer.** The dermis is underlain by subcutaneous fatty connective tissue called the **hypodermis (subcorium).** The dermis differentiates to its definitive form in the second and third trimesters, although it is thin at birth and thickens progressively through infancy and childhood.

The pattern of external ridges and grooves produced in the skin by the dermal papillae varies from one part of the body to another. The palmar and plantar surfaces of the hands and feet carry a familiar pattern of whorls and loops; the eyelids have a diamond-shaped pattern, and the ridges on the upper surface of the trunk resemble a cobweb. The first skin ridges to appear are the whorls on the palmar and plantar surfaces of the digits, which develop in the 11th and 12th weeks. The entire system of surface patterns is established early in the fifth month of fetal life. Thereafter, each patch of skin retains its characteristic pattern even if it is transplanted to a different part of the body.

Blood vessels form within the subcutaneous mesenchyme, deep to the developing dermis, in the fourth week. These branch to form a single layer of vessels in the dermis by the late sixth week and two parallel planes of vessels by the eighth week. Branches of these vessels follow nerves within the dermis and enter the papillary layer to become associated with the hair follicles. These branches may disappear and reappear during different stages of hair follicle differentiation.

It is estimated that the skin of the neonate contains 20 times more blood vessels than it needs to support its own metabolism. This excess is required for thermoregulation in the neonate. Much of the definitive vasculature of the skin develops in the first few weeks after birth.

The integument produces specialized structures including hair, epidermal glands, and nails

The skin contains a large number of specialized structures, including the hair, the sebaceous, sweat, and mammary glands; the nails of the fingers and toes; and the teeth.

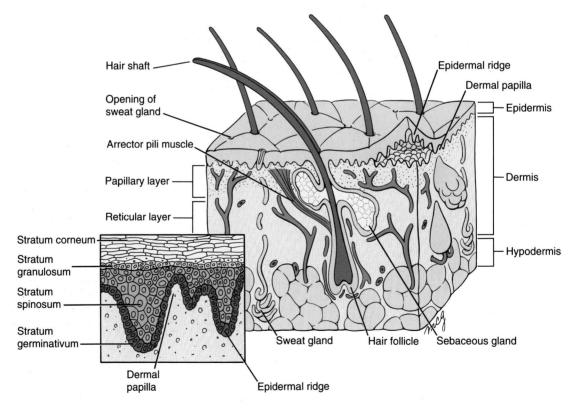

Fig. 14-4. Definitive organization of the dermis and epidermis. The patterns of interdigitating dermal papillae and epidermal ridges first develop during the third month. Sebaceous glands develop from the epidermal lining of the hair follicles, appearing about 1 month after a given hair bud is formed. (Modified from Williams PL, Warwick R, Dyson M, Bannister LH. 1989. Gray's Anatomy. Churchill Livingstone, Edinburgh, with permission.)

In addition, the ectodermal placodes discussed in the preceding two chapters can be regarded as skin derivatives.

Hair follicles are formed by the epidermis and dermis together

Hair follicles first appear at the end of the second month on the eyebrows, eyelids, upper lip, and chin. Hair follicles do not appear in other regions until the fourth month. Most if not all hair follicles are present by the fifth month, and it is believed that novel hair follicles do not form after birth. About 5 million hair follicles develop in both males and females. The differences between the two sexes in the distribution of various kinds of hairs is caused by the different concentrations of circulating sex steroid hormones.

The hair follicle first appears as a small concentration of ectodermal cells called a **hair germ** in the basal layer of the primitive, two-layered epidermis (Fig. 14-5A). Hair germs are thought to be induced by the underlying dermis. The hair germ proliferates to form a rodlike **hair peg** that pushes down into the dermis (Fig. 14-5B–F). Within the dermis, the tip of the hair peg expands, forming a **bulbous hair peg,** and the dermis cells just beneath the tip of the bulb proliferate to form a small hillock called the **dermal papilla.** About 4 weeks after the hair germ begins to grow, the dermal papilla invaginates into the expanded base of the hair bulb (Fig. 14-5D, E). Except in the case of the eyebrows and eyelashes, the dermal root sheath of the follicle becomes associated with a bundle of smooth muscle cells called the **arrector pili** muscle, which functions to erect the hair (making "gooseflesh") (Fig. 14-4).

The layer of proliferating ectoderm that overlies the dermal papilla in the base of the hair bulb becomes the **germinal matrix.** The germinal matrix is responsible for producing the hair shaft (Fig. 14-5D–F): proliferation of the germinal matrix produces cells that undergo a specialized process of keratinization and are added to the base of the hair shaft. The growing hair shaft is thus pushed outward through the follicular canal. If the hair is to be colored, the maturing keratinocytes incorporate pigment pro-

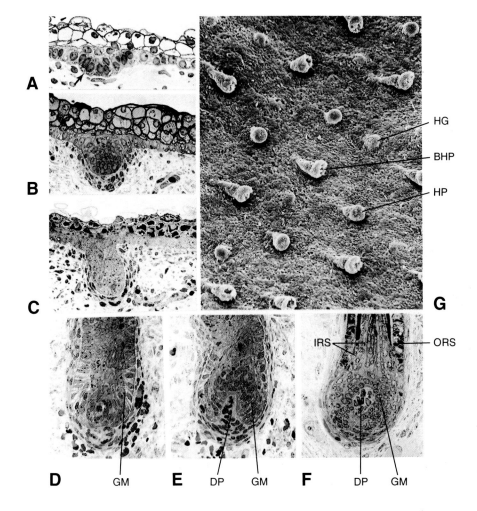

Fig. 14-5. Development of the hair follicle. (**A**) Hair germ at 80 days; (**B**) elongating hair germ later in the first trimester, (**C**) hair peg in the second trimester. (**D–F**) Development of the follicle base from the elongated hair peg stage to the bulbous hair peg stage. The dermal papilla (DP) invaginates into the base of the developing follicle, inducing the germinal matrix (GM). In Fig. F, the hair shaft can be seen growing up the center of the follicle, and the inner and outer epidermal root sheaths (IRS and ORS) are differentiating. (**G**) Scanning electron micrograph of the undersurface of the developing epidermis, showing hair germs (HG), hair pegs (HP), and bulbous hair pegs (BHP) growing into what originally was the dermis. (From Holbrook KA. 1988. Structural abnormalities of the epidermally derived appendages in skin from patients with ectodermal dysplasia: insight into developmental errors. Birth Defects Orig Artic Ser 24:15, with permission; photos courtesy of Dr. Karen Holbrook.)

duced by the melanocytes of the hair bulb. The epidermal cells lining the follicular canal constitute the **inner** and **outer epidermal root sheath.**

The first generation of hairs formed are fine and unpigmented and are called **lanugo.** These hairs first appear during the 12th week. They are mostly shed before birth and are replaced by coarser hairs during the perinatal period. At puberty, the rising levels of sex hormones cause the fine body hair to be replaced by coarser hairs on some parts of the body: the axilla and pubis of both sexes and the face and (in some races) the chest and back of males.

Sebaceous, sweat, and apocrine glands are produced by downgrowths of the epidermis

Several types of glands are produced by downgrowth of the epidermis. Three types of glands—the sebaceous glands, apocrine glands, and sweat glands—are widespread over the body. The milk-producing mammary glands represent a specialized type of epidermal gland.

The **sebaceous glands** produce the oily **sebum** that lubricates the skin and hair. Over most of the body, these glands form as diverticulae of the hair follicle shafts, budding from the side of the epidermal root sheath about 4 weeks after the hair germ begins to elongate. In some areas of hairless skin—such as the glans penis of males and the labia minora of females—sebaceous glands develop as independent downgrowths of epidermis. The bud grows into the dermis tissue and branches to form a small system of ducts ending in expanded secretory acini (alveoli) (Fig. 14-4). The acini secrete by a **holocrine** mechanism; that is, entire secretory cells filled with vesicles of secretory products break down and are shed. The basal layer of the acinar epidermis consists of proliferating stem cells that constantly renew the supply of maturing secretory cells.

Mature sebaceous glands are present on the face by 6 months of development. Sebaceous glands are highly active in the fetus, and the sebum they produce combines with desquamating epidermal cells and remnants of the periderm to form a waterproof protective coating for the fetus called the **vernix caseosa.** After birth the sebaceous glands become relatively inactive, but at puberty they again begin to secrete large quantities of sebum in response to the surge in circulating sex steroids.

The **apocrine glands** are highly coiled, unbranched glands that develop in association with hair follicles. They initially form over most of the body, but in the later months of fetal development they are lost except in certain areas, such as the axillae, mons pubis, prepuce, scrotum, and labia minora. They begin to secrete at puberty, producing a complex mix of substances that are modified by bacterial activity into odorous compounds. These

compounds may function primarily in social and sexual communication. The secretory cells lining the deep half of the gland secrete their products by an **apocrine** mechanism: small portions of cytoplasm containing secretory vesicles pinch off and are released into the lumen of the gland.

The **sweat glands** first appear at about 20 weeks as buds of stratum germinativum that grow down into the underlying dermis to form unbranched, highly coiled glands (Fig. 14-6). The central cells degenerate to form the gland lumen, and the peripheral cells differentiate into an inner layer of secretory cells and an outer layer of **myoepithelial cells,** which are innervated by sympathetic fibers and contract to expel sweat from the gland (Fig. 14-6). The secretory cells secrete fluid directly across the plasma membrane (**eccrine** secretion). Sweat glands form over the entire body surface except for a few areas such as the nipples. Large sweat glands develop as buds of the epithelial root sheath of hair follicles, superficial to the buds of sebaceous glands, in the axilla and areola.

Sweat glands fail to develop in the X-linked genetic disorder **hypohydrotic ectodermal dysplasia.** Infants with this disorder are vulnerable to potentially lethal hyperpyrexia (extremely high fever). The disease is also associated with abnormal dermal papillae. An apparently homologous condition in the mouse can be "cured" by administering epidermal growth factor after birth.

The mammary glands are modified apocrine glands that arise along mammary ridges on either side of the body

In the fourth week, a pair of epidermal thickenings called the **mammary ridges** develop along either side of the body from the area of the future axilla to the future inguinal region and medial thigh (Fig. 14-7). In humans, these ridges normally disappear except at the site of the breasts. The remnant of the mammary ridge produces the **primary bud** of the mammary gland in the fifth week (Fig. 14-7A, B). This bud grows down into the underlying dermis. In the tenth week the primary bud begins to branch, and by the 12th week several **secondary buds** have formed (Fig. 14-7C). These buds lengthen and branch throughout the remainder of gestation, and the resulting ducts canalize by the coalescence of small lumina (Fig. 14-7D, E). At birth, the mammary glands consist of 15 to 25 **lactiferous ducts,** which open onto a small superficial depression called the **mammary pit** (Fig. 14-7D, E). Proliferation of the underlying mesoderm usually converts this pit to an everted nipple within a few weeks after birth, although occasionally the nipple remains depressed (**inverted nipple**). The skin surrounding the nipple also proliferates to form the areola.

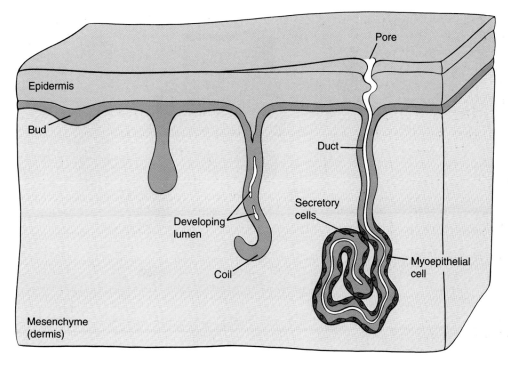

Fig. 14-6. Development of sweat glands. Sweat glands first appear as elongated downgrowths of the epidermis at about 20 weeks. The outer cells of the downgrowth develop into a layer of smooth muscle, while the inner cells become the secretory cells of the gland.

It is not very infrequent for one or more supernumerary nipples (**polythelia**) or supernumerary breasts (**polymastia**) to form along the line of the mammary ridges. The most common location is just below the normal breast. Supernumerary nipples are about as common in males as in females. More rarely, an ectopic nipple forms off the line of the mammary ridge as a consequence of migration of mammary tissue. Supernumerary breasts are often discovered at puberty or during pregnancy, when they enlarge or even lactate in response to stimulatory hormones.

The fingernails and toenails form from epidermis on the palmar and plantar surface of the digits

The nail anlagen first appear as epidermal thickenings on the palmar and plantar surfaces of the tips of the digits (Fig. 14-8A). These thickenings form at about 10 weeks on the fingers and at about 14 weeks on the toes. Almost immediately, the nail anlagen migrate to the dorsal surface of the digits, dragging branches of the palmar and plantar nerves along with them. On the dorsal surface the nail anlage forms a shallow depression called the **primary nail field,** which is surrounded laterally and proximally by ectodermal **nail folds** (Fig. 14-8A, B). The stratum germinativum of the proximal nail fold proliferates

to become the **formative zone** or **root** that produces the horny **nail plate** (Fig. 14-8C). Like a hair, the nail plate is made of compressed keratinocytes. A thin layer of epidermis called the **eponychium** initially covers the nail plate, but this layer normally degenerates except at the nail base. The growing nails reach the tips of the fingers by the eighth month and the tips of the toes by birth.

The teeth are formed by ectoderm and neural crest-derived mesenchyme

In the sixth week, a U-shaped ridge of epidermis called the **dental lamina** appears on the upper and lower jaws (Fig. 14-9A). In the seventh week, 10 centers of epidermal cell proliferation develop at intervals on each dental lamina and grow down into the underlying mesenchyme. A concentration of mesenchyme appears under and around each of these 20 ingrowths. The composite structure consisting of the dental lamina ingrowth and the mesenchymal concentration is called a **tooth bud** (Fig. 14-9A).

Experiments in which dental laminae and mesenchymal concentrations have been cultured with and without each other have shown that tooth development requires both components. Moreover, the concentration of mesenchymal tissue actually consists of neural crest-derived cells mi-

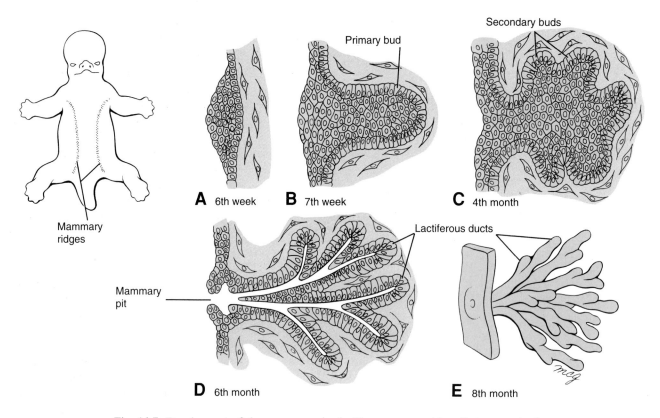

Fig. 14-7. Development of the mammary glands. The mammary ridges first appear in the fourth week as thickened lines of epidermis that extend from the thorax to the medial thigh. (**A, B**) In the region of the future mammary glands, the mammary ridge ectoderm begins to proliferate in the fifth week to form the primary mammary buds. (**C, D**) Secondary buds form during the third month and become canalized to form lactiferous ducts during the last 3 months of fetal life. (**E**) Organization of lactiferous ducts around the developing nipple in the eighth month.

grating from the caudal region of the mesencephalon and the cranial region of the metencephalon. These neural crest cells may be guided by signals (including a variety of extracellular matrix molecules) generated by the presumptive centers of tooth development in the epidermis.

It was also suggested at one point that the tooth buds are induced by the sensory branch of the trigeminal nerve that reaches the site of each presumptive tooth bud just before the tooth bud forms. However, experiments in which the epidermal and mesenchymal precursors of the tooth buds were cultured with and without the trigeminal ganglion demonstrated that tooth development depends only on the ectodermal and mesenchymal precursors.

During the eighth week, instructive influences from the epidermis cause the mesenchymal condensation to invade the base of the dental lamina ingrowth, forming a hillock-shaped mesenchymal **dental papilla** (Fig. 14-9A). This stage of tooth development is called the **cap stage** because the dental lamina invests the top of the papilla like a cap.

The mesenchyme surrounding the papilla and its dental lamina cap condense to form an enclosure called the **dental sac** (Fig. 14-9A). By 10 weeks, the dental papilla has deeply invaginated the dental lamina and constitutes the core of the developing tooth. This is called the **bell stage** of tooth development, because the dental lamina looks like a bell resting over the dental papilla (Fig. 14-9B).

During the bell stage, the outermost cells of the dental papilla become organized into a layer just adjacent to the inner enamel epithelium. These cells differentiate into the **odontoblasts,** which will produce the dentin of the teeth (Fig. 14-9B). In the seventh month these cells begin to secrete the nonmineralized matrix of the dentin, called **predentin,** which later progressively calcifies to form **dentin.** Production of predentin begins at the junction with the inner enamel epithelium and moves inward. The odontoblasts migrate inward as the dentin matrix is laid down, but they spin out behind them long cell processes (**odontoblastic processes**) that extend through the thick-

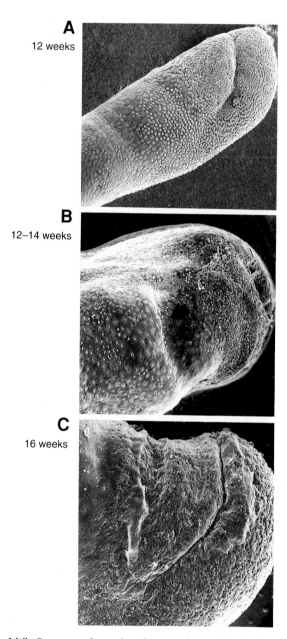

Fig. 14-8. Sequence of scanning electron micrographs showing the development of the nails between 12 and 16 weeks. (**A**) At first the surface of the nail bed is covered with periderm. (**B**) The margin of the dorsal nail fold (arrow) is clearly defined by 12 to 14 weeks. (**C**) The nail plate is apparent by 16 weeks. (From Holbrook KA. 1988. Structural abnormalities of the epidermally derived appendages in skin from patients with ectodermal dysplasia: insight into developmental errors. Birth Defects Orig Artic Ser 24:15, with permission.)

ness of the dentin. The inner mesenchyme of the dental papilla becomes the tooth pulp.

During the bell stage the dental lamina differentiates to form the **enamel organ,** which will produce the enamel layer of the tooth. First, the dental lamina becomes a three-layered structure, consisting of an **inner enamel epithelium** overlying the dental papilla, a middle **enamel** or **stellate reticulum** of star-shaped cells dispersed in an extracellular layer, and an **outer enamel epithelium.** As soon as mineralized dentin is formed, cells of the inner epithelium differentiate into enamel-producing **ameloblasts** and begin to secrete rod-shaped enamel prisms between themselves and the underlying dentin (Fig. 14-9B, C). It is thought that prior production of mineralized dentin is necessary for the induction of enamel secretion by the ameloblasts.

The 20 tooth buds give rise directly to the **primary (deciduous** or **milk) teeth,** consisting in each half-jaw of two incisors, one canine, and two premolars. Early in the bell stage, however, the dental lamina superficial to each tooth bud produces a small diverticulum that migrates to the base of the primary tooth bud and becomes the bud of the **secondary (permanent)** tooth that will replace it (Fig. 14-9C). The buds of the permanent molars, which do not have a deciduous precursor, arise during postnatal life from a pencil-like extension of the dental lamina that burrows back into the posterior jaw from the hindmost primary tooth buds. The full human dentition consists of 32 teeth, including three molars, but the third molars (wisdom teeth) often fail to develop or to erupt.

The roots of the teeth begin to form in late fetal and early postnatal life. At the base of the tooth crown, the confluence of the inner and outer enamel epithelia elongate to form the **epithelial root sheath** (Fig. 14-9D). The mesenchyme just internal to the epithelial sheath differentiates into odontoblasts, which produce dentin. Each root contains a narrow canal of dental pulp, by which nerves and blood vessels enter the tooth (Fig. 14-9D).

The tooth roots are enclosed in extensions of the mesenchymal dental sac. The inner cells of this portion of the dental sac differentiate into **cementoblasts,** which secrete a layer of **cementum** to cover the dentin of the root. At the neck of the tooth root, the cementum meets the enamel at a **cementoenamel junction** (Fig. 14-9C, D). The outermost cells of the dental sac participate in bone formation as the jaws ossify and also form the **periodontal ligament** that holds the tooth to its bony socket or **alveolus.**

Experimental studies suggest that the formation of the primary teeth is enhanced by vitamin D_3 and that the specific morphology of each tooth crown is regulated by interactions with the surrounding mesenchyme. The eruption of the primary teeth, starting at about 6 months after birth, is due to the lengthening of the tooth roots. Mandibular teeth

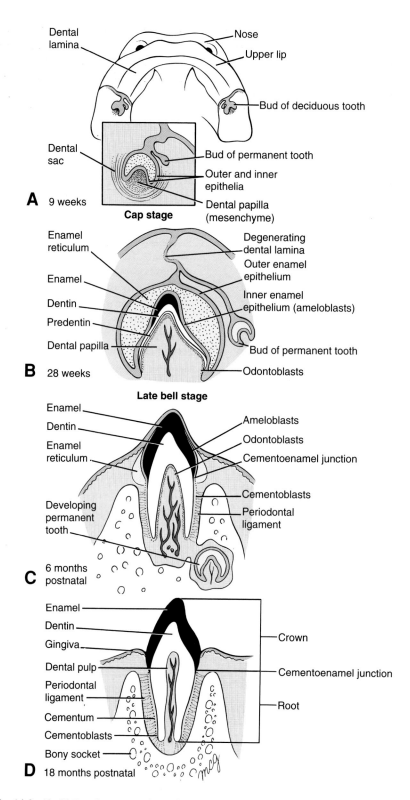

Fig. 14-9. (A–D) Development and eruption of the primary dentition. Notice that the ectodermal lamina gives rise to the enamel organ, which secretes the enamel of the tooth, whereas the neural crest cells that initially form the dental papilla differentiate into the odontoblasts, which secrete the dentin.

usually erupt earlier than the corresponding maxillary teeth. The primary dentition is usually fully erupted by 2 years. At about age 6 to 8, the primary teeth begin to be shed and are replaced by the permanent teeth.

The formation of enamel or dentin is affected by a number of congenital disorders, such as **amelogenesis** **imperfecta** and **dentinogenesis imperfecta.** Recent work shows that these disorders are caused by mutations in regulatory or structural genes involved in the synthesis of enamel or dentin. A combination of genetic, molecular, and developmental studies promises to bring rapid advances in the diagnosis and treatment of these conditions.

15

Fetal Development and the Fetus as Patient

The Fetal Period; Development and Functioning of the Placenta; Teratogenesis and Fetal Infections; Fetal Diagnosis; Fetal Surgery and Gene Therapy

SUMMARY

The **gestation period** of humans from fertilization to birth is usually 266 days (38 weeks). The first 8 weeks constitute the **embryonic period.** The remainder of gestation constitutes the **fetal period.** The 9-month gestation period is divided into three 3-month **trimesters.** Fetuses born between weeks 22 and 28 have grave difficulty in surviving, mainly because of the immaturity of the lungs (see Ch. 6). From the end of the third week until birth, the fetus receives nutrients and eliminates its metabolic wastes via the placenta. The placenta also secretes hormones, including **sex steroids** that maintain pregnancy. **Maternal antibodies** also cross the placenta to provide protection against fetal and neonatal infections. Unfortunately, however, **teratogenic compounds** and some **microorganisms** can cross the placenta.

Development of the placenta begins when the implanting blastocyst induces the **decidual reaction** in the maternal endometrium, causing the endometrium to become a nutrient-packed, vascular tissue called the **decidua.** By the second month, the growing embryo bulges into the uterine lumen. Villi originally cover the entire chorion, but by the end of the third month they are restricted to the area of the embryonic pole that becomes the site of the mature placenta. The villi continue to grow and branch throughout gestation, and the intervillous space is subdivided into 15 to 25 partially separated compartments, called **cotyledons. Human twins** form either by the fertilization of two oocytes (**dizygotic twins**) or, less often, by the splitting of a single early embryo (**monozygotic twins**). Dizygotic twins implant separately, and each develops its own set of fetal membranes (amnion, chorion, and placenta). Depending on when monozygotic twins separate, they may implant together and share some or all of these fetal membranes. The placenta grows with the fetus; at birth it weighs about one-sixth as much as the fetus.

Advances in the safety and sophistication of **techniques for sampling fetal tissues** and the use of **novel imaging techniques** to examine the fetus are rapidly providing new approaches to the **prenatal diagnosis** and **treatment of congenital disorders.** As more is learned about the **molecular biology** and **molecular genetics** of development, it may become possible to devise treatments to **correct developmental deficiencies** such as the absence of sweat glands or lung surfactant. Moreover, the development of **gene therapy techniques** (see Ch. 1) may make it possible to correct many heritable disorders at the genetic level in utero. Our increasing ability to diagnose and treat diseases in utero and in very premature infants raises **ethical and legal questions** that require thoughtful debate. Questions of this nature have always arisen at the forefront of new medical techniques. What is somewhat unusual in this case is the extreme speed with which both our understanding of human developmental biology and our clinical practice are advancing and the fact that the decisions and solutions to the resulting medical questions affect **a new category of patient: the unborn fetus.**

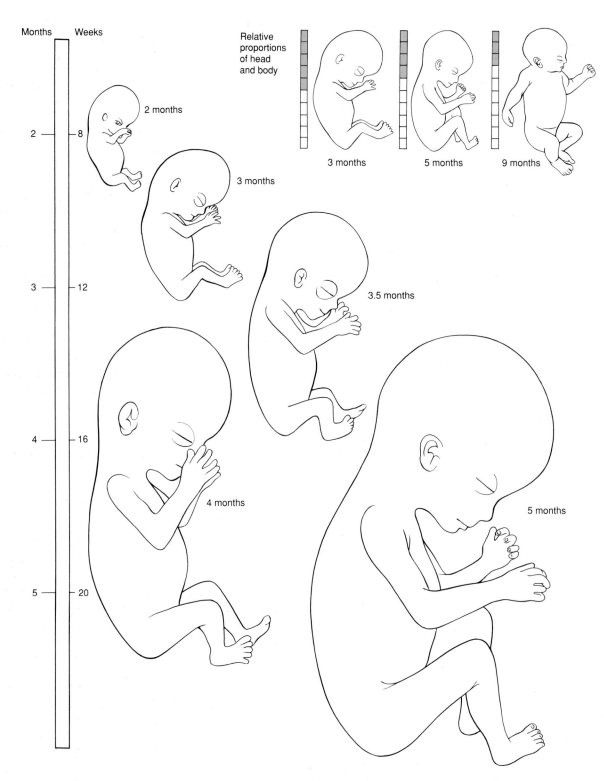

Timeline. Fetal development.

During the fetal period, the embryonic organ systems mature and the fetus grows

Most of the preceding text has concentrated on the **embryonic period,** from the late third through the eighth weeks, the period during which the organs and systems of the body are formed. The succeeding **fetal period,** from 8 weeks to birth at about 38 weeks, is devoted to the maturation of these organ systems and to growth. The fetus grows from 8 g at 8 weeks to about 3,400 g at birth, a 425-fold increase. Most of this weight is put on in the third trimester (7 to 9 months), although the fetus grows in length mainly in the second trimester (4 to 6 months). The growth of the fetus is accompanied by drastic changes in proportion: at 9 weeks the head of the fetus represents about half of its **crown–rump length** (the "sitting height" of the fetus), whereas at birth it represents about one-fourth of the crown–rump length.

Although all the organ systems are present by 8 weeks, few of them are functional. The most prominent exceptions are the heart and blood vessels, which begin to circulate blood during the fourth week. Even so, the reconfiguration of the fetal circulatory system described in Chapter 8 is not complete until 3 months. The sensory systems also lag. The auditory ossicles are not free to vibrate until just before birth, for example, and, although the neural retina of the eye differentiates during the third and fourth months, the eyelids remain closed until 5 to 7 months, and the eyes cannot focus properly until several weeks after birth.

A number of organs do not finish maturing until after birth. The most obvious example is the reproductive system and associated sexual characteristics, which, as in most animals, do not finish developing until the individual is old enough to be likely to reproduce successfully. In humans, a relatively large number of other organs are also immature at birth. This accounts for the prolonged helpless infancy of humans compared with many mammals. The slowest-maturing organ of humans, and the one that largely sets the pace of infancy and childhood, is the brain. The cerebrum and cerebellum are both quite immature at birth.

Fetal life is supported by the placenta, an organ with maternal and fetal components

The placental tissues are derived from the maternal decidua basalis and the fetal chorion

As the blastocyst implants, it stimulates a response in the uterine endometrium called the **decidual reaction** (Fig. 15-1). The cells of the endometrial **stroma** (the fleshy layer of endometrial tissue that underlies the endometrial epithelium lining the uterine cavity) accumulate lipid and glycogen and are then called **decidual cells.** The stroma thickens and becomes more highly vascularized, and the endometrium as a whole is then called the **decidua.**

Late in the embryonic period, the **abembryonic** side of the growing embryo (the side opposite to the **embryonic** pole where the germ disc and connecting stalk attach) begins to bulge into the uterine cavity (Fig. 15-2). This protruding portion of the embryo is covered by a thin capsule of endometrium called the **decidua capsularis.** The embedded, embryonic pole of the embryo is underlain by a zone of decidua called the **decidua basalis,** which will participate in forming the mature placenta. The remaining areas of decidua are called the **decidua parietalis.** In the third month, as the growing fetus begins to fill the womb, the decidua capsularis is pressed against the decidua parietalis, and in the fifth and sixth months the decidua capsularis disintegrates.

Development of the uteroplacental circulatory system begins late in the second week as cavities called **trophoblastic lacunae** form in the syncytiotrophoblast of the chorion and anastomose with maternal capillaries. At the end of the third week, fetal blood vessels begin to form in the connecting stalk and extraembryonic mesoderm. Meanwhile, as described in Chapter 2, the extraembryonic mesoderm lining the chorionic cavity proliferates to form **tertiary stem villi** that project into the blood-filled trophoblastic lacunae. By the end of the fourth week, tertiary stem villi cover the entire chorion.

The villi disappear from the chorion laeve and lengthen in the chorion frondosum

As the embryo begins to bulge into the uterine lumen during the second month, the villi on the protruding, abembryonic side of the chorion disappear (Fig. 15-2). This region of the chorion is now called the **smooth chorion** or **chorion laeve,** whereas the portion of the chorion associated with the decidua basalis retains its villi and is called the **chorion frondosum** (from Latin *frondosus,* leafy).

The placental villi continue to grow during most of the remainder of gestation. Starting in the ninth week, the tertiary stem villi lengthen by the formation of terminal **mesenchymal villi,** which originate as sprouts of syncytiotrophoblast **(trophoblastic sprouts)** similar in cross section to primary stem villi (see Ch. 2) (Fig. 15-3). These terminal extensions of the teritary stem villi reach their maximum length in the 16th week and are called **immature intermediate villi.** The cells of the cytotrophoblastic layer become more disapersed in these villi, leaving gaps in that layer of the villus wall.

Starting near the end of the second trimester, the tertiary stem villi also form numerous slender side branches called

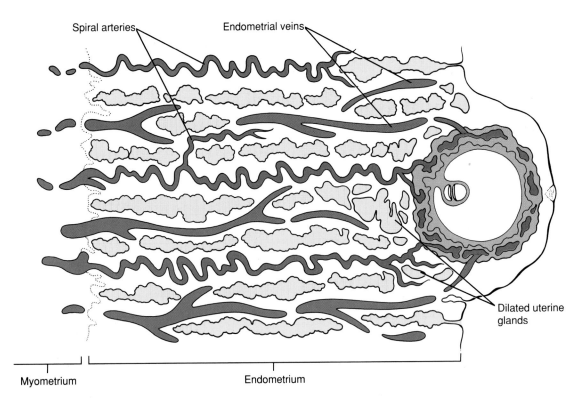

Spiral arteries

Endometrial veins

Dilated uterine glands

Myometrium

Endometrium

Fig. 15-1. The decidua. As the blastocyst implants in the uterine wall, the endometrial stroma thickens to form the decidua. The endometrial glands enlarge, the stromal cells become engorged with lipid and glycogen, and endometrial veins and spiral arteries make connections with the trophoblastic lacunae. (Modified from Williams PL, Warwick R, Dyson M, Bannister LH. 1989. Gray's Anatomy. Churchill Livingstone, Edinburgh, with permission.)

mature intermediate villi. The first-formed mature intermediate villi finish forming by week 32 and then begin to produce small, nodulelike secondary branches called **terminal villi.** These terminal villi complete the structure of the **placental villous tree.** It has been suggested that the terminal villi are formed not by active outgrowth of the syncytiotrophoblast but rather by coiled and folded villous capillaries that bulge against the villus wall.

Because the blood-filled **intervillous space** into which the villi project is formed from trophoblastic lacunae that grow and coalesce, it is lined on both sides with syncytiotrophoblast (see Fig. 15-3B). The maternal face of the placenta, called the **basal plate,** consists of this syncytiotrophoblast lining plus a supporting layer of decidua basalis. On the fetal side, the layers of the chorion form the **chorionic plate** of the placenta.

The placenta is subdivided into cotyledons by the wedgelike placental septa

During the fourth and fifth months, wedgelike walls of decidual tissue called **placental (decidual) septa** grow into the intervillous space from the maternal side of the placenta, separating the villi into 15 to 25 groups called **cotyledons** (Fig. 15-3). Since the placental septa do not fuse with the chorionic plate, maternal blood can flow freely from one cotyledon to another.

Respiratory gases, nutrients, waste products, and antibodies are exchanged between maternal and fetal blood in the placenta

Maternal blood enters the intervillous spaces of the placenta through about 100 **spiral arteries,** bathes the villi, and leaves again via **endometrial veins** (Fig. 15-1). The placenta contains approximately 150 ml of maternal blood, and this volume is replaced about three or four times per minute. Nutrients and oxygen pass from the maternal blood across the layers of the villus wall into the fetal blood and waste products such as carbon dioxide, urea, uric acid, and bilirubin (a breakdown product of hemoglobin) reciprocally pass from the fetal blood to the maternal blood.

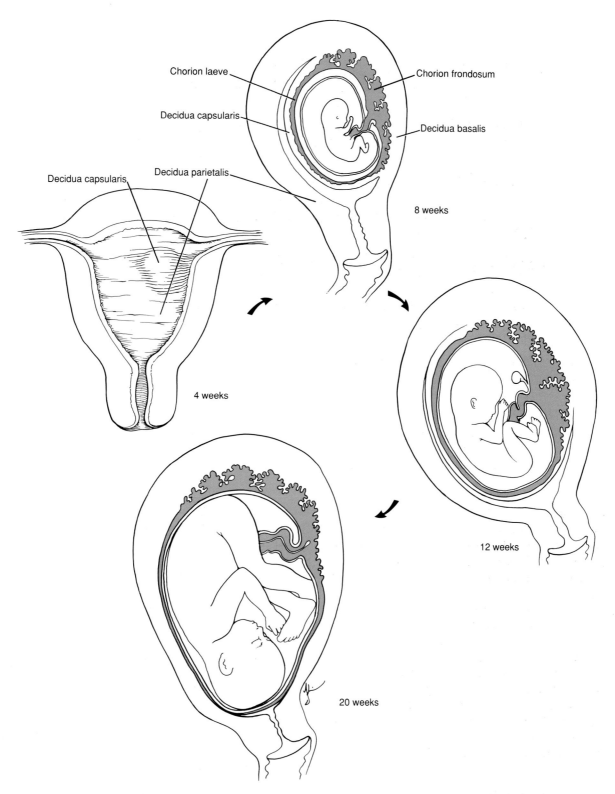

Fig. 15-2. Development of the chorion and decidua during the first 5 months. The decidua is divided into three portions: the decidua capsularis overlying the growing conceptus; the decidua basalis underlying the placenta; and the decidua parietalis lining the remainder of the uterus.

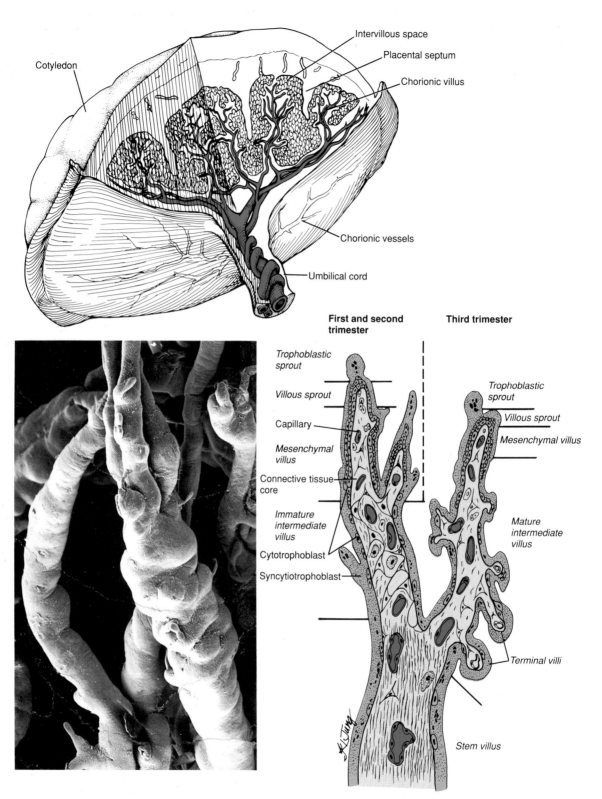

Fig. 15-3. Development of the placenta. (From Castellucci M, Scheper M, Scheffen I et al. 1990. The development of the human villous tree. Anat Embryol 181:117, with permission.)

Antibodies also cross the placenta to enter the fetal circulation, and in this way the mother gives the fetus limited passive immunity against a variety of infections, such as diphtheria and measles. These antibodies persist in the infant's blood for several months after birth, guarding the infant against infectious diseases until its own immune system matures.

Erythroblastosis fetalis is caused by the passage of anti-Rh antibodies from an Rh⁻ mother to an Rh⁺ fetus

There is one fairly common instance in which the transfer of antibodies from the mother to the fetus is not beneficial: when the antibodies are directed against an Rh factor on the fetal red blood cells and cause hemolysis (dissolution) of the fetal red blood cells. The **Rh factors** are a group of genetically determined surface molecules that are present on the plasma membrane of red blood cells in most, but not all, individuals. Individuals whose blood cells carry an Rh factor are **Rh⁺**; individuals whose blood cells lack one are **Rh⁻.** Rh factors provoke a strong immune response in RH⁻ individuals. If an Rh⁻ mother carries an Rh⁺ fetus and fetal blood leaks into the maternal circulation, the mother will manufacture antibodies against the fetal red blood cells. Significant leaks of fetal blood across the placenta into the maternal circulation normally occur only at birth, so the resulting antibodies do not form in time to harm the fetus that first induces them. However, if the same mother bears a second Rh⁺ fetus, her anti-Rh antibodies can cross the placenta and destroy fetal red blood cells, causing anemia in the fetus and newborn. This condition is called **hemolytic disease of the newborn** or **erythroblastosis fetalis.** The latter name comes from the fact that the destruction of red blood cells stimulates a compensatory production of large numbers of immature nucleated fetal red blood cells called **erythroblasts.** Another, sometimes fatal, consequence of the disease is **hydrops**—the accumulation of water in the fetus. Moreover, the destruction of red blood cells releases large amounts of bilirubin (a breakdown product of hemoglobin) into the fetal circulation. This substance can be deposited in the developing brain, leading to cerebral damage and, in some cases, to death.

The effects of erythroblastosis fetalis can be prevented by giving transfusions of Rh⁻ blood to the fetus in utero and to the newborn, so that the maternal antibodies find fewer cells to destroy. A more economical preventive approach is to administer anti-Rh antibodies to the RH⁻ mother immediately after the birth of each Rh⁺ baby. These antibodies destroy the fetal Rh⁺ red blood cells in her circulation before they stimulate her own immune system; this prevents her from manufacturing anti-Rh antibodies.

The placenta also allows the passage of some viral and bacterial pathogens

Although the placenta is fairly impermeable to microorganisms, a number of viruses and bacteria can cross it and infect the fetus. Because the fetus has no functioning immune system and relies solely on maternal antibodies for protection, it is often inept at fighting infections. Therefore, a disease that is mild in the mother may damage or kill the fetus. Viruses that can cross the placenta and infect the fetus include rubella virus (the agent of rubella or German measles), varicella-zoster virus (the agent of varicella or chickenpox), cytomegalovirus (the agent of mononucleosis), and coxsackievirus (the agent of various diseases, usually mild, in the adult). Cytomegalovirus causes one of the most common viral infections of the fetus. If this virus infects the embryo early in development, it may induce abortion; infection occurring later may cause a wide range of congenital abnormalities, including blindness, microcephaly, and mental retardation. One bacterium that has recently come to unpleasant prominence as a cause of congenital infections in American children is *Treponema pallidum,* the agent of syphilis. The incidence of syphilis among Americans has increased steadily since the 1950s, and the bacterium readily crosses the placenta.

HIV can be transmitted across the placenta, during parturition, or in breast milk

Human immunodeficiency virus (HIV) is the agent of human immune deficiency syndrome (AIDS) and related syndromes. This virus can sometimes cross the placenta from an infected mother to infect the unborn fetus. It is commonly transmitted during the birth process or in the mother's milk during breast-feeding. Infants infected perinatally with HIV may appear to be healthy at birth, but they usually come down with AIDS by the time they are 3 years old. As in adults, the disease slowly destroys a crucial component of the immune system and leaves the infant vulnerable to repeated infections. Parotid gland infections, diarrhea, bronchitis, and chronic middle ear infections are common in infants with AIDS. Pneumonia caused by the protozoan *Pneumocystis carinii,* a characteristic infection of adults with AIDS, is a particularly alarming symptom in infants: the mean survival time of infants diagnosed with AIDS and *Pneumocystis carinii* pneumonia is 1 to 3 months. HIV-1 infection is also correlated with an increased rate of low birthweight, intrauterine fetal death, and preterm birth.

The incidence of transmission of HIV from mother to infant in the United States was estimated to be 1.5 per thousand population in 1989; the incidence in the state of New

York for that year was estimated as 5.8 per thousand. In the late 1980s, about 1,800 HIV-infected babies were born per year in the United States. However, the World Health Organization estimates that by the year 2000, 10 million infants worldwide will have acquired HIV from their mothers.

Teratogens reach the fetus by crossing the placenta

Many previous chapters have alluded to the role of teratogens in causing various specific congenital abnormalities. Other teratogens may not cause a specific malformation but may nevertheless result in **intrauterine growth retardation (IUGR).** Teratogens reach the fetus by crossing the placenta.

It is not always easy to identify a compound as a teratogen. Two approaches are used: **epidemiologic studies,** which attempt to relate antenatal exposure to a suspect compound with the occurrence of various congenital anomalies; and studies in which the compound is administered to pregnant experimental animals and the offspring are checked for abnormalities. It is often difficult to gather enough epidemiologic data to yield a clear result, however, and findings from animal studies are not necessarily applicable to humans. These difficulties are compounded by the complicated nature of teratogenesis. As discussed in previous chapters, most congenital deformities are multifactorial in etiology: that is, their pathogenesis depends on the genetic makeup of the individual as well as on exposure to the teratogen. An identical dose of a teratogen may cause severe anomalies in one individual and have no effect on another. In addition, malformations of a given structure can usually be caused only during the **sensitive period,** when that structure is undergoing morphogenesis. The timeline illustrations at the beginning of each chapter in this book generally define the sensitive periods of the corresponding tissues and organ systems. Since the major events of organogenesis take place during the first 8 weeks of development, that is the period during which the fetus is most vulnerable to teratogens.

Many therapeutic drugs are known to be teratogenic; these include retinoids (vitamin A and analogs), the anticoagulant warfarin, the anticonvulsants trimethadione and phenytoin, and a number of the chemotherapeutic agents used to treat cancer. Most teratogenic drugs exert their main effects during the embryonic period. However, care must be exercised in administering certain anesthetics and other drugs even late in pregnancy or at term, since they may endanger the health of the fetus.

Some recreational drugs are also teratogenic; these include tobacco, alcohol, and cocaine. Cocaine, ingested by alarming numbers of pregnant women (the drug affected 300,000 to 400,000 newborns in 1990 in the United

States), readily crosses the placenta and may cause addiction in the developing fetus. In some of the major cities of the United States, as many as 20 percent of babies are born to mothers who abuse cocaine. Unfortunately, fetal cocaine addiction may have permanent effects on the individual, although studies suggest that early intervention with intensive emotional and educational support in the first few years of life may be helpful.

Pregnant women who use cocaine have higher frequencies of fetal morbidity (disease) and mortality (death) than pregnant women who do not. Cocaine use is associated not only with low birthweight but also with some specific developmental anomalies, including infarction of the cerebral cortex and a variety of cardiovascular malformations. It is often difficult to isolate cocaine as the teratogen responsible for a given effect, however, since women who abuse cocaine often abuse other drugs as well, including marijuana, alcohol, tobacco, and heroin.

Children of cocaine-abusing mothers may be born premature as well as addicted: cocaine-using mothers have a very high frequency of **preterm labor.** Preterm labor occurs in 25 percent of women who test positive for cocaine on a urine test at admission to the hospital for labor and delivery, but in only 8 percent of women who do not test positive for cocaine at admission. Two mechanisms have been proposed by which cocaine could cause preterm labor. On the one hand, cocaine, which is a potent constrictor of blood vessels, may cause abruption of the placental membranes (premature separation of the placenta from the uterus) by partly shutting off the flow of blood to the placenta. On the other hand, there is evidence that cocaine directly affects the contractility of the uterine myometrium (muscle layer), perhaps making it hypersensitive to signals that initiate labor.

The placenta produces steroid and protein hormones and prostaglandins

The placenta is an extremely prolific producer of hormones. Two of its major products are the steroid hormones **progesterone** and **estrogen,** which are responsible for maintaining the pregnant state and preventing spontaneous abortion or preterm labor. As discussed in Chapter 1, the corpus luteum produces progesterone and estrogen during the first weeks of pregnancy. By the 11th week, however, the corpus luteum degenerates and the placenta assumes its role.

During the first 2 months of pregnancy, the syncytiotrophoblast of the placenta produces the glycoprotein hormone **human chorionic gonadotropin,** which supports the secretory activity of the corpus luteum. Because this hormone is produced only by fetal tissue and is excreted in the mother's urine, it is used as the basis for pregnancy tests. However, it is also produced abundantly by hydatidiform moles, and persistence of the hormone beyond 2 months of gestation may indicate a molar pregnancy.

The placenta produces an extremely wide range of other protein hormones, including, to name a few, placental lactogen, human chorionic thyrotropin, human chorionic corticotropin, insulinlike growth factors, prolactin, relaxin, corticotropin-releasing hormone, and endothelin. In fact, it is becoming increasingly clear that the placenta makes many of the hormones also manufactured by the hypothalamus and pituitary.

In addition, placental membranes synthesize **prostaglandins,** a family of compounds that perform a range of functions in various tissues of the body. Placental prostaglandins appear to be intimately involved in the maintenance of pregnancy and onset of labor. The signal that initiates labor seems to be a reduction in the ratio of progesterone to estrogen, but the effect of this signal may be mediated by an elevation in the levels of prostaglandins produced by the placenta.

The production and resorption of amniotic fluid are normally in close balance

As described in Chapter 6, embryonic folding transforms the amnion from a small bubble on the dorsal side of the germ disc to a sac that completely encloses the embryo. By the eighth week, the expanding amniotic sac completely fills the old chorionic cavity and fuses with the chorion. The expansion of the amnion is due largely to an increase in the amount of **amniotic fluid.** The volume of amniotic fluid increases through the seventh month and then decreases somewhat in the last two months. At birth the volume of amniotic fluid is typically about 1 L.

Amniotic fluid, which is very similar to blood plasma in composition, is initially produced by the transport of fluid across the amniotic membrane itself. After about 16 weeks, fetal urine also makes an important contribution to the amniotic fluid. If the fetus does not excrete urine—either because of bilateral renal agenesis (absence of both kidneys) or because the lower urinary tract is obstructed (obstructive uropathy)—the volume of amniotic fluid will be too low (the condition called **oligohydramnios**) and the amniotic cavity, in consequence, will be too small. A small amniotic cavity can cramp the growth of the fetus and cause various congenital malformations, notably pulmonary hypoplasia.

Because amniotic fluid is constantly produced, it must also be constantly resorbed. This is accomplished mainly by the fetal gut, which absorbs the fluid drunk by the fetus. Excess fluid is then returned to the maternal circulation via the placenta. Malformations that make it impossible for the fetus to drink—for example, esophageal atresia or anencephaly result in an overabundance of amniotic fluid, a condition called **hydramnios** or **polyhydramnios.**

The degree to which monozygotic twins share fetal membranes indicates the stage at which they separated

Twins that form by the splitting of a single original embryo are called **monozygotic** or **identical** twins. These twins share an identical genetic makeup and therefore look alike as they grow up. **Dizygotic** or **fraternal** twins, in contrast, arise from separate oocytes produced during the same menstrual cycle. Dizygotic twin embryos implant separately and develop separate fetal membranes (amnion, chorion, and placenta). Monozygotic twins, in contrast, may share none, some, or all of their fetal membranes, depending on how late in development the original embryo splits to form twins.

If the splitting occurred during cleavage—for example, if the two blastomeres produced by the first cleavage division become separated—the monozygotic twin blastomeres will implant separately, like dizygotic twin blastomeres, and will not share fetal membranes (Fig. 15-4). Alternatively, if the twins are formed by splitting of the inner cell mass within the blastocyst, they will occupy the same chorion but will be enclosed by separate amnions and will use separate placentae, each placenta developing around the connecting stalk of its respective embryo (Fig. 15-4). Finally, if the twins are formed by splitting of a bilaminar germ disc, they will occupy the same amnion (Fig. 15-4).

Because fetal membranes fuse when they are forced together by the growth of the fetus, it may not be immediately obvious whether the membranous septum separating a pair of twins represents just amniotic membranes (meaning that the twins share a chorion) or fused amnions and chorions (meaning that the twins originally did not share fetal membranes). The clue is the thickness and opacity of the septum: amniotic membranes are thin and almost transparent, whereas chorionic membranes are thicker and somewhat opaque.

Chorionic vessels in the placentae of monozygotic twins may become connected and may cause problems for the fetuses

Monozygotic placentae usually become connected by anastomosis of chorionic vessels, usually arteries. This shared circulation usually poses no problem, but if one twin dies late in gestation or if the blood pressure of one twin drops significantly, the remaining twin is at risk. If

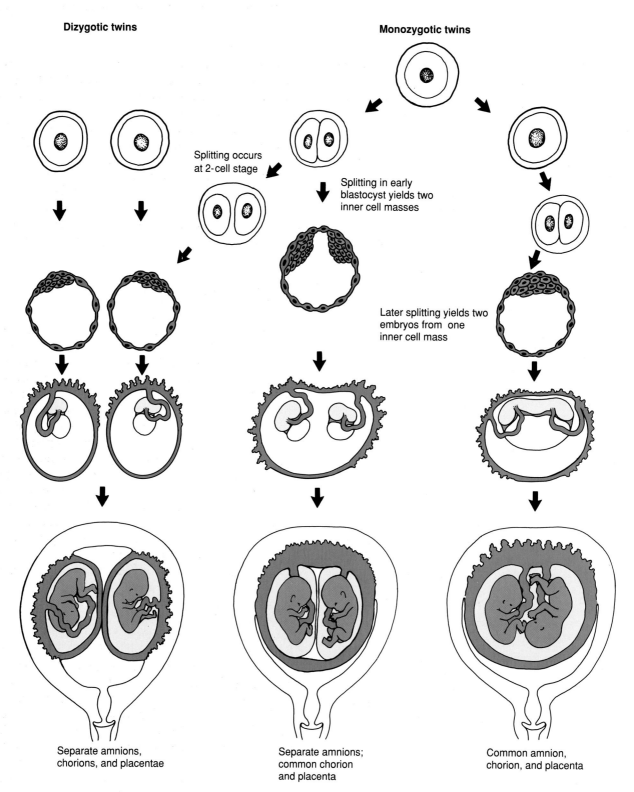

Dizygotic twins

Monozygotic twins

Splitting occurs
at 2-cell stage

Splitting in early
blastocyst yields two
inner cell masses

Later splitting yields two
embryos from one
inner cell mass

Separate amnions,
chorions, and placentae

Separate amnions;
common chorion
and placenta

Common amnion,
chorion, and placenta

Fig. 15-4. Uterine disposition of various types of twins. The degree to which monozygotic twins share placental membranes depends on the stage of development at which the originally single embryo separates: if the splitting occurs at the two-cell stage of cleavage, the twins will develop as separately as dizygotic twins; if the splitting yields a blastocyst with two inner cell masses, then the embryos will share a single chorion and placenta but occupy separate amnions; if the splitting occurs after the formation of the inner cell mass, the embryos will occupy a single amnion.

one twin dies, the other twin may be killed by an **embolism** (blocked blood vessel) caused by bits of tissue that break off in the dead twin and enter the shared circulation. If the blood pressure of one twin falls sharply, the other twin may suffer heart failure as its heart attempts to fill both circulatory systems at once.

Until recently, the only treatment for these situations was to wait until the healthy twin was old enough to have a chance of surviving outside the womb and then to perform a cesarean section. Surgical techniques are being developed, however, that may allow routine removal of the dead or diseased twin, allowing the other twin to develop normally. This procedure is technically difficult, however, because fetal operations have a tendency to induce preterm labor.

Modern diagnostic techniques make it possible to assess the health of the unborn

Three diagnostic techniques have begun to revolutionize the diagnosis of embryonic and fetal malformations and genetic diseases. These are **amniocentesis, chorionic villus sampling,** and **ultrasonography.**

In amniocentesis, amniotic fluid is aspirated and examined

In amniocentesis, amniotic fluid is aspirated from the amniotic cavity (usually between 14 and 16 weeks gestation) through a needle inserted via the abdominal wall and is examined for various clues to fetal disease. Amniotic fluid contains metabolic byproducts of the fetus as well as cells sloughed from the fetus (possibly the lungs) and amniotic membrane. The protein α-fetoprotein, for example, is a useful indicator. Elevated levels of this protein may indicate the presence of an open neural tube defect, such as anencephaly or other open defects such as gastroschisis. Fetal cells in the amniotic fluid can be cultured and karyotyped to determine the sex of the fetus and to detect chromosomal anomalies. The technique of Southern blotting can be used to screen the genome for the presence or absence of specific mutations that cause heritable diseases. Amniocentesis has limitations early in gestation, however, both because it is difficult to perform when the volume of amniotic fluid is small and because a small sample may not yield enough cells for Southern blotting.

Chorionic villus sampling yields larger cell samples than amniocentesis

In chorionic villus sampling, a small sample of tissue (10–40 mg) is removed from the chorion by a catheter inserted through the cervix or with a needle inserted through the abdominal wall. This tissue may be directly karyotyped or karyotyped after culture. Chorionic villus sampling can be performed early in gestation and yields enough tissue for Southern blotting. A complication of this technique, however, is that maternal tissue may be mistaken for fetal tissue. This error could lead to an incorrect diagnosis or sex determination and, in the worst case, could lead to a decision to abort a fetus that was actually normal. This risk is avoided by growing cells from the sample in culture and comparing them with fetal cells obtained by amniocentesis. This use of chorionic villus sampling or amniocentesis is usually recommended for mothers older than 35 years.

Ultrasonography can be used to view the fetus in utero

In ultrasonography, the inside of the body is scanned with a beam of ultrasound (sound with a frequency of 3 to 10 MHz), and a computer is used to analyze the pattern of returning echoes. Because tissues of different density reflect sound differently, revealing tissue interfaces, the pattern of echoes can be used to decipher the inner structure of the body. The quality of the images yielded by ultrasonography is rapidly improving, and it is now possible to visualize the structure of the developing fetus and to identify many malformations. Ultrasonography is also now used to guide the needles or catheters used for amniocentesis and chorionic villus sampling. These procedures were formerly performed unguided, with a higher consequent risk of piercing the fetus. There is as yet no evidence that ultrasound harms fetal tissues.

Various types of "display modes," or ways of analyzing and displaying ultrasound data, are used, each with particular advantages. **M-mode** ultrasonography shows the changes in position of a structure with time. **B-mode** ultrasonography (such as **two-dimensional echocardiography**) shows the anatomy of a two-dimensional plane of scanning and can be performed in real time. **Doppler ultrasonography** yields flow information and can be used to study the pattern of flow within the heart and developing blood vessels. The miniaturization of ultrasound electronics has led to the development of **endosonography,** in which a miniature ultrasound probe is inserted into a body orifice such as the vagina and is thus brought close to the structure of interest, permitting a higher resolution image.

Real-time B-mode ultrasonography is the type most often used to examine the fetus. A wide variety of fetal anomalies can be seen and diagnosed by this technique, including craniofacial defects, limb anomalies, diaphragmatic hernias, caudal dysgenesis syndromes, teratomas, spina bifida, and renal agenesis (Fig. 15-5). Abnormalities of the fetal heart and heartbeat can be analyzed.

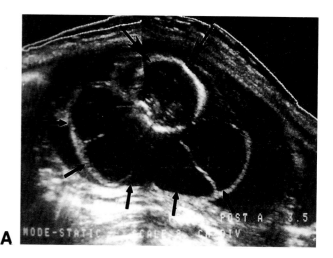

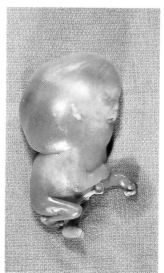

Fig. 15-5. Cystic hygroma detected by ultrasound. (**A**) Ultrasound scan showing the fetus in the uterine cavity. The smaller circular structure (long arrows) is the fetal skull; the large, thin-walled, cushionlike structure posterior to it (short arrows) is a cystic hygroma in the cervical region. (**B**) The stillborn fetus. (Photos courtesy of Dr. Tariq Siddiqi.)

Improving techniques of fetal diagnosis and surgery pose new questions for parent and physician

If amniocentesis or chorionic villus sampling reveals that a fetus has a significant genetic anomaly, should the fetus be aborted? If ultrasonography shows a malformation serious enough to kill or deform the fetus, should corrective fetal surgery be attempted? The answers to these questions involve many factors, including (1) the risk to the mother of continuing the pregnancy, (2) the availability of surgeons and resources for fetal surgery, (3) the risk of the operation to the fetus and the mother, (4) the severity of the anomaly or disease, and (5) the advantage of correcting the defect in utero instead of after birth.

A wide range of fetal anomalies could potentially be corrected operatively. For example, a diaphragmatic hernia that would result in pulmonary hypoplasia has been corrected by opening the uterus, restoring the herniated viscera to the abdominal cavity, and repairing the fetal diaphragm (Fig. 15-6). Hydrocephalus caused by stenosis of the cerebral aqueduct of Sylvius (see Ch. 13) can be corrected by inserting a ventriculoamniotic shunt through the skull into the forebrain ventricle. This shunt has a one-way pressure valve that allows excess cerebrospinal fluid to vent into the amniotic cavity. The brain is then free to develop normally. Obstructive uropathy (constriction of the lower urinary tract, which prevents the urine produced by the kidneys from escaping) results in oligohydramnios and consequent fetal malformations, including pulmonary hypoplasia and defects of the face and limbs, and also in damage to the developing kidneys because of the backpressure of urine in the kidney tubules. Repair of the obstruction prevents these problems.

The anomalies in these examples would all cause death or major malformation if left uncorrected until birth. What about the case of a defect, such as cleft lip, that is not life-threatening? Cleft lips are routinely repaired after

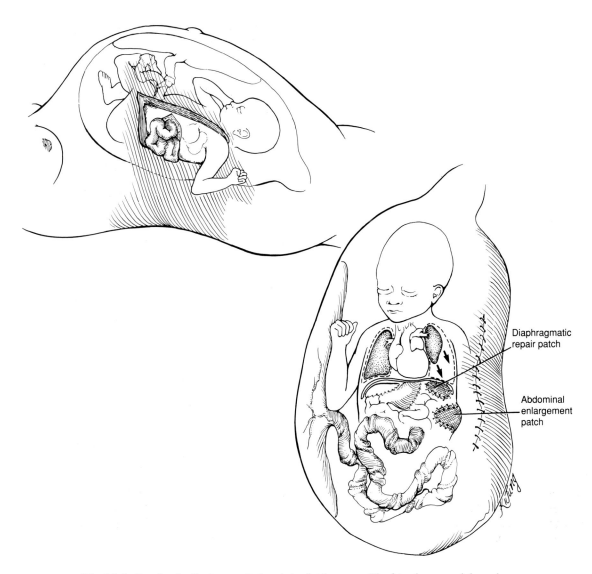

Fig. 15-6. Repair of a diaphragmatic hernia by fetal surgery. The fetus is exposed through an incision in the uterine and abdominal walls. The fetal viscera are retracted from the left pleural cavity, and the hole in the diaphragm is repaired with a Gore-Tex patch. The left lung now has room to grow normally. Since the fetal abdominal cavity is too small for the restored viscera, a second Gore-Tex enlargement patch is placed in the fetal abdominal wall. (Modified from Harrisson MR, Adzik NS, Longaker MT et al. 1990. Successful repair in utero of a fetal diaphragmatic hernia after removal of herniated viscera from the left thorax. N Engl J Med 322:1582, with permission.)

birth, but the result is not perfect; it has been argued that correction in utero would prevent scarring and give a cosmetically perfect result. Is the potential value of this outcome to parents and child worth the risk and expense of the procedure? These are questions under current debate.

Gene therapy of the fetus may be possible

As discussed above, modern techniques such as amniocentesis, chorionic villus sampling, and Southern blotting

make it possible to detect mutations and chromosomal anomalies in the fetus. Is there any way to correct these errors at the genetic level before birth so that development can be normal? The answer to this question is: possibly yes.

The technique of insertional mutagenesis has been used successfully to cure genetic diseases in experimental animals, for example, in mice with a dominant mutation that impairs normal blood cell differentiation and causes anemia. In this experiment, primitive hematopoietic (blood cell-producing) stem cells were removed from a mutant mouse and the wild-type, normal gene was introduced (transfected) into these cells via a retrovirus vector. The "cured" stem cells were then introduced back into the mutant mouse, which in the meantime had been subjected to high-dose irradiation to destroy all its hematopoietic stem cells. The "cured" stem cells repopulated the mouse's bone marrow and proceeded to produce genetically normal blood cells.

Not all genetic disease are good candidates for gene therapy. It has been suggested that a candidate disease should meet the following criteria: (1) it should be a recessive disease caused by the absence of a normally functioning copy of the gene; (2) its gene should be amenable to cloning; (3) its gene should encode a single polypeptide; (4) the polypeptide should not require either a specific cellular environment or precise regulation to be expressed and perform its function; (5) it should be cured if the polypeptide is expressed by a cell type other than the affected tissue; and (6) it should be feasible to insert the gene into a tissue that can safely be removed from and then replaced into the body. These sound like daunting criteria, but in fact a long list of genetic diseases apparently meet them, including adenosine deaminase deficiency, argininosuccinic aciduria, citrullinemia, Gaucher disease type I, phenylketonuria, and some autoimmune diseases.

It may be feasible to apply the technique of gene therapy to correct some of the human genetic blood diseases by using a procedure called **fetal liver transplant.** In a preliminary experiment, this procedure was used to treat fetuses that were diagnosed with diseases that severely cripple the white blood cells of the immune system (such as the disease suffered by the "boy in the bubble") or with thalassemia (a blood disease caused by a genetic error that prevents the synthesis of a protein involved in the production of hemoglobin). In these cases, cells from the fetal liver (the first major hematopoietic organ) were obtained from normal aborted fetuses and were infused via an ultrasound-guided needle into the umbilical vein of the affected fetus. These cells successfully colonized the liver of the developing fetus and proceeded to manufacture the missing protein, alleviating the disease. It is easy to transplant cells from one fetus to another because the immature fetal immune system does not reject foreign tissue. It is also possible to utilize umbilical cord blood for transplants such as these since this is an excellent source of hematopoietic stem cells. Moreover, since in some disorders there may be advantages to using gene therapy to correct an infant's own cells, the infants own umbilical cord may provide cells that can be appropriately transfected, grown up, and reintroduced without rejection. Advantages of the use of cord blood (compared to bone mar-

row or fetal liver), include (1) lack of discomfort during collection, (2) high recovery of viable stem cells, (3) rapid expansion of stem cells in culture, (4) high rate of recovery of viable stem cells after **cryopreservation,** (5) reduced graft vs host disease, and (6) efficiency of transfection with "corrected" genes. Umbilical cord blood has already been used in many human patients to treat diseases potentially curable with bone marrow transplants including **severe combined immunodeficiency.**

The field of human developmental biology is advancing at a dazzling rate

The fields of embryology and genetics have made steady progress since the days of Brooks, Whitman, Spemann, and Mangold in the early 20th century. Our understanding of animal and plant development began to make much more rapid strides, however, as the disciplines of embryology, genetics, biochemistry, and cytology began to merge into the science that Paul Weiss first called **developmental biology** in the early 1950s. Many of the advances of the last half century have led to an understanding of fundamental developmental mechanisms and have established the conceptual framework for modern developmental biology.

More recently, the study of mammalian development (including the genetics and development of humans) has made impressive progress. The project of mapping the entire human genome is underway; within one or two decades the location of virtually every human gene may be known. Recombinant DNA technology and transgenic techniques are rapidly leading to an understanding of the genomic control of development and of the pathogenesis of many human congenital anomalies.

These advances, along with the findings of previous decades, have begun to answer the questions of how the development of humans and other mammals is regulated on the molecular level. It is especially exciting to witness our emerging understanding of the significance of master genes, such as the *Hox* genes and other well-conserved regulatory genes, that play a key role in morphogenesis. These insights, in turn, have made it feasible to address the clinical correction of human congenital abnormalities. Optimism in this area is also supported by the staggering development of sophisticated technologies, including computers, diagnostic techniques, and fetal surgical methods. This explosive increase in our understanding of human development will produce countless practical applications over the next 10 to 20 years. We must carefully consider how this knowledge can be applied so that suffering can be alleviated.

Suggested Reading

CHAPTER 1

Descriptive Embryology

Aitken RJ. 1995. The complexities of conception. Science 269:39

Archer DF, Zeleznik AJ, Rockette HE. 1988. Ovarian follicular maturation in women. II. Reversal of estrogen inhibited ovarian folliculogenesis by human gonadotropin. Fertil Steril 50:555

Byskov AG. 1986. Differentiation of the mammalian embryonic gonad. Physiol Rev 66:71

Clermont Y. 1972. Kinetics of spermatogenesis in mammals: seminiferous epithelium cycle and spermatogonial renewal. Physiol Rev 52:198

DeSousa PA, Valdimarsson G, Nicholson BJ, Kidden GM. 1993. Connexin trafficking and the control of gap junction assembly in mouse preimplantation embryos. Development 117:1355

Eddy EM, Clark JM, Gong D, Fenderson BA. 1981. Origin and migration of primordial germ cells in mammals. Gamete Res 4:333

Enders AC, Hendrickx AG, Schlake S. 1983. Implantation in the rhesus monkey: initial penetration of the endometrium. Am J Anat 167:275

Gilman J. 1948. The development of the gonads in man, with consideration of the role of fetal endocrines and the histogenesis of ovarian tumors. Contrib Carnegie Inst 32:81

Hammen R. 1944. Studies on Impaired Fertility in Man with Special Reference to the Male. p. 206. Munksgaard and Milford, Copenhagen

Hertig AT, Rock J, Adams EC. 1956. A description of 34 human ova within the first 17 days of development. Am J Anat 98:435

Lawson KA, Hage J. 1994. Clonal analysis of the origin of primordial germ cells in the mouse. CIBA Symp. 182. Germline Development. John Wiley and Sons, New York

Luckett WP. 1978. Origin and differentiation of the yolk sac and extraembryonic mesoderm in presomite human and rhesus monkey embryos. Am J Anat 152:59

O'Rahilly R. 1973. Developmental stages in human embryos. A. Embryos of the first three weeks (stages 1–9). Carnegie Inst Wash Publ, p. 531

Pedersen RA, Wu K, Balakier H. 1986. Origin of the inner cell mass in mouse embryos: cell lineage analysis by microinjection. Dev Biol 117:581

Pincus G, Enzmann EV. 1935. The comparative behavior of mammalian eggs in vivo and in vitro. I. The activation of ovarian eggs. J Exp Med 62:665

Russell LD. 1980. Sertoli-germ cell interactions: a review. Gamete Res 3:179

Schultz RM, Endo Y, Mattei P et al. 1988. Egg induced modifications of the mouse zona pellucida. Prog Clin Biol Res 284:77

Smith C, Moore HDM, Hearn JP. 1987. The ultrastructure of early implantation in the marmoset monkey (*Callitrix jacchus*). Anat Embryol 175:399

Tarkowski AK, Wroblewska J. 1967. Development of blastomeres of mouse eggs isolated at the 4- and 8-cell stage. J Embryol Exp Morphol 18:155

Wasserman PM. 1991. Elements of Mammalian Fertilization. Vol. I. Basic Concepts. CRC Press, Boca Raton, FL

Witschi E. 1948. Migration of the germ cells of human embryos from the yolk sac to the primitive gonadal folds. Contrib Embryol Carnegie Inst 32:67

Applications to Clinical Practice

Alvarez F, Brache V, Fernandez E et al. 1988. New insights on the mode of action of intrauterine contraceptive devices in women. Fertil Steril 49:768

Capecchi MR. 1989. The new mouse genetics: altering the genome by gene targeting. Trends Genet 5:70

Comhaire FH. 1994. Male contraception: hormonal, mechanical and other. Hum Reprod 9:22

Connell EB. 1989. Barrier contraceptives. Clin Obstet Gynecol 32:377

de Grouchy J, Turleau C. 1984. Clinical Atlas of Human Chromosomes. John Wiley & Sons, New York

Devroey P, Staessen C, Camus M et al. 1989. Zygote intrafallopian transfer as a successful treatment for unexplained fertility. Fertil Steril 52:246

Diczfalusy E, Bygdeman M (eds). 1987. Fertility Regulation Today and Tomorrow. Raven Press, New York

Djerassi C. 1989. The bitter pill. Science 245:356

Doetschman TC. 1989. Gene targeting in embryonic stem cells. p. 89. In First N, Haseltine FP (eds): Transgenic Animals in Medicine and Agriculture (The Biotechnology Series). Butterworth, Stoneham, MA

Doetschman T, Gregg RG, Maeda N et al. 1987. Targeted correction of a mutant HPRT gene in mouse embryonic stem cells. Nature (London) 330:576

Edward RG. 1994. Implantation interception and contraception. Hum Reprod 9:73

Frohman MA, Martin GR. 1989. Cut, paste, and save: new approaches to altering specific genes in mice. Cell 56:145

Gordon JW. 1989. Transgenic animals. Int Rev Cytol 115:171

Groner Y, Elroy-Stein O, Bernstein Y et al. 1986. Molecular genetics of Down's syndrome: overexpression of transfected human Cu/Zn-superoxide dismutase gene and the consequent physiological changes. Cold Spring Harbor Symp Quant Biol L1:381

Hook EB. 1989. Issues pertaining to the impact and etiology of trisomy 21 and other aneuploidy in humans: a consideration of evolutionary implications, maternal age mechanisms, and other matters. Prog Clin Biol Res 311:1

Jaenisch R. 1988. Transgenic animals. Science 240:1468

Jones KL. 1988. Smith's Recognizable Patterns of Human Malformations. WB Saunders, Philadelphia

Ketting E, Visser AP. 1994. Contraception in the Netherlands: the low abortion rate explained. Patient Counseling Education 23:161

Kim HS, Smithies O. 1988. Recombinant fragment assay for gene targeting based on the polymerase chain reaction. Nucleic Acids Res 16:8887

Korenberg JR, Chen XN, Schipper R et al. 1994. Down syndrome phenotypes: the consequence of chromosomal imbalance. Proc Natl Acad Sci USA 91:4997

McFarlan D (ed). 1991. Guinness Book of World Records. p. 14. Bantam, New York

McKusick VA. 1989. Mapping and sequencing the human genome. N Engl J Med 320:910

McLaren A. 1988. The IVF conceptus: research today and tomorrow. Ann NY Acad Sci 541:639

Morton NE, Chiu D, Holland C et al. 1987. Chromosome anomalies as predictors of recurrence risk for spontaneous abortion. Am J Med Genet 28:353

Prather RS, Hageman LJ, First NL. 1989. Preimplantation mammalian aggregation and injection chimeras. Gamete Res 22:233

Robertson E, Bradley A, Kuehn M, Evans MJ. 1986. Germ-line transmission of genes introduced into cultured pluripotential cells by a retroviral vector. Nature (London) 323:445

Silvestre L, Dubois C, Renault M et al. 1989. Voluntary interruption of pregnancy with mifepristone (RU 486) and a prostaglandin analogue: a large scale French experience. N Engl J Med 322:645

Steptoe PC, Edwards RG. 1978. Birth after the implantation of a human embryo. Lancet ii:366

Tarkowski AK. 1961. Mouse chimeras developed from fused eggs. Nature (London) 190:857

Temmerman M. 1994. Sexually transmitted diseases and reproductive health. Sexually Transmitted Diseases 21:555

Verlinsky Y, Kuliev A. 1994. Human preimplantation diagnosis: needs, efficiency and efficacy of genetic and chromosome analysis. [Review.] Baillieres Clin Obstet Gynecol 8:177

Wapner RJ, Jackson L. 1988. Chorionic villous sampling. Clin Obstet Gynecol 31:328

Wilcox AJ, Weinberg CR, O'Connor JF et al. 1988. Incidence of early loss of pregnancy. N Engl J Med 319:189

Wood EC. 1988. The future of in vitro fertilization. Ann NY Acad Sci 541:715

Wu FCW. 1988. Male contraception: current status and future prospects. Clin Endocrinol 29:443

Zipursky A, Poon A, Doyle J. 1992. Leukemia in Down syndrome: a review. Pediatr Hematol Oncol 9:139

CHAPTER 2

Descriptive Embryology

Cross JC, Werb Z, Fisher SJ. 1994. Implantation and the placenta: key pieces of the developmental puzzle. Science 266:1508

Enders AC, King B. 1988. Formation and differentiation of extraembryonic mesoderm in rhesus monkey. Am J Anat 181:327

Fleming TP. 1987. A quantitative analysis of cell allocation to trophectoderm and inner cell mass of the mouse. Dev Biol 119:520

Gardner RL. 1983. Origin and differentiation of extraembryonic tissues in the mouse. Int Rev Exp Pathol 24:63

Hertig AT. 1935. Angiogenesis in the early human chorion and in the primary placenta of the macaque monkey. Contrib Embryol Carnegie Inst 25:37

Hertig AT, Rock J. 1941. Two human ova of the previllous stage, having a developmental age of about eleven and twelve days respectively. Contrib Embryol Carnegie Inst 29:127

Hertig AT, Rock J. 1945. Two human ova of the previllous stage, having a developmental age of about seven and nine days respectively. Contrib Embryol Carnegie Inst 31:65

Hertig AT, Rock J. 1949. Two human ova of the previllous stage, having a developmental age of about eight and nine days respectively. Contrib Embryol Carnegie Inst 33:169

Hertig AT, Rock J, Adams EC. 1956. A description of 34 human ova within the first seventeen days of development. Am J Anat 98:435

Hertig AT, Rock J, Adams EC, Menkin MC. 1959. Thirty-four fertilized human ova, good, bad, and indifferent, recovered from 210 women of known fertility. Pediatrics 23:202

Lawson KA, Meneses JJ, Pedersen RA. 1986. Cell fate and cell lineage in the presomite mouse embryo, studied with an intracellular tracer. Dev Biol 115:325

Lawson KA, Pedersen R. 1992. Clonal analysis of cell fate during gastrulation and early neurulation in the mouse. CIBA Symp. 165.

Postimplantation Development in the Mouse. John Wiley & Sons, New York

Luckett WP. 1971. The origin of the extraembryonic mesoderm in the early human and rhesus monkey embryos. Anat Rec 169:369

Luckett WP. 1973. Amniogenesis in the early human and rhesus monkey embryos. Anat Rec 175:375

Luckett WP. 1975. The development of primordial and definitive amniotic cavities in early rhesus monkey and human embryos. Am J Anat 144:149

Luckett WP. 1978. Origin and differentiation of the yolk sac and extraembryonic mesoderm in presomite human and rhesus monkey embryos. Am J Anat 152:59

Streeter GL. 1942. Developmental horizons in human embryos. Description of age group XI, 13 to 20 somites, and age group XII, 21 to 29 somites. Contrib Embryol Carnegie Inst 30:211

Vogler H. 1987. Human blastogenesis. Formation of the extraembryonic cavities. Bibl Anat 30:1

Applications to Clinical Practice

Barlow DP. 1995. Gametic imprinting in mammals. Science 270:1610

Bracken MB. 1987. Incidence and aetiology of hydatidiform mole: an epidemiological review. Br J Obstet Gynaecol 94:1123

Cassidy SB. 1995. Uniparental disomy and genomic imprinting as causes of human genetic disease. Environ Mol Mutagen 25:13

Chatkupt S, Antonowicz M, Johnson WG. 1995. Parents do matter: genomic imprinting and parental sex effects in neurological disorders. J Neurol Sci 130:1

Hadchoucl M, Farza H, Simon D, Tillais P, Pourecl C. 1987. Maternal inhibition of hepatitis B surface antigen gene expression in transgenic mice correlates with de novo methylation. Nature 329:454

Kajii T, Ohama K. 1977. Androgenetic origin of hydatidiform mole. Nature 264:633

Lawler SD, Fisher RA. 1987. Genetic studies in hydatidiform mole with clinical correlations. Placenta 8:77

Leighton PA, Saam JS, Ingram RD, Tilghman SM. 1996. Genomic imprinting in mice: its function and mechanism. Biol Reprod 54:273

Lewis JL Jr. 1993. Diagnosis and management of gestational trophoblastic disease. Cancer 71:1639

Li E, Beard C, Jaenisch R. 1993. Role for DNA methylation in genomic imprinting. Nature 366:362

Lyon MF. 1993. Epigenetic inheritance in mammals. TIG 9:123

McGrath J, Solter D. 1984. Completion of mouse embryogenesis requires both the maternal and paternal genomes. Cell 37:179

Reik W. 1989. Genomic imprinting and genetic disorders in man. Trends Genet Sci. 5:331

Rose PG. 1995. Hydatidiform mole: diagnosis and management. Semin Oncol 22:149

Sapienza C. 1990. Parental imprinting of genes. Sci Am 263:52

Strain L, Warner JP, Johnston T, Bonthron DT. 1995. A human parthenogenetic chimera. Nature Genet 11:164

Surani MAH, Barton SC, Norris ML. 1984. Development of reconstituted mouse eggs suggests imprinting of the genome during gametogenesis. Nature 308:548

Swain JL, Stewart TA, Leder P. 1987. Parental legacy determines methylation and expression of an autosomal transgene: a molecular mechanism for parental imprinting. Cell 50:719

Szulman AE. 1987. Clinicopathologic features of partial hydatidiform mole. J Reprod Med 32:640

Tartoff KD, Bremer M. 1990. Mechanisms for the construction and developmental control of heterochromatin formation and imprinted chromosome domains. Development (Suppl):35

CHAPTER 3

Descriptive Embryology

Bellairs R. 1986. The primitive streak. Anat Embryol 174:1

Meier S, Tam PPL. 1982. Metameric pattern development in the embryonic axis of the mouse. I. Differentiation of cranial segments. Differentiation 21:95

Müller F, O'Rahilly R. 1983. The first appearance of the major divisions of the human brain at stage 9. Anat Embryol 168:419

O'Rahilly R. 1973. Developmental Stages in Human Embryos. Part A. Embryos of the First 3 Weeks (Stages 1–9). Carnegie Institute of Washington, Washington, DC

Snow MHL. 1981. Growth and its control in early mammalian development. Br Med Bull 37:221

Tam PPL, Beddington RSP. 1987. The formation of mesodermal tissues in the mouse embryo during gastrulation and early organogenesis. Development 99:109

Tam PPL, Meier S, Jacobson A. 1982. Differentiation of the metameric pattern in the embryonic axis of the mouse. II. Somitomeric organization of the presomitic mesoderm. Differentiation 21:109

Applications to Clinical Practice

Barnes JD, Crosby JL, Jones CM et al. 1994. Embryonic expression of *Lim-1*, the mouse homolog of *Xenopus Xlim-1,* suggests a role in lateral mesoderm differentiation and neurogenesis. Dev Biol 161:168

Bennett D. 1975. The *T*-locus of the mouse. Cell 6:441

Duhamel B. 1961. From the mermaid to anal imperforation: the syndrome of caudal regression. Arch Dis Child 36:152

Faust C, Magnuson T. 1993. Genetic control of gastrulation in the mouse. Curr Opin Genet Dev 3:491

Graff JM, Bansal A, Melton DA. 1996. Xenopus Mad proteins transduce distinct subsets of signals for the TGF-β superfamily. Cell 85:479

Hahn SA, Schutte M, Hoque AT, Moskaluk CA, da Costa LT, Rozenblum E, Weinstein CL, Fischer A, Yeo CJ, Hruban RH, Kern SE. 1996. DPC4, a candidate tumor suppressor gene at human chromosome 18q21.1. Science 271:350

Herrmann BG, Labeit S, Poustka A et al. 1990. Cloning of the *T* gene required in mesoderm formation in the mouse. Nature 343:617

Hogan B, Blessing M, Winnier GE et al. 1994. Growth factors in development: the role of TGF-β related polypeptide signalling molecules in embryogenesis. Development (suppl) 53–60

Holley SA, Jackson PD, Sasai Y et al. 1995. A conserved system for dorsal-ventral patterning in insects and vertebrates involving sog and chordin. Nature 376:249

Ivens A, Moore G, Williamson R. 1988. Molecular approaches to dysmorphology. J Med Genet 25:473

Kallen B, Winberg J. 1974. Caudal mesoderm pattern of anomalies: from renal agenesis to sirenomelia. Teratology 9:99

Kalter H. 1993. Case reports of malformations associated with maternal diabetes: a history and critique. Clin Genet 43:174

Kessler DS, Melton DA. 1994. Vertebrate embryonic induction: mesoderm and neural patterning. Science 266:596

Khoury MJ, Cordero JF, Greenberg F et al. 1983. A population study of the VACTERL association: evidence for its etiological heterogeneity. Pediatrics 71:815

Knecht AK, Good PJ, Dawid IB et al. 1995. Dorsal-ventral patterning and differentiation of nogin-induced neural tissue in the absence of medoderm. Development 121:1927

Krumlauf R. 1993. *Hox* gene and pattern formation in the branchial region of the vertebrate head. TIG 9:106

Liu F, Hata A, Baker JC, Doody J, Carcamo J, Harlan PM, Massague J. 1996. A human Mad protein acting as a BMP-regulated transcriptional activator. Nature 381:620

Moos M Jr, Wang S, Krinks M. 1995. Anti-dorsalizing morphogenetic protein is a novel TGF-β homolog expressed in the Spemann organizer. Development 121:4293

Niehrs C, Steinbeisser H, De Robertis EM. 1994. Mesodermal patterning by a gradient of the vertebrate homeobox gene goosecoid. Science 263:817

Nieto MA, Sargent MG, Wilkinson DG, Cooke J. 1994. Control of cell behavior during vertebrate development by slug, a zinc finger gene. Science 264:835

Nüsslein-Volhard C. 1994. Of flies and fishes. Science 266:572

O'Reilly MA, Smith JC, Cunliffe V. 1995. Patterning of the mesoderm in *Xenopus:* dose dependent and synergistic effects of brachyury and Pintallavis. Development 121:1351

Quan L, Smith DW. 1973. The VATER association. J Pediatr 82:104

Rashbass P, Wilson V, Rosen B, Beddington RS. 1994. Alterations of gene expression during mesoderm formation and axial patterning in brachyury (*T*) embryos. Int J Dev Biol 38:35

Russell LJ, Weaver DD, Bull MJ. 1981. The axial mesoderm aplaysia syndrome. Pediatrics 67:176

Schmidt J, Francois V, Bier E, Kimelman D. 1995. *Drosophila* short gastrulation induces an ectopic axis in *Xenopus:* evidence for conserved mechanisms of dorsal-ventral patterning. Development 121:4319

Shawlot W, Behringer RR. 1995. Requirement for *Lim1* in head-organizer function. Nature 374:425

Shin HS. 1989. The *T/T* complex and the genetic control of mouse development. p. 443. In Litwin SD (ed): Human Immunogenetics: Basic Principles and Clinical Relevance. Marcel Dekker, Inc., New York

Smith WC, Knecht AK, Wu M, Harland RM. 1993. Secreted noggin protein mimics the Spemann organizer in dorsalizing *Xenopus* mesoderm. Nature 361:547

Smith WC, McKendry R, Ribisi S Jr, Harland RM. 1995. A nodal-related gene defines a physical and functional domain within the Spemann organizer. Cell 82:37

Stott D, Kispert A, Herrman BG. 1993. Rescue of the tail defect in brachyury mice. Genes Dev 7:197

Taira M, Otani H, Saint-Jeannet JP, Dawid IB. 1994. Role of the *LIM* class homeodomain protein Xlim-1 in neural and muscle induction by the Spemann organizer in *Xenopus*. Nature 372:677

Toyama R, O'Connell ML, Wright CV et al. 1995. Nodal induces ectopic goosecoid and lim1 expression and axis duplication in zebrafish. Development 121:383

Watanabe T, Kim S, Candia A et al. 1995. Molecular mechanisms of Spemann's organizer formation: conserved growth factor synergy between *Xenopus* and mouse. Genes Dev 9:3038

Wilkinson DG, Bhatt S, Herrmann BG. 1990. Expression pattern of the mouse *T* gene and its role in mesoderm formation. Nature 343:657

Wilson V, Manson L, Skarnes WC, Beddington RSP. 1995. The *T* gene is necessary for normal mesodermal morphogenetic movements during gastrulation. Development 121:877

Yamada G, Mansouri A, Torres M et al. 1995. Targeted mutation of the murine goosecoid gene results in craniofacial defects and neonatal death. Development 121:2917

CHAPTER 4

Descriptive Embryology

Bronner-Fraser M. 1982. Distribution of latex beads and retinal pigment epithelial cells along the ventral neural crest pathway. Dev Biol 91:50

Christ B, Jacob M, Jacob HJ. 1983. On the origin and development of the ventrolateral abdominal muscles in the avian embryo. Anat Embryol 166:87

Christ B, Ordahl CP. 1995. Early stages of chick somite formation. Anat Embryol 191:381

Grasser RF. 1979. Evidence that sclerotomal cells do not migrate medially during normal embryonic development in the rat. Am J Anat 154:509

Jacobson A. 1988. Somitomeres: mesodermal segments of vertebrate embryos. Development 104:209

Jacobson A, Tam PPL. 1982. Cephalic neurulation in the mouse embryo analyzed by SEM and morphometry. Anat Rec 203:375

Karfunkel P. 1974. Mechanisms of neural tube formation. Int Rev Cytol 38:245

Lash JW, Ostrovsky D. 1986. On the formation of somites. p. 547. In Browder LW (ed): Developmental Biology, A Comprehensive Synthesis. Vol. 2. The Cellular Basis of Morphogenesis. Plenum Press, New York

Le Douarin NM. 1980. The ontogeny of the neural crest in avian embryo chimeras. Nature 286:663

Meier S. 1984. Somite formation and its relationship to metameric patterning of the mesoderm. Cell Differ 14:235

Morriss-Kay GM. 1981. Growth and development of pattern in the cranial neural epithelium of rat embryos during neurulation. J Embryol Exp Morphol 65:225

Müller F, O'Rahilly R. 1980. The early development of the nervous system in staged insectivore and primate embryos. J Comp Neurol 193:741

Müller F, O'Rahilly R. 1987. The development of the human brain, the closure of the cranial neuropore, and the beginning of secondary neurulation at stage 12. Anat Embryol 176:413

Noden DM. 1980. The migration and cytodifferentiation of cranial neural crest cells. p. 3. In Pratt RM, Christiansen RL (eds): Current Research Trends in Prenatal Craniofacial Development. Elsevier/North Holland, New York

O'Rahilly R, Müller F. 1986. The meninges in human development. J Neuropathol Exp Neurol 45:588

O'Rahilly R, Müller F. 1989. Bidirectional closure of the rostral neuropore. Am J Anat 184:259

Sanes JR. 1983. Roles of extracellular matrix in neural development. Annu Rev Physiol 45:581

Schoenwolf G. 1984. Histological and ultrastructural studies of secondary neurulation in mouse embryos. Am J Anat 169:361

Tam PPL. 1984. The histogenetic capacity of tissues in the caudal end of the embryonic axis of the mouse. J Embryol Exp Morphol 82:253

Tamarin A. 1983. Stage 9 macaque embryos studied by scanning electron microscopy. J Anat 137:765

Applications to Clinical Practice

Campbell LR, Dayton DH, Sohal GS. 1986. Neural tube defects: a review of human and animal studies on the etiology of neural tube defects. Teratology 34:171

Chidabaram A, Goldstein AM, Gailani MR, Gerrard B, Bale SJ, DiGiovanna JJ, Bale AE, Dean M. 1996. Mutations in the human homolog of the *Drosophila* patched gene in Caucasian and African-American nevoid basal cell carcinoma syndrome patients. Cancer Res 56:4599

Conlon RA. 1995. Retinoic acid and pattern formation in vertebrates. TIG 11:314

Fan C-M, Tessier-Lavigne M. 1994. Patterning of mammalian somites by surface ectoderm and notochord: evidence for sclerotome induction by a hedgehog homolog. Cell 79:1175

Fan C-M, Porter JA, Chiang C et al. 1995. Long-range sclerotome induction by sonic hedgehog: direct role of the aminoterminal cleavage product and modulation by the cyclic AMP signaling pathway. Cell 81:457

Günther T, Struwe M, Aguzzi A, Schughart K. 1994. Open brain, a new mouse mutant with severe neural tube defects, shows altered gene expression patterns in the developing spinal cord. Development 120:3119

Hamburger V. 1988. The Heritage of Experimental Embryology. Hans Spemann and the Organizer. Oxford University Press, New York

Hol FA, Hamel BCJ, Geurds MPA et al. 1995. A frameshift mutation in the gene for *Pax 3* in a girl with spina bifida and mild signs of Waardenburg syndrome. J Med Genet 32:52

Hunt P, Krumlauf R. 1992. *Hox* codes and positional specification in vertebrate embryonic axes. Annu Rev Cell Biol 8:277

Jacobson AG, Sater A. 1988. Features of embryonic induction. Development 104:341

Jessell TM, Melton DA. 1992. Diffusible factors in vertebrate embryonic induction. Cell 68:257

Johnson R, Rothman AL, Xie J, Goodrich LV, Bare JW, Bonifas JM, Quinn AG, Myers RM, Cox DR, Epstein Jr EH, Scott MP. 1996. Human homolog of patched, a candidate gene for basal cell nevus syndrome. Science 272:1668

Kessel M, Balling R, Gruss P. 1990. Variations in cervical vertebrae after expressions of *Hoxl.l* transgene in mice. Cell 61:301

Kostic D, Capecchi MR. 1994. Targeted disruptions of the murine *Hoxa-4* and *Hoxa-6* genes result in homeotic transformations of components of the vertebral column. Mech Dev 45:231

Lammer EJ, Sever LE, Oakley GP Jr. 1987. Teratogen update: valproic acid. Teratology 35:465

LeMouellic H, Lallemand Y, Brûlet P. 1992. Homeosis in the mouse induced by a null mutation in the *HOX-3.1* gene. Cell 69:251

Mansouri A, Stoykova A, Gruss P. 1994. *Pax* genes in development. J Cell Sci Suppl 18:35

Marigo V, Scott MP, Johnson RL, Goodrich LV, Tabin CJ. 1996. Conservation in hedgehog signaling: induction of a chicken patched homolog by sonic hedgehog in the developing limb. Development 122:1225

Marti E, Takada R, Bumcrot DA et al. 1995. Distribution of sonic hedgehog peptides in the developing chick and mouse embryo. Development 121:2537

Monsoro-Burg A-H, Bontoux M, Teillet M-A, LeDouarin N. 1994. Heterogeneity in the development of vertebrae. Proc Nati Acad Sci USA 591:10435

Müller F, O'Rahilly R. 1984. Cerebral dysraphia (future anencephaly) in a human twin embryo at stage 13. Teratology 30:167

Nau H. 1994. Valproic Acid-Induced Neural Tube Defects. Neural Tube Defects. CIBA Symp. 181. John Wiley & Sons, New York, p. 144

Roelink H, Augsburger A, Heemskerk J et al. 1994. Floor plate and motor neuron induction by Vhh-1, a vertebrate homolog of hedgehog expressed by the notochord. Cell 76:761

Shewmon DA, Capron AM, Peacock WJ, Schulman B. 1989. The use of anencephalic infants as organ sources: a critique. JAMA 261:1773

Tam PPL, Trainor PA. 1993. Specification and segmentation of the paraxial mesoderm. Anat Embryol 189:275

Tassabehji M, Newton VE, Leverton K et al. 1994. *PAX3* gene structure and mutations: close analogies between Waardenburg syndrome and the Splotch mouse. Hum Mol Genet 3:1069

Yamada T, Pfaff SL, Edlund T, Jessell TM. Control of cell pattern in the neural tube: motor neuron induction by diffusible factors from notocord and floor plate. Cell 73:673

CHAPTER 5

Descriptive Embryology

Altman J, Bayer S. 1985. The development of the rat spinal cord. Adv Anat Embryol Cell Biol 85:1

Bronner-Fraser M. 1993. Environmental influences on neural cell migration. J Neurobiol 24:233

Davies AM. 1990. Ontogeny of the somatosensory system. Annu Rev Neurosci 13:61

Erickson CA. 1988. Control of pathfinding by the avian neural crest. Development (Suppl) 103:63

Fearon ER, Cho KR, Nigro JM et al. 1990. Identification of a chromosome 18q gene that is altered in colorectal cancers. Science 247:49

Goodman CS. 1996. Mechanisms and molecules that control growth cone guidance. Annu Rev Neurosci 19:341

Henion PD, Weston JA. 1994. Retinoic acid selectively promotes the survival and proliferation of neurogenic precursors in cultured neural crest cell populations. Dev Biol 161:243

Kazuko K-M, Masu M, Hink L et al. 1996. Deleted in Colorectal Cancer (DCC) encodes a netrin receptor. Cell 87:175

Kennedy TE, Serafini T, de la Torre J et al. 1994. Netrins are diffusible chemotropic factors for commissural axons in the embryonic spinal cord. Cell 78:425

Keynes R, Cook G, Davies J et al. 1990. Segmentation and the development of the vertebrate nervous system. J Physiol Paris 84:27

Levi-Montalcini R. 1987. The nerve growth factor: thirty-five years later. EMBO J 6:1145

Tosney KW. 1988. Somites and axon guidance. Scanning Electron Microsc 2:427

Vielmetter J, Kayyem JF, Roman JM et al. 1994. Neogenin, an avian cell surface protein expressed during terminal neuronal differentiation, is closely related to the human tumor suppressor molecule. Deleted in Colorectal Cancer. J Cell Biol 127:2009

Applications to Clinical Practice

Baynash AG, Hosoda K, Gia A et al. 1994. Interaction of endothelin-3 with endothelin-B receptor is essential for development of epidural melanocytes and enteric neurons. Cell 79:1277

Besmer P, Manova K, Duttlinger R et al. 1993. The c-kitgard (steel factor) and its receptor c-kit/w pleiotropic roles in gene to genesis and melanogenesis. Development (Suppl.) 125

Bronner-Fraser M. 1995. Origins and developmental potential of the neural crest. Exp Cell Res 218:405

Cable J, Jackson I, Steel K. 1995. Mutations of the *W* locus affect survival of neural crest-derived melanocytes in the mouse. Mech Dev 50:139

Carcassonne M, Guys JM, Monsson-Lacombe G, Kreitman B. 1989. Management of Hirschsprung's disease: curative surgery before 3 months of age. J Pediatr Surg 24:1032

Dow E, Cross S, Wolgemuth J et al. 1994. Second locus for Hirschsprung's disease/Waardenburg syndrome in a large Mennonite kindred. Am J Med Genet 53:75

Edery P, Lyonnet S, Mulligan L et al. 1994. Mutations of the RET proto-oncogene in Hirschsprung's disease. Nature 367:378

Gershon MD, Clalazonitis A, Rothman TP. 1993. From neural crest to bowel: development of the enteric nervous system. J Neurobiol 24:199

Horstadius S. 1950. The Neural Crest. Its Properties and Derivatives in the Light of Experimental Research. Oxford University Press, London

Hosoda K, Hammer RE, Richardson JA et al. 1994. Targeted and natural (piebald-lethal) mutations of endothelin-B receptor gene produce megacolon associated with spotted coat color in mice. Cell 79:1267

Kinashi T, Springer T. 1994. Steel factor and c-kit regulate cell-matrix adhesion. Blood 83:1033

Le Douarin NM, Smith J. 1988. Development of the peripheral nervous system from the neural crest. Annu Rev Cell Biol 4:375

Morrison-Graham K, Weston JA. 1989. Mouse mutants provide new insights into the role of extracellular matrix in cell migration and differentiation. Trends Genet 5:116

Paran WJ, Liddell RA, Wright A et al. 1995. A high resolution linkage map of the lethal spotting locus: a mouse model for Hirschsprung's disease. Mammalian Genome 6:1

Payette RP, Tennyson VM, Pomeranz HD et al. 1988. Accumulation of components of basal laminae: association with the failure of neural crest cells to colonize the presumptive aganglionic bowel of *ls/ls* mutant mice. Dev Biol 125:341

Puffenberger EG, Hosoda K, Washington SS et al. 1994. A missense mutation of the endothelin-B receptor gene in multigenic Hirschsprung's disease. Cell 79:1259

Rothman TP, Gershon MD. 1984. Regionally defective colonization of the terminal bowel by precursors of enteric neurons in lethal spotted mutant mice. Neuroscience 12:1293

Serbedzija G, Bronner-Fraser M, Fraser S. 1994. Developmental potential of trunk neural crest cells in mouse. Development 120:1709

Swenson O. 1989. My early experience with Hirschsprung's disease. J Pediatr Surg 24:839

Vogel K, Marusich M, Weston JA. 1993. Restriction of neurogenic ability during neural crest migration. J Neurobiol 24:162

Wehrle-Haller B, Weston J. 1995. Soluble and cell-bound forms of steel factor activity play distinct roles in melanocyte precursor dispersal and survival on the lateral neural crest migration pathway. Development 121:731

Weston JA. 1970. The migration and differentiation of neural crest cells. Adv Morphol 8:41

CHAPTER 6

Descriptive Embryology

Bucher U, Reid L. 1961. Development of the intrasegmental bronchial tree: the pattern of branching and development of cartilage at various stages of intrauterine life. Thorax 16:207

Burri PH. 1984. Fetal and postnatal development of the lung. Annu Rev Physiol 46:617

Frank L. 1990. Preparation for birth. p. 1141. In Massaro D (ed.): Lung Cell Biology. Marcel Dekker, Inc., New York

Gattone VH, Morse DE. 1984. Pleuroperitoneal canal closure in the rat. Anat Rec 208:445

Heuser CH, Corner GW. 1957. Developmental horizons in human embryos. Description of age group X, 4–12 somites. Contrib Embryol 244:29

Hilfer SR, Rayner RM, Brown JW. 1985. Mesenchymal control of branching in fetal mouse lung. Tissue Cell 17:523

Hislop A, Howard S, Fairweather DVI. 1984. Morphometric studies on the structural development of the lung in *Macaca fascicularis* during fetal and postnatal life. J Anat 138:95

Langston C, Kida K, Reed M, Thurlbeck WM. 1984. Human lung growth in late gestation and in the neonate. Am Rev Respir Dis 129:607

Müller F, O'Rahilly R. 1983. The first appearance of the major divisions of the human brain at stage 9. Anat Embryol 168:419

O'Rahilly R, Müller F. 1984. Respiratory and alimentary relations in staged human embryos. Ann Otol Rhinol Laryngol 93:421

Pringle KC. 1986. Human fetal lung development and related animal models. Clin Obstet Gynecol 29:502

Searles RL. 1986. A description of caudal migration during growth leading to the formation of the pericardial and pleural coeloms, the caudal movement of the aortic arches, and the development of the shoulder. Am J Anat 77:271

Tyler WS. 1983. Small airways and terminal units. Comparative subgross anatomy of lungs. Am Rev Respir Dis 128:S32

Wigglesworth JS. 1988. Lung development in the second trimester. Br Med Bull 44:894

Zeltner TB, Burri PH. 1987. The postnatal development and growth of the human lung. II. Morphometry. Respir Physiol 67:269

Applications to Clinical Practice

Avery ME, Taeusch HW. 1984. Disorders of the diaphragm. p. 189. In Schaffer AJ (ed): Schaffer's Diseases of the Newborn. WB Saunders, Philadelphia

Cardoso WV. 1995. Transcription factors and pattern formation in the developing lung. Am J Physiol 269:2429

Clark JC, Wert S, Bachurski C et al. 1995. Targeted disruption of the surfactant protein B gene disrupts surfactant homeostasis causing respiratory failure in newborn mice. Proc Natl Acad Sci USA 92:7794

Fujiwara T, Maeta H, Chida S et al. 1980. Artificial surfactant therapy in hyaline membrane disease. Lancet ii:55

Glasser SW, Korthagen TR, Wert SE, Whitsett JA. 1994. Transgenic models for study of pulmonary development and disease. Am J Physiol 267:2489

Hilfer SR. 1996. Morphogenesis of the lung: control of embryonic and fetal lung branching. Annu Rev Physiol 58:93

Hislop A, Fairweather DVI, Blackwell RJ, Howard S. 1984. The effect of amniocentesis and drainage of amniotic fluid on lung development in *Macaca fascicularis*. Br J Obstet Gynaecol 91:835

Kitterman JA. 1984. Fetal lung development. J Dev Physiol 6:67

Lawrence S, Rosenfeld CR. 1986. Fetal pulmonary development and abnormalities of amniotic fluid volume. Semin Perinatol 10:142

Nogee LM, Garnier G, Dietz HC et al. 1994. A mutation in the surfactant B gene responsible for fatal neonatal respiratory disease in multiple kindreds. J Clin Invest 93:1860

Notter RH. 1988. Biophysical behavior of lung surfactant: implications for respiratory physiology and pathophysiology. Semin Perinatol 12:180

O'Rahilly R, Müller F. 1984. Respiratory and alimentary relations in staged human embryos. Ann Otol Rhinol Laryngol 93:421

Peters SK, Werner S, Liao X et al. 1994. Targeted expression of a dominant negative FGF receptor blocks branching morphogenesis and epithelial differentiation of the mouse lung. EMBO J 13:3296

Rice W. 1995. Developmental aspects of surfactant. Semin Respir Crit Care Med. 16:11

Singer DB. 1984. Morphology of hyaline membrane disease and its pulmonary sequelae. p. 63. In Stern L (ed). Hyaline Membrane Disease, Pathogenesis and Pathophysiology. Grune & Stratton, New York

Whitsett JA. 1991. Pulmonary surfactant and respiratory distress syndrome in the premature infant. p. 1723. In Crystal RG, Est JB, Barren PJ et al (eds): The Lung. Vol II (Section 6). Raven Press, New York

Whitsett JA, Korfhagen TR. 1996. Regulation of gene transcription in respiratory epithelial cells. Am J Respir Cell Mol Biol 14:118

CHAPTER 7

Descriptive Embryology

Anderson RH, Becker AE, Tranum-Jensen J, Janse MJ. 1981. Anatomico-electrophysiological correlations in the conduction system—a review. Br Heart J 45:67

Anderson RH, Wilkinson JL, Becker AE. 1978. The bulbus cordis—a misunderstood region of the developing human heart: its significance to the classification of congenital cardiac malformations. Birth Defects XIV:1

Bartelings MM, Gittenberger-de Groot AC. 1989. The outflow tract of the heart—embryologic and morphologic correlations. Int J Cardiol 22:289

Cooper MH, O'Rahilly R. 1971. The human heart at seven postovulatory weeks. Acta Anat 79:280

De Haan RL. 1965. Morphogenesis of the vertebrate heart. p. 377. In De Haan RL, Ursprung H (eds): Organogenesis. Holt Rinehart and Winston, New York

Dieterlen-Lieve F, Pardanaud L, Yassine F, Cormier F. 1988. Early haemopoietic stem cells in the avian embryo. J Cell Sci Suppl 10:29

Hay DA. 1978. Development and fusion of the endocardial cushions. Birth Defects XIV:69

Hiruma T, Hirakow R. 1989. Epicardial formation in embryonic chick heart: computer-aided reconstruction, scanning, and transmission electron microscopy studies. Am J Anat 184:129

Kirby ML. 1988. Role of extracardiac factors in heart development. Experientia 44:944

Manasek FJ. 1969. Embryonic development of the heart. II. Formation of the epicardium. J Embryol Exp Morphol 22:333

Manasek FJ. 1972. Early cardiac morphogenesis is independent of function. Dev Biol 27:584

Maron BJ, Hutchins GM. 1974. The development of the semilunar valves in the human heart. Am J Pathol 74:331

Netter FH. 1969. Heart. p. 112. In Yonkman FF (ed): The CIBA Collection of Medical Illustrations. Vol. 5 CIBA, New York

O'Rahilly R. 1971. The timing and sequence of events in human cardiogenesis. Acta Anat 79:70

Pexieder T. 1978. Development of the outflow tract of the embryonic heart. Birth Defects XIV:29

Pexieder T, Janecek P. 1984. Organogenesis of the human embryonic and early fetal heart as studied by microdissection and SEM. p. 401. In Nora JJ, Takao A (eds). Congenital Heart Disease: Causes and Processes. Futura Publishing Co, Mount Kisco, NY

Satin J, Fujii S, DeHaan RL. 1988. Development of the cardiac beat rate in early chick embryos is regulated by regional cues. Dev Biol 129:103

Shimada Y, Ho E, Toyota N. 1981. Epicardial covering over myocardial wall in the chicken embryo as seen with the scanning electron microscope. Scanning Microsc 11:275

Steding G, Seidl W. 1984. Cardiac septation in normal development. p. 481. In Nora JJ, Takao A (eds): Congenital Heart Disease: Causes and Processes. Futura Publishing Co, Mount Kisco, NY

Teal SI, Moore W, Hutchins GM. 1986. Development of aortic and mitral valve continuity in the human embryonic heart. Am J Anat 176:447

Viragh SZ, Challice CE. 1981. The origin of the epicardium and the embryonic myocardial circulation of the mouse. Anat Rec 201:157

Viragh SZ, Challice CE. 1983. The development of the early atrioventricular conduction system in the embryonic heart. Can J Physiol Pharmacol 61:775

Wenink ACG. 1976. Development of the human cardiac conducting system. J Anat 121:617

Wenink ACG. Gittenberger-de Groot AC. 1986. Embryology of the mitral valve. Int J Cardiol 11:75

Applications to Clinical Practice

Anderson RH, Tynan. 1988. Tetralogy of Fallot—a centennial review. Int J Cardiol 21:219

Anderson RH, Wenink ACG. 1988. Thoughts on concepts of development of the heart in relation to the morphology of congenital malformations. Experientia 44:951

Ando M, Takao A, Yutani C et al. 1984. What is cardiac looping? Consideration based on morphologic data. p. 553. In Nora JJ, Takao A (eds): Congenital Heart Disease: Causes and Processes. Futura Publishing Co, Mt. Kisco, NY

Behrman RE, Vaughan VC III. 1983. Congenital heart disease. p. 1121. In Nelson W (ed): Nelson Textbook of Pediatrics. 12th Ed. WB Saunders Co, Philadelphia

Brueckner M, D'eustachio P, Horwich AL. 1989. Linkage mapping of a mouse gene, iv, that controls left-right asymmetry of the heart and viscera. Proc Natl Acad Sci USA 86:5035

Chultheiss TM, Xydas S, Lassar AB. 1995. Induction of avaian cardiac myogenesis by anterior endoderm. Development 121:4203

Clark EB. 1987. Mechanisms in the pathogenesis of cardiac malformations. p. 3. In Pierpont MEM, Moller JH (eds): Genetics of Cardiovascular Disease. Martinus Nijhoff Publishing, Boston

Clark EB. 1987. Mechanisms in the pathogenesis of congenital cardiac malformations. p. 3. In Pierpont MEM Moller JH (eds): Genetics of Cardiovascular Disease Martinus Nijhoff Publishing, Boston

Dyson E, Sucov HM, Kubalak SW et al. 1995. Atrial-like phenotype is associated with embryonic ventricular failure in retinoid x receptor 2–/–mice. Proc Natl Acad Sci USA 92:7386

Eisenberg LM, Markwald RR. 1995. Molecular regulation of atrioventricular valvuloseptal morphogenesis. Circ Res 77:1

Evans SM, Yan W, Murillo MP et al. 1995. Tinman, a *Drosophila* homeobox gene required for heart and represented by a family of genes in vertebrates: XNKx-2.3, a second vertebrate homolog of tinman. Development 121:3889

Fuller SJ, Chien KR. 1994. Genetic engineering of cardiac muscle cells: in vitro and in vivo. Genet Eng 16:17

Geisterfer-Lowrance AAT, Christe M, Corner DA et al. 1996. A mouse model of familial hypertrophic cardiomyopathy. Science 272:731

Grace AA, Chien KR. 1995. Congenital long QT syndromes. Toward molecular dissection of arrhythmia substrates. Circulation 92:2786

Hooper C. 1991. Decoding the secrets of the heart. J NIH Res 3:69

Hunter JJ, Tanaka N, Rockman HA et al. 1995. Ventricular expression of a *MLC-2v-ras* fusion gene induces cardiac hypertrophy and selective diastolic dysfunction in transgenic mice. J Biol Chem 270:23173

Keating MT, Sanguinetti MC. 1996. Molecular genetic insights into cardiovascular disease. Science 272:681

Kirby ML. 1987. Cardiac morphogenesis—recent research advances. Pediatr Res 21:219

Kirby ML. 1989. Plasticity and predetermination of mesencephalic and trunk neural crest transplanted into the region of the cardiac neural crest. Dev Biol 134:402

Kirby ML, Cheng G, Stadt H, Hunter G. 1995. Differential expression of the 110 ribosomal protein during heart development. Biochem Biophys Res Commun 212:461

Krug EL, Mjaavedt CH, Markwald RR. 1987. Extracellular matrix from embryonic myocardium elicits an early morphogenetic event in cardiac endothelial differentiation. Dev Biol 120:348

Layton WM, Manasek FJ. 1980. Cardiac looping in early *iv/iv* mouse embryos. p. 109. In Van Praagh R, Takao A (eds): Etiology and Morphogenesis of Congenital Heart Disease. Futura Publishing Co, Mt. Kisko, NY

McKenna WJ. 1993. Hypertrophic cardiomyopathy: an update. Cardiologia 38:277

Mendelson C, Lohnes D, Decimo D et al. 1994. Function of the retinoic acid receptors (RARs) during development (II). Multiple abnormalities at various stages of organogenesis in RAR double mutants. Development 120:2749

Morrison-Graham K, Schattman GC, Bork T et al. 1992. A PDGF receptor mutation in the mouse (patch) perturbs the development of a non-neuronal subset of neural crest-derived cells. Development 115:113

Ojeda JL, Hurle JM. 1981. Establishment of the tubular heart. Role of cell death. p. 101. In Pexieder T (ed): Mechanisms of Cardiac Morphogenesis and Teratogenesis. Perspectives in Cardiovascular Research. Vol. 5. Raven Press, New York

Olson EN, Srivastava D. 1996. Molecular pathways controlling heart development. Science 272:671

Payne RM, Johnson MC, Grant JW, Strauss AW. 1995. Toward a molecular understanding of congenital heart disease. Circulation 91:494

Pierpont MEM, Moller JH. 1987. Congenital cardiac malformations. p. 13. In Pierpont MEM, Moller JH (eds): Genetics of Cardiovascular Disease. Martinus Nijhoff Publishing, Boston

Rindt H, Knotts S, Robbins J. 1995. Segregation of cardiac and skeletal muscle-specific regulatory elements of the β-myosin heavy chain gene. Proc Natl Acad Sci USA 92:1540

Reanne AG, deSousa PA, Kulkarni S et al. 1995. Cardiac malformation in neonatal mice lacking connexin 43. Science 267:1831

Roden DM, George AL Jr, Bennett PB. 1995. Recent advances in understanding the molecular mechanisms of the long QT syndrome. J Cardiovasc Electron Physiol 6:1023

Rosenquist TH, McCoy JR, Waldo KL, Kirby ML. 1988. Origin and propagation of elastogenesis in the developing cardiovascular system. Anat Rec 221:860

Schilhaur MW, Oosterwegel MA, Moerer P et al. 1996. Defects in cardiac outflow tract formation and pro-B-lymphocyte expansion in mice lacking *Sox-4*. Nature 380:711

Shiojima I, Komuro I, Inazawa J et al. 1995. Assignment of cardiac homeobox gene *csx* to human chromosome 5q3r. Genomics 27:204

Tanigawa G, Jarcho JA, Kass S et al. 1990. A molecular basis for familial hypertrophic cardiomyopathy: an a/B cardiac myosin heavy chain hybrid gene. Cell 62:991

Wenink ACG, Zevallos JC. 1988. Developmental aspects of atrioventricular septal defects. Int J Cardiol 18:65

Yutzey KE, Bader D. 1995. Diversification of cardiomyogenic cell lineages during early heart development. Circ Res 77:216

CHAPTER 8

Descriptive Embryology

Aikawa E, Kawano J. 1982. Formation of coronary arteries sprouting from the primitive aortic sinus wall of the chick embryo. Experientia 38:816

Anderson RH, Ashley GT. 1974. Growth and development of the cardiovascular system—anatomical development. p. 165. In Davis JA, Dobbing J (eds): Scientific Foundations of Pediatrics. WB Saunders, Philadelphia

Coceani F, Olley PM. 1988. The control of cardiovascular shunts in the fetal and neonatal period. Am J Physiol Pharmacol 66:1129

Coffin D, Poole TJ. 1988. Embryonic vascular development: immunohistochemical identification of the origin and subsequent morphogenesis of the major vessel primordia of quail embryos. Development 102:735

Congdon ED. 1922. Transformation of the aortic arch system during the development of the human embryo. Carnegie Contrib Embryol 14:46

Evans HM. 1909. On the development of the aortae, cardinal and umbilical veins, and the other blood vessels of vertebrate embryos from capillaries. Anat Rec 3:498

Hirakow R. 1983. Development of the cardiac blood vessels in staged human embryos. Acta Anat 115:220

Hutchins GM, Kessler-Hanna A, Moore GW. 1988. Development of the coronary arteries in the embryonic human heart. Circulation 77:1250

Netter FH. 1969. Embryology. p. 112. In Yonkman FF (ed): The CIBA Collection of Medical Illustrations. CIBA, Summit, NJ

Noden DM. 1989. Embryonic origins and assembly of blood vessels. Annu Rev Respir Dis 140:1097

Noden DM. 1990. Origins and assembly of avian embryonic blood vessels. Ann NY Acad Sci 588:236

Poole TJ, Coffin JD. 1989. Vasculogenesis and angiogenesis: two distinct mechanisms establish embryonic vascular pattern. J Exp Zool 251:224

Applications to Clinical Practice

Adkins RB, Maples MD et al. 1986. Dysphagia associated with aortic arch anomaly in adults. Am Surg 52:238

Anderson RH, Ashley GT. 1974. Growth and development of the cardiovascular system. p. 165. In Davis JA, Dobbing J (eds): Scientific Foundations of Pediatrics. WB Saunders, Philadelphia

Angelini P. 1989. Normal and anomalous coronary arteries: definitions and classifications. Am Heart J 117:418

Carmeliet P, Ferreira V, Breier G et al. 1996. Abnormal blood vessel development and lethality in embryos lacking a single VEGF allele. Nature 380:435

Chen C, Parangi S, Tolentino MJ, Folkman J. 1995. A strategy to discover circulating angiogenesis inhibitors generated by human tumors. Cancer Res 55:4230

Clark EB. 1987. Mechanisms in the pathogenesis of congenital cardiac malformations. p. 3. In Pierpont MEM, Moller JH (eds): The Genetics of Cardiovascular Disease. Martinus Nijhoff Publishing, Boston

Conte G, Pellegrini A. 1984. On the development of the coronary arteries in human embryos stages 14–19. Anat Embryol 169:209

Cudennec CA, Thiery J-P, Le Dourarin NM. 1981. In vitro induction of adult erythropoiesis in early mouse yolk sac. Proc Natl Acad Sci USA 78:2410

D'Amato RJ, Loughnan MS, Flynn E, Folkman J. 1994. Thalidomide is an inhibitor of angiogenesis. Proc Natl Acad Sci USA 91:4082

Drake CJ, Little CD. 1995. Exogenous vascular endothelial growth factor induces malformed and hyperfused vessels during embryonic neovascularization. Proc Natl Acad Sci USA 92:7657

Dumont DJ, Fong GH, Puri MC et al. 1995. Vascularization of the mouse embryo: a study of flk-1, tek, tie, and vascular endothelial growth factor expression during development. Dev Dynam 203:80

Dumont DJ, Gradwohl G, Fong GH et al. 1994. Dominant-negative and targeted null mutations in the endothelial receptor tyrosine kinase, tek, reveal a critical role in vasculogenesis of the embryo. Genes Dev 8:1897

Dumont DJ, Yamaguchi TP, Conlon RA et al. 1992. tek, a novel tyrosine kinase gene located on mouse chromosome 4, is expressed in endothelial cells and their presumptive precursors. Oncogene 7:1471

Dzierzak E, Medvinsky A. 1995. Mouse embryonic hematopoiesis. Trends Genet 11:359

Enebstein J, Waleh NS, Kramer RH. 1992. Basic FGF and TGF-β differentially modulate integrin expression of human microvascular endothelial cells. Exp Cell Res 203:499

Ezekowitz RA, Mulliken JB, Folkman J. 1992. Interferon α-2a therapy for life-threatening hemangiomas of infancy. N Engl J Med 326:1456

Fan TP, Jaggar R, Bicknell R. 1995. Controlling the vasculature: angiogenesis, antiangiogenesis and vascular targeting of gene therapy. Trends Pharmacol Sci 16:57

Fennie C, Cheng J, Dowbenko D et al. 1995. CD34+ endothelial cell lines derived from murine yolk sac induce the proliferation and differentiation of yolk sac CD34+ hematopoietic progenitors. Blood 86:4454

Ferrar N, Carver-Moore K, Chen H et al. 1996. Heterozygous embryonic lethality induced by targeted inactivation of the VEGF gene. Nature 380:439

Flamme I, Breier G, Risau W. 1995. Vascular endothelial growth factor (VEGF) and VEGF receptor 2 (flk-1) are expressed during vasculogenesis and vascular differentiation of the quail embryo. Dev Biol 169:699

Flamme I, von Reutern M, Drexler HC et al. 1995. Overexpression of vascular endothelial growth factor in the avian embryo induced hypervascularization and increased vascular permeability without alterations of embryonic pattern formation. Dev Biol 171:399

Folkman J. 1995. Angiogenesis in cancer, vascular, rheumatoid and other disease. Nature Med 1:27

Folkman J. 1995. The influence of angiogenesis research on management of patients with breast cancer. Breast Cancer Res Treat 36:109

Fong GH, Rossant J, Gertsenstein M, Breitman ML. 1995. Role of the Flt-1 receptor tyrosine kinase in regulating the assembly of vascular endothelium. Nature 376:66

Freedom RM, Cullam JAG, Moss CAF. 1984. Angiocardiography of Congenital Heart Disease. Macmillan, New York

Friesel RE, Maciag T. 1995. Molecular mechanisms of angiogenesis: fibroblast growth factor signal transduction. FASEB J 9:919

George EL, Georges-Labouesse EN, Patel-King RS et al. 1993. Defects in mesoderm, neural tube and vascular development in mouse embryos lacking fibronectin. Development 119:1079

Hartman AF, Goldring D, Strauss AW et al. 1977. Coarctation of the aorta. p. 199. In Moss AJ, Adams FH, Emmanouilides GC (eds): Heart Diseases in Infants, Children, and Adolescents. Williams & Wilkins, Baltimore

Haywood GA, Ward DE. 1989. Anomalous origins of left anterior descending and circumflex coronary arteries from separate orifices in the right coronary sinus. Int J Cardiol 24:373

Huang E, Nocka K, Beier DR et al. 1990. The hematopoietic growth factor KL is encoded by the Sl locus and is the ligand of the c-kit receptor, the gene product of the W locus. Cell 63:225

Huang H, Zettergren LD, Auerbach R. 1994. In vitro differentiation of B cells and myeloid cells from the early mouse embryo and its extraembryonic yolk sac. Exp Hematol 22:19

Huang L, Turck CW, Rao P, Peters KG. 1995. GRB2 and SH-PTP2: potentially important endothelial signalling molecules downstream of the TEK/TIE2 receptor tyrosine kinase. Oncogene 11:2097

Huyhn A, Dommergues M, Izac B et al. 1995. Characterization of hematopoietic progenitors from human yolk sacs and embryos. Blood 86:4474

Jakeman LB, Armanini M, Phillips HS, Ferrara N. 1993. Developmental expression of binding sites and messenger ribonucleic acid for vascular growth factor suggests role for this protein in vasculogenesis and angiogenesis. Endocrinology 133:848

Kallianpur AR, Jordan JE, Brandt SJ. 1994. The SCL/TAL-1 gene is expressed in progenitors of both hematopoietic and vascular systems during embryogenesis. Blood 83:1200

Kolch W, Martiny-Baron G, Kieser A, Marme D. 1995. Regulation of the expression of the VEGF/VPS and its receptors: role in tumor angiogenesis. Breast Cancer Res Treat 36:139

Korhonen J, Polvi A, Partanen J, Alitalo K. 1994. The mouse tie receptor tyrosine kinase gene: expression during embryonic angiogenesis. Oncogene 9:395

Lawson KA, Pedersen R. 1992. Clonal analysis of cell fate during gastrulation and early neurulation in the mouse. CIBA Symp. 165. Postimplantation Development in the Mouse. John Wiley & Sons, New York

Lawson KA, Hage WJ. 1994. Clonal analysis of the origin of primordial germ cells in the mouse. CIBA Symp. 182. Germline Development. John Wiley & Sons, New York

Matsui Y, Zsebo KM, Hogan BLM. 1990. Embryonic expression of a hematopoietic growth factor encoded by the Sl locus and the ligand for c-kit. Nature 347:667

Millauer B, Wizigmann-Voos S, Schnurch H. 1993. High affinity VEGF binding and developmental expression suggest Flk-1 as a major regulator of vasculogenesis and angiogenesis. Cell 72:835

Moller JH. 1987. Vascular abnormalities. p. 339. In Pierpont MEM, Moller JH (eds): The Genetics of Cardiovascular Disease. Martinus Nijhoff Publishing, Boston

Muller AM, Medvinsky A, Strouboulis J et al. 1994. Development of hematopoietic stem cell activity in the mouse embryo. Immunity 1:291

Nakano T, Kodama H, Honjio T. 1996. In vitro development of primitive and definitive erythrocytes from different precursors. Science 272:722

O'Reilly MS, Brem H, Folkman J. 1995. Treatment of murine hemangioendotheliomas with the angiogenesis inhibitor AGM-1470. J Pediatr Surg 30:325

O'Reilly MS, Holmgren L, Shing Y et al. 1994. Angiostatin: a novel angiogenesis inhibitor that mediates the suppression of metastases by a Lewis lung carcinoma. Cell 79:315

Peschle C, Mavilio F, Care A et al. 1985. Haemoglobin switching in human embryos. Nature 313:235

Pierpont MEM, Moller JH. 1987. Congenital cardiac malformations. p. 13. In Pierpont MEM, Moller JH (eds): The Genetics of the Cardiovascular System. Martinus Nijhoff Publishing, Boston

Plate KH, Risau W. 1995. Angiogenesis in malignant gliomas. Glia 15:339

Rak J, Mitsuhashi Y, Bayko L et al. 1995. Mutant *ras* oncogenes upregulate VEGF/VPF expression: implications for induction and inhibition of tumor angiogenesis. Cancer Res 55:4575

Rich IN. 1995. Primordial germ cells are capable of producing cells of the hematopoietic system in vitro. Blood 86:463

Sato TN, Qin Y, Kozak CA, Audus KL. 1993. Toe-1 and tie-2 define another class of putative receptor tyrosine kinase genes expressed in early embryonic vascular system. Proc Natl Acad Sci USA 90:9355

Shalaby F, Rossant J, Yamaguchi TP et al. 1995. Failure of blood-island formation and vasculogenesis in Klk-1-deficient mice. Nature 376:62

Smith BR, Johnson GA, Groman EV, Linney E. 1994. Magnetic resonance microscopy of mouse embryos. Proc Natl Acad Sci USA 91:3530

Soto B, Pacifico AD. 1990. Angiocardiography in Congenital Heart Malformations. Futura Publishing Company, Inc, Mount Kisco, NY

Tavian M, Coulombel L, Luton D et al. 1996. Aorta-associated CD34+ hematopoietic cells in the early human embryo. Blood 87:67

Wagner EF, Risau W. 1994. Oncogenes in the study of endothelial cell growth and differentiation. Semin Can Biol 5:137

Yamaguchi TP, Dumont DJ, Conlon RA et al. 1993. flk-1, an flt-related receptor tyrosine kinase is an early marker for endothelial cell precursors. Development 118:489

CHAPTER 9

Descriptive Embryology

Alpert S, Hanahan D, Teitelman G. 1988. Hybrid insulin genes reveal a developmental lineage for pancreatic endocrine cells and imply a relationship with neurons. Cell 53:295

Gordon JI. 1989. Intestinal epithelial differentiation: new insights from chimeric and transgenic mice. J Cell Biol 108:1187

Kanagasuntherum R. 1957. Development of the human lesser sac. J Anat 91:188

Le Douarin NM. 1988. On the origin of pancreatic exocrine cells. Cell 53:169

Moutsouris C. 1966. The "solid stage" and congenital intestinal atresia. J Pediatr Surg 1:446

O'Rahilly R. 1978. The timing and sequence of events in the development of the human digestive system and associated structures during the embryonic period proper. Anat Embryol 153:123

O'Rahilly R, Müller F. 1987. Developmental stages in human embryos. Carnegie Inst Wash Publ 637:1

Reddy S, Elliot RB. 1988. Ontogenic development of peptide hormones in the mammalian fetal pancreas. Experientia 44:1

Severn CB. 1972. A morphological study of the development of the human liver. I. Development of the hepatic diverticulum. Am J Anat 131:133

Severn CB. 1972. A morphological study of the human liver. II. Establishment of liver parenchyma, extrahepatic ducts, and associated venous channels. Am J Anat 133:85

Stephens FD. 1988. Embryology of the cloaca and anorectal malformations. Birth Defects Orig Artic Ser 24:177

Vellguth S, van Gaudecker B, Muller-Hermelink H-K. 1985. The development of the human spleen. Cell Tissue Res 242:579

Yokoh Y. 1970. Differentiation of the dorsal mesentery in man. Acta Anat 76:56

Applications to Clinical Practice

Afzelius BA. 1976. A human syndrome caused by immotile cilia. Science 193:317

Agatstein E, Stabile B. 1984. Peritonitis due to intraperitoneal perforation of infected urachal cysts. Arch Surg 119:1269

Akintan B, Adekunle A. 1985. A fatal case of ruptured infected urachal cyst. Int Urol Nephrol 17:133

Almirantis Y. 1995. Left-right asymmetry in vertebrates. Bioessays 17:79

Brown CK, Olshaker JS. 1988. Meckel's diverticulum. Am J Emerg Med 6:157

Brown NA, Hoyle C, McCarthy A, Wolpert L. 1989. The development of asymmetry: the sidedness of drug induced limb abnormalities is reversed in situs inversus mice. Development 107:637

Brown NA, Lander A. 1993. On the other hand. . . . . Nature 363:303

Brown NA, Wolpert L. 1990. The development of handedness in left/right symmetry. Development 109:1

Brueckner M, D'Eustachio P, Horwich AL. 1989. Linkage mapping of a mouse gene, *iv*, that controls left-right asymmetry of the heart and viscera. Proc Natl Acad Sci USA 86:5035

Collignon J, Varlet I, Robertson EJ. 1996. Relationship between asymmetric nodal expression and the direction of embryonic turning. Nature 381:155

Collins RL. 1975. When left-handed mice live in right-handed worlds. Science 187:181

Cooke, J. 1995. Vertbrate embryo handedness. Nature 374:681

Danos MC, Jost HJ. 1995. Linkage of cardiac left-right asymmetry and dorsal-anterior development in *Xenopus*. Development 121:1467

de Vries PA. 1980. The pathogenesis of gastroschisis and omphalocele. J Pediatr Surg 15:245

Dott NM. 1923. Anomalies of intestinal rotation and fixation: their embryology and surgical aspects; with report of five cases. Br J Surg 2:251

Estrada RL. 1958. Anomalies of Intestinal Rotation and Fixation. p. 1. Charles C Thomas, Springfield, IL

Ewing T. 1993. Genetic "master switch" for left-right asymmetry found. Science 260:624

Frazer JE, Robbins RH. 1915. On the factors concerned in causing rotation of the intestine in man. J Anat Physiol 50:75

Klar AJS. 1994. A model for specification of the left-right axis in vertebrates. TIG 10:392

Layton WM. 1976. Random determination of a developmental process. J Hered 67:336

Levin M, Johnson RL, Stern CD et al. 1995. A molecular pathway determining left-right asymmetry in chick embryogenesis. Cell 82:803

Lowe L, Supp DM, Sampath K et al. 1996. Conserved left/right asymmetry of nodal expression and alteration in situs inversus. Nature (in press)

Mall FP. 1898. Development of the human intestine and its position in the adult. Bull Johns Hopkins Hosp 9:197

Marshall VF, Muecke EC. 1962. Variations in exstrophy of the bladder. J Urol 88:766

Meno C, Saijoh Y, Fujii H et al. 1996. Left-right asymmetric expression of the TGFβ-family member lefty in mouse embryos. Nature 381:151

Muecke EC. 1964. The role of the cloacal membrane in exstrophy: the first successful experimental study. J Urol 92:659

Pringle KC. 1988. Abdominal wall defects and obstructive uropathies. Fetal Ther 3:67

Reyes HM, Meller JL, Loeff D. 1989. Neonatal intestinal obstruction. Clin Perinatol 16:85

Roush W. 1995. Embryos travel forking path as they tell left from right. Science 269:1514

Siebert JR, Machin GA, Sperber GH. 1989. Anatomic findings in dicephalic conjoined twins: implications for morphogenesis. Teratology 40:305

Stalsberg H. 1970. Mechanism of dextral looping of the embryonic heart. Am J Cardiol 25:265

Synder WH, Chaffin L. 1954. Embryology and pathology of the intestinal tract: presentation of 40 cases of malrotation. Ann Surg 140:368

Torfs C, Curry C, Roeper P. 1990. Gastroschisis. J Pediatr 116:1

Vane DW, West KW, Grosfeld JL. 1987. Vitelline duct anomalies. Arch Surg 122:542

Wolpert L, Brown NA. 1995. Hedgehog keeps to the left. Nature 377:103

Yokoyama T, Copeland N, Jenkins NA et al. 1993. Reversal of left-right asymmetry: a situs inversus mutation. Science 260:679

Yost HJ. 1992. Regulation of vertebrate left-right asymmetries by extracellular matrix. Nature 357:158

CHAPTER 10

Descriptive Embryology

Buehr M, Gu S, McLaren A. 1993. Mesonephric contribution to testis differentiation in the fetal mouse. Development 117:273

Byskov AG. 1986. Differentiation of mammalian embryonic gonad. Physiol Rev 66:71

Cate RL, Mattaliano RJ, Hession C et al. 1986. Isolation of the bovine and human genes for Müllerian inhibiting substance and expression of the human gene in animal cells. Cell 45:685

Ekblom P, Sariola H, Karkinen-Jaaskelainen M, Saxen L. 1982. The origin of the glomerular endothelium. Cell Differ 11:35

Fine H. 1982. The development of the lobes of the metanephros and fetal kidney. Acta Anat 113:93

Grobstein C. 1955. Inductive interaction in the development of the mouse metanephros. J Exp Zool 130:319

Huston JM, Beasely SW. 1988. Embryological controversies in testicular descent. Semin Urol 6:68

Jost A, Magre S. 1988. Control mechanisms of testicular differentiation. Philos Trans R Soc Lond Ser B 322:55

Kluth D, Lambrecht W, Reich P. 1988. Pathogenesis of hypospadias—more questions than answers. J Pediatr Surg 23:1095

Marshall FF. 1978. Embryology of the lower genitourinary tract. Urol Clin North Am 5:3

McLaren A. 1988. Somatic and germ-cell sex in mammals. Philos Trans R Soc Lond Ser B 322:3

McLaren A. 1990. What makes a man a man? Nature (London) 346:216

Merchant-Larios H, Moreno-Mendoza N, Buehr M. 1993. The role of the mesonephros in cell differentiation and morphogenesis of the mouse fetal testis. Int J Dev Biol 37:407

O'Rahilly R. 1977. The development of the vagina in the human. Birth Defects Orig Artic Ser 13:123

O'Rahilly R. 1977. Prenatal human development. p. 35. In Wynn RM (ed): Biology of the Uterus. Plenum Press, New York

O'Rahilly R. 1983. The timing and sequence of events in the development of the human reproductive system during the embryonic period proper. Acta Embryol 166:247

Potter EL. 1972. Normal and Abnormal Development of the Kidney. Year Book Medical Publishers, Chicago

Satoh M. 1991. Histogenesis and organogenesis of the gonad in human embryos. J Anat 177:85

Saxen L, Sariola H, Lehtonen E. 1986. Sequential cell and tissue interactions governing organogenesis of the kidney. Anat Embryol 175:1

Spaulding MH. 1921. The development of the external genitalia in the human embryo. Contrib Embryol Carnegie Inst 13:67

Stephens FD. 1988. Embryology of the cloaca and embryogenesis of anorectal malformations. Birth Defects Orig Artic Ser 24:177

Wensing CGJ. 1988. The embryology of testicular descent. Horm Res 30:144

Williams HG. 1983. Regulatory features of seminal vesicle development and function. Curr Top Cell Regul 22:201

Applications to Clinical Practice

Bain J. 1986. Hypogonadal states in the male. Compr Ther 12:39

Bard JBL, McConnell JE, Davies JA. 1994. Towards a genetic basis for kidney development. Mech Dev 48:3

Behringer RR. 1994. The in vivo roles of Müllerian-inhibiting substance. Curr Top Devel Biol 29:171

Behringer RR, Finegold MJ, Cate RL. 1994. Müllerian inhibiting substance function during mammalian sexual development. Cell 79:415

Berry AC, Chantler C. 1986. Urogenital malformations and disease. Br Med Bull 42:181

Bogan JS, Page D. 1994. Ovary? Testis?—a mammalian dilemma. Cell 76:603

Burgoyne PS, Buehr M, Koopman P, Rossant J. 1988. Cell autonomous action of the testis-determining gene: Sertoli cells are exclusively XY in XX-XY chimeric mouse testes. Development 102:443

Burris TP, Guo W, Le T, McCabe ER. 1995. Identification of a putative steroidogenic factor-1 response element in the DAX-1 promoter. Biochem Biophys Res Commun 214:576

Chahnazarian A. 1988. Determinants of the sex ratio at birth: review of recent literature. Soc Biol 35:214

Cherfas J. 1991. Sex and the single gene. Science 252:782

Churchill BM, Abara EO, McLorie GA. 1987. Ureteral duplication, ectopy, and ureteroceles. Manag Princ Pediatr Urol 34:1273

de la Chapelle A. 1986. Genetic molecular studies on 46,XX and 45,X males. Cold Spring Harbor Symp Quant Biol 51:249

deVries PA. 1984. The surgery of anorectal anomalies: its evolution, with evaluations of procedures. p. 1. In Ravitch MM (ed): Current Problems in Surgery. Year Book Medical Publishers, Chicago

Dey BR, Sukhatme VP, Roberts AB et al. 1994. Repression of the transforming growth factor-β 1 gene by the Wilms' tumor suppressor gene product. Mol Endocrinol 8:595

Dressler GR. 1995. The genetic control of renal development. Curr Opin Nephrol Hypertension 4:253

Drummond IA, Madden SL, Rohwer-Nutter P et al. 1992. Repression of the insulinlike growth factor II gene by the Wilms tumor suppressor WT1. Science 257:674

Eccles MR, Yun K, Reeve AE, Fidler AE. 1995. Comparative in situ hybridization analysis of *PAX2, PAX8* and *WT1* gene transcription in human fetal kidney and Wilms' tumors. Am J Pathol 146:40

Ford CE. 1970. Cytogenetics and sex determination in man and mammals. J Biosocial Sci Suppl 2:7

Ford CE, Hammerton JL. 1956. The chromosomes of man. Nature (London) 178:1020

Ford CE, Jones KW, Polani P et al. 1959. A sex chromosome anomaly in a case of gonadal dysgenesis (Turner's syndrome). Lancet i:711

Graves JA. 1995. The evolution of mammalian sex chromosomes and the origin of sex determining genes. Philos Trans R Soc Ser B Biol Sci 350:305

Grubb GR, Yun K, Williams BR et al. 1994. Expression of WT1 protein in fetal kidneys and Wilms tumors. Lab Invest 71:472

Gubbay J, Collignon J, Koopman P et al. 1990. A gene mapping to the sex-determining region of the mouse Y chromosome is a member of a novel family of embryologically expressed genes. Nature (London) 346:245

Haber DA, Sohn RL, Buckler AJ et al. 1991. Alternative splicing and genomic structure of the Wilms' tumor gene *WT1.* Proc Natl Acad Sci USA 88:9618

Hastie ND. 1992. Dominant negative mutations in Wilms tumor (*WT1*) gene cause Denys-Drash syndrome—proof that a tumor-suppressor gene plays a crucial role in normal geni-tourinary development. Hum Mol Genet 1:293

Haqq CM, King CY, Ukiyama E et al. 1994. Molecular basis of mammalian sexual determination: activation of Müllerian inhibiting substance gene expression by SRY. Science 266:1994

Ingraham HA, Lala DS, Ikeda Y et al. 1994. The nuclear receptor steroidogenic factor 1 acts at multiple levels of the reproductive axis. Genes Dev 8:2302

Jacobs PA, Ross A. 1966. Structural analyses of the Y chromosome in man. Nature (London) 210:352

Jacobs PA, Strong JA. 1959. A case of human intersexuality having a possible XXY sex determining mechanism. Nature (London) 183:302

Knudson AG, Strong LC. Mutation and cancer: a model for Wilms' tumor of the kidney. J Natl Cancer Inst 48:313

Koopman P, Gubbay J, Vivian N et al. 1991. Male development of chromosomally female mice transgenic for Sry. Nature (London) 351:117

Korach K. 1994. Insights from the study of animals lacking functional estrogen receptor. Science 266:1524

Kreidberg JA, Sariola H, Loring JM et al. 1993. WT-1 is required for early kidney development. Cell 74:679

Kubota T, Saitoh S, Matsumoto T et al. 1994. Excess functional copy of allele at chromosomal region (11p15) may cause Wiedemann-Beckwith (EMG) syndrome. Am J Med Genet 49:378

Lala DS, Ikeda Y, Luo X et al. A cell-specific nuclear receptor regulates the steroid hydroxylases. Steroids 60:10

Little MH, Prosser J, Condie A et al. 1992. Zinc finger point mutations within the *WT1* gene in Wilms' tumor patients. Proc Natl Acad Sci USA 89:4791

Luo XN, Reddy JC, Yeyati PL et al. 1995. The tumor suppressor gene *WT1* inhibits *ras*-mediated transformation. Oncogene 11:743

McElreavey K, Vilain E, Abbas N et al. 1993. A regulatory cascade hypothesis for mammalian sex determination: SRY represses a negative regulator of male development. Proc Natl Acad Sci USA 90:3368

McLaren A. 1990. What makes a man a man? Nature (London) 346:216

Mittwoch U. 1992. Sex determination and sex reversal: genotype, phenotype, dogma and semantics. Hum Genet 89:467

Moffat DB. 1982. Developmental abnormalities of the urogenital system. p. 357. In Chisholm GD, and Williams DI (eds): Scientific Foundations of Urology. Year Book Medical Publishers, Chicago

Montesano R, Schaller G, Orci L. 1991. Induction of epithelial tubular morphogenesis in vitro by fibroblast-derived soluble factors. Cell 66:697

Moyer JH, Lee-Tischler MJ, Kwon H-Y et al. 1994. Candidate gene associated with a mutation causing recessive polycystic kidney disease in mice. Science 264:1329

Müller U. 1987. Mapping of testis-determining locus on Yp by the molecular analysis of XX males and XY females. Development 101:52

Mundlos S, Pelletier J, Darveau A et al. 1993. Nuclear localization of the protein encoded by the Wilms' tumor gene *WT1* in embryonic and adult tissues. Development 119:1329

Nomura M, Bartsch S, Nawata H et al. 1995. An E box element is required for the expression of the *ad4bp* gene, a mammalian homolog of *ftz-f1* gene, which is essential for adrenal and gonadal development. J Biol Chem 270:7453

Page DC, Fisher EMC, McGillivray B, Brown LG. 1990. Additional deletion in sex-determining region of human Y chromosome resolves paradox of X,t(Y,22) female. Nature (London) 346:279

Patterson LT, Dressler GR. 1994. The regulation of kidney development: new insights from an old model. Curr Opin Genet Dev 4:696

Perantoni AO, Dove LF, Karanova I. 1995. Basic fibroblast growth factor can mediate the early inductive events in renal development. Proc Natl Acad Sci USA 92:4696

Pontiggia A, Whitfield S, Goodfellow PN et al. 1995. Evolutionary conservation in the DNA-binding and -binding properties of HMG-boxes from SRY proteins of primates. Gene 154:277

Pritchard-Jones K, Fleming S, Davidson D et al. 1990. The candidate Wilms' tumor gene is involved in genitourinary development. Nature 346:194

Richards JS, Fitzpatrick SL, Clemens JW et al. 1995. Ovarian cell differentiation: a cascade of multiple hormones, cellular signals, and regulated genes. Recent Prog Hormone Res 50:223

Rimini R, Pontiggia A, Spada F et al. 1995. Interaction of normal and mutant Sry proteins with DNA. Philos Trans R Soc Ser B Biol Sci 350:215

Rosier MF, Goguel AF, Martin A et al. 1994. A 1. 7-Mb YAC contig around the human BDNF gene (11p13): integration of the physical, genetic and cytogenetic maps in relation to WARG syndrome. Genomics 24:69

Ryner LC, Swain A. 1995. Sex in the '90s. Cell 81:483

Saxen L, Karkinen-Jaaskelainen M, Lehtonen E et al. 1976. Inductive tissue interactions. p. 331. In Poste G, Nicholson GL (eds): The Cell Surface in Animal Embryogenesis and Development. Elsevier/North Holland, Amsterdam.

Schuchardt A, D'Agati V, Larsson-Blomberg L et al. 1994. Defects in the kidney and enteric nervous system of mice lacking the tyrosine kinase receptor Ret. Nature 367:380

Shen W-H, Moore CCD, Ikeda Y et al. 1994. Nuclear receptor steroidogenic factor 1 regulates the Müllerian inhibiting substance gene: a link to the sex determination cascade. Cell 77:651

Sinclaire AH, Berta P, Palmer MS et al. 1990. A gene from the human sex-determining region encodes a protein with homology to a conserved DNA-binding motif. Nature (London) 346:240

Smith ED. 1988. Incidence, frequency of types, and etiology of anorectal malformations. Birth Defects Orig Artic Ser 24:231

Stephens FD. 1988. Embryology of the cloaca and embryogenesis of anorectal malformations. Birth Defects Orig Artic Ser 24:177

Telerman A, Dodemont H, Degraef C et al. 1992. Identification of the cellular protein encoded by the Wilms' tumor (WT1) gene. Oncogene 7:2545

Thomas DFM. 1989. Cloacal malformations: embryology, anatomy and principles of management. Prog Pediatr Surg 23:135

Tommerup N, Schempp W, Meinecke P et al. 1993. Assignment of an autosomal sex reversal locus (SRA1) and campomelic dysplasia (CMPD1) to 17q24.3-q25.1. Nature Genet 4:170

van Niekerk WA, Retief AE. 1981. The gonads of human true hermaphrodites. Hum Genet 58:117

Wada M, Seeger RC, Mizoguchi H, Koeffler HP. 1995. Maintenance of normal imprinting of H19 and IGF2 genes in neuroblastoma. Cancer Res 55:3386

Werner H, Shen-Orr Z, Rauscher FJ 3rd et al. 1995. Inhibition of cellular proliferation by the Wilms' tumor suppressor WT1 is associated with suppression of insulin-like growth factor I receptor gene expression. Mol Cell Biol 15:3516

CHAPTER 11

Descriptive Embryology

Bardeen CR, Lewis WH. 1901. Development of the limbs, body wall, and back in man. Am J Anat 1:1

Brookes M. 1955. The vascularization of long bones in the human fetus. J Anat 92:261

Carrington JL, Fallon JF. 1988. Initial budding is independent of apical ectodermal ridge activity: evidence from a limbless mutant. Development 104:361

Chevallier A, Kieny M, Mauger A. 1977. Limb-somite relationship: origin of the limb musculature. J Embryol Exp Morphol 41:245

Christ B, Jacob HJ. 1980. Origin, distribution, and determination of chick limb bud mesenchymal cells. p. 67. In Merker H-J, Nau H, Neubert D (eds): Teratology of the Limbs. Walter D. Gruyter, Berlin

Christ B, Jacob HJ, Jacob M, Brand B. 1986. Principles of hand ontogenesis in man. Acta Morphol Neerl-Scand 24:249

Gardner E. 1968. The embryology of the clavicle. Clin Orthop 58:9

Hinrichsen KV, Jacob HJ, Jacob M et al. 1994. Principles of ontogenesis of leg and foot in man. Ann Anat 176:121

Honig MG, Lance-Jones C, Landmesser L. 1986. The development of sensory projection patterns in embryonic chick hindlimb under experimental conditions. Dev Biol 118:532

Jacob M, Christ B, Jacob HJ. 1980. On the migration of myogenic stem cells into the prospective wing region of chick embryos. Anat Embryol (Berl) 153:179

Kelley RO. 1985. Early development of the vertebrate limb: an introduction to morphogenetic tissue interactions using scanning electron microscopy. Scanning Microsc II:827

Kelly RO, Fallon JF. 1981. The developing limb: an analysis of interacting cells and tissues in a model morphogenetic system. p. 49. In Connelly TG, Brinkley LL, and Carlson BM (eds): Morphogenesis and Pattern Formation. Raven Press, New York

Kieny M, Chevallier A. 1979. Anatomy of tendon development in the embryonic chick wing. J Embryol Exp Morphol 49:153

Landmesser L. 1988. Peripheral guidance cues and the formation of specific motor projections in the chick. p. 121. In Easter SS Jr., Berald KF, Carlson BM (eds): From Message to Mind. Sinauer Associates, Inc, Sunderland, MA

Noback CR, Robertson GG. 1951. Sequences of appearance of ossification centers in the human skeleton during the first five prenatal months. Am J Anat 89:1

O'Rahilly R, Gray DJ, Gardner E. 1957. Chondrification in the hands and feet of staged human embryos. Contrib Embryol Carnegie Inst 36:183

O'Rahilly R, Meyer DB. 1956. Roentgenographic investigation of the human skeleton during early fetal life. Am J Roentgenol 76:455

O'Rahilly R, Muller F. 1987. Development stages in human embryos. Carnegie Inst Wash Publ 637:1

Rubin L, Saunders JW Jr. 1972. Ectodermal-mesodermal interactions in the growth of limb buds in the chick embryo: constancy and temporal limits of the ectodermal induction. Dev Biol 28:94

Rutz R, Haney C, Hauschka S. 1982. Spatial analysis of limb bud myogenesis: a proximodistal gradient of muscle colony-forming cells in chick embryo leg buds. Dev Biol 90:399

Saunders JW. 1948. The proximo-distal sequence of origin of the parts of the chick wing and the role of the ectoderm. J Exp Zool 108:363

Saunders JW, Gasseling MT. 1983. New insights into the problem of pattern regulation in the limb bud of the chick embryo. p. 67. In Fallon JF, Caplan AI (eds): Limb Development and Regeneration. Part A. Alan R Liss, New York

Solursh M, Drake C, Meier S. 1987. The migration of myogenic cells from the somites at the wing level in avian embryos. Dev Biol 121:389

Stephens TD, Beier RLW, Bringhurst DC et al. 1989. Limbness in the early chick embryo lateral plate. Dev Biol 133:1

Summerbell D, Honig LS. 1982. The control of pattern across the antero-posterior axis of the chick limb bud by a unique signaling region. Am Zool 22:105

Tosney K, Landmesser LT. 1984. Pattern and specificity of axonal outgrowth following varying degrees of chick limb bud ablation. J Neurosci 4:2518

Wachtler F, Christ B, Jacob HJ. 1982. Grafting experiments on determination and migratory behavior of presomitic, somitic, and somatopleural cells in avian embryos. Anat Embryol (Berl) 164:369

Wolpert L. 1978. Pattern formation in biological development. Sci Am 239:154

Applications to Clinical Practice

Bhat BV, Ashok BA, Puri RK. 1987. Lobster claw hand and foot deformity in a family. Indian Pediatr 24:675

Bitgood MJ, McMahon AP. 1995. Hedgehog and BMP genes are co-expressed at many diverse sites of cell-cell interaction in the mouse embryo. Dev Biol 172:126

Brown KS, Cranley RE, Greene R et al. 1981. Disproportionate micromelia (*Dmm*): an incomplete dominant mouse dwarfism with abnormal cartilage matrix. J Embryol Exp Morphol 62:165

Bryant SV. 1996. Digit induction by Henson's node and notochord involves the expression of shh but not RAR-β 2. Dev Biol 173:318

Chan DC, Laufer E, Tabin C, Leder P. 1995. Polydactylous limbs in Strong's Luxoid mice result from ectopic polarizing activity. Development 121:1971

Chan DC, Wynshaw-Boris A, Leder P. 1995. Formin isoforms are differentially expressed in the mouse embryo and are required for normal expression of fgf-4 and shh in the limb bud. Development 121:3151

Charite J, de Graaff W, Shen S, Deschamps J. 1994. Ectopic expression of *Hoxb-8* causes duplication of the ZPA in the forelimb and homeotic transformation of axial structures. Cell 78:589

Chen Y, Dong D, Kostetskii I, Zile MH. 1996. Henson's node from viamin A-deficient quail embryo induces chick limb bud duplication and retains its normal symmetric expression of sonic hedgehog (Shh). Dev Biol 173:256

Cohn MJ, Izpisua-Belmonte JC, Abud H et al. 1995. Fibroblast growth factors induce additional limb development from the flank of chick embryos. Cell 80:739

Collins MD, Fradkin R, Scott WJ. 1990. Induction of postaxial forelimb ectrodactyly with anticonvulsive agents in A/J mice. Teratology 41:61

Crossley PH, Martin GR. 1995. The mouse *Fgf8* gene encodes a family of polypeptides and is expressed in regions that direct outgrowth and patterning in the developing embryo. Development 121:439

Cusic AM, Dagg CP. 1985. Spontaneous and retinoic acid-induced postaxial polydactyly in mice. Teratology 31:49

D'Amato RJ, Loughnan MS, Flynn E, Folkman J. 1994. Thalidomide is an inhibitor of angiogenesis. Proc Natl Acad Sci USA 91:4082

Davis AP, Capecchi MR. 1994. Axial homeosis and appendicular skeleton defects in mice with a targeted disruption of *hoxd-11*. Development 120:2187

Davis AP, Witte DP, Hsieh-Li Hm et al. 1995. Absence of radius and ulna in mice lacking *hoxa-11* and *hoxd-11*. Nature 375:791

Dealy CN, Kosher RA. 1996. IGF-I, insulin and FGFs induce outgrowth of the limb buds of amelic chick embryos. Development 122:1323

Duboule D. 1993. The function of *Hox* genes in the morphogenesis of the vertebrate limb. Ann Genet 36:24

Ehninger G, Eger K, Stuhler A, Schuler U. 1993. Thalidomide—the need for a new clinical evaluation of an old drug. Bone Marrow Transplant 12(Suppl 3):S26

Eichele G, Tickle C, Alberts BW. 1984. Microcontrolled release of biologically active compounds in chick embryo: beads of 200 µm-diameter for the local release of retinoids. Anal Biochem 142:542

Elmer WA, Pennybacker MF, Knudsen TB, Kwasigroch TE. 1988. Alterations in cell surface galactosyltransferase activity during limb chondrogenesis in *Brachypod* mutant mouse embryos. Teratology 38:475

Fawcett D, Pasceri P, Fraser R et al. 1995. Postaxial polydactyly in forelimbs of CRABP-II mutant mice. Development 121:671

Francis PH, Richardson MK, Brikell PM, Tickle C. 1994. Bone morphogenetic proteins and a signalling pathway that controls patterning in the developing chick limb. Development 120:209

Gould SE, Upholt WB, Kosher RA. 1995. Characterization of chicken syndecan-3 as a heparan sulfate proteoglycan and its expression during embryogenesis. Dev Biol 168:438

Graham JM. 1985. The association between limb anomalies and spatially-restricting uterine environments. Prog Clin Biol Res 163c:99

Haramis AG, Brown JM, Zeller R. 1995. The limb deformity mutation disrupts the SHH/FGF-4 feedback loop and regulation of 5' *HoxD* genes during limb pattern formation. Development 121:4237

Hardy A, Richardson MK, Francis-West PH et al. 1995. Gene expression, polarising activity skeletal patterning in reaggregated hind limb mesenchyme. Development 121:4329

Hartwig NG, Vermeij-Keers C, De Vies HE et al. 1989. Limb body wall malformation complex: an embryologic etiology? Hum Pathol 20:1071

Hayamizu TF, Bryant SV. 1994. Reciprocal changes in *Hox D13* and RAR-beta 2 expression in response to retinoic acid in chick limbs. Dev Biol 166:123

Helms J, Thaller C, Eichele G. 1994. Relationship between retinoic acid and sonic hedgehog, two polarizing signals in the chick wing bud. Development 120:3267

Higginbottom MC, Jones KL, Hall BD, Smith DW. 1979. The amniotic band disruption complex: timing of amniotic rupture and variable spectra of consequent defects. J Pediatr 95:544

Izpisua-Belmonte JC, Duboule D. 1992. Homeobox genes and pattern formation in the vertebrate limb. Dev Biol 152:26

Jaeggi E, Kind C, Morger R. 1990. Congenital scalp and skull defects with terminal transverse limb anomalies (Adams-Oliver syndrome): report of three additional cases. Eur J Pediatr 149:565

Klein KL, Scott WJ, Wilson JG. 1981. Aspirin-induced teratogenesis: a unique pattern of cell death and subsequent polydactyly in the rat. J Exp Zool 216:107

Knudsen TB, Kochhar DM. 1981. The role of morphogenetic cell death during abnormal limb-bud outgrowth in mice heterozygous for the dominant mutation *He-mimelia-extra toe (Hmx)*. J Embryol Exp Morphol 65:289

Kochhar DM. 1973. Limb development in mouse embryos. I. Analysis of teratogenic effects of retinoic acid. Teratology 7:289

Kochhar DM. 1985. Cellular expression of a mutant gene (*cmd/cmd*) causing limb and other defects in mouse embryos. Prog Clin Biol Res 163c:131

Laufer E, Nelson CE, Johnson RL et al. 1994. Sonic hedgehog and FGF-4 act through a signaling cascade and feedback loop to integrate growth and patterning of the developing limb bud. Cell 79:993

Lenz W. 1988. A short history of thalidomide embryopathy. Teratology 38:203

Lenz W, Knapp K. 1962. Foetal malformation due to thalidomide. German Med Monthly 7:253

Lohnes D, Mark M, Mendelsohn C et al. 1994. Function of the retinoic acid receptors (RARs) during development (I) Craniofacial and skeletal abnormalities in RAR double mutants. Development 120:2723

Lopez-Martinez A, Chang DT, Chiang C et al. 1995. Limb-patterning activity and restricted posterior localization of the amino-terminal product of the Sonic hedgehog cleavage. Curr Biol 5:791

Luo J, Pasceri P, Conlon RA et al. 1995. Mice lacking all isoforms of retinoic acid receptor beta develop normally and are susceptible to the teratogenic effects of retinoic acid. Mech Dev 53:61

Lyons KM, Hogan BL, Robertson EJ. 1995. Colocalization of BMP 7 and BMP 2 RNAs suggests that these factors cooperatively mediate tissue interactions during murine development. Mech Dev 50:71

Maas RL, Zeller R, Woychik RP et al. 1990. Disruption of formin-encoding transcripts in two mutant limb deformity alleles. Nature (London) 346:853

MacCabe JA, Errick J, Sauders JW. 1974. Ectodermal control of the dorsoventral axis of the leg bud of the chick embryo. Dev Biol 39:69

Mahmud R, Bresnick J, Hornbruch A et al. 1995. A role for FGF-8 in the initiation and maintenance of vertebrate limb bud out-growth. Curr Biol 5:797

Marigo V, Roberts DJ, Lee SM et al. 1995. Cloning, expression, and chromosomal location of SHH and IHH: two human homologues of the *Drosophila* segment polarity gene hedgehog. Genomics 28:44

Masuya H, Sagai T, Wakana S et al. 1995. A duplicated zone of polarizing activity in polydactylous mouse mutants. Genes Dev 9:1645

McNeisch JD, Scott WJ, Potter SS. 1988. Legless, a novel mutation found in PHT1-1 transgenic mice. Science 241:837

Mendelsohn C, Lohnes D, Decimo D et al. 1994. Function of the retinoic acid receptors (RARs) during development (II) Multiple abnormalities at various stages of organogenesis in RAR double mutants. Development 120:2749

Merker H-J. 1977. Considerations of the problem of critical period during development of the limb skeleton. Birth Defects Orig Artic Ser 13:179

Mima T, Ohuchi H, Noji S, Mikawa T. 1995. FGF can induce outgrowth of somatic mesoderm both inside and outside of limb-forming regions. Dev Biol 167:617

Morgan BA, Tabin C. 1994. *Hox* genes and growth: early and late roles in limb bud morphogenesis. Development (Suppl) 181

Mundlos S, Mulliken JB, Abramson DL et al. 1996. Genetic mapping of cliedocranial dysplasia and evidence of a microdeletion in one family. Hum Mol Genet 4:71

Muragaki Y, Mudlos S, Upton J, Olsen B. 1996. Altered growth and branching patterns in synpolydactyly caused by mutations in *HOXD13*. Science 272:548

Neubert R, Hinz N, Thiel R, Neubert D. 1995. Down-regulation of adhesion receptors on cells of primate embryos as a probable mechanism of the teratogenic action of thalidomide. Life Sci 58:295

Niswander L, Jeffery S, Martin GR, Tickle C. 1994. A positive feedback loop coordinates growth and patterning in the vertebrate limb. Nature 371:609

Niswander L, Tickle C, Vogel A et al. 1993. FGF-4 replaces the apical ectodermal ridge and directs outgrowth and patterning of the limb. Cell 75:579

Noji S, Nohno T, Koyama E et al. 1991. Retinoic acid induces polarizing activity but is unlikely to be a morphogen in the chick limb bud. Nature (London) 350:83

Ohuchi H, Yoshioka H, Tanaka A et al. 1994. Involvement of androgen-induced growth factor (FGF-8) gene in mouse embryogenesis and morphogenesis. Biochem Biophys Res Commun 204:882

Olsen B. 1995. Mutations in collagen genes resulting in metaphyseal and epiphyseal dysplasias. Bone 17:45S

O'Rahilly R. 1985. The development and classification of anomalies of the limbs in the human. Prog Clin Biol Res 163c:85

Parr BA, McMahon AP. 1995. Dorsalizing signal Wnt-7a required for normal polarity of D-V and A-P axes of mouse limb. Nature 374:350

Perrimon N. 1995. Hedgehog and beyond. Cell 80:517

Regemorter NV, Milare J, Ramet J et al. 1982. Familial ectrodactyly and polydactyly: variable expressivity of one single gene—embryological considerations. Clin Genet 22:206

Reid L. 1990. From gradients to axes, from morphogenesis to differentiation. Cell 63:875

Riddle RD, Ensini M, Nelson C et al. 1995. Induction of the *LIM* homeobox gene *Lmxl* by Wnt7a establishes dorsoventral pattern in the vertebrate limb. Cell 83:631

Riddle RD, Johnson RL, Laufer E, Tabin C. 1993. Sonic hedgehog mediates the polarizing activity of the ZPA. Cell 75:1401

Robert B, Sassoon D, Jacq B et al. 1989. *Hox-7*, a mouse homeobox gene with a novel pattern of expression during embryogenesis. EMBO J 8:91

Ruffing L. 1977. Evaluation of thalidomide children. Birth Defects Orig Artic Ser 13:287

Rutledge JC, Shourbaji AG, Hughes LA et al. 1994. Limb and lower-body duplications induced by retinoic acid in mice. Proc Natl Acad Sci USA 91:5436

Satre MA, Kochhar DM. 1989. Elevations in the endogenous levels of the putative morphogen retinoic acid in embryonic mouse limb-buds associated with limb dysmorphogenesis. Dev Biol 133:529

Savage MP, Fallon JF. 1995. FGF-2 mRNA and its antisense message are expressed in a developmentally specific manner in the chick limb bud and mesonephros. Dev Dynam. 202:343

Scadding SR, Maden M. 1994. Retinoic acid gradients during limb regeneration. Dev Biol 162:608

Scott WJ. 1985. Asymmetric limb malformations induced by drugs or mutant genes. Prog Clin Biol Res 163c:111

Scott WJ Jr, Walter R, Tzimas G et al. 1994. Endogenous status of retinoids and their cytosolic binding proteins in limb buds of chick vs mouse embryos. Dev Biol 165:397

Silengo MC, Biagli M, Bell GL et al. 1987. Triphalangeal thumb and brachyectrodactyly syndrome. Clin Genet 31:13

Simeone A, Acampora D, Arcioni L et al. 1990. Sequential activation of *HOX2* homeobox genes by retinoic acid in human embryonal carcinoma cells. Nature (London) 346:763

Small KM, Potter SS. 1993. Homeotic transformations and limb defects in *Hoxa-11* mutant mice. Genes Dev 7:2318

Smith SM, Pang K, Sundin O et al. 1989. Molecular approaches to vertebrate limb morphogenesis. Development (Suppl) 107:121

Storm EE, Huynh TV, Copeland NG et al. 1994. Limb alterations in brachipodism mice due to mutations in a new member of the TGF-beta-superfamily. Nature 368:639

Sucov HM, Izpisua-Belmonte JC, Ganan Y, Evans RM. 1995. Mouse embryos lacking RXR alpha are resistant to retinoic-acid-induced limb defects. Development 121:3997

Sulik K, Dehart DB. 1988. Retinoic-acid-induced limb malformations resulting from apical ectodermal ridge death. Teratology 37:527

Tabin C. 1995. The initiation of the limb bud: growth factors, *Hox* genes, and retinoids. Cell 80:671

Tanaka EM, Gann AF. 1995. Limb development. The budding role of FGF. Curr Biol 5:594

Thaller C, Eichele G. 1988. Characterization of retinoic acid metabolism in the developing chick wing bud. Development 103:473

Tickle C. 1995. Vertebrate limb development. Curr Opin Genet Dev 5:478

Tickle C, Alberts B, Wolpert L, Lee J. 1982. Local application of retinoic acid to the limb bud mimics the action of the polarizing region. Nature (London) 296:564

Tickle C, Lee J, Eichele G. 1985. A quantitative analysis of the effect of all-trans-retinoic acid on the pattern of chick wing development. Dev Biol 109:82

Tickle C, Summerbell D, Wolpert L. 1975. Positional signalling and specification of digits in chick limb morphogenesis. Nature (London) 254:199

Torpin R. 1968. Amniochorionic mesoblastic fibrous strings and amniotic bands. Am J Obstet Gynecol 91:65

Van Allen MI, Curry C, Gallagher L. 1987. Limb body wall complex. I. Pathogenesis. Am J Med Genet 28:529

Viljoen DL, Kidson SH. 1990. Mirror polydactyly: morphogenesis based on a morphogen gradient theory. Am J Med Genet 35:229

Vogel A, Roberts-Clarke D, Niswander L. 1995. Effect of FGF on gene expression in chick limb bud cells in vivo and in vitro. Dev Biol 171:507

Vogel A, Rodriguez, Warnken W, Belmonte JCI. 1996. Dorsal cell fate specified by chick *Lmxl* during vertebrate limb development. Nature 378:716

Wang Y, Sassoon D. 1995. Ectoderm-mesenchyme and mesenchyme-mesenchyme interactions regulate *Msx-1* expression and cellular differentiation in the murine limb. Dev Biol 168:374

Weaver T, Scott WJ. 1984. Acetazolamide teratogenesis: interaction of maternal metabolic and respiratory acidosis in the induction of ectrodactyly in C57BL/6J mice. Teratology 30:195

Wulfsberg EA, Mirkinson LJ, Meister SJ. 1993. Autosomal dominant tetramelic postaxial oligodactyly. Am J Med Genet 46:579

Yamaguchi TP, Rossant J. 1995. Fibroblast growth factors in mammalian development. Curr Opin Genet Dev 5:485

Yang Y, Niswender L. 1995. Interaction between the signaling molecules WNT7a and SHH during vertebrate limb development: dorsal signals regulate anteroposterior patterning. Cell 80:939

Yokouchi Y, Nakzato S, Yamamoto M et al. 1995. Misexpression of *Hoxa-13* induces cartilage homeotic transformation and changes cell adhesiveness in chick limbs. Genes Dev 9:2509

Yuan H, Corbi N, Basilico C, Dailey L. 1995. Developmental-specificity activity of the FGF-4 enhancer requires the synergistic action of *Sox2* and *Oct-3*. Genes Dev 9:2635

Zeller R, Jackson-Grusby L, Leder P. 1989. The limb deformity gene is required for apical ectodermal ridge differentiation and antero-posterior limb pattern formation. Genes Dev 3:1481

Zou H, Niswander L. 1996. Requirement for BMP signaling in interdigital apoptosis and scale formation. Science 272:738

CHAPTER 12

Development of the Head and Neck

Ballabio M, Nicolini U, Jowett T et al. 1989. Maturation of thyroid function in normal human fetuses. Clin Endocrinol 31:565

Ferguson MWJ. 1988. Palate development. Development 103(Suppl): 41

Friedberg J. 1989. Pharyngeal cleft sinuses and cysts, and other benign neck lesions. Pediatr Clin North Am 36:1451

Gans C. 1987. The neural crest: a spectacular invention. p. 361. In Maderson PFA (ed): Developmental and Evolutionary Aspects of the Neural Crest. John Wiley, New York

Gans C. 1988. Craniofacial growth, evolutionary questions. Development 103(Suppl):3

Hengerer AS. 1984. Embryological development of the sinuses. Ear Nose Throat J 63:134

Le Douarin NM, Ziller C, Couly GF. 1993. Patterning of neural crest derivatives in the avain embryo: in vivo and in vitro studies. Dev Biol 159:24

Lobach DF, Haynes BF. 1987. Ontogeny of the human thymus during fetal development. J Clin Immunol 7:81

Margriples U, Laitman JT. 1987. Developmental change in the position of the fetal human larynx. Am J Phys Anthropol 72:463

Marion M, Hinojosa R, Khan AA. 1985. Persistence of the stapedial artery: a histopathologic study. Otolaryngol Head Neck Surg 93:298

Merida-Velasco JA, Garcia-Garcia JD, Espin-Ferra J, Linares J. 1989. Origin of the ultimobranchial body and its colonizing cells in human embryos. Acta Anat 136:325

Muller F, O'Rahilly R, Tucker J. 1985. The human larynx at the end of the embryonic period proper. 2. The laryngeal cavity and the innervation of its lining. Ann Otol Rhinol Laryngol 94:607

Noden DM. 1984. Craniofacial development: new views on old problems. Anat Rec 208:1

Noden DM. 1988. Interactions and fates of avian craniofacial mesenchyme. Development 103(Suppl):121

O'Rahilly R. 1978. The timing and sequence of events in the development of the human digestive system and associated structures during the embryonic period proper. Anat Embryol 153:123

O'Rahilly R, Muller F. 1984. The early development of the hypoglossal nerve and occipital somites in staged human embryos. Am J Anat 169:237

O'Rahilly R, Muller F. 1987. Developmental stages in human embryos. Carnegie Inst Wash Publ 637:1

Swarts JD, Rood SR, Doyle WJ. 1986. Fetal development of the auditory tube and paratubal musculature. Cleft Palate J 23:289

Tan SS, Morriss-Kay GM. 1986. Analysis of cranial neural crest cell migration and early fates in postimplantation rat chimeras. J Embryol Exp Morphol 98:21

Thorogood P. 1988. The developmental specification of the vertebrate skull. Development 103(Suppl):141

Trainer PA, Tam PP. 1995. Cranial paraxial mesoderm and neural crest cells of the mouse embryo: co-distribution in the craniofacial mesenchyme but distinct segregation in branchial arches. Development 121:2569

Van der Linden EJ, Burdi A, de Jonge HJ. 1987. Critical periods in the prenatal morphogenesis of the human lateral pterygoid muscle, the mandibular condyle, the articular disk, and medial articular capsule. Am J Orthod Dentofac Orthop 91:22

von Gaudecker B. 1986. The development of the human thymus microenvironment. p. 1. In Muller-Hermelink HK (ed): The Human Thymus, Histophysiology and Pathology. Springer-Verlag, Berlin

von Gaudecker B. 1988. Development and functional anatomy of the human tonsilla palatina. Acta Otolaryngol Suppl 454:28

Wachtler F, Jacob M. 1986. Origin and development of the cranial skeletal muscles. Bibl Anat 29:24

Wedden SE, Ralphs JR, Tickle C. 1988. Pattern formation in the facial primordia. Development 103(Suppl):31

Wong G, Weinberg S, Symington JM. 1985. Morphology of the developing articular disc of the human temporomandibular joint. J Oral Maxillofac Surg 43:565

Zaw-Tun HA. 1985. Reexamination of the origin and early development of the human larynx. Acta Anat 122:163

Development of the Eyes

Barnstable CJ. 1987. A molecular view of vertebrate retinal development. Mol Neurobiol 1:9

Jacobson AG, Sater AK. 1988. Features of embryonic induction. Development 104:341

O'Rahilly R. 1966. The early development of the eye in staged human embryos. Contrib Embryol Carnegie Inst 38:1

O'Rahilly R. 1983. The timing and sequence of events in the development of the human eye and ear during the embryonic period proper. Anat Embryol 168:87

Noden D. 1983. The role of the neural crest in patterning of avian cranial skeletal, connective, and muscle tissues. Dev Biol 96:144

Saha MS, Spann C, Grainger RM. 1989. Embryonic lens induction: more than meets the optic vesicle. Cell Differ Dev 28:153

Sevel D. 1988. A reappraisal of development of the eyelids. Eye 2:123

Tam P. 1989. Regionalization of the mouse embryonic ectoderm: allocation of prospective ectodermal tissues during gastrulation. Development 107:55

Wachtler F. 1984. The extrinsic ocular muscles in birds are derived from the prechordal plate. Naturwissenschaften 71:379

Development of the Ears

Declau F, Jacob W, Dorrine W et al. 1989. Early ossification within the human fetal otic capsule: morphological and microanalytical findings. J Laryngol Otol 103:1113

Gilbert P. 1957. The origins and development of the human extrinsic ocular muscles. Contrib Embryol Carnegie Inst 246:61

Mallo M, Gridley T. 1996. Development of the mammalian ear: coordinate regulation of formation of the tympanic ring and the external acoustic meatus. Development 122:173

Marquet JE, DeClau F, De Cock M et al. 1988. Congenital middle ear malformations. Acta Oto-Rhino-Laryngol Belg 42:117

McPhee JR, Van De Water TR. 1986. Epithelial-mesenchymal tissue interactions guiding otic capsule formation: the role of the otocyst. J Embryol Exp Morphol 97:1

Michaels L. 1988. Origin of congenital cholesteatoma from a normally occurring epidermoid rest in the developing middle ear. Int J Pediatr Otorhinolaryngol 15:51

Moro J, Pastor F, Gato A, Barbosa E. 1990. Patterns of epithelial cell death during early development of the human inner ear. Ann Otol Rhinol Laryngol 99:482

O'Rahilly R. 1963. The early development of the otic vesicle in staged human embryos. J Embryol Exp Morphol 11:741

Van De Water TR. 1988. Tissue interactions and cell differentiation: neurone-sensory cell interaction during otic development. Development 103(Suppl):185

Van De Water TR. 1980. The morphogenesis of the middle and the external ear. Birth Defects: Orig Artic Ser 16:147

Applications to Clinical Practice

Akam M. 1989. *Hox* and *HOM*: homologous gene clusters in insects and vertebrates. Cell 57:347

Alberch P, Kollar E. 1988. Strategies of head development: workshop report. Development 103(Suppl):25

al-Ghamdi S, Freedman A, Just N et al. 1992. Fourth branchial cleft cyst. J Otolaryngol 21:447

Ali F, Persaud TVN. 1988. Mechanisms of fetal alcohol effects: role of acetaldehyde. Exp Pathol 33:17

Anneren G, Gustafsson J, Sunnegardh J. 1989. DiGeorge syndrome in a child with partial monosomy of chromosome 22. Uppsala J Med Sci 94:47

Balling R, Mutter G, Gruss P, Kessel M. 1989. Craniofacial abnormalities induced by ectopic expression of the homeobox gene *Hox-1.1* in transgenic mice. Cell 58:337

Barnes JD, Crosbey JL, Jones CM et al. 1994. Embryonic expression of *Lim-1*, the mouse homolog of *Xenopus XLim-1*, suggest a role in lateral mesoderm differentiation and neurogenesis. Dev Biol 161:168

Belloni E, Muenke M, Roessler E et al. 1996. Identification of Sonic Hedgehog as a candidate gene responsible for holoprosencephaly. Nature Genet 14:353

Bockman DE, Kirby ML. 1985. Neural crest interactions in the development of the immune system. J Immunol 135:766s

Burdi AR, Kusnetz AB, Venes JL, Gebarski SS. 1986. The natural history and pathogenesis of the cranial coronal ring articulations: implications in understanding the pathogenesis of the Crouzon craniostenotic defects. Cleft Palate 23:28

Chiang G, Litingtung Y, Lee E, Young KE, Cordon JF, Westphal H, Beachy PA. 1996. Cyclopia and defective axial patterning in mice lacking sonic hedgehog gene function. Nature 383:407

Ciment G, Weston JA. 1985. Segregation of developmental abilities in neural-crest-derived cells: identification of partially restricted intermediate cell types in the branchial arches of avian embryos. Dev Biol 111:73

Couly GF, LeDouarin N. 1987. Mapping of the early neural primordium in quail-chick chimeras. II. The prosencephalic neural plate and neural folds: implications for the genesis of cephalic human congenital abnormalities. Dev Biol 120:198

Cozzi F, Myers NA, Piacenti S et al. 1993. Maturational dysautonomia and facial anomalies associated with esophageal atresia: support for neural crest involvement. J Pediatr Surg 28:798

Cserjesi P, Brown D, Lyons GE et al. 1995. Expression of the novel basic helix-loop-helix gene *eHAND* in neural crest derivatives and extraembryonic membranes during mouse development. Dev Biol 170:664

Dean M. 1996. Polarity, proliferation and the hedgehog pathway. Nature Genet 14:245

Dolle P, Lufkin T, Krumlauf et al. 1993. Local alterations of *Krox20* and *Hox* gene expression in the hindbrain suggest lack of rhombomers 4 and 5 in homozygote null *Hoxa-1* (*Hoxa-1.6*) mutant embryos. Proc Natl Acad Sci U S A 90:7666

Ferguson MWJ. 1987. Palate development: mechanisms and malformations. Ir J Med Sci 156:309

Frasch M, Chen X, Lufkin T. 1995. Evolutionary-conserved enhancers direct region-specific expression of the murine *Hoxa-1* and *Hoxa-2* loci in both mice and *Drosophila*. Development 121:957

Fraser S, Keynes R, Lumsden A. 1990. Segmentation in the chick embryo hindbrain is defined by cell lineage restrictions. Nature (London) 344:431

Frohman MA, Martin GR, Cordes SP et al. 1993. Altered rhombomere-specific gene expression and hyoid bone differentiation in the mouse segmentation mutan, kreisler (kr). Development 117:925

Gaunt SJ, Sharpe PT, Duboule D. 1988. Spatially restricted domains of homeo-gene transcripts in mouse embryos: relation to a segmented body plan. Development 103(Suppl):169

Gendron-Maguire M, Mallo M, Zhang M et al. 1993. *Hoxa-2* mutant mice exhibit homeotic transformation of skeletal elements derived from cranial neural crest. Cell 75:1317

Goodrich ES. 1930. Studies on the Structure and Development of Vertebrates. Macmillan, London

Granstrom G, Kullaa-Mikkonen A. 1990. Experimental craniofacial malformations induced by retinoids and resembling branchial arch syndromes. Scand J Plast Reconstr Hand Surg 24:3

Hall BK. 1982. Mandibular morphogenesis and craniofacial malformations. J Craniofac Genet Dev Biol 2:309

Hanneman EH, Trevarrow B, Metcalfe W et al. 1988. Segmental pattern of development of the hindbrain and spinal cord of the zebrafish embryo. Development 103(Suppl):49

Hart P, Krumlauf R. 1991. Deciphering the *Hox* code: clues to patterning branchial regions of the head. Cell 66:1075

Hinojosa R, Green JD, Brecht K et al. 1996. Otocephalus: histopathology and three- dimensional reconstruction. Otolaryngol Head Neck Surg 114:44

Holland PWH. 1988. Homeobox genes and the human head. Development 103(Suppl):117

Hunt P, Ferretti P, Krumlauf F et al. 1995. Restoration of normal *Hox* code and branchial arch morphogenesis after extensive deletion of hindbrain neural crest. Dev Biol 168:584

Irving D, Willhite C, Burk D. 1986. Morphogenesis of isotretinoin-induced microcephaly and micrognathia studied by scanning electron microscopy. Teratology 34:141

Jacobson AG. 1993. Somitomeres: mesodermal segments of the head and trunk. In Hanken J, Hall BH (eds): The Skull. University of Chicago Press, Chicago

Kirby M. 1989. Plasticity and predetermination of mesencephalic and trunk neural crest transplanted into the region of the cardiac neural crest. Dev Biol 134:402

Krumlauf R. 1994. *Hoxgenes* in vertebrate development. Cell 78:191

Krumlauf R, Marshall H, Studer M et al. *Hox* homeobox genes and regionilization of the nervous system. J Neurobiol 24:1328

Kurtani SC, Eichele G. 1993. Rhombomere transplantation repatterns the segmental organization of cranial nerves and reveals cell-autonomous expression of a homeodomain protein. Development 117:105

LeDouarin N, Smith J. 1988. Development of the peripheral nervous system from the neural crest. Annu Rev Cell Biol 4:375

Lee YM, Osumi-Yamashita N, Ninomiya Y et al. 1995. Retinoic acid stage dependently alters the migration pattern and identity of hindbrain neural crest cells. Development 121:825

Lewis J. 1989. Genes and segmentation. Nature (London) 341:382

Lohnes D, Mark M, Mendelsohn C et al. 1995. Developmental roles of the retinoic acid receptors. J Steroid Biochem Mol Biol 53:475

Lumsden A, Sprawson N, Graham A. 1991. Segmental origin and migration of neural crest cells in the hindbrain region of the chick embryo. Development 113:1281

Lyn S, Giguere V. 1994. Localization of CRABP-I and CRABP-II mRNA in the early mouse embryo by whole-mount in situ hybridization: implications for teratogenesis and neural development. Dev Dynam 199:280

Mahmood R, Flanders KC, Morriss-Kay GM. 1992. Interactions between retinoids and TGF-β s in mouse morphogenesis. Development 116:67–74

Mahmood R, Kiefer P, Guthrie S et al. 1995. Multiple roles for FGF-3 during cranial neural development in the chicken. Development 121:1399

Manley NR, Cappecchi MR. 1995. The role of *Hoxa-3* in mouse thymus and thyroid development. Development 121:1989

Mark M, Lufkin T, Vonesch JL et al. 1993. Two rhombomers are altered in *Hoxa-1* mutant mice. Development 119:39

Marshall H, Nonchev S, Sham MH et al. Retinoic acid alters hindbrain *Hox* code and induces transformation of rhombomeres 2/3 into a 4/5 identity. Nature 360:737

McKay IJ, Muschamore I, Krumlauf R et al. 1994. The kreisler mouse: a hindbrain segmentation mutant that lacks two rhombomeres. Development 120:2199

McNutt TL, Harris C. 1994. Lindane embryotoxicity and differential alteration of cysteine and glutathione levels in rat embryos and visceral yolk sacs. Reprod Toxicol 8:351

Meier S. 1981. Development of the chick embryo mesoblast: morphogenesis of the prechordal plate and cranial segments. Dev Biol 83:49

Mendelsohn C, Lohnes D, Decimo D et al. 1994. Function of the retinoic acid receptors (RARs) during development (II). Multiple abnormalities at various stages of organogenesis in RAR double mutants. Development 120:2749

Moore G, Ivens A, Chambers J et al. 1988. The application of molecular genetics to detection of craniofacial abnormality. Development 103(Suppl):233

Moro Balbas JA, Gato A, Alonso Revuelta MI et al. 1993. Retinoic acid induces changes in the rhomboencephalic neural crest cells migration and extracellular matrix composition in chick embryos. Teratol 48:197

Morrison-Graham K, Schatteman GC, Bork T et al. 1992. A PDGF receptor mutation in the mouse (Patch) perturbs the development of a nonneuronal subset of neural crest-derived cells. Development 115:133

Nieto MA, Sechrist J, Wilkinson DG et al. 1995. Relationship between spatially restricted *Krox-20* gene expression in branchial neural crest and segmentation of the chick embryo hindbrain. EMBO J 14:1697

Murphy P, Davidson D, Hill RE. 1989. Segment-specific expression of a homeobox-containing gene in the mouse hindbrain. Nature (London) 341:156

Noden D. 1980. The migration and cytodifferentiation of cranial neural crest cells. p. 3. In Pratt RM, Christiansen RL (eds): Current Research Trends in Prenatal Craniofacial Development. Elsevier/North-Holland, New York

Noden DM. 1986. Patterning of avian craniofacial muscles. Dev Biol 116:347

Noden D. 1988. Interactions and fates of avian craniofacial mesenchyme. Development 103(Suppl):121

Nucci P, Manitto MP, Faiella A et al. 1994. Balanced translocation (t 2q; 10p) and ocular anomalies. A possible *Hox* gene defect. Ophthal Gen Z 15:129

Osumi-Yamashita N, Ninomiya Y, Doi H et al. 1994. The contribution of both forebrain and midbrain crest cells to the mesenchyme in the frontonasal mass of mouse embryos. Dev Biol 164:409

Pannese M, Polo C, Andreazzoli M et al. 1995. The *Xenophus* homolog of *Otx2* is a maternal homeobox gene that demarcates and specifies anterior body regions. Development 121:707

Popperl H, Bienz M, Studer M et al. 1995. Segmental expression of *Hoxb-1* is controlled by a highly conserved autoregulatory loop dependent upon *exd/pbx*. Cell 81:1031

Porter JA, Young KE, Beachy PA. 1996. Cholesterol modification of hedgehog signalling proteins in animal development. Science 274:255

Poswillo D. 1988. The aetiology and pathogenesis of craniofacial deformity. Development 103(Suppl):207

Prince V, Lumsden A. 1994. *Hoxa-2* expression in normal and transposed rhombomeres: independent regulation in the neural tube and neural crest. Development 120:911

Qiu M, Bulfone A, Martinez S et al. 1995. Null mutation of *Dlx-2* results in abnormal morphogenesis of proximal first and second branchial arch derivatives and abnormal differentiation in the forebrain. Genes Dev 9:2523

Raju K, Tang S, Dube ID et al. 1993. Characterization and developmental expression of *Tlx-1*, the murine homolog of *HOX11*. Mech Dev 44:51

Rijli FM, Mark M, Lakkaraju S et al. 1993. A homeotic transformation is generated in the rostral branchial region of the head by disruption of *Hoxa-2*, which acts like a selector gene. Cell 75:1333

Robinson GW, Mahon KA. 1994. Differential and overlapping expression domains of *Dlx-2* and *Dlx-3* suggest distinct roles for Distal-less homeobox genes in craniofacial development. Mech Dev 48:199

Roessler E, Belloni E, Gaudenz K et al. 1996. Mutations in the human Sonic Hedgehog gene cause holoprosencephaly. Nat Gen 14:357

Rutledge JC. 1989. Recent advances in prenatal craniofacial development: report of a conference and review of topics. Pediatr Pathol 9:613

Sechrist J, Scheron T, Bronner-Fraser M. 1994. Rhombomere rotation reveals that multiple mechanisms contribute to the segmental pattern of hindbrain neural crest migration. Development 120:1777

Sechrist J, Serbedzija GN, Scherson T et al. 1993. Segmental migration of the hindbrain neural crest does not arise from its segmental generation. Development 189:691

Sham MH, Vesque C, Nonchev S et al. 1993. The zinc finger gene *Krox20* regulates *HoxB2* (*Hox2.8*) during hindbrain segmentation. Cell 72:183

Shawlot W, Behringer R. 1995. Requirement for *Lim1* in head organization function. Nature 374:425

Shean ML, Duester G. 1993. The role of alcohol dehydrogenase in retinoic acid homeostasis and fetal alcohol syndrome. Alcohol Alcohol 2(suppl):51

Shum L, Sakakura Y, Bringas P Jr et al. 1993. EGF abrogation-induced fusilli-form dysmorphogenesis of Meckel's cartilage during embryonic mouse mandibula morphogenesis in vitro. Development 118:903

Simeone A, Acampora D, Arcioni L et al. 1990. Sequential activation of *HOX2* homeobox genes by retinoic acid in human embryonal carcinoma cells. Nature (London) 346:763

Simeone A, Avantaggiato V, Moroni MC et al. 1995. Retinoic acid induces stage-specific antero-posterior transformation of rostral central nervous system. Mech Dev 51:83

Slavkin HC. 1993. Rieger syndrome revisited: experimental approaches using pharmacologic and antisense strategies to abrogate EGF and TGF-alpha functions resulting in dysmorphogenesis during embryonic mouse craniofacial mophogenesis (review). Am J Med Genet 47:689

Snodgrass SR. 1994. Cocaine babies: a result of multiple teratogenic influences. J Child Neurol 9:227

Solazza L, Madaro E, De Gionni PP et al. 1994. Dermoid cysts of the oral floor. A clinical case report and review of the literature. Minerva Stomatol 43:171 Sperber GH, Honoré LH, Machin GA. 1989. Microscopic study of holoprosencephalic facial anomalies in trisomy 13 fetuses. Am J Med Genet 32:443

Sperber GH, Johnson ES, Honoré L, Machin GA. 1987. Holoprosencephalic synopthalmia (cyclopia) in an 8 week fetus. J Craniofac Genet Dev Biol 7:7

Studer M, Popperl H, Marshall H et al. 1994. Role of conserved retinoic acid response element in rhombomere restriction of *Hoxb-1*. Science 265:1728

Sulik KK, Cook CS, Webster WS. 1988. Teratogens and craniofacial malformations: relationships to cell death. Development 103 (Suppl):213

Sulik KK, Johnston MC, Daft PA et al. 1986. Fetal alcohol syndrome and DiGeorge anomaly: critical ethanol exposure periods for craniofacial malformations as illustrated in an animal model. Am J Med Genet 2(Suppl):97

Sulik KK, Johnston MC, Smiley SJ et al. 1987. Mandibulofacial dysostosis (Treacher Collins syndrome): a new proposal for pathogenesis. Am J Med Genet 27:359

Tan S, Morriss-Kay G. 1985. The development and distribution of the cranial neural crest in the rat embryo. Cell Tissue Res 240:403

Taylor LE, Bennett GD, Finnel RH. 1995. Altered gene expression in murine branchial arches following in utero exposure to retinoic acid. J Craniofac Genet Dev Biol 15:13

Tissier-Seta JP, Mucchielli ML, Mark M et al. 1995. *Barxl,* a new mouse homeodomain transcription factor expressed in craniofacial ectomesenchyme and the stomach. Mech Dev 51:3

Tongiori E, Bernhardt RR, Zinn K et al. 1995. Tenascin-C mRNA is expressed in cranial neural crest cells, in some placodal derivatives, and in discrete domains of the embryonic zebrafish brain. J Neurobiol 28:391

Trainor PA, Pam PP. 1995. Cranial paraxial mesoderm and neural crest cells of the mouse embryo: co-distribution of the craniofacial mesenchyme but distinct segregation in branchial arches. Development 121:2569

Tuckett F, Lim L, Morriss-Kay G. 1985. The ontogenesis of cranial neuromeres in the rat embryo. I. A scanning electron microscope and kinetic study. J Embryol Exp Morphol 87:215

Van Mierop LHS, Kutsche LM. 1986. Cardiovascular anomalies in DiGeorge syndrome and importance of neural crest as a possible pathogenetic factor. Am J Cardiol 58:133

Walker PJ, Edwards MJ, Petroff V et al. 1995. Agnathia (severe micrognathia), aglossia and choanal atresia in an infant. J Pediatr Child Health 31:358

Waterson EJ, Murray-Lyon IM. 1990. Preventing alcohol related birth damage: a review. Soc Sci Med 30:349

Webster WS, Lipson AH, Sulik KK. 1988. Interference with gastrulation during the third week of pregnancy as a cause of some facial abnormalities and CNS defects. Am J Med Genet 31:505

Wedden SE. 1987. Epithelial-mesenchymal interactions in the development of chick facial primordia and the target of retinoid action. Development 99:341

West JR, Chen WJ, Pantzis NJ. 1994. Fetal alcohol syndrome: the vulnerability of the developing brain and possible mechanisms of damage. Metab Brain Dis 9:291

Willhite C, Hill RM, Irving D. 1986. Isotretinoin-induced craniofacial malformations in humans and hamsters. J Craniofac Genet Dev Biol 2(Suppl):193

Zhang M, Kim HJ, marshall H et al. 1994. Ectopic *Hoxa-1* induces rhombomere transformation in mouse hindbrain. Development 120:2431

CHAPTER 13

Descriptive Embryology

Bossy J. 1980. Development of olfactory and related structures in staged human embryos. Anat Embryol 161:225

Brunjes PC, Frazier LL. 1986. Maturation and plasticity in the olfactory system of vertebrates. Brain Res Rev 11:1

Couly G, Le Douarin NM. 1988. The fate map of the cephalic neural primordium at the presomitic to the 3-somite stage in the avian embryo. Development 103(suppl.):101

D'Amico-Martel A. 1982. Temporal patterns of neurogenesis in avian cranial sensory and autonomic ganglia. Am J Anat 163:351

D'Amico-Martel A. 1983. Contributions of placodal and neural crest cells to avian cranial peripheral ganglia. Am J Anat 166:445

Davies AM. 1990. NGF synthesis and NGF receptor expression in the embryonic mouse trigeminal system. J Physiol (Paris) 84:100

Davies AM, Lumsden A. 1990. Ontogeny of the somatosensory system: origins and early development of primary sensory neurons. Annu Rev Neurosci 13:61

Didier YR, Gilbert W. 1990. Pioneer neurons in the mouse trigeminal sensory system. Proc Natl Acad Sci USA 87:923

Fontaine-Perus J, Chanconie M, Le Douarin NM. 1988. Developmental potentialities in the nonneuronal population of quail sensory ganglia. Dev Biol 128:359

Gilbert MS. 1935. Some factors influencing the early development of the mammalian hypophysis. Anat Rec 62:337

Herrup K. 1987. Roles of cell lineage in the developing mammalian brain. Curr Top Dev Biol 21:65

Hinrichsen K, Mestres P, Jacob HJ. 1986. Morphological aspects of the pharyngeal hypophysis in human embryos. Acta Morphol Neerl-Scand 24:235

Jacobson AG. 1981. Morphogenesis of the neural plate and tube. p. 233. In Connally TJ, Brinkley LL, Carlson BM (eds): Morphogenesis and Pattern Formation. Raven Press, New York

Jacobson M. 1984. Cell lineage analysis of neural induction: origins of cells forming the induced nervous system. Dev Biol 102:122

Jacobson M. 1985. Clonal analysis and cell lineages of the vertebrate central nervous system. Annu Rev Neurosci 8:71

Katz DM. 1990. Trophic regulation of nodose ganglion cell development: evidence for an expanded role of nerve growth factor during embryogenesis in the rat. Exp Neurol 110:1

Katz MJ. 1983. Ontophyletics of the nervous system: development of the corpus callosum and the evolution of axon tracts. Proc Natl Acad Sci USA 80:5936

Le Douarin N, Fontaine-Perus J, Couly G. 1986. Cephalic ectodermal placodes and neurogenesis. Trends Neurosci 9:175

Lefebve PP, Leprince P, Weber T et al. 1990. Neuronotrophic effect of developing otic vesicle on cochleo-vestibular neurons: evidence for nerve growth factor involvement. Brain Res 507:254

Lemire RJ, Loeser JD, Leech RW, Alvord EC. 1975. Normal and Abnormal Development of the Human Nervous System. Harper & Row, Hagerstown, MD

McKay RDG. 1989. The origins of cellular diversity in the mammalian central nervous system. Cell 58:815

Morriss-Kay G, Tuckett F. 1987. Fluidity of the neural epithelium during forebrain formation in rat embryos. J Cell Sci 8:433

Müller F, O'Rahilly R. 1980. The early development of the nervous system in staged insectivore and primate embryos. J Comp Neurol 193:741

Müller F, O'Rahilly R. 1986. The development of the human brain and the closure of the rostral neuropore at stage 11. Anat Embryol 175:205

Müller F, O'Rahilly R. 1986. The development of the human brain from a closed neural tube at stage 13. Anat Embryol 177:203

Müller F, O'Rahilly R. 1988. The first appearance of the future cerebral hemispheres of the human embryo at stage 14. Anat Embryol 177:495

Müller F, O'Rahilly R. 1989. The human brain at stage 17, including the appearance of the future olfactory bulb and the amygdaloid nuclei. Anat Embryol 180:353

Nichols DH. 1986. Formation and distribution of neural crest mesenchyme to the first pharyngeal arch region of the mouse embryo. Am J Anat 176:221

Noden D. 1984. Craniofacial development: new views on old problems. Anat Rec 208:1

Noden D. 1986. Origins and patterning of craniofacial mesenchymal tissues. J Craniofac Genet Dev Biol 2(suppl.):15

Northcutt RG, Gans C. 1983. The genesis of neural crest and epidermal placodes: a reinterpretation of vertebrate origins. Q Rev Biol 58:1

O'Rahilly R, Gardner E. 1971. The timing and sequence of events in the development of the human nervous system during the embryonic period proper. Z Anat Entwicklungsgesch 134:1

O'Rahilly R, Müller F. 1981. The first appearance of the human nervous system at stage 8. Acta Embryol 163:1

O'Rahilly R, Müller F. 1984. The early development of the hypoglossal nerve and occipital somites in staged human embryos. Am J Anat 169:237

O'Rahilly R, Müller F. 1984. Embryonic length and cerebral landmarks in staged human embryos. Anat Rec 209:265

O'Rahilly R, Müller F. 1986. The meninges in human development. J Neuropathol Exp Neurol 45:588

Rakic P. 1984. Organizing principles for development of primate cerebral cortex. p. 21. In Sharma SC (ed): Organizing Principles of Neural Development. Plenum Press, New York

Rakic P. 1984. Emergence of neuronal and glial cell lineages in primate brain. p. 29. In Black IB (ed): Cellular and Molecular Biology of Neural Development. Plenum Press, New York

Rubenstein JLR, Martinez S, Shinamura K, Puelles L. 1994. The embryonic forebrain: the prosomeric model. Science 266:576

Sakai Y. 1987. Neurulation in the mouse. I. The ontogenesis of neural segments and the determination of topographical regions in a central nervous system. Anat Rec 218:450

Schoenwolf G. 1982. On the morphogenesis of the early rudiments of the developing central nervous system. Scanning Electron Microsc 1:289

Sidman RL, Rakic P. 1973. Neuronal migration, with special reference to developing human brain: a review. Brain Res 62:1

Tam P. 1989. Regionalization of the mouse embryonic ectoderm: allocation of prospective ectodermal tissues during gastrulation. Development 107:55

Tan SS, Morriss-Kay G. 1985. The development and distribution of the cranial neural crest in the rat embryo. Cell Tissue Res 240:403

Van de Water TR. 1988. Tissue interactions and cell differentiation: neuron-sensory cell interaction during otic development. Development 103(suppl.):185

Walicke PA. 1989. Novel neurotrophic factors, receptors, and oncogenes. Annu Rev Neurosci 12:103

Williams RW, Herrup K. 1988. The control of neuron cell number. Annu Rev Neurosci 11:423

Wilson-Pauwels L, Akesson EJ, Stewart PA. 1988. Cranial Nerves: Anatomy and Clinical Comments. BC Decker Inc, Toronto

Windle W. 1970. Development of neural elements in human embryos of four to seven weeks gestation. Exp Neurol (Suppl) 5:44

Applications to Clinical Practice

Bovolenta P, Dodd J. 1990. Guidance of commissural growth cones at the floor plate in embryonic rat spinal cord. Development 109:435

Burden-Gulley SM, Payne HR, Lemmon V. 1995. Growth cones are actively influenced by substrate-bound adhesion molecules. J Neurosci 15:4370

Caddy KWT, Sidman RL, Eicher EM. 1981. Stumbler, a new mutant mouse with cerebellar disease. Brain Res 208:251

Calof AL, Campanero MR, O'Rear JJ et al. 1994. Domainspecific activation of neuronal migration and neurite out-growth-promoting activities of laminin. Neuron 13:117

Chou SM, Gilbert EF, Chun RWM et al. 1990. Infantile olivopontocerebellar atrophy with spinal muscular atrophy (infantile OPCA + SMA). Clin Neuropathol 9:21

Clarkson TW. 1993. Mercury: major issues in environmental health. Environ Health Perspect 100:31

Cohen A, Bray GM, Aquayo AJ. 1994. Neurotrophin-4/5 (NT-4/5) increases adult rat retinal ganglion cell survival and neurite outgrowth in vitro. J Neurobiol 25:953

Colello RJ, Guillery RW. 1990. The early development of retinal ganglion cells with uncrossed axons in the mouse: retinal position and axonal course. Development 108:515

Cook JE. 1991. Correlated activity in the CNS: a role on every time scale? Trends Neurosci 14:397

Drescher U, Dremoser C, Handwerker C et al. 1995. In vitro guidance of retinal ganglion cell axons by RAGs, a 25 kDa tectal protein related to ligands for Egh receptor tyrosine kinases. Cell 87:359

Goshima Y, Nakamura F, Strittmatter P, Strittmatter SM. 1995. Collapsin-induced growth cone collapse mediated by an intracellular protein related to UNC-33. Nature 376:509

Gottmann K, Lux HD. 1995. Growth cone calcium ion channels: properties, clustering, and functional roles (review). Perspect Dev Neurobiol 2:371

Gouw LG, Digre KB, Harris CP et al. 1994. Autosomal dominant cerebellar ataxia with retinal degeneration: clinical neuropathological and genetic analysis of a large kindred. Neurology 44:1441

Halfter W, Yip, YP, Yip JW. 1994. Axonin 1 is expressed primarily in subclasses of avian sensory neurons during outgrowth. Brain Res 78:87

Hankin MH, Lagenaur CF. 1994. Cell adhesion molecules in the early developing mouse retina: retinal neurons show preferential outgrowth in vitro on L1 but not N-CAM. J Neurobiol 25:472

Hanks M, Wurst W, Anson-Cartwright L et al. 1995. Rescue of the *En-1* mutant phenotype by replacement of *En-1* by *En-2*. Science 269:679

Harding BN, Dunger DB, Grant DB, Erdohazi M. 1988. Familial olivopontocerebellar atrophy with neonatal onset: a recessively inherited syndrome with systemic and biochemical abnormalities. J Neurol Neurosurg Psychiatry 51:385

Hatten ME, Liem RKH, Mason CA. 1984. Defects in specific associations between astroglia and neurons occur in microcultures of weaver mouse cerebellar cells. J Neurosci 4:1163

Hatten ME, Liem RKH, Mason CA. 1986. Weaver mouse cerebellar granule neurons fail to migrate on wild-type astroglial processes *in vitro*. J Neurosci 6:2676

Herrup K, Sunter K. 1987. Numerical matching during cerebellar development: quantitative analysis of granule cell death in staggerer mouse chimeras. J Neurosci 7:829

Isaacs KR, Abbott LC. 1992. Development of the paramedian lobule of the cerebellum in wild-type and tottering mice. Dev Neurosci 14:386

Kater SB, Rehder V. 1995. The sensory-motor role of growth cone filopedia (review). Curr Opin J Neurobiol 5:68

Kolodkin AL, Matthes DJ, Goodman CS. 1993. The semaphorin genes encode a family of transmembrane and secreted growth cone guidance molecules. Cell 75:1389

Kumar D. 1986. Genetic aspects of congenital cerebellar ataxia. Indian J Pediatr 53:761

Leone M, Brignolio F, Rosso MG et al. 1990. Friedrich's ataxia: a descriptive epidemiological study in an Italian population. Clin Genet 38:161

Lin CH, Forscher P. 1993. Cytoskeletal remodeling during growth cone-target interactions. J Cell Biol 121:1369

McMahon AP, Bradley A. 1990. The *Wnt-1(int-1)* protooncogene is required for development of a large region of the mouse brain. Cell 62:1073

O'Leary. 1991. Development (suppl.) 2:123

O'Leary DDM, Fawcett JW, Cowan WM. 1986. Topographic targeting errors in the retinocollicular projection and their elimination by selective ganglion cell death. J Neurosci 6:3692

O'Rahilly R. 1983. The timing and sequence of events in the development of the human eye and ear during the embryonic period proper. Anat Embryol 168:87

O'Rourke NA, Fraser SE. 1990. Dynamic changes in optic fiber terminal arbors lead to retinotopic map formation: an in vivo confocal microscopic study. Neuron 5:159

Pallas SL, Roe AW, Sur M. 1990. Visual projections induced into the auditory pathway of ferrets. I. Novel inputs to primary auditory cortex (AI) from the LP/pulvinar complex and the topography of the MGN-AI projection. J Comp Neurol 298:50

Puschel AW, Adams RH, Betz H. 1995. Murine semaphorin D/collapsin is a member of a diverse gene family and creates domains inhibitory for axonal extension. Neuron 14:941

Rader C, Stoeckli ET, Ziegler U et al. 1993. Cell-cell adhesion by homophilic interaction of the neuronal recognition molecule axonin-1. Eur J Biochem 214:133

Roberts CW, Sonder AM, Lumsden A, Korsmeyer SJ. 1995. Development expression of *Hox11* and specification of splenic cell fate. Am J Pathol 146:1089

Salinas PC, Fletcher C, Copeland NG et al. 1994. Maintenance of Wnt-3 expression in Purkinje cells of the mouse cerebellum depends on interactions with granule cells. Development 120:1277

Sandib M, Rao Y, Siu CH. 1994. The homophilic binding site of the neural cell adhesion molecule NCAM is directly involved in promoting neurite outgrowth from cultured neural retinal cells. J Biol Chem 269:14841

Schiller F. 1995. Staggering gait in medical history. Ann Neurol 37:127

Sidman RL, Conover CS, Carson JH. 1985. Shiverer gene maps near the distal end of chromosome 18 in the house mouse. Cytogenet Cell Genet 39:241

Sidman RL, Green MC, Appel SH. 1965. Catalog of the Neurological Mutants of the Mouse. Harvard University Press, Cambridge, MA

Sidman RL, Willinger M, Margolis DM. 1983. Mouse weaver mutation affects granule cell neurite growth *in vitro*. Birth Defects Orig Artic Ser 19:189

Simon H, Gurthrie S, Lumsden A. 1994. Rebulation of SCI/Dm-GRASP during the migration of motor neurons in the chick embryo brain stem. J Neurobiol 25:1129

Sonmez E, Herrup K. 1984. Role of staggerer gene in determining cell number in cerebellar cortex. II. Granule cell death and persistence of external granule cell layer in young mouse chimeras. Dev Brain Res 12:271

Sperry RW. 1963. Chemoaffinity in the orderly growth of nerve fiber patterns and connections. Proc Natl Acad Sci USA 50:703

Sretavan DW, Feng L, Pure E, Reichert LF. 1994. Embryonic neurons of the developing optic chiasm express L1 qand CD44, cell surface molecules with opposing effects on retinal axon growth. Neuro 12:957

Stoecki ET, Landmesser LT. 1995. Axonin-1, Nr-CAM, and Ng-CAM play different roles in the in vivo guidance of chick commissural neurons. Neuron 14:1165

Strittmatter SM, Igarashi M, Fishman MC. 1994. Gap-43 amino terminal peptides modulate growth cone morphology and neurite outgrowth. J Neurosci 14:5503

Strittmatter SM, Fankauser C, Huang PL et al. 1995. Neuronal pathfinding is abnormal in mice lacking the neuronal growth cone protein GAP-43. Cell 80:445

Superneau D, Wertelecki W, Zellweger H. 1985. Letter to the editor: the Marinesco-Sjögren syndrome described a quarter of a century before Marinesco. Am J Genet 22:647

Sussman DJ, Klingensmith J, Salinas P et al. 1994. Isolation and characterization of a mouse homolog of the *Drosophila* segment polarity gene dishevelled. Dev Biol 166:73

Thomas KR, Capecchi MR. 1990. Targeted disruption of the murine *int-1* proto-oncogene resulting in sever abnormalities in midbrain and cerebellar development. Nature (London) 346:847

Thomas KR, Musci TS, Neumann PE, Capecchi MR. 1991. Swaying is a mutant allele of the proto-oncogene *Wnt-1*. Cell 67:969

Vaughan L, Weber P, D'Alessandri L et al. 1994. Tenascin-contactin/F11 interactions: a clue for a developmental role? Perspect Dev Neurobiol 2:43

Weimar WR, Lane PW, Sidman RL. 1982. Vibrator *(vb):* a spinocere-bellar system degeneration with autosomal recessive inheritance in mice. Brain Res 251:357

Wurst W, Auerbach AB, Joyner AL. 1994. Multiple developmental defects in Engrailed-1 mutant mice: an early mid-hindbrain dele-tion and patterning defects in forelimbs and sternum. Development 120:2065

Zheng JQ, Felder M, Conner JA, Poo MM. 1994. Turning of the nerve growth cones induced by neurotransmitters (see comments). Nature 368:140

Zheng JQ, Wan JJ, Poo MM. 1996. Essential role of filopodia in chemotactic turning of nerve growth cone induced by glutamate gradient. J Neurosci 16:1140

CHAPTER 14

Barnhill RL, Wolf JE. 1987. Angiogenesis and the skin. J Am Acad Dermatol 16:1226

Biggs PJ, Wooster R, Ford D et al. 1995. Familial cylindromatosis (turban tumour syndrome) gene localized to chromosome 16q12–q13: evidence for its role as a tumor suppressor gene. Na-ture Genet 11:441

Blecher SR, Kapalanga J, LaLonde D. 1990. Induction of sweat glands by epidermal growth factor in murine X-linked anhidrotic ectodermal dysplasia. Nature (London) 345:542

Byrne C, Tainsky M, Fuchs E. 1994. Programming gene expression in developing epidermis. Development 120:2369

Chang JC, Smith LR, Froning KJ et al. 1995. CD8+ T-cells in psori-atic lesions preferentially use T-cell receptors V beta 3 and/or V beta 13.1 genes. Ann NY Acad Sci 756:370

Chiego DJ Jr. 1995. The early distribution and possible role of nerves during odontogenesis. Int J Dev Biol 39:191

Epstein EH Jr. 1993. The morbid cutaneous anatomy of the human genome. Arch Dermatol 129:1417

Foster C, Bertram JF, Holbrook KA. 1988. Morphometric and statisti-cal analyses describing the *in utero* growth of human epidermis. Anat Rec 222:201

Foster C, Holbrook KA. 1989. Ontogeny of Langerhans cells in human embryonic and fetal skin: cell densities and phenotypic ex-pression relative to epidermal growth. Am J Anat 184:157

French LE, Chonn A, Ducrest D et al. 1993. Murine clusterin: molecular cloning and mRAN localization of a gene associated with epithelial differentiation processes during embryogenesis. J Cell Biol 122:1119

Fuchs E. 1990. Epidermal differentiation: the bare essentials. J Cell Biol 111:2807

Gans C. 1988. Craniofacial growth, evolutionary questions. Develop-ment 103(suppl.):3

Hahn H, Wicking C, Zaphiropoulos PG, Cjailani MR, Shanley S, Chidambaram A et al. 1996. Mutations of the human homolog of Drosophila patched in the nevoid basal cell carcinoma syndrome. Cell. 85:841

Heikinheimo K. 1994. Stage-specific expression of decapentaplegic-Vg-related genes 2,4, and 6 (bone morphogenetic proteins 2, 4, and 6) during human tooth development. J Dent Res 73:590

Helder MN, Ozkaynak E, Sampath KT et al. 1995. Expression pattern of osteogenic protein-1 (bone morphogenetic protein-7) in human and mouse development. J Histochem Cytochem 43:1035

Holbrook KA. 1988. Structural abnormalities of the epidermally derived appendages in skin from patients with ectodermal dysplasia: insight into developmental errors. Birth Defects Orig Artic Ser 24:15

Holbrook K. 1989. Biologic structure and function: perspectives on morphologic approaches to the study of the granular layer ker-atinocyte. J Invest Dermatol 92:84S

Holbrook KA, Dale BA, Smith LT et al. 1987. Markers of adult skin expressed in the skin of the first trimester fetus. Curr Probl Derma-tol 16:94

Holbrook K, Smith LT. 1981. Ultrastructural aspects of human skin during the embryonic, fetal, premature, neonatal, and adult periods of life. Birth Defects Orig Artic Ser 17:9

Holbrook KA, Underwood RA, Vogel AM et al. 1989. The appear-ance, density, and distribution of melanocytes in human embryonic and fetal skin revealed by the anti-melanoma monoclonal anti-body, HMB-45. Anat Embryol 180:443

Holbrook K, Vogel AM, Underwood RA, Foster CA. 1988. Mela-nocytes in human embryonic and fetal skin: a review and new find-ings. Pigm Cell Res 1 (suppl.):6

Johnson CL, Holbrook KA. 1989. Development of human embryonic and fetal dermal vasculature. J Invest Dermatol 93:10s

Kollar EJ. 1981. Tooth development and dental patterning. p. 87. In Connelly TJ, Brinkley LL, Carlson BM (eds): Morphogenesis and Pattern Formation. Raven Press, New York

Krey AK, Moshell AN, Dayton DH et al. 1987. Morphogenesis and malformations of the skin. NICHD/NIADDK Research Workshop. J Invest Dermatol 88:464

Lumsden AGS. 1988. Spatial organization of the epithelium and the role of neural crest cells in the initiation of the mammalian tooth germ. Development 103(suppl.):155

Lumsden AGS, Buchanan JAG. 1986. An experimental study of timing and topography of early tooth development in the mouse embryo with an analysis of the role of innervation. Arch Oral Biol 31:301

Mina M, Kollar EJ. 1987. The induction of odontogenesis in non-dental mesenchyme combined with early murine mandibular arch epithelium. Arch Oral Biol 32:123

Moore K. 1988. The Developing Human. WB Saunders, Philadelphia

Moynahan EJ. 1974. The developmental biology of the skin. p. 526. In Davis JA, Dobbing J (ed): Scientific Foundations of Paediatrics. WB Saunders, Philadelphia

Newman M. 1988. Supernumerary nipples. Am Fam Physician 38:183

Nieukoop PD, Johnen AG, Albers B. 1985. The Epigenetic Nature of Early Chordate Development. p. 249. Cambridge University Press, Cambridge

Niswander L, Martin GR. 1992. Egf-4 expression during gastrulation, myogenesis, limb and tooth development in the mouse. Develop-ment 114:755

Nordlund J. 1986. The lives of pigment cells. Dermatol Clin 4:407

Nordlund JJ, Abdel-Malek ZA, Boissy R, Rheins LA. 1989. Pigment cell biology: an historical review. J Invest Dermatol 92:53S

Pablos JL, Everett ET, Harley R et al. 1995. Transforming growth factor-β 1 and collagen gene expression during postnatal skin de-velopment and fibrosis in tight skin mouse. Lab Invest 72:670

Perkins T, Trickler DP, Shklar G. 1988. Improvement of dental devel-opment in osteopetrotic mice by maternal vitamin D_3 sulfate ad-ministration. J Craniofac Genet Dev Biol 8:83

Polakowska RR, Haake AR. 1994. Apoptosis: the skin from a new perspective. Death Differ 1:19

Price ML, Griffiths WAD. 1985. Normal body hair—a review. Clin Exp Dermatol 10:87

Ranta R. 1986. A review of tooth formation in children with cleft lip/plate. Am J Orthod Dentofac Orthop 90:11

Salinas CF. 1981. Orodental findings and genetic disorders. Birth Defects Orig Artic Ser 18:79

Satokata I, Maas R. 1994. Msx1 deficient mice exhibit cleft palate and abnormalities of craniofacial and tooth development, Nature Genet 6:348

Sasaki S, Shimokawa H. 1995. The amelogenin gene. Int J Dev Biol 39:127

Scott G, Ewing J, Ryan D, Abboud C. 1994. Stem cell factor regulates human melanocyte-matrix interactions. Pigment Cell Res 7:44

Slavkin HC. 1987. Gene regulation in the development of oral tissues. J Dent Res 67:1142

Slavkin HC, MacDougall M, Zeichner-David M et al. 1988. Molecular determinants of cranial neural crest-derived odontogenic estomesenchyme during dentinogenesis. Am J Med Genet 4:7

Slootweg PJ, de Weger RA. 1994. Immunohistochemical demonstration of bc1-2 protein in human tooth germs. Arch Oral Biol 39:545

Smith LT, Holbrook KA. 1986. Embryogenesis of the dermis in human skin. Pediatr Dermatol 3:271

Spritz RA, Ho L, Strunk KM. 1994. Inhibition of proliferation of human melanocytes by a KIT antisense oligodeoxynucleotide: implications for human piebaldism and mouse dominant white spotting (W). J Invest Dermatol 103:148

Takahashi J, Ikeda T. 1995. Molecular cloning and expression of rat and mouse B16 gene: implications on organogenesis. Oncogene 11:879

Turner EP. 1974. The growth and development of the teeth. p. 420. In Davis JA, Dobbing J (eds): Scientific Foundations of Paediatrics. WB Saunders, Philadelphia

van Oostrom CT, de Vries A, Verbeek, SJ et al. 1994. Cloning and characterization of the mouse *XPAC* gene. Nucleic Acids Res 22:11

CHAPTER 15

Almici C, Carlo-Stella C, Wagner JE, Rizzoli V. 1995. Umbilical cord blood as a source of hematopoietic stem cells: from research to clinical application. Hematologica 80:473

Bernischke K, Driscoll SG. 1967. The placenta in multiple pregnancy. Handb Pathol Histol 7:187

Bordignon C, Notarangelo LD, Nobili N et al. 1995. Gene therapy in peripheral blood lymphocytes and bone marrow for ADA-immunodeficient patients. Science 270:470

Brambati B, Tului L, Simoni G, Travi M. 1991. Genetic diagnosis before the eighth gestational week. Obstet Gynecol 77:318

Brundin P, Bjorklund A, Lindvall O. 1990. Practical aspects of the use of human fetal brain tissue for intracerebral grafting. Prog Brain Res 82:707

Burton DJ, Filly RA. 1991. Sonographic analysis of the amniotic band syndrome. AJR 156:555

Caldwell MB, Rodgers MF. 1991. Epidemiology of pediatric HIV infection. Pediatr Clin North Am 38:1

Castellucci M, Scheper M, Scheffen I et al. 1990. The development of the human villous tree. Anat Embryol 181:117

Champetier J, Yver R, Tomasella T. 1989. Functional anatomy of the liver of the human fetus: applications of ultrasonography. Surg Radiol Anat 11:53

Chiriboga CA, Vibbert M, Malouf R et al. 1995. Neurological correlates of fetal cocaine exposure: transient hypertonia of infancy and early childhood. Pediatrics 96:1070

Christ JE. 1990. Plastic surgery for the fetus. Plast Reconstr Surg 86:1238

Crombleholme TM, Langer JC, Harrison MR, Zanjani ED. 1991. Transplantation of fetal cells. Am J Obstet Gynecol 164:218

Dado DV, Kernahan DA, Gianopoulos JG. 1990. Intra-uterine repair of cleft lip: what's involved. Plast Reconstr Surg 85:461

Dick JE, Magli MC, Huszar D et al. 1985. Introduction of a selectable gene into primitive stem cells capable of long-term reconstitution of the hemopoietic system of *W/W* mice. Cell 42:71

Doran TA. 1990. Chorionic villus sampling as the primary diagnostic tool in prenatal diagnosis. J Reprod Med 35:935

Dunbar CE, Emmons RV. 1994. Gene transfer into hematopoietic progenitor and stem cells: progress and problems. Stem Cells 12:563

Editorial. 1990. Editorial comments. J Am Osteopathol Assoc 90:970

European Collaborative Study. 1991. Children born to women with HIV-1 infection: natural history and risk of transmission. Lancet 337:253

Evans MI. 1989. Fetal surgery in the 1990's. Am J Dis Child 143:1431

Evans RG (ed). Council on Scientific Affairs. 1991. Medical diagnostic ultrasound instrumentation and clinical interpretation. Report of the Ultrasonography Task-force. JAMA 265:1155

Fox DA. 1995. Biological therapies: a novel approach to the treatment of autoimmune disease. Am J Med 99:82

Goldsmith MF. 1988. Anencephalic organ donor program suspended; Loma Linda report expected to detail findings. JAMA 260:1671

Gwinn M, Pappaioanou M, George JR et al. 1990. Prevalence of HIV infection in childbearing women in the United States. JAMA 265:1704

Hallock GG. 1990. In defense of intrauterine repair of cleft lip. Plast Reconstr Surg 86:801

Hanania EG, Kavanagh J, Hortobagyi G et al. 1995. Recent advances in the application of gene therapy to human disease. Am J Med 99:537

Harrison MR, Adzik NS, Longaker MT et al. 1990. Successful repair in utero of a fetal diaphragmatic hernia after removal of herniated viscera from the left thorax. N Engl J Med 322:1582

Hepper PG. 1995. Human fetal behavior and maternal cocaine use: a longitudinal study. Neurotoxicology 16:139

Holloway M. 1990. Experimental surgery may feed ethical debates. Sci Am 263:46

Jones KL, Bernischke K. 1983. The developmental pathogenesis of structural defects: the contribution of monozygotic twins. Semin Perinatol 7:239

Jones SA, Challis JRG. 1990. Effects of corticotropin releasing hormone and adenocorticotropin on prostaglandin output by human placenta and fetal membranes. Gynecol Obstet Invest 29:165

Kaplan P, Normandin J, Wilson GN et al. 1990. Malformations and minor anomalies in children whose mothers had prenatal diagnosis: comparison between CVS and amniocentesis. Am J Med Genet 37:366

Karson EM. 1990. Prospects for gene therapy. Biol Reprod 42:39

Kohn DB, Weinberg KI, Nolta JA, Heiss LN, Lenarsky C, Crooks GM, Hanley ME, Annett G, Brooks JS, el-Koureiy A et al. 1995. Engraftment of gene modified umbilical cord blood cells in neonates with adenosine deaminase deficiency. Nature Med 1:1017

Kumar RM, Uduman SA, Khurranna AK. 1995. Impact of maternal HIV-1 infection on perinatal outcome. Int J Gynecol Obstet 49:137

Leach RE, Ory SJ. 1989. Modern management of ectopic pregnancy. J Reprod Med 34:324

Livingston RA, Hutton N, Halsey NA et al. 1995. Human immunodeficiency virus-specific IgA in infants born to human immunodeficiency virus-seropositive women. Arch Pediatr Adol Med 149:503

Lipshultz SE, Frssica JJ, Orav EJ. 1991. Cardiovascular abnormalities in infants prenatally exposed to cocaine. J Pediatr 118:44

Longaker MT, Golbus MS, Filly R et al. 1991. Maternal outcome after open fetal surgery. A review of the first 17 human cases. JAMA 265:737

Lu L, Shen RN, Broxmeyer HE. 1996. Stem cells from bone marrow, umbilical cord blood and peripheral blood for clinical application: current status and future application. [Review]. Crit REv Oncol-Hemat 22:61

Luebke HJ, Reiser CA, Pauli RM. 1990. Fetal disruptions: assessment of frequency, heterogeneity, and embryological mechanisms in a population referred to a community-based stillbirth assessment program. Am J Med Genet 36:56

Marshall E. 1995. Gene therapy's growing pains. Science 269:1050

Moore KL. 1988. The Developing Human. Clinically Oriented Embryology. WB Saunders, Philadelphia

Olsen GD. 1995. Potential mechanisms of cocaine-induced developmental neurotoxicity: a minireview. Neurotoxicology 16:159

Orrell RW, Lilford RJ. 1990. Chorionic villus sampling and rare side effects: will a randomised controlled trial detect them? Int J Gynecol Obstet 32:29

Peabody JL, Emery JR, Aswal S. 1989. Experience with anencephalic infants as prospective organ donors. N Engl J Med 321:344

Quinn NP. 1990. The clinical application of cell grafting techniques in patients with Parkinson's disease. Prog Brain Res 82:619

Ray JG. 1995. Lues-lues: maternal and fetal considerations of syphilis. Obstet Gynecol Surv 50:845

Reynolds DW, Stagno S, Alford CA. 1986. Congenital cytomegalovirus infection. p. 93. In Sever JL, Brent RL (eds): Teratogen Update: Environmentally Induced Birth Defect Risks. Alan R Liss, New York

Rosenfeld MA, Chu CS, Seth P et al. 1994. Gene transfer to freshly isolated human repsiratory epithelial cells in vitro using replication-deficient adenovirus containing the human cystic fibrosis transmembrane conductance regulator cDNA. Hum Gene Ther 5:331

Rothenberg LS. 1990. The anencephalic neonate and brain death: an international review of medical, ethical, and legal issues. Transplant Proc 22:1037

Sachs ES, Jahoda MGJ, Los FJ et al. 1990. Interpretation of chromosome mosaicism and discrepancies in chorionic villous studies. Am J Med Genet 37:268

Santulli TV. 1990. Fetal echocardiography: assessment of cardiovascular anatomy and function. Clin Perinatol 17:911

Schlesinger C, Raabe G, Ngo T, Miller K. 1990. Discordant findings in chorionic villus direct preparation and long term culture—mosaicism in the fetus. Prenatal Diagn 10:609–612

Slavkin HC. 1995. Molecular biology experimental strategies for craniofacial-oral-dental dysmorphology. Connect Tissue Res 32:233

Snodgrass SR. 1994. Cocaine babies: a result of multiple teratogenic influences. J Child Neurol 9:227

Stolar CJH. 1990. Repair in utero of a fetal diaphragmatic hernia. N Engl J Med 323:1279

Taylor BJ, Chadduck WM, Kletzel M et al. 1990. Anencephalic infants as organ donors: the medical, legal, moral, and economic issues. J Arkansas Med Soc 87:184

Thompson MW. 1986. Genetics in Medicine. 4th Ed. WB Saunders, Philadelphia

Touraine JL, Raudrant D, Royo C et al. 1991. In utero transplantation of hemopoietic stem cells in humans. Transplant Proc 23:1706

Wapner RJ, Jackson L. 1988. Chorionic villus sampling. Clin Obstet Gynecol 31:328

Ward H. 1990. Review of the development and current status of techniques for monitoring embryonic and fetal development in the first trimester of pregnancy. Am J Med Genet 35:157

Warwick R, Williams PL. 1990. Gray's Anatomy. 36th Ed. Churchill Livingstone, Edinburgh

Werler MM, Pober BR, Holmes LB. 1986. Smoking and pregnancy. p. 131. In Sever JL, Brent RL (eds): Teratogen Update: Environmentally Induced Birth Defect Risks. Alan R Liss, New York

Glossary

A

Abdominal foregut Segment of the gastrointestinal tract that is vascularized by the celiac trunk; includes the abdominal esophagus, stomach, and upper half of the duodenum.

Abducent nerve (VI) Possesses only motor functions and innervates the lateral rectus muscles of the eyeball.

Abembryonic Away from the embryo.

Achrodolichomelia Disproportionately large hands and feet.

Acoustic (cochlear) ganglion of nerve VIII Neurons of this ganglion (serving special sense of hearing) arise from ectoderm within the otic placode.

Adactyly Absence of all the digits on a limb.

Adenohypophysis Anterior lobe of the pituitary formed by invagination of stomodeal ectoderm (Rathke's pouch); produces small peptide hormones including prolactin, luteinizing hormone, and follicle-stimulating hormone in response to blood-borne releasing factors produced by the hypothalamus.

Alar (dorsal) columns Pair of columns of the spinal cord and brain stem formed by gray matter of the dorsal regions of the neural tube; cells give rise to association neurons.

Alisphenoid bone Bone of the orbit that arises from the palatopterygoquadrate bar.

Allantois Ventral diverticulum of the hindgut that becomes a superior extension of the primitive urogenital sinus after partitioning of the cloaca; forms the urachus or median umbilical ligament.

Alveolus See **Mature alveoli.**

Alveolus (of tooth) Bony socket of the tooth formed by mesenchyme of the dental sac; teeth are anchored to it by the periodontal ligament.

Ambisexual stage (also **Indifferent phase**) Course of genital development in male and female embryos is virtually identical until the seventh week.

Amelia Absence of one or more limbs.

Ameloblasts Ectodermal cells that differentiate from the inner enamel epithelium; secrete the enamel of the tooth.

Amnioblasts Cells differentiated from epiblast cells that form the amniotic membrane.

Amniocentesis Aspiration of amniotic fluid for analysis, usually through a needle inserted into the amnion via the abdominal wall; typically done between 14 and 16 weeks of gestation.

Amnion (amniotic cavity) Appears on day 8 as fluid begins to collect between epiblast cells; eventually fills with amniotic fluid for protection and space for growth of embryo and fetus.

Amniotic fluid Dialysate of blood, first secreted by the amniotic membrane; by 16 weeks of gestation fetal urine is a major contributor to volume.

Amniotic membrane Surrounds the amnion; inner layer is composed of amnioblasts while the outer layer is extraembryonic somatopleuric mesoderm.

Ampulla Structures that form at tips of bifurcating ureteric buds; ultimately induce the metanephric intermediate mesoderm to form nephrons.

Anal membrane Formed at about 7 weeks, along with the urogenital membrane, as the cloacal membrane is divided by the urorectal septum.

Anal pit (proctodeum) Ectoderm-lined invagination formed by proliferation of mesenchyme surrounding the anal membrane; forms the lower one-third of the anorectal canal.

Anencephaly Anomaly caused by failure of the neuropore to close; brain may be completely missing or reduced to an exposed dorsal mass of undifferentiated neural tissue.

Angioblastic cords Short blind-ended cords formed as angiocysts coalesce.

Angioblastic plexuses Formed as angioblastic cords coalesce into complex interconnected vascular networks.

Angioblasts Vessel-forming cells that may arise from any kind of mesoderm except prechordal plate mesoderm.

Angiocysts Vesicles formed by angioblasts during the process of vasculogenesis.

Angiogenesis Mechanism whereby pre-existing vessels lengthen or branch by sprouting.

Anterior cardinal veins Bilaterally symmetric, paired veins that drain blood from the head and neck into their respective common cardinal veins during early fourth week; distal ends give rise to internal jugular veins; proximal right end becomes the superior vena cava.

Anterior commissure Fiber tract that develops within the lamina terminalis at the most cranial end of the telencephalon to connect olfactory centers in the left and right cerebral hemispheres.

Anterior lobe (of the pituitary) See **Adenohypophysis.**

Anti-müllerian hormone (AMH) Member of the TGF-β family; produced by pre-Sertoli cells following expression of the sex-determining region of the Y chromosome; causes regression of the paramesonephric ducts (also termed **Müllerian-inhibiting substance [MIS]**).

Aortic arches Paired arteries derived from arteries surrounding the pharynx of piscine progenitors; correspond to arches 1, 2, 3, 4, and 6 of the ancestral fish but have become highly modified to form the great vessels of the thorax.

Aortic sac Aortic arches (2, 3, 4, and 6) sprout from this most distal specialization of the truncus arteriosus; forms part of the arch of the aorta and the brachiocephalic artery.

Aortic valve See **Semilunar valves.**

Apical ectodermal ridge Thickening at the distal end of the limb bud that induces underlying mesodermal core to grow distally; type of segment produced from the mesodermal core depends on a *HOX* gene combinatorial code.

Apocrine glands Coiled glands that develop with hair follicles; later lost except in the regions of the mons pubis, axilla, prepuce, scrotum, and labia minora; at puberty they produce complex secretions modified by bacterial activity into odorous compounds that may function in social and sexual communication.

Appendix epididymis Small remnant of the degenerate cranial end of the mesonephric duct in males.

Appendix testis Small remnant of the proximal end of the paramesonephric duct in males.

Arrector pili muscle Smooth muscle within the papillary layer of the dermis attached to the dermal root sheath of the hair follicle; raises the hair shaft, causing "goose flesh."

Ascending aorta Most proximal segment of the aorta derived from the truncus arteriosus.

Association neurons Cells of the dorsal column that develop to interconnect the motor neurons of the ventral columns with neuronal processes.

Associational nuclei (of the cranial nerves) Neuronal concentrations formed by gray matter of the alar columns of the brain stem; serve cranial nerves V, VII, VIII, IX, and X.

Astrocytes Neuroglial cells of the central nervous system; one of many kinds of non-neuronal "supporting" cells of the central nervous system; formed by glioblasts arising from cells of the ventricular layer of the neural tube.

Atrioventricular node (AVN) Secondary pacemaker region within the superior endocardial cushion that receives impulses from the sinoatrial node (SAN) to regulate beating of the ventricles.

Atrioventricular sulcus Constriction that demarcates the primitive atrium and primitive ventricle in the third week.

Atrioventricular (AV) valves Prevent backflow into the atria during systole; their cusps, chordae tendineae, and papillary muscles are sculpted from ventricular muscle; two-cusped AV valve of the left ventricle is the **bicuspid (mitral) valve;** three-cusped AV valve of the right ventricle is the **tricuspid valve.**

Auditory ossicles Three small bones (incus, malleus, and stapes) suspended in the middle ear in mammals to transduce vibrations from the eardrum to the oval window of the cochlea.

Aural (auricular) cysts and fistulae May be formed as regions of the first pharyngeal cleft are enclosed during formation of the external auditory meatus; may drain into the external auditory meatus or preauricular region via an auricular fistula.

Autonomic nervous system Composed of two-neuron pathways that constitute the sympathetic and parasympathetic nervous systems; systems operate "autonomously" to effect contractions of smooth muscle and glands throughout the body.

Axis arteries Central arteries of the limbs derived from the seventh intersegmental arteries (upper limb) and fifth lumbar intersegmental arteries (lower limb).

Axon Processes that usually conduct impulses away from the neuronal cell body; usually synapse with other neurons or with effector organs.

B

Basal (ventral) columns Pair of columns of the spinal cord and brain stem formed by gray matter of the ventral regions of the neural tube; cells give rise to somatic motor neurons.

Basal layer (of the dermis) Underlying layer of the periderm consisting of proliferating cells; gives rise to the germinative layer of the mature epidermis.

Basal nuclei (of the cerebral hemispheres) Heterogeneous nuclear masses located subcortically within the cerebral hemispheres; include the amygdaloid body, caudate, and lentiform nuclei.

Basket neuroblasts Neuroblasts of the cerebellar cortex; formed during the initial wave of neuroblast production by the external germinal layer of the cerebellum.

Bell stage (of tooth) Stage of tooth development attained by 10 weeks when the dental papilla invaginates deeply into the core of the bud of the developing tooth.

Bicuspid (mitral) valve See **Atrioventricular valves.**

Bilaminar germ disc Embryo following differentiation of the epiblast and hypoblast.

Bladder Arises from the primitive urogenital sinus; formed as an anterior division of the cloaca by the urorectal septum.

Blood islands Cysts of angioblasts containing hemoblasts; coalesce to form blood vessels in the yolk sac and also form the coronary vasculature.

Bone collar Arises by ossification of the periphery of the shaft of long bones from the primary ossification center.

Bony socket (of tooth) See **Alveolus (of tooth).**

Bowman's capsule Distal, thin-walled expansion of the renal vesicle that surrounds the glomerulus to form the renal corpuscle.

Brachial plexus Mixture of ventral primary rami of spinal nerves C5 to T1; innervates the upper extremity.

Brain stem Cranial extension of the spinal cord; includes the myelencephalon, pons of the metencephalon, and mesencephalon.

Branchial arches Gill bars of fish; homologous structures of humans are pharyngeal arches.

Branchial efferent Refers to motor nuclei and pathways innervating striated muscles derived from pharyngeal (branchial) arch mesoderm (cranial nerves V, VII, IX, and X).

Broad ligament (of uterus) Formed as peritoneal folds are swept toward the midline of the pelvic cavity as the paramesonephric ducts zipper together to form the superior vagina and uterus.

Bronchial bud First three branchings of respiratory diverticulum are primary, secondary, and tertiary bronchial buds that respectively form the primary bronchi, lung lobes, and bronchopulmonary segments.

Buccopharyngeal membrane Region of fusion of epiblast and hypoblast apparent early in the third week; breaks down in the fourth week, opening the oral cavity to the pharynx.

Bulbourethral glands Endodermal diverticula of the pelvic urethra in the male that form just inferior to the prostate between weeks 10 and 12; formed under the influence of dihydrotestosterone.

Bulbous hair peg Formed from a rod-like hair peg as the dermal papilla invaginates into its tip.

Bulboventricular sulcus Constriction that demarcates the superior end of the primitive ventricle (presumptive left ventricle) and inferior end of the bulbus cordis (presumptive right ventricle) in the third week.

Bulbus cordis Segment of primitive heart tube that is first apparent at the end of the third week; inferior end forms much of the **right ventricle;** superior end forms an outflow channel, the **conotruncus,** which then forms the proximal **conus cordis** and distal **truncus arteriosus,** which later divides into ascending aorta and pulmonary trunk.

Bundle of His Specialized myocytes that comprise a conduction pathway that carries impulses from the atrioventricular node to the ventricles; right and left branches serve the right and left ventricles, respectively.

C

Calvaria Dermal bones that constitute the cranial vault, skull cap, or roof of the skull.

Cap stage (of tooth development) Is initiated as neural crest-derived mesenchymal dental papillae invade the tooth buds in the eighth week.

Cardiac jelly Acellular secretion of the myocardium that plays a central role in septation of the heart and formation of the atrioventricular canals but later disappears.

Cardinal system of veins Drains the head and neck, body wall, and extremities of the embryo; consists of anterior and posterior cardinal veins; posterior cardinals are replaced by subcardinal and supracardinal veins during the second month.

Cardiogenic area Forms between the septum transversum and neural plate on day 19; cardiogenic angioblasts coalesce into vascular cords and later into lateral endocardial tubes; lateral endocardial tubes fold and fuse to form the primitive heart tube.

Cartilage Dense avascular connective tissue containing chondrocyte surrounded by an extracellular matrix (mainly collagen type II and proteoglycans).

Caudal and cranial neuropores Openings produced by the initial formation of the neural tube; as the neural tube closes, both become progressively smaller, closing on day 24 and day 26, respectively.

Cementoblasts Cells that differentiate from the inner layer of mesenchyme of the dental sac adjacent to the tooth root; secrete a layer of cementum to cover the tooth root dentin.

Cementoenamel junction Region at the neck of the tooth root that marks the boundary between cementum of the root and enamel of the crown.

Cementum Mineralized secretion (modified bone) of the cementoblasts that covers the dentin of the tooth root.

Central canal (of spinal cord) Arises from the neural canal; formed within the neural tube during neurulation; contains cerebrospinal fluid and is continuous with the brain ventricles.

Central sulcus Groove within the cerebrum separating frontal and parietal lobes.

Central tendon of the diaphragm Forms as the diaphragm differentiates and myoblasts of the septum transversum migrate into its periphery and into pleuroperitoneal membranes.

Cephalocaudal folding Stiff dorsal midline structures (notochord, neural plate, and somites) overgrow cranial and caudal ends of the embryo; both flexible ends fold sharply under to form three-dimensional vertebrate form.

Cerebellar hemispheres Formed by the cerebellar primordia of the rhombic lips; connected by the vermis.

Cerebellar nuclei (dentate, globose, emboliform, fastigial) Pairs of neuronal nuclei of the cerebellum formed by the internal granular layer; relay all cerebellar input.

Cerebellar primordia (plates) Lateral swellings of the rhombic lips; give rise to the cerebellar hemispheres.

Cerebellum Higher center formed by alar plates of the metencephalon; controls posture, balance, and smooth execution of movements.

Cerebral aqueduct Formed from narrowing of primitive ventricle of mesencephalon; transports cerebrospinal fluid produced by the choroid plexuses to the fourth ventricle; constriction may result in hydrocephalus.

Cerebral cortex Multilayered stratum of gray matter within the cerebrum; formed by the differentiation of the cortical plate and subplate during cytodifferentiation of the cerebral hemispheres.

Cerebral hemispheres Bubble-like outpouchings of the telencephalon; first appear at day 32 and expand rapidly to cover the diencephalon; initially smooth walled but begin to form folds (gyri) separated by grooves (sulci) in the fourth month that continue to form throughout fetal life; most evolutionarily advanced part of the brain.

Cerebrospinal fluid Produced by the choroid plexuses of the lateral, third, and fourth ventricles; intraventricular pressure is maintained through a balance between synthesis and reabsorption through venous plexuses within the spinal cord and cranial sinuses; supports and protects the brain and spinal cord.

Cervical cysts Produced by enclosure of the second, third, and fourth pharyngeal clefts by overgrowth of the second arch; typically transitory lateral cervical sinus does not disappear; may drain to the skin through an external cervical fistula; typically drains to the palatine tonsil through an internal cervical fistula.

Cervical flexure Second of three flexures that develop between the fifth and eighth weeks to bend the brain ventrally at the junction between the spinal cord and the myelencephalon.

Cervical nephrotomes Primitive excretory structures that arise in the cervical intermediate mesoderm during the early part of the fourth week; nonfunctional.

Chain ganglion (also Sympathetic chain ganglion) Formed as neural crest cells collect on both sides of the developing spinal cord at almost every level; contain peripheral neurons of the sympathetic nervous system.

Chemoaffinity hypothesis Axonal growth cones exhibit differential adherence to molecules specifically distributed within the extracellular matrix.

Chondrification Process by which dense mesenchymal precursors of the skeleton are converted into cartilage.

Chondrocranium Endochondral enclosure composing skulls of protochordates and early fishes; most primitive part of the skull in humans; now composes bones of the skull base.

Chondrocytes Cells that differentiate from dense condensation of lateral plate mesoderm; form the bones of limbs in response to growth factors.

Chorda tympani Branch of the facial nerve that carries special afferent fibers innervating taste buds on the anterior two-thirds of the tongue.

Chordae tendineae See **Atrioventricular valves.**

Chorion Outermost fetal membrane consisting of three kinds of tissues: syncytiotrophoblast, cytotrophoblast, and extraembryonic somatopleuric mesoderm.

Chorion frondosum Region of the chorionic wall that becomes associated with the decidua basalis; in the region of implantation retains its "leaf-like" chorionic villi.

Chorion laeve Abembryonic wall of the chorion loses its chorionic villi during the second month to become smooth walled.

Chorionic cavity Separates the embryo with its attached amnion and yolk sac from the chorion; by the end of the eighth week growth of the amniotic cavity obliterates it as layers of amniotic membrane and chorion loosely fuse together.

Chorionic villous sampling A small amount of tissue is removed from the chorion via a catheter inserted through the cervix or a needle inserted via the abdominal wall.

Choroid plexus Specialization of ependyma and vasculature that produces cerebrospinal fluid within the lateral, third, and fourth ventricles.

Ciliary ganglion Parasympathetic ganglion of the third cranial nerve; contains peripheral neurons of the parasympathetic pathway innervating the sphincter pupillae muscle of the iris and smooth muscles of the ciliary body.

Circumventricular organs Specializations of the third ventricle ependyma; include the subfornical organ, organum vasculosum of the lamina terminalis, and median eminence; may secrete material from the nervous tissues or vasculature into the cerebrospinal fluid.

Clitoris Arises from the genital tubercle in females.

Cloacal folds Develop in both male and female embryos just lateral to the cloacal membrane early in the fifth week; later divide into anterior urethral (urogenital) folds and posterior anal folds.

Cloacal membrane Caudal membrane that disintegrates in the seventh week to form the inferior boundary of the urinary system and gastrointestinal tract.

Coagulation plug A fibrin coagulum that forms at the site of the invading blastocyst in the endometrial lining of the uterus.

Cochlear ganglion (VIII) See **Acoustic ganglion.**

Collecting tubules (ducts) One to three million develop within the metanephroi from the last 10 or 11 generations of branchings of the ureteric buds.

Collodion baby   Baby is born with a persistent periderm "cocoon" that may slough after birth or may be removed by the physician.

Combined superior ganglion of cranial nerves VII and VIII   Contain sensory neurons derived from both the neural crest of the rhombencephalon and ectoderm from the first epibranchial placode; serve taste and general sensory functions (cranial nerve VII) and balance and hearing (cranial nerve VIII).

Common cardinal veins   Short vessel segments that drain blood into the right and left horns of the sinus venosus, respectively; the confluence of the anterior and posterior cardinal veins.

Compaction   Polarization and adhesion of blastomeres within the morula maximizing cell-to-cell contact; facilitated by cytoskeletal and cytomuscular elements.

Conduction system   Myocytes within the developing heart tube develop a more rapid rate of depolarization to produce two pacemaker regions, the sinoatrial node (regulating atrial rhythm) and atrioventricular node connected by a myocardial conduction pathway to coordinate ventricular rhythmicity via the bundle of His; a primitive conduction system develops as early as day 22.

Connecting stalk   A broad mass of extraembryonic somatopleuric mesoderm connecting the amnion to the cytotrophoblast that later forms the umbilical cord.

Conotruncus   Region of the bulbus cordis that forms the conus cordis and the truncus arteriosus.

Contact guidance theory   Axonal growth cones are guided by physical characteristics of the extracellular matrix.

Conus cordis   Segment of the outflow tract that is derived from the conotruncus and remodeled to form outflow regions (conus arteriosus or infundibulum) of the definitive right ventricle and part of the left ventricle.

Copula   Median swelling of the second pharyngeal arch is overgrown by the hypopharyngeal eminence of the third and fourth arches.

Cornua of the hyoid   Greater and lesser horns of the hyoid that provide attachment sites for muscles and the stylohyoid ligament; lesser cornua and upper rim of the hyoid are derived from the second pharyngeal arch cartilage (Reichert's cartilage); lower rim and greater cornua are derived from the third arch cartilage.

Coronary sinus   Vestige of the left horn of the sinus venosus that completely detaches from the left anterior cardinal vein; in conjunction with cardiac veins, forms venous system that will drain the myocardium.

Coronary sulcus (of the phallus)   A shallow depression that demarcates the glans from the shaft.

Coronary vessels   Form from epicardium as subepicardial plexuses fuse with sprouts of the aorta and coronary sinus; form the coronary arteries and coronary veins, respectively.

Corpora bigemina   Longitudinal swellings of the mesencephalon that are precursors of the inferior and superior colliculi.

Corpus callosum   Large fiber tract that connects the neocortices of the left and right cerebral hemispheres.

Corpus striatum   Neuronal aggregations within the floor of the cerebral hemispheres; form some of the basal nuclei of the cerebrum.

Cortical plate   See **Cerebral cortex.**

Cortical sex cords (secondary)   Secondary sex cords at the cortex of the developing genital ridges surround the primordial germ cells in the female gonad to become follicle cells.

Cotyledons   Formed during the fourth and fifth months as placental septa grow into the intervillous space, separating the villi into 15 to 25 groups.

Cranial (mesencephalic) flexure   Initial flexure of the brain; bends the prosencephalon ventrally between the fourth and eighth weeks of development in the region of the mesencephalon.

Cranial nerve sensory ganglia   Comparable to the dorsal root ganglia of the spinal cord; form in association with cranial nerves V, VII, VIII, IX, and X; contain peripheral sensory neuronal cell bodies that receive input from sensory organs in the head and pharynx for relay to associational nuclei within the brain stem.

Cranial nerves   Twelve pairs develop in humans in association with the brain stem; serve diverse functions; motor, sensory, somatic, or mixed; mainly innervate structures and tissues of the head and pharynx; vagus nerve (X) provides parasympathetic preganglionic fibers to thoracic and abdominal viscera.

Cranial (rostral) neuropore   See **Caudal and cranial neuropores.**

Cribriform plate (of the ethmoid bone)   Perforated bone formed from ossification around fibers from the developing olfactory bulbs.

Cricoid cartilage   Complete cartilaginous ring at the base of the larynx that may be derived from cartilage arising within sixth pharyngeal arch.

Crista terminalis   Ridge of tissue that demarcates the boundary between the sinus venarum (definitive atrium) and right primitive atrium (right auricle); contains a conduction pathway connecting the sinoatrial node and atrioventricular node.

Crown (of the tooth)   Covered with enamel and extends into the jaw to the level of the cementoenamel junction.

Crura of the diaphragm   Muscular bands formed of condensed mesenchyme that attach to vertebral bodies L1 to L3 (on the right) and L1 and L2 (on the left).

Cumulus expansion   Following ovulatory stimulus cumulus cells secrete a hyaluronic acid-rich extracellular matrix; resultant mucoid mass adheres to the oocyte during ovulation and may aid in transport of the cumulus-oocyte complex into the oviduct.

Cystic diverticulum   Endodermal outgrowth that appears about day 26 just inferior to the hepatic diverticulum on the ventral wall of the duodenum; forms the gallbladder, cystic duct, and part of the common bile duct.

Cytoplasmic maturation (of gametes)   Cytoplasmic changes occurring during the process of gametogenesis within the male and female germ cell line, converting them into mature gametes.

Cytotrophoblast   Cells of the trophoblast that retain their cell membranes and enclose the blastocyst cavity.

D

Decidua basalis   Zone of decidual tissue in the wall of the uterus underlying the embedded embryonic pole of the embryo.

Decidua capsularis   Zone of decidua overlying the part of the embryo that protrudes into the lumen of the uterus.

Decidual cells   Formed as cells of the endometrial stroma within the wall of the uterus differentiate in response to the implanting embryo by accumulating lipid and glycogen.

Decidual parietalis   Does not directly cover the embryo (like the decidua basalis and capsularis).

Decidual reaction   In response to implantation endometrial stromal cells accumulate lipid and glycogen; the endometrium thickens, endometrial glands enlarge, and endometrial veins and spiral arteries make connections with trophoblastic lacunae.

Decidual (placental) septa   Wedge-like walls of decidual tissue that grow into the intervillous spaces to separate the villi into 15 to 25 cotyledons.

Decision-making point   Nerve fibers leave nerve trunk to innervate end organs at a specific point; divergence of the nerve may occur in response to a chemoattractant or tropic substance or result from the growth cone's unique capacity to follow structural or molecular cues present in the substrate.

Deep ring (of inguinal canal)   Site of weakening and evagination of the transversalis fascia produced by the evagination of the processus vaginalis.

Definitive (secondary) endoderm Germ layer of the trilaminar embryo arising from the epiblast during gastrulation; forms the gastrointestinal tract and its derivatives.

Definitive left atrium Heart chamber formed by incorporation of pulmonary veins into the posterior wall of the primitive atrium.

Definitive left ventricle Heart chamber primarily derived from the primitive ventricle; in part formed by left wall of the conus cordis.

Definitive oocyte or definitive spermatocyte (spermatid) The definitive haploid (lN); spermatocyte and oocyte have completed both meiotic divisions.

Definitive pericardial cavity An anterior cavity containing the heart that forms, along with the pleural cavities, as the primitive pericardial cavity (in which developing heart is suspended) is divided by two coronal pleuropericardial folds in the fifth week; folds fuse at the midline, and, with esophageal mesoderm, form the pericardial sac.

Definitive right atrium Heart chamber formed by incorporation of the sinus venosus into the posterior wall of the primitive atrium.

Definitive right ventricle Heart chamber primarily derived from the inferior end of the bulbus cordis; also incorporates part of the right wall of the conus cordis and primitive ventricle.

Definitive urogenital sinus Lower expanded region of the primitive urogenital sinus; gives rise to the vestibule of the vagina in the female and the penile urethra in the male.

Dendrite Short neuronal processes, often highly branched; usually conduct impulses toward the neuronal cell body and its axon and form synapses with the axons of other neurons.

Dental laminae U-shaped ridges of surface ectoderm that appear on the upper and lower jaws in the seventh week; each forms the ectodermal component of ten primary tooth buds.

Dental papilla Concentrations of mesenchyme, derived from migrating neural crest cells, form under the surface ectoderm of the upper and lower jaw, respectively, stimulating ten centers of ingrowth from each dental lamina; together with each ingrowth, forms a primary tooth bud.

Dental pulp A canal within the core of the mature tooth that transports nerves and blood vessels into the tooth.

Dental sac Mesenchymal investment that encloses the tooth bud at the end of the second month; forms cementoblasts and the periodontal ligament and contributes to the alveolus.

Dermal papilla of dermis Evaginations of the papillary layer of the dermis that interdigitate with overlying epidermal ridges to form the pattern of external ridges and grooves of the skin.

Dermal papilla of hair follicle Mesenchyme that invaginates into the tips of hair pegs, converting them to bulbous hair pegs; layer of proliferating ectoderm overlying it forms the germinal matrix that forms the hair shaft.

Dermatome Formed as a dermomyotome splits; contributes to development of the dermis.

Dermis (corium) Derived from both lateral plate mesoderm and the dermatomes of the somites; consists of two layers: a papillary layer just underlying the epidermis and a deeper, dense, irregular layer (reticular layer).

Dermomyotome Portion of the somite that remains in place after the sclerotome migrates medially; quickly splits into a myotome and a dermatome.

Dextrocardia Condition resulting from an opposite "dextral" looping of the primary heart tube displacing the apex of the left ventricle to the right.

Diaphragm Chief respiratory muscle of humans; derivative of four embryological structures: septum transversum, pleuroperitoneal membranes, paraxial mesoderm of the body wall, and lateral plate mesoderm.

Diaphysis Shaft of the long bone.

Diarthroidal (synovial) joint See **Synovial joint.**

Diencephalon (between-brain) One of two secondary brain vesicles formed by the prosencephalon (forebrain); gives rise to the epithalamus and its derivatives and to the thalamus and the hypothalamus.

Dihydrotestosterone Androgen that is produced by conversion of testosterone by the enzyme 5-α-reductase; responsible for male development of the prostate, bulbourethral glands, seminal vesicles, and male differentiation of the external genitalia during embryonic and fetal life.

Distal tongue buds (lateral lingual swellings) Overgrow the median tongue bud to give rise to most of the anterior two-thirds of the tongue.

Dizygotic (fraternal) twins Arise from two separate oocytes; do not share any fetal membranes.

Doppler ultrasonography Ultrasound mode that allows visualization and analysis of blood flow within the fetal heart and blood vessels.

Dorsal mesentery Thin peritoneal membrane that suspends abdominal viscera in the coelomic cavity; forms mesentery of the abdominal esophagus, mesogastrium, greater omentum, small intestines, and transverse and sigmoid colons.

Dorsal mesocardium Dorsal mesentery of the primitive heart tube that ruptures in the fourth week to form the transverse pericardial sinus.

Dorsal nucleus of the vagus Contains preganglionic parasympathetic neurons that innervate the viscera via the vagus nerve.

Dorsal pancreatic bud Sprouts from the dorsal duodenal wall to form the head, body, and tail of the pancreas after fusion with the ventral pancreatic bud.

Dorsal primary ramus Dorsal branch of any spinal nerve that innervates skin and deep muscles of the back; contains motor, sensory, and sympathetic fibers.

Dorsal root Comprised of the dorsal root ganglion and its centripetal and centrifugal fibers.

Dorsal root ganglion Formed from concentrations of neural crest cells that collect just lateral to the second cervical to first coccygeal segments of the spinal cord.

E

Ectoderm Descends from epiblast cells following completion of gastrulation; differentiates into surface ectoderm (forms the epidermis) and neural epithelium (forms neurons, supporting cells, neural crest cells, and ependyma of the central nervous system).

Ectodermal placodes Ectodermal thickenings including the nasal and otic placodes, trigeminal placode, and four epibranchial (epipharyngeal) placodes; all play major roles in producing neurons within several of the sensory ganglia associated with the cranial nerves.

Ectodactyly Absence of any number of fingers or toes.

Edinger-Westphal nucleus Contains preganglionic parasympathetic neurons that innervate postganglionic neurons within the ciliary ganglia that innervate the sphincter pupillae muscle of the iris and the smooth muscle cells of the ciliary body.

Efferent ductules (ductuli efferentes) Formed as epigenital mesonephric tubules unite with the presumptive rete testis; provide pathway for sperm from seminiferous and rete testis tubules to the vas deferens.

Embryoblast Arises from inner cell mass of the morula during first week of development and gives rise to the embryo proper.

Embryonic period Typically described as the period when most of the organ systems are developing, between the late third week and the eighth week.

Embryonic stem cells   Arise from the inner cell mass during in vitro culture of blastocysts removed from a fertilized genital tract; totipotent; produce injection chimeras when introduced into a normal blastocyst.

Enamel   Mineralized secretion of the ameloblasts (derived from the inner enamel epithelium of the enamel organ) that covers the dentin of the crown of the mature tooth.

Enamel organ   Differentiates from the dental lamina; consists of an inner and outer enamel epithelium with a middle enamel or stellate reticulum of star-shaped cells embedded in an extracellular matrix; inner enamel epithelium secretes enamel.

Endocardial cushions   Thickenings in the atrioventricular canal are regions of thickened cardiac jelly.

Endocardium   Lining of the heart tube derived from the lateral endocardial tubes; consists of endothelium and thin subendothelial connective tissue.

Endochondral ossification   Ossification of a cartilaginous precursor.

Endometrial stroma   Fleshy part of the uterine wall immediately underlying the endometrial epithelium.

Endometrium   Consists of an epithelial lining of the uterine lumen and a mesodermal stroma (lamina propria) containing vasculature and endometrial glands.

Endosonography   Miniature ultrasound probe is inserted into a body orifice to visualize internal structures.

Endothelial cells   Arise from angioblasts to form initial vascular network; provide endothelial lining for the entire cardiovascular system.

Enteric ganglia   Ganglia embedded within the walls of the gastrointestinal tract derived from vagal and sacral neural crest cells.

Ependyma   Cellular membrane lining the ventricles of the brain and the central canal of the spinal cord; arises directly from the ventricular layer; may participate in the development of the choroid plexuses and specialized circumventricular organs that produce cerebrospinal fluid.

Ependymal cell   Last cells to differentiate from the ventricular layer of the brain and spinal cord; form an ependymal lining of the neural canal.

Epiblast   Sheet of cells that appears with the hypoblast as the embryoblast differentiates to form the bilaminar embryo; eventually gives rise to all cells and tissues of the amnion and the embryo proper.

Epibranchial (epipharyngeal) placodes   Four regions of ectoderm located just dorsal to the pharyngeal arches; produce neurons that form more distal sensory ganglia of the cranial nerves.

Epicardium (visceral pericardium)   Outer tunic of thin serous membrane that covers the myocardium; derived from splanchnopleuric mesoderm; forms the coronary vessels.

Epidemiologic studies   Examination of the spread and prevalence of diseases in communities.

Epidermal ridges   Invaginations of epidermis that interdigitate with the dermal papillae to produce the distinctive ridges and grooves of the skin.

Epididymis   Convoluted region of the vas deferens attached to the posterior side of the testis that serves as a reservoir for spermatozoa.

Epigenital mesonephric tubules   Degenerates in females to form a remnant called the epoophoron; in males, 5 to 12 of these give rise to the efferent ductules.

Epiglottis   Covers the opening of the trachea during swallowing; formed within the region of the fourth arch.

Epimere   Formed from splitting of myotomes; gives rise to the deep epaxial muscles of the back, including the erector spinae and transversospinalis groups.

Epiphyseal plate   Cartilaginous segments at the base of the epiphysis at both ends of long bones; provide a mechanism for the elongation of the long bones until about the 20th year.

Epiphysis   Part of a long bone that develops from a site of secondary ossification, usually at the end of a bone.

Epiploic foramen of Winslow   Narrow canal just posterior to the lesser omentum formed from reduction of the communication of the lesser and greater sacs of the peritoneal cavity as the stomach, liver, and lesser omentum are repositioned during the sixth week.

Epithalamus   Forms the pineal gland; also forms the trigonum habenulae, including the habenular nucleus and the posterior and habenular commissures.

Epithelial root sheath (of the tooth)   Epithelium immediately overlying the dentin of the tooth root; formed by the confluence of inner and outer enamel epithelium.

Eponychium   Thin layer of epidermis initially covering the nail plate.

Epoophoron   Vestiges of the epigenital mesonephric tubules scattered in the mesovarium.

Erythroblastosis fetalis   If a mother who lacks Rh factors bears an Rh⁺ baby and fetal blood leaks across the placenta into the maternal circulation (usually at birth), the mother may make antibodies against these factors; if she bears a second Rh⁺ fetus, the anti-Rh antibodies cross into the fetal circulation and destroy the fetus' red blood cells; the fetus then overproduces red blood cells; the number of immature nucleated erythroblasts increases within the fetal circulation.

Ethmoid sinuses   Paranasal air sinuses; begin to form within the ethmoid bone, communicating with the nasal passages through the middle meatus; complete their growth during puberty.

Exocoelomic cavity (primary yolk sac)   Formed as cells at the periphery of the hypoblast proliferate and migrate out onto the cytotrophoblast to line the blastocyst cavity.

Exocoelomic membrane (Heuser's membrane)   Arises from hypoblast cells that line the primary yolk sac (exocoelomic cavity).

Exocoelomic vesicles   Collection of vesicles at the abembryonic pole arising from disintegration of the primary yolk sac, which also ultimately disintegrate.

External auditory meatus   Derivative of the first pharyngeal cleft consisting of a channel from the pinna to the tympanic membrane.

External germinal (granular) layer (of the cerebellum)   Forms superficial to the marginal layer during the third month; beginning in the fourth month its neuroblasts successively give rise to basket neuroblasts, granule neuroblasts, and stellate neuroblasts.

Extraembryonic coelom   See **Chorionic cavity.**

Extraembryonic endoderm   Cells arising from the periphery of the hypoblast (primary endoderm) that form the exocoelomic membrane and secrete the extraembryonic reticulum; a second wave of hypoblast proliferation forms the extraembryonic endoderm that lines the secondary yolk sac.

Extraembryonic mesoderm   Lines the primary and secondary yolk sacs during the second week and is said to arise from the epiblast at the caudal end of the bilaminar germ disc; migrates out to form two layers that gradually separate the amnion from the cytotrophoblast.

Extraembryonic reticulum   Acellular matrix secreted between exocoelomic membrane and cytotrophoblast by the exocoelomic membrane; vacuoles form within it during the second week that coalesce to form the chorionic cavity.

F

Facial nerve (VII)   Contains branchial efferent, sensory, and visceral efferent fibers; grows into the second pharyngeal arch where it innervates muscles of facial expression and provides sensory innervation to the soft palate.

Facial skeleton (viscerocranium)   Supports pharyngeal arches and their derivatives; evolved from skeletal elements of the branchial arches; in humans, much of the original branchial arch skeleton of the upper jaw has been replaced by dermal bones.

False ribs   Includes ribs 8 to 12, which do not articulate directly with the sternum ventrally (see **True ribs**).

Fate map   Diagram of the differentiation of epiblast cells showing developmental fate of each of its regions constructed using cell tracing and lineage studies.

Fertilization   A spermatozoon penetrates the cumulus mass and zona pellucida, causing fusion of spermatozoon and secondary oocyte membranes; fusion of male and female pronuclei form a diploid, 2N zygote.

Fetal liver transplant   Fetal liver cells, suspended in a culture medium, are injected into the umbilical vein of a fetus to colonize the fetal liver, providing stem cells for hemopoiesis.

Fetal period   From end of the 8th through 38th week of gestation; characterized by growth and maturation of the organ systems.

Fibrocartilage   Type of cartilage usually occurring between bones, ligaments, or tendons; composes structures such as the menisci of the knee or shoulder joint.

Filopodia   Cellular extensions thought to be responsible for motility of axonal growth cones.

First meiotic division   Involves DNA replication and recombination and yields two haploid 2N daughter cells; produces two secondary spermatocytes in the male and a secondary oocyte and the first polar body in the female.

First trimester   First 3 months of gestation.

Fissuration   Process (along with the process of foliation) producing fissures within the cerebellar cortex.

Flocculonodular lobes   Most posterior (and primitive) lobes of the cerebellum; separated from the more cranial vermis and cerebellar hemispheres by a posterolateral fissure.

Floor plate   Formed as the ventral midline of the neural plate thins; becomes a hinge allowing the lateral lips of the developing neural folds to rise and meet in the dorsal midline during neurulation.

Foliation   See **Fissuration.**

Follicle cells   Nurse cells of the oocyte that develop from secondary cortical sex cords; form the cumulus oophorus and membrana granulosa cells.

Follicular canal   Canal lined by the inner and outer epidermal root sheath of the hair follicle; contains the outgrowing hair shaft.

Foramen cecum   Endodermal pit lying in the midline of the tongue within the terminal sulcus; gives rise to the thyroglossal duct (transient) and thyroid gland.

Foramen ovale   Inferior opening in the septum secundum that allows blood to flow from the right to left atrium during embryonic and fetal life.

Foregut   Develops from the cranial end of the primitive gut tube to form the pharyngeal foregut, thoracic esophagus, and abdominal foregut (abdominal esophagus, stomach, and superior half of duodenum).

Formative zone (root; of nail plate)   Arises from the stratum germinative of the proximal nail fold; produces the horny nail plate.

Fossa ovalis   Formed as foramen ovalis closes as septum primum and septum secundum fuse following birth.

Fourth ventricle   Forms by expansion of the neural canal in the region of the rhombencephalon.

Fraternal (dizygotic) twins   Arise from two separate oocytes and therefore do not share any of the fetal membranes.

Frontal lobes   Large superoventral lobes of the cerebral hemispheres separated from the more posterior parietal lobes by a groove called the central sulcus; each consists of two major regions, the prefrontal (largely "association" cortex) and precentral (sensorimotor) regions.

Frontal sinuses   Paranasal air sinuses; appear at fifth or sixth postnatal year; comprised of two separate cavities within the frontal bone—an extension of the ethmoid sinus and an independent invagination of the middle meatus.

Frontonasal prominence   One of five processes that give rise to the face (with two maxillary swellings and two mandibular swellings); forms the skull and forehead; gives rise to the nasal placodes that form the medial and lateral nasal processes.

Fundus   Superoposterior expansion of the stomach that is superior to a horizontal plane drawn through the apex of the cardiac incisure.

G

Ganglion   A discrete cell body composed of a concentration of neurons of the peripheral nervous system.

Gartner's cysts   Vestiges of the inferior end of the mesonephric duct located in the wall of the vagina.

Gastrulation   Process of epiblast ingress through the primitive streak forming the primary germ layers, namely, the definitive endoderm and mesoderm.

Gene therapy   Genetically defective stem cells are removed and then "cured" at the genetic level by gene targeting techniques and reintroduced into the individual.

General afferent   Refers to that part of the nervous system involved in the reception of impulses of general sensation: served by the trigeminal (V) and facial (VII) nerves and pharyngeal and laryngeal cavities (V, IX, X).

Genetic screening (of polar bodies)   Polar bodies contain DNA that can be screened to obtain genetic information about a female's germ cell line.

Genital ridge   Primordial gonad formed by germ cell migration just medial to the mesonephroi (embryonic kidneys).

Germ line   Cells originating within primary ectoderm that migrate into the yolk sac and differentiate into primordial germ cells during early weeks of embryonic development; cells then migrate to genital ridge, where they differentiate into gametes.

Germinal matrix   See **Dermal papilla of hair follicle.**

Germinal vesicle   Large, watery nucleus formed during the dictyotene stage of the first meiotic prophase in the primary oocyte that may protect genetic material within the primary oocyte from destructive effects of teratogens or irradiation.

Germinal vesicle breakdown   Reinitiation of nuclear maturation in primary oocytes resulting in disintegration of germinal vesicle membrane.

Germinative layer (stratum germinativum)   Layer of the mature epidermis derived from the basal proliferating layer of surface ectoderm; contains stem cells that differentiate into the keratinized cells of overlying layers that proliferate to replenish its own stem cell population.

GIFT (Gamete intrafallopian transfer)   Technique often employed for anovulatory syndrome or suboptimal spermatozoa motility; male and female gametes are collected and then separately reintroduced through a catheter into oviduct for fertilization (see also **ZIFT**).

Glans (of clitoris; of penis)   Distal end of the clitoris and penis demarcated from the shaft by the coronary sulcus.

Glioblast   Produced after the formation of neuroblasts ceases by the ventricular neuroectoderm of the neural tube; differentiate into glial cells.

Glomerulus   Small bundle of capillaries surrounded by the Bowman's capsule of the metanephric tubule; form the renal corpuscle.

Glossopharyngeal nerve (IX)   Innervates structures that develop from tissues within the third pharyngeal arch; contains branchial and visceral efferent fibers; provides general sensory innervation to most of the posterior one-third of the tongue, pharyngeal cavity, and superior esophagus; also contains special (taste) fibers that conduct impulses from the vallate papillae; innervates the stylopharyngeus muscle.

Gonocyte   Cells of the germ line of males or females during meiosis, including primary, secondary, and definitive oocytes or spermatocytes.

Granular layer Stratum of the cerebellum composed of granule cells and some stellate and basket cells that arise within and migrate from the external germinal layer.

Granule neuroblasts Formed during the second wave of neuroblasts formation by the external germinal layer of the cerebellar cortex; migrate inward to establish the granular layer.

Gray matter Regions of the central nervous system containing neuronal cell bodies; initially organized into a marginal layer, then into ventral and dorsal columns that may further differentiate into motor and associational nuclei, respectively.

Gray ramus communicans Diminutive bundle of neuronal fibers connecting the sympathetic chain ganglion to the spinal nerve; contain postganglionic sympathetic fibers only.

Greater omentum Fold of the dorsal mesogastrium that encloses the lower recess of the lesser sac; forms a repository of fat in the adult.

Greater sac Remainder of the peritoneal cavity after formation of the lesser sac.

Greater splanchnic nerve Comprised of preganglionic fibers originating from central neurons located in the intermediolateral columns at spinal cord levels T5 to T12; collect into a single nerve that innervates the celiac ganglia.

Growth cone Develops at the advancing end of elongating axons and is thought to provide locomotory force required for axonal growth; capable of sensing chemical and physical characteristics of the extracellular matrix and mesenchyma.

Gubernaculum Ligamentous cord that condenses in the seventh week to effect descent of the testes in males; forms the round ligaments of the uterus and ovarian ligaments in females.

H

Hair follicles Formed from the epidermis and dermis; form the hair shafts and sebaceous glands; first evident as concentrations of epidermal cells (hair germs) in the basal layer of the primitive two-layered epidermis that elongate to form hair pegs.

Hair germ Ectodermal concentrations arising in the basal layer of the primitive epidermis; form hair follicles.

Hair peg Rod-like structure formed from elongation of the hair germ.

Hair shaft Specialized aggregations of keratinocyte generated by the germinal matrix of the hair follicle and pushed outward through the follicular canal.

Hard palate Formed subsequent to fusion of the palatine shelves when mesenchyme within the anterior region ossifies.

Harlequin fetus Results from defect of the mechanism that bundles the keratin fibers in the stratum granulosum; keratinocytes cannot be sloughed; these babies usually die shortly after birth.

Hematopoietic stem cell Arise in primary ectoderm; migrate to yolk sac, liver, and (possibly) to aorta-gonad-mesonephros (AGM) region to form blood cells that ultimately seed adult hematopoietic organs (spleen, thymus, and bone marrow).

Hemimelia Reduction or stunting of distal limb segments.

Hemivertebra Lopsided vertebra produced when the notochord fails to induce the ventral sclerotome on one side; may result in lateral curvature of the spinal column (scoliosis).

Hepatic diverticulum Endodermal outgrowth of the duodenum; forms on day 22 on the ventral wall of the descending segment of the duodenum; grows into the ventral mesentery, where it forms liver parenchyma (hepatocytes), bile canaliculi, and hepatic ducts.

Higher centers More complex structures of the brain (cerebellum, diencephalon, and cerebral hemispheres); retain very few traces of spinal cord organization.

Hindgut Segment formed from the caudal end of the primitive gut tube; vascularized by the inferior mesenteric artery; forms left one-third of the transverse colon, the descending colon, and rectum.

Hippocampal (fornix) commissure Fiber tract that develops within the lamina terminalis; connects left and right hippocampi of the cerebral hemispheres.

Horny layer (stratum corneum) Outermost layer of the mature epidermis produced as lytic enzymes are released; metabolic activity ceases in cells of the outer layer of the stratum granulosum, producing flattened, scale-like, terminally differentiated keratinocytes.

Horny nail plate Compressed keratinocytes produced by the formative zone or root of the nail plate.

Horseshoe kidney Fusion of the inferior poles of the metanephroi during their ascent from the sacral region may result in formation of a horsehoe-shaped kidney that may be caught under the inferior mesenteric artery.

Hydramnios (oligohydramnios) Insufficient amounts of amniotic fluid within the amnion; may be caused by renal agenesis or an obstructive uropathy that prevents fetus from urinating into the amnion.

Hydrops Accumulation of water in the fetus.

Hymen Endodermal membrane that initially partitions the lumen of the inferior vagina from the vestibule; usually partially ruptured after the fifth fetal month but remnants may persist.

Hyoid bone Ossifies from cartilage of the second pharyngeal arch (Reinchert's cartilage) and the third pharygeal arch; stabilizes the tongue and the larynx.

Hypoblast (primary endoderm) Sheet of cells that appears with the epiblast as the embryoblast laminates; it eventually forms the extraembryonic endoderm.

Hypodermis (subcorium) Subcutaneous fatty connective tissue underlying the dermis.

Hypoglossal nerve (XII) Develops in association with occipital somites and innervates all of the intrinsic muscles of the tongue except the palatoglossus; exclusively motor in function.

Hypomere Formed from splitting of myotomes; gives rise to the deep hypaxial muscles of the lateral and ventral body wall in the thorax and abdomen.

Hypopharyngeal (hypobranchial) eminence Swelling on the floor of the pharynx in the region of the third and fourth pharyngeal arches; gives rise to the posterior one-third of the tongue.

Hypophyseal cartilages Forms the body of the sphenoid bone of the chondrocranium.

Hypothalamic sulcus Groove that demarcates the boundary between the thalamus and the hypothalamus.

Hypothalamus Inferoventral swelling of the diencephalon; regulates endocrine activity of the pituitary and many autonomic responses; also functions in the limbs system, which controls/regulates emotion and sleep/waking mechanisms.

I

Identical (monozygotic) twins Arise from the same oocyte, which may split at the two-cell stage or at later stages of development; possess the same genetic makeup; may or may not share fetal membranes.

Immature intermediate villi Extensions of the stem villi formed during the first and second trimester by development of trophoblastic and villous sprouts; contain a core of connective tissue and blood vessels, within an incomplete jacket of cytotrophoblast, covered by a complete layer of syncytiotrophoblast; do not possess terminal villous branches.

In situ vesicle formation and fusion   See **Vasculogenesis.**

Incus bone   Auditory ossicle arising from the palatopterygoquadrate bar.

Indifferent phase   See **ambisexual stage.**

Inferior colliculi   Develop from alar plate neuroblasts that migrate into the mesencephalic roof plate; relay information from the cochlea to auditory areas of the cerebral cortex.

Inferior (geniculate) ganglion of cranial nerve VII   Formed by neural crest cells and cells of the first epibranchial (epipharyngeal) placode; relays impulses of general sensation to the brain stem from the skin of the auricular concha, small patch of skin behind the ear, and external tympanic membrane; also conveys sensation of taste from the anterior two-thirds of the tongue and from the hard and soft palates to the nucleus of the tractus solitarius.

Inferior (nodose) ganglion of cranial nerve X (vagus)   Neurons within this ganglion arise from third and fourth epibranchial placodes; relay general and special (taste) sensations to the general afferent column and the nucleus of the tractus solitarius, respectively.

Inferior (petrosal) ganglion of cranial nerve IX (glossopharyngeal)   Neurons within this ganglion are derived from the second epibranchial placode; relay general and special (taste) sensations to the general afferent column and the nucleus of the tractus solitarius, respectively.

Inferior vena cava   Vessel that returns systemic blood from the trunk and lower extremities to the right atrium; formed from the right vitelline, subcardinal, supracardinal, and posterior cardinal veins.

Infundibulum   Evagination of the floor of the diencephalon formed in the third week; forms the posterior pituitary gland (neurohypophysis).

Inguinal canal   Defect occurring in both males and females formed in the anterior abdominal wall by the processus vaginalis as it forces thin sock-like extensions of transversalis fascia, internal oblique muscle, and external oblique muscle into the labioscrotal swelling.

Inner cell mass (embryoblast)   Blastomeres arising from first cells to divide during early cleavages that segregate within the center of the morula and differentiate into the embryo (outer cells differentiate into placental membranes).

Inner enamel epithelium   Derived from the ectoderm of the dental lamina; differentiates into the ameloblasts that secrete the enamel of the root crown.

Inner epidermal root sheath (of the hair follicle)   Directly lines the follicular canal.

Insemination   Deposition of seminal fluid within the vagina, during coitus, or with a catheter as in "artificial" insemination.

Insula   Portion of the cerebral cortex forming the floor of the lateral cerebral fossa; eventually covered by the temporal lobe.

Intermaxillary process   Formed by the growth and fusion of the inferior regions of the left and right medial nasal processes; forms the philtrum of the upper lip and the primary palate.

Intermediate layer (of the dermis)   Produced in the 11th week by the basal layer of the epidermis; gives rise to outer layers of the mature epidermis.

Intermediate mesoderm   Lies between paraxial mesoderm and lateral plate mesoderm from the cervical to sacral regions; forms embryonic and definitive kidneys and part of the male genital system.

Intermediate zone   Formed between the ventricular and marginal zone; neuroblasts within it and the ventricular zone migrate outward to form the cortical plate; eventually forms white matter of the cerebral hemispheres.

Intermediolateral cell columns   Collections of gray matter containing central (preganglionic) neurons of the sympathetic nervous system (T1 to L2).

Internal capsule   Massive fiber bundle that carries fibers from the thalamus to the cerebral cortex and from the cerebral cortex to lower regions of the brain and spinal cord.

Internal germinal layer   Neuroblast-producing layer of the cerebellum; arises from the ventricular layer to form primitive nuclear neuroblasts (form the cerebellar nuclei), primitive Purkinje neuroblasts, and Golgi neuroblasts.

Intersegmental artery   Paired intersegmental arteries that sprout from the dorsal aorta; vascularize all of the derivatives of the somites and the extremities (see **Axis artery**).

Interthalamic adhesions   May form as the thalami expand into the third ventricle.

Interventricular foramen of Munro   Openings that allow passage of cerebrospinal fluid between the third ventricle and lateral ventricles.

Intervillous space   Blood-filled cavities within the placenta arising from the trophoblastic lacunae.

Interzone   Region of fibroblastic tissue, within the rod-like bone precursor, that will form the joint.

Intraembryonic coelomic cavity   Formed as cavities between splanchnopleuric and somatopleuric lateral plate mesoderm on the left and right sides coalesce during embryonic folding; forms the definitive pericardial, left and right pleural, and peritoneal cavities.

Intraperitoneal (organ)   Suspended within the peritoneal cavity by a mesentery.

Intrauterine growth retardation (IUGR)   Effects of some toxins, teratogens, or disease states of the mother may lead to an inhibition of fetal growth.

Intrinsic muscles of the larynx   Move laryngeal parts; change the length and tension of the vocal folds and the space between the vocal folds; except for the cricothyroid muscle, innervated by the recurrent laryngeal branch of the vagus nerve.

K

Karyotype   Description of the composition of the genome with respect to the number and condition of autosomes and sex chromosomes or a preparation of condensed chromosomes that may be viewed with a microscope.

Keratinocytes   Cells of the epidermis produced by the stratum germinative forming three additional superficial layers: the stratum spinosum, the stratum granulosum, and the stratum corneum (in order of maturation); contain keratin proteins.

L

Labia minora   Medial swellings of the female external genitalia that border the vestibule of the vagina and arise from the urethral folds; homologous to the corpus spongiosum (spongy or penile urethra) of the penis.

Labioscrotal swellings   Develop lateral to the urethral (urogenital) folds in both males and females; form the labia majora in females and the scrotum in males.

Lamellar ichthyosis   Excessive keratinization of the skin; skin may scale off in flakes; babies are usually viable.

Lamina terminalis   Point of final closure of the cranial neuropore; extends from the dorsal region of the optic chiasm to rostrum of the corpus callosum; includes the anterior and hippocampal commissures.

Langerhans cells   Formed within the bone marrow; migrate to the epidermis (initially in the seventh week) to form the macrophage immune cells of the skin.

Larynx Formed from cartilage arising from lateral plate mesoderm of the fourth and sixth pharyngeal arches; musculature formed from cranial paraxial mesoderm of these arches.

Lateral apertures (foramina of Luschka) Facilitate transfer of cerebrospinal fluid from the fourth ventricle to the subarachnoid space of the brain stem and spinal cord.

Lateral cerebral fossa See **Lateral cerebral sulcus.**

Lateral cerebral sulcus Formed as the lateral cerebral fossa becomes a deeper, elongated cleft.

Lateral cervical sinuses See **Cervical cysts.**

Lateral endocardial tubes Paired tubes that form within the lateral regions of the cardiogenic area by vasculogenesis; fuse to form the primitive heart tube.

Lateral folding Results in fusion of the lateral edges of the ectoderm, somatopleuric mesoderm, presumptive coelomic cavities, splanchnopleuric mesoderm, and endoderm in the 4- to 5-week embryo; cylindrical vertebrate body is formed with its integument, musculature, and gut tube.

Lateral nasal process Form from the lateral regions of the nasal placodes of the frontonasal prominence; give rise to the lateral regions of the nose.

Lateral plate mesoderm Mesodermal sheet lateral to the intermediate mesoderm; splits into somatopleuric mesoderm (forms parietal serous lining of body cavities) and splanchnopleuric mesoderm (forms serous membrane ensheathing visceral organs).

Lateral ventricles Two cavities within the cerebral hemispheres arising from expansion of the neural canal within the telencephalon; initially occupy most of the volume of the cerebral hemispheres, but are gradually constricted by growth and thickening of the cerebral cortex; communicate with the third ventricle through the interventricular foramina of Munro.

Least splanchnic nerve Composed of preganglionic sympathetic axons originating from central sympathetic neurons at spinal cord level T12; innervates peripheral neurons within ganglia associated with the superior mesenteric artery.

Left brachiocephalic vein Develops from thymic and thymus veins to connect the distal end of the left anterior cardinal vein with the right; drains blood from the left side of the head and neck to the superior vena cava.

Lesser omentum Mesentery between the liver and lesser curvature of the stomach derived from the ventral mesentery; includes the hepatogastric and hepatoduodenal ligaments.

Lesser sac Portion of the peritoneal cavity posterior to the stomach; partially segregated by rotation of the stomach and secondary fixation of the duodenum to the posterior body wall.

Lesser splanchnic nerve Composed of sympathetic preganglionic fibers originating from central sympathetic neurons located within the intermediolateral columns at spinal cord levels T10 and T11; innervates peripheral neurons located within the aorticorenal ganglia.

Leydig (interstitial) cells Differentiate in response to the protein encoded by the sex-determining region of the Y chromosome from mesenchymal stroma in the genital ridge; secrete male steroid hormones.

Limb bud Formed as somites in the limb regions (C5 to C8, L3 to L5) induce somatopleuric lateral plate mesoderm within the flank to proliferate; upper extremity limb buds appear at about 24 days; lower extremity limb buds appear at about 28 days.

Lobes (of the cerebellum) Initial subdivisions of the cerebellum; consist of the anterior, middle, and flocculonodular.

Lumbar splanchnic nerve Composed of sympathetic preganglionic axons originating from central neurons located within the intermediolateral columns at spinal cord levels L1 to L2; innervates peripheral neurons located in the diffuse inferior mesenteric ganglia or plexus.

Lung bud Endodermal foregut diverticulum that bifurcates into primary bronchiole buds; forms the bronchioles and alveoli of the lungs; also called respiratory diverticulum and pulmonary diverticulum.

M

Major calyces Calyces of the metanephric collecting system formed after formation of the renal pelvis as the next four generations of ureteric bud bifurcations coalesce.

Malleus bone Auditory ossicle arising from Meckel's cartilage.

Mammary glands Modified apocrine glands; develop within a pair of epidermal thickenings (mammary ridges) that extend from the axilla to the inguinal region; two primary buds of the mammary glands appear by the seventh week; numerous secondary buds appear by the fourth month that become canalized to form lactiferous ducts by the sixth month; each mammary gland consists of 15 to 25 lactiferous ducts by birth.

Mammary pit Depression that is the opening to the lactiferous ducts of the mammary gland that form in the sixth month.

Mammary ridges See **Mammary glands.**

Mandible bone Formed largely of dermal elements that have invested the Meckel's cartilage within the mandibular swelling of the first pharyngeal arch.

Mandibular swellings Inferior divisions of the first pharyngeal arch that give rise to the lower jaw and lip; contain Meckel's cartilage.

Mantle layer Layer of gray matter peripheral to the ventricular layer formed by differentiating neuroblasts of the neural tube.

Marginal layer Most peripheral layer of white matter of the developing neural tube composed of nerve cell fibers that emanate from the neuronal cell bodies of the mantle layer.

Maternal sinusoids Expanded maternal capillaries within the endometrium that become connected to trophoblastic lacunae to establish uteroplacental circulation.

Mature alveoli Differentiate from branches of respiratory bronchioles (immature alveoli or terminal sacs); first appear at about week 28, produced through year 8; differentiation involves thinning of squamous epithelial lining of terminal sacs and production of surfactant.

Mature intermediate villi Slender side branches of the tertiary stem villi that begin to form near the end of the second trimester; produce small nodular secondary branches called terminal villi.

Maxilla bone In primitive jawed fishes, formed largely from cartilage within the palatopterygoquadrate bar; in humans, formed largely of dermal bone.

Maxillary sinuses Paranasal air sinuses that form within the maxilla during the third fetal month; grow larger during childhood.

Maxillary swellings Superior divisions of the first pharyngeal arch that give rise to the upper jaw and lip.

Meckel's cartilage Cartilaginous element that forms from neural crest cells within the mandibular swelling of the first pharyngeal arch; forms the malleus in humans; a remnant of this cartilage may be evident within the core of the mandible.

Medial nasal processes Formed from the medial regions of the nasal placodes; from the medial region of the nose and the intermaxillary process.

Median aperture (foramen of Magendie) Single median opening in the roof plate of the fourth ventricle allows cerebrospinal fluid to flow from the fourth ventricle to the subarachnoid space of the brain stem and spinal cord.

Median sulcus Groove that demarcates the medial line of fusion of the distal tongue buds.

Median tongue bud (tuberculum impar) Medial swelling of the first pharyngeal arch that is largely overgrown by distal tongue buds; forms a small part of the posterior region of the anterior two-thirds of the tongue.

Medulla oblongata Most caudal region of the rhombencephalon; arises from the myelencephalon and is most like the spinal cord in organization; most of the cranial nerve nuclei are formed within this part of the brain; acts as a relay between higher centers and the spinal cord; regulates respiration, heartbeat, reflex movements, and several other functions.

Medullary sex cords Primitive sex cords in the medullary region of the genital ridge that differentiate into pre-Sertoli cells to form testis cords; at puberty these cords become canalized to form the seminiferous tubules; also form the rete testis tubules that connect the seminiferous tubules to the efferent ductules.

Meiotic arrest in the female germ line, first stage Cells of the female germ line initiate meiosis during late embryonic or early fetal life, synthesize DNA, and enter the prophase stage of the first meiotic division; chromosomes condense during the dictyotene stage, meiotic progress is suspended, and the nucleus swells with fluid, producing the germinal vesicle.

Meiotic arrest in the female germ line, second stage Meiotic arrest of the primary oocyte at the first meiotic prophase is overcome following an ovulatory stimulus producing a secondary oocyte arrested at the second meiotic metaphase; secondary oocyte does not resume meiotic progress unless fertilized.

Meiotic maturation Changes in the chromosomes and DNA that occur during both meiotic divisions.

Melanocytes Neural crest-derived cells that migrate from the neural tube into the epidermis by the sixth to seventh week; become the pigment cells of the integument.

Membrane bones (of skull) Arise from the dermal armor of the armored fishes; form the cranial vault, including frontal, parietal, and superior regions of the occipital squamata; have also overgrown cartilages of the facial skeleton to form most of the maxilla, zygomatic bone, squamata of the temporal bone, and mandible.

Membranous ossification Bony tissue that develops within mesenchymal tissue in the absence of a cartilaginous precursor.

Membranous urethra Arises from the pelvic urethra of the primitive urogenital sinus in the region of the developing sphincter urethra muscle.

Membranous ventricular septum Develops from migrating neural crest cells; failure of neural crest cell migration into the heart may result in ventricular septal defects.

Meningocele Type of spina bifida in which the meninges evaginate through a dorsal defect of the vertebral canal.

Meningohydroencephalocele Anomaly of the occipital region in which part of the brain (ventricle and meninges) evaginate through a defect resulting from inadequate ossification of the cranial vault.

Meningomyelocele Severe example of spina bifida in which a sac or cele (including meninges and a segment of spinal cord) protrude through a defect in the vertebral canal.

Meniscus (of joint) Crescent-shaped fibrocartilaginous structure serving to increase the concavity of the joint.

Merkel cells Contain keratin and form desmosomes with adjacent keratinocytes; lie at the base of the epidermis and are associated with nerve endings where they function as pressure-sensing mechanoreceptors; found only in palmar or plantar regions.

Mesencephalic (cranial) flexure Initial flexure of the brain that develops at the level of the future mesencephalon on day 22.

Mesencephalon (midbrain) One of the three primary brain vesicles; also one of the five secondary brain vesicles; primarily a relay center but also contains cranial nerve nuclei, visual and auditory centers, and other structures.

Mesoderm "Middle" layer of trilaminar embryo arising from the epiblast by gastrulation during the third week; classified as paraxial, intermediate, or lateral plate mesoderm.

Mesodermal core Precursor of the limb buds; lateral plate mesoderm (the mesodermal core) and a cap of ectoderm.

Mesonephric (wolfian) ducts First function in elimination of urine; sprout ureteric buds that form the collecting system of the metanephroi; exstrophy into the posterior wall of the bladder to form trigone of the bladder; degenerate in females; form the spermatic ducts (vasa deferentia) in males.

Mesonephric excretory unit Renal corpuscle and its connection to the mesonephric duct.

Mesonephric tubules First function to form the urine of the mesonephros and transport it to mesonephric ducts; degenerate in females to form the epoophoron and paroophoron; 5 to 12 of these persist in males to form efferent ductules.

Mesonephroi "Middle" kidneys that develop from intermediate mesoderm in the thoracic and lumbar regions; functional from the 6th to the 10th week.

Metanephric excretory unit Includes the renal corpuscle (Bowman's capsule enclosing a glomerulus), proximal convoluted tubule, loops of Henle, and distal convoluted tubule.

Metanephroi Definitive kidneys that arise through inductive interactions between the ureteric bud and metanephric blastema in the sacral region; ascend to superior lumbar levels.

Metaphysis Growing region of the long bone located between the epiphyseal plate (physis) and the shaft (diaphysis).

Metencephalon (behind-brain) Cranial region of the rhombencephalon; gives rise to the pons and the cerebellum.

Midgut Region of the primitive gut tube vascularized by the superior mesenteric artery; communicates directly with the cavity of the yolk sac via the vitelline duct; gives rise to portions of the duodenum, jejunum, ileum, ascending colon, and transverse colon.

Minor calyces Formed after formation of the major calyces as an additional four generations of ureteric bud bifurcations coalesce; each drains a tree of collecting ducts (renal pyramid) that converge to form a renal papilla.

Molecular layer Layer of the cerebellar cortex formed primarily by Purkinje and basket neuroblasts and the dendritic trees of the Golgi and granule cells in the underlying granular layer.

Monosomy Absence of one chromosome of a single pair of chromosomes in an otherwise genotypically normal embryo.

Monozygotic (identical) twins See **Identical twins.**

Mosaic (embryo) Composed of a mixture of cells with different karyotypes; chromosome 21 nondisjunction may occur in a single embryonic cell during cleavage; resulting fetus develops as a mosaic of normal and trisomy 21 cells.

Motor neurons Develop within the gray matter of the ventral gray columns of the spinal cord and brain stem; innervated by axons of association neurons and in turn sprout axons that exit the spinal cord via the ventral roots.

Müllerian-inhibiting substance (MIS) See **Anti-müllerian hormone.**

Müllerian tubercle Remnant of the inferior end of the paramesonephric duct in males.

Muscles of facial expression Formed from the paraxial mesoderm (from somitomere 6) in the second pharyngeal arch.

Muscles of mastication Formed from the paraxial mesoderm (from somitomere 4) in the first pharyngeal arch.

Muscular ventricular septum Septation of the ventricles is initiated by growth of this thickened ridge of musculature; anterior trabeculated region is the primary ventricular fold (septum); smooth posterior region is the inlet septum; demarcated by the septomarginal trabecula or moderator band.

Myelencephalon (medulla brain) Caudal region (secondary brain vesicle) of the rhombencephalon; gives rise to the medulla oblongata and is most like the spinal cord in organization.

Myelin sheath Lamellar covering of nerve axons of the peripheral nervous system produced by Schwann cells; those investing axons of the central nervous system are formed by oligodendrocytes.

Myocardium Cardiac muscle arising from splanchnopleuric mesoderm that invests the primary heart tube; secretes cardiac jelly and gives rise to the conduction system.

Myoepithelial cells Muscle cells of epidermal origin form the outer layer of the sweat glands; innervated by sympathetic fibers that stimulate contractions to expel sweat from the gland.

Myotome Formed as the dermomyotome splits; further splits into epimeres and hypomeres and also gives rise to myoblasts that form upper and lower extremity musculature.

N

N number Applied to descriptions of meiotic or mitotic cells; the number of copies of each unique DNA strand within the cell.

Nail folds Two lateral ectodermal folds and a single proximal ectodermal fold surround the nail field; proximal nail fold produces the formative zone or root of the nail plate.

Nasal fin Thickened floor of the nasal sac; vacuolates and thins to form the oronasal membrane, which breaks down to form an opening between the nasal sac and oral cavity (primitive choana).

Nasal pits Shallow depressions that form within the central regions of the nasal placodes in the sixth week; posterior regions fuse together to form a single nasal sac.

Nasal placodes Ectodermal thickenings on the ventral surface of the frontonasal prominence that appear in the fourth week; form medial and lateral nasal processes.

Nasal sac See **Nasal pits.**

Nasolacrimal duct Ectodermal duct that forms through the invagination of the nasolacrimal groove; invested by bone during ossification of maxilla; drains lacrimal secretions from the conjunctival sac into the nasal cavity.

Nasolacrimal groove See **Nasolacrimal duct.**

Nephric (renal) vesicle (nephrotome) Derived from intermediate mesoderm of the mesonephroi and metanephroi; form nephric tubules.

Nephric tubules General term denoting the mesonephric and metanephric tubules derived from intermediate mesoderm; form the nephrons of the mesonephroi and metanephroi, respectively.

Neural canal A lumen formed within the neural tube during neurulation that becomes the central canal of the spinal cord and the ventricles of the brain.

Neural cord Solid midline structure formed from the caudal eminence during secondary neurulation; fuses with the caudal end of the neural tube; neural canal develops within it; forms the caudal end of the spinal cord and pia and dura of the filum terminale.

Neural crest Population of cells arising from the lateral lips of the neural plate that detach during formation of the neural tube and migrate to form a variety of structures.

Neural groove Thin longitudinal midline groove that bisects the neural plate into presumptive right and left neural folds.

Neural plate Begins to form on day 18 in epiblast along the midsagittal axis cranial to the primitive pit; undergoes neurulation in the fourth week to form the neural tube (precursor of the central nervous system).

Neurenteric canal Formed as ventral floor of hollow notochordal process degenerates; facilitates communication between amniotic cavity and yolk sac through the primitive pit.

Neuroblasts Formed as neuroepithelial cells within the central nervous system divide and differentiate; subsequently elongate and migrate to form the mantle layer of the neural tube.

Neuroectoderm Neural epithelium arising from the ectoderm within the neural plate.

Neurohypophysis (posterior pituitary) Region of the pituitary gland formed by the infundibulum of the diencephalon.

Neuromere Transitory subdivisions of the brain first evident on day 20 as transverse sulci separate the presumptive brain into small segments; nine such segments (rhombomeres) may form in the presumptive rhombencephalon.

Neuronal fibers Nerve cell axons and their accompanying glial investment.

Neurosensory cells of the olfactory epithelium Produced by cells of the nasal placode; cell bodies located within the olfactory epithelium of the nasal cavity; axons penetrate the cribriform plate of the ethmoid bone to synapse with secondary neurosensory cells within the olfactory bulb.

Neurulation Process of folding of the neural plate and closure of the cranial and caudal neuropores to form the neural tube.

Notochord A solid cylinder formed as the notochordal plate detaches from the endoderm; later induces the spinal cord and vertebral bodies.

Notochordal plate Flattened midventral bar of mesoderm formed from the hollow notochordal process.

Notochordal process One of the first mesodermal structures to arise by gastrulation as cells surround the primitive pit, forming hollow tube extending cranially in the axial midline; elongates as cells are added at its caudal end.

Nuclear maturation (of gamete) Process of nuclear remodeling and changes in DNA content and chromosome number occurring during meiosis without regard to cytoplasmic changes.

Nucleus ambiguus Located in the caudal hindbrain; provides branchial efferent fibers for cranial nerves IX, X, and XI.

Nucleus habenulae Formed within the epithalamus; may function as a relay for olfactory, somatic, and visceral afferent pathways.

Nucleus pulposus Central region of the intervertebral disc arising directly from the notochord; original tissue may be replaced by cells of the annulus fibrosis in early childhood.

Nutrient artery Single dominant artery that supplies the medullary cavity of a long bone.

O

Oblique vein of the left atrium Drains the wall of the left atrium; arises from the distal end of the left sinus horn and is directly connected to the coronary sinus.

Occipital lobes Posterior lobes of the cerebral hemispheres demarcated from the parietal lobes by the occipital sulcus; contains visuosensory areas that interpret visual information passed from the lateral geniculate bodies.

Occipital sulcus See **Occipital lobes.**

Oculomotor nerve (III) Supplies motor innervation to the following extrinsic muscles of the eye: levator palpebrae superioris, superior rectus, medial rectus, inferior rectus, and inferior oblique and parasympathetic innervation to the sphincter pupillae and ciliary muscles.

Odontoblast Neural crest-derived cells arising from the dental papilla; secrete the nonmineralized matrix of the dentin (predentin) in the seventh month; predentin calcifies to form the dentin.

Olfactory bulb Outgrowth of the telencephalon that appears in the sixth week as axons of primary sensory neurons differentiating within the nasal placodes begin to synapse with neurons; neurons become secondary sensory neurons of the olfactory system; axons of the secondary olfactory neurosensory cells elongate, forming a stalk-like olfactory tract; these synapse within olfactory centers of the cerebral hemispheres; olfactory bulbs and tracts are also called the olfactory nerve (I).

Olfactory epithelium Arises from the nasal placode to form the primary olfactory neurosensory cells.

Olfactory nerve (I) See **Olfactory bulb.**

Olfactory tract See **Olfactory bulb.**

Oligodendrocytes Supporting cells within the central nervous system; arise from glioblasts that arise from the ventricular layer; form sheet-like processes that wrap around axons to form myelin sheaths within the central nervous system.

Oligohydramnios See **Hydramnios.**

Olivary nuclei Rhombencephalic nuclei formed by alar column gray matter that migrate into ventral regions of the rhombencephalon, reeling their axons out behind them.

Oogonium Differentiates directly from a primordial germ cell; constitutes the stem cells of the female germ line.

Optic nerve (II) Composed of the axons of ganglion cells in the anterior layer of the neural retina that pass from the eyeball at the optic disc as the optic nerve; convey visual sensation from the retina to the lateral geniculate bodies.

Oronasal membrane See **Nasal fin.**

Ostium primum Opening in the septum primum that closes as the septum primum fuses with the septum intermedium.

Ostium secundum Develops by programmed cell death (apoptosis) within the superior region of the septum primum as the ostium primum closes.

Otic ganglion Parasympathetic ganglion of the glossopharyngeal nerve; houses peripheral neurons whose postganglionic fibers innervate the parotid gland.

Outer cell mass (trophoblast) Formed by "late-dividing" cells of the morula that remain at the periphery and serve as the primary source for placental membranes.

Outer enamel epithelium Derived from the ectoderm of the dental lamina.

Outer epidermal root sheath Constitutes the outer epidermal wall of the root canal of the hair follicle.

P

Palatine shelves Medial growths of the maxillary processes that form the secondary palate.

Palatine tonsils Lymphoid structures that form from endoderm of the second pharyngeal pouch and mesoderm of the second pharyngeal membrane.

Palatopterygoquadrate bar (maxillary process) Forms from neural crest cells within the maxillary swellings of the first pharyngeal arch; gives rise to the alisphenoid bone of the orbit and the incus bone of the middle ear.

Papillary muscles Muscular specializations of the ventricular walls that anchor the chordae tendineae of the atrioventricular valves.

Papillary region (of the dermis) Superficial layer elaborated into ridge-like dermal papillae that interdigitate with the epidermal ridges.

Parachordal cartilages Gives rise to the base of the occipital bone.

Paradidymis Remnants of the degenerate paragenital mesonephric tubules in the male genital system (see **Paragenital mesonephric tubules**).

Parafollicular (C) cells Calcitonin-secreting cells of the thyroid that arise from the telopharyngeal (ultimobranchial) body of the fifth pouch.

Paragenital mesonephric tubules Adjacent to the developing gonad; degenerate to form the paradidymis; degenerate in females to form the paroophoron.

Paramesonephric (müllerian) ducts Paired ducts that develop in the early seventh week; degenerate in males, leaving the appendix, testis, and müllerian tubercle; form superior end of the vagina, the uterus, and fallopian tubes (oviducts) in females.

Parasympathetic ganglia Peripheral neurons of the parasympathetic nervous system are housed in one of four cranial ganglia (ciliary [III], sphenopalatine and submandibular [VII], and otic [IX]) or numerous small ganglia embedded within the walls of the viscera of the thorax, abdomen, and pelvis (vagus [X]).

Parasympathetic nervous system Two-neuron subdivision of the autonomic nervous system that includes central motor neurons within nuclei of the brain stem and intermediolateral columns of the spinal cord (S2 to S4); sprouts preganglionic fibers that synapse with motor neurons of peripheral ganglia in the head and in the walls of trunk viscera that in turn sprout postganglionic fibers that innervate end organs; termed a craniosacral system and is involuntarily active during periods of peace and relaxation.

Parietal lobes Lobes of the cerebral hemispheres bounded anteriorly by the central sulcus from the frontal lobe and posteriorly by the occipital sulcus from the occipital lobe; contain motor and somatosensory areas and a speech area; function largely in discrimination and interpretation.

Paroophoron Remnants of the paragenital mesonephric tubules in females; scattered in the mesovarium.

Parotid (salivary) glands Develop from ectoderm within the groove formed by fusion of the maxillary and mandibular swellings.

Pelvic kidney Metanephric kidney that fails to ascend between the sixth and ninth weeks; remains within the pelvis.

Pelvic splanchnic nerves Formed by parasympathetic preganglionic fibers emerging from the ventral surface of the sacral cord (S2 to S4); innervates ganglia of target viscera.

Pelvic urethra Constricted region of the primitive urogenital sinus at the base of the presumptive bladder; gives rise to the membranous urethra in females and the membranous and prostatic urethras in males.

Penile urethra Part of the urethra in males enclosed within the corpora spongiosum of the penis; derived from the definitive urogenital sinus.

Penis Male phallus derived from the genital tubercle and the fusion of urethral folds.

Pericardioperitoneal canals Facilitate communication between the superior primitive pericardial cavity and inferior peritoneal cavity through the septum transversum.

Periderm During the fourth week the surface ectoderm proliferates to produce this superficial epidermal cell layer; usually sloughed by the 21st week; with sebaceous gland secretions, produces a waterproof covering called the vernix caseosa.

Periodontal ligaments Derivatives of the inner layer of the dental sac that anchor the root of the tooth to the alveolus.

Periotic (petromastoid) bones Arise from mesenchyme of the otic capsule to form the bony labyrinth enclosing the inner ear.

Peritoneal cavity Derived from the region of the intraembryonic coelomic cavity inferior to the diaphragm; forms the abdominal and pelvic cavities.

Permissive pathways Pathways for growth cones of elongating nerves; most notably devoid of dense mesenchyme or glycosaminoglycans.

Phallus (indifferent stage) Gives rise to the clitoris in the female and the penis in the male.

Pharyngeal arches Paired structures in human embryos evolved from branchial arches 1, 2, 3, 4, and 6 of primitive fishes to form facial and pharyngeal structures.

Pharyngeal clefts Outer grooves between the pharyngeal arches.

Pharyngeal membranes Thin, three-layered membranes consisting of ectoderm, mesoderm, and endoderm; separate the pharyngeal pouches from the pharyngeal clefts; first pharyngeal membrane forms the tympanic membrane or eardrum.

Pharyngeal pouches Inner grooves within the pharynx; separate the pharyngeal arches but also give rise to important cavities and glands.

Philtrum Medial groove of the upper lip; formed from the inferior region of the intermaxillary process.

Phocomelia Shortened limbs may lack several intermediary segments, taking the form of seal-like appendages.

Pineal gland Small pine-cone-shaped gland; develops from an evagination of the epithalamus.

Pioneer axon Provides pathway along which other axons may grow.

Pituitary Formed from the roof of the stomodeum (Rathke's pouch) and the infundibulum (floor of the diencephalon); Rathke's pouch gives rise to the anterior lobe and pars intermedia and the infundibulum forms the posterior pituitary (neurohypophysis).

Placenta Derived from the maternal decidua basalis and the fetal chorion; provides a mechanism to exchange oxygen, nutrients, carbon dioxide, and wastes between the fetal and the maternal circulations.

Pleural cavities Formed along with the definitive pericardial cavity by division of the primitive pericardial cavity by the pleuropericardial folds.

Pleuropericardial folds Coronal folds of the lateral body wall that grow into the primitive pericardial cavity during the fifth week; folds fuse together in the midline and, with esophageal mesoderm, form the left and right pleural cavities and an anterior definitive pericardial cavity; forms the parietal pericardium, mediastinal pleura, and fibrous pericardium.

Pleuroperitoneal membranes Grow from the posterolateral body walls in the plane of the septum transversum to seal off the pericardioperitoneal canals.

Ploidy Number of copies of distinct chromosomes within a cell nucleus; haploid cell nucleus contains 23 chromosomes; diploid cell nucleus contains a pair of 23 chromosomes (46 chromosomes).

Polar body Three minute, nonfunctional products of unequal meiotic divisions in the female germ line.

Polydactyly Existence of extra fingers or toes.

Polyhydramnios An excess of amniotic fluid; may occur if the fetus is not able to swallow amniotic fluid as in cases of esophageal atresia or anencephaly.

Pons Functions to relay signals between the spinal cord and the cerebral and cerebellar cortices; composed largely of white matter; also contains pontine nuclei that relay input from the cerebrum to the cerebellum.

Pontine flexure Third flexure of the brain; begins bending the cerebellum back upon the myelencephalon in the fifth week of development at the level of the metencephalon.

Pontine nuclei Formed by alar column gray matter that migrates into the ventral region of the brain stem.

Portal system Specialized system of veins that drains the gastrointestinal tract into the liver for processing of nutrients; arises from right and left vitelline veins and their median anastomoses.

Posterior and habenular commissures Fiber tracts that connect the left and right epithalami and, with the nucleus habenulae, form the trigonum habenulae.

Posterior cardinal veins Bilateral paired vessels that drain the trunk and lower extremities between the fourth and eighth weeks; superseded by the subcardinal and supracardinal systems.

Posterior lobe (of pituitary) See **Neurohypophysis.**

Postganglionic fibers See **Preganglionic fibers** and **Parasympathetic nervous system.**

Pre-Sertoli cell Formed by medullary sex cord cells that differentiate during the sixth or seventh week of development and then give rise to Sertoli cells.

Prechordal cartilages Form the ethmoid bone of the chondrocranium.

Prechordal plate Small block of mesoderm that forms just cranial to the tip of the notochordal process; induces cranial midline structures such as the brain.

Predentin Nonmineralized matrix of the dentin; first secreted by the odontoblasts in the seventh month.

Preganglionic fibers Sympathetic or parasympathetic autonomic fibers emanating from central neurons that innervate neurons in peripheral ganglia.

Prevention of polyspermy Contents of cortical granules are released into the perivitelline space (between oocyte membrane and zona pellucida) as the first spermatozoon fuses with the oocyte membrane, preventing further binding of additional sperm.

Prevertebral (preaortic) ganglion Peripheral sympathetic ganglia that house the second neuron of the two-neuron sympathetic pathway innervating the abdominal viscera; associated with major abdominal branches of the descending aorta.

Primary brain vesicles From upon complete closure of the cranial neuropore; expansions that form each vesicle are apparent within the neural tube.

Primary buds (of mammary glands) Paired ingrowths of mammary ridge epidermis; precursors of the mammary glands.

Primary endoderm See **Hypoblast.**

Primary intestinal loop During the fifth week the midgut forms this hairpin loop that herniates into the umbilicus.

Primary oocyte or **spermatocyte** During preparatory stage of the first meiotic division oogonium and spermatogonium are converted to the primary oocyte or primary spermatocyte respectively.

Primary palate Short dorsal extension of the intermaxillary process; fuses with the palatine shelves (secondary palate) in the region of the incisive foramen.

Primary sensory cells of the olfactory system See **Olfactory epithelium** and **Olfactory bulb.**

Primary (deciduous) teeth Ten are formed within both upper and lower dental laminae; in each half-jaw will form two incisors, one canine, and two premolars; begin to erupt in the sixth month; fully erupted by 2 years of age; replaced by secondary or permanent teeth.

Primary yolk sac Formed by transformation of the blastocyst cavity; is later pushed toward abembryonic pole and degenerates to form exocoelomic vesicles and cysts.

Primitive atrium Appears as a small expansion of the primitive heart tube early in the fourth week; forms right auricle as it is displaced on the right side by incorporation of the right sinus venosus and left auricle as it is displaced on the left side by intussusception of the pulmonary veins.

Primitive groove Shallow groove running from the primitive pit to the caudal end of the primitive streak.

Primitive (primary) heart tube Formed by fusion of the lateral endocardial tubes.

Primitive node Lip of ectoderm around the primitive pit at the cranial end of the primitive streak forming the notochordal process.

Primitive nuclear neuroblasts Formed by the inner germinal layer of the cerebellum in the fourth month; migrate and give rise to the deep cerebellar nuclei.

Primitive pericardial cavity See **Definitive pericardial cavity.**

Primitive pit Depression surrounded by the primitive node at the cranial end of the primitive streak.

Primitive sex cords Form within the presumptive gonads (genital ridges) in response to arrival of the primordial germ cell; arise from cells of the coelomic epithelium and possibly cells of the mesonephros.

Primitive streak Composed of the primitive node, primitive pit, and primitive groove; forms at beginning of third week and provides the mechanism for gastrulation.

Primitive urogenital sinus Formed from the ventral region of the cloaca as it is divided by the urorectal septum; gives rise to the bladder, pelvic urethra, and definitive urogenital sinus.

Primitive ventricle Expansion of the primitive heart tube apparent early in the fourth week; mainly forms the definitive left ventricle; small portion contributes to formation of the definitive right ventricle.

Processus vaginalis Evagination of the peritoneum that plays an active role in formation of the inguinal canal; normally obliterated in females; distal remnant in the male is the tunica vaginalis; in both sexes, may remain intact and give rise to a congenital indirect hernia.

Pronucleus Chromosomes and nucleoplasm of definitive oocyte and definitive spermatocyte become separately enclosed within their own nuclear envelopes during fertilization to form female and male pronuclei, respectively.

Prosencephalon (forebrain) Region of neural plate forming this primary brain vesicle is apparent even prior to closure of the cranial neuropore; will form two secondary brain vesicles: the cranial telencephalon and diencephalon.

Prostate Male gland formed from five endodermal lobes that sprout from the pelvic urethra at the base of the bladder in the 10th week; smooth muscle and connective tissue components are derived from the splanchnopleuric mesoderm that initially covers the hindgut; formed under influence of dihydrotestosterone.

Prostatic urethra Segment of the pelvic urethra that becomes enclosed within the developing prostate gland.

Proximal nail fold See **Nail folds.**

Psoriasis Hyperproliferative skin disease; may be caused by overproduction of transforming growth factor-α

Pulmonary diverticulum See **Lung bud.**

Pulmonary trunk Outflow tract of the right ventricle that develops from the truncus arteriosus.

Pulmonary valve See **Semilunar valves.**

Purkinje neuroblasts Formed by the internal germinal layer of the cerebellum and, with the basket neuroblasts formed by the external germinal layer, contribute to formation of the molecular layer of the cerebellum.

Q

Quail–chick chimera system Experimental model (originally developed by Le Douarin) in which small pieces of chick embryo tissue are removed and replaced with tissue obtained from a quail embryo; the quail cells may differentiate and/or migrate and, due to their distinctive nucleoli, may be followed throughout their subsequent development.

R

Rachischisis Synonym for spina bifida; craniorachischisis may refer to anencephaly.

Rathke's pouch Ectodermal evagination of the roof of the stomodeum; forms the anterior lobe of the pituitary and the pars intermedia.

Recurrent laryngeal branch of the vagus nerve Provides motor innervation to the intrinsic muscles of the larynx and also includes sensory fibers that innervate the mucous membrane of the larynx below the vocal cords; also possesses general visceral efferent fibers innervating the mucous membrane of the trachea.

Reichert's cartilage Cartilage of the second pharyngeal arch formed by neural crest cells.

Renal (Malpighian) corpuscle Comprised of the Bowman's capsule and glomerulus.

Renal papilla Convergence of collecting ducts from a single renal pyramid at the minor calyx.

Renal pelvis Large expansion of the hilus of the developing kidney formed from the initial bifurcation of the ureteric bud.

Renal pyramid Pyramidal grouping of collecting ducts extending from the tip of each minor calyx (from the renal papilla) to connect with metanephric excretory units within the renal cortex.

Respiratory bronchial Sprout from terminal bronchials between 16 and 28 weeks; branch to form terminal sacs.

Respiratory diverticulum See **Lung bud.**

Rete testis Thin-walled tubules that connect the seminiferous tubules with the efferent ductules formed as the deepest medullary sex cords differentiate.

Reticular layer Thick layer of dense irregular connective tissue; deep layer of the dermis.

Retroperitoneal (organ) Embedded within the subserous fascia of the peritoneum lining the body wall and located behind the parietal peritoneum from a point of view within a body cavity.

Rh factor Genetically determined surface molecules present on the plasma membranes of red blood cells in most but not all individuals (see **Erythroblastosis fetalis**).

Rhombencephalon (hindbrain) Region of the neural plate forming this primary brain vesicle is evident prior to closure of the cranial neuropore; will form two secondary brain vesicles: the metencephalon and myelencephalon.

Rhombic lips (of the hindbrain) Arise as thickenings of the alar columns; form the cerebellar primordia that in turn give rise to the cerebellum; some of the gray matter within it migrates into the ventral floor of the hindbrain to form the pontine and olivary nuclei.

Rhombomere Neuromeres of the rhombencephalon (see **Neuromere**).

Roof plate Thin dorsal wall of the spinal cord and brain stem.

Root of nail plate See **Formative zone (root; of nail plate.**

Root of the tooth Region deep to the boundary of the cementoenamel junction; embedded within the alveolus and covered with cementum.

S

Sacral plexus Large plexus of nerves (anterior to the pyriformis muscle and the sacrum) composed of ventral primary rami of the lumbosacral trunk (L4, L5) and S1 to S4.

Salivatory nuclei Innervate the salivary and lacrimal glands via nerves VII and IX.

Schwann cells See **Myelin sheath.**

Sclerotome Results from differentiation of somites; ventromedial and loose core cells migrate and surround the notochord and neural tube to eventually form the vertebrae.

Scoliosis Curvature of the spine often caused by unequal development or growth of the left and right halves of a vertebral body (see **Hemivertebra**).

Scrotum Contains the testes in the male; homologous to the labia majora of the female; arises from the labioscrotal swellings.

Sebaceous glands   Usually form as diverticula of the hair follicles within 4 weeks after the hair germ begins to elongate; formed in most regions of the body; branch into a small system of ducts that expand into small terminal acini that secrete sebum through a holocrine mechanism.

Second meiotic division   Double-stranded chromosomes divide within secondary gonocyte yielding two haploid 1N daughter cells; two definitive spermatocytes or spermatids in males and a definitive oocyte and polar body in females.

Second trimester   Fourth through sixth months of gestation.

Secondarily retroperitoneal (organ)   Appears to be retroperitoneal; initially an intraperitoneal organ that became secondarily fused to the body wall.

Secondary buds (of mammary glands)   See **Mammary glands.**

Secondary endoderm   See **Definitive (secondary) endoderm.**

Secondary neurosensory cells of the olfactory system   See **Olfactory bulb.**

Secondary neurulation   Process resulting in formation of the caudal spinal cord and filum terminale by the caudal eminence.

Secondary oocyte or **Secondary spermatocyte**   Products of the first meiotic division that are haploid and 2N.

Secondary teeth   See **Primary (deciduous) teeth.**

Secondary yolk sac   Forms first blood vessels and blood cells; typically disappears, but may form anomalous Meckel's diverticulum.

Semilunar (trigeminal) ganglion of cranial nerve V   Sensory ganglion of the fifth cranial nerve; comprised of neurons arising from the neural crest as well as from the trigeminal placode; serves general afferent functions of the trigeminal nerve.

Semilunar valves   Valves of the aortic and pulmonary outflow tracts that arise as cell death foci sculpt cusps from the left and right truncoconal septa, a minor anterior truncus swelling (a cusp of the pulmonary valve), and a minor posterior swelling (a cusp of the aortic valve).

Seminal vesicles   Diverticula of the mesonephric ducts; form convoluted glands that contribute secretions to the seminal fluid that nourish and protect sperm following ejaculation.

Seminiferous tubules   Derived from the cells of the primitive medullary sex cords; form pre-Sertoli cells and then Sertoli cells that differentiate at puberty.

Sensitive period   Period in which an organ or organ system is sensitive to effects of teratogens.

Sensory capsules   Evolved from primitive ossification centers to protect the nasal epithelium, eyeball, and ear.

Sensory neurons   Arise from neural crest cells that then collect lateral to the spinal cord within dorsal root ganglia; form both axons and dendritic processes that innervate the association neurons of the dorsal gray columns and target organs, respectively; may also be applied to neurons within the cranial sensory ganglia associated with cranial nerves V, VII, IX, and X and to the special sensory neurons of the retina, the nose, and the ears; may also be loosely applied to the association neurons within the dorsal (sensory) gray columns of the spinal cord and brain stem.

Septum intermedium   Divides the single atrioventricular canal into right and left atrioventricular canals as the superior and inferior endocardial cushions meet and fuse during the sixth week.

Septum primum   Membranous interatrial septum that forms adjacent to the left atrium; first contains an **Ostium primum,** which closes when the septum fuses with the **Septum intermedium; Ostium secundum** then forms in its superior region.

Septum secundum   Grows from the atrial roof just to the right of the septum primum; forms the foramen ovale.

Septum transversum   Cranial block of mesoderm apparent at the leading edge of the trilaminar germ disc on about day 22; translo-

cated inferiorly and ventrally to the region of the presumptive diaphragm during embryonic folding; becomes innervated by cervical nerves C3, C4, and C5 and gives rise to the central tendon of the diaphragm.

Sertoli cells   Arise through differentiation of medullary sex cord cells in male embryos and actively participate in nuclear and cytoplasmic maturation of male germ cells; differentiation is not complete until puberty, when they form seminiferous tubules.

Sex determination   The male sex is determined by presence of a Y sex chromosome (XY), and female sex is determined by absence of a Y sex chromosome (XX).

Sex-determining region of the Y chromosome (SRY)   Gene in the 1A1 region of the Y chromosome that encodes a transcription factor (the SRY protein) with a pivotal role in male sex determination and development.

Shaft (of the clitoris; of the penis)   Short shaft of the female clitoris arises from the proximal end of the genital tubercle; longer shaft of the male penis is derived from the proximal end of the genital tubercle and the fusing urethral folds.

Sinus venarum   Smooth-walled region of the definitive right atrium formed by intussusception of the right horn of the sinus venosus.

Sinus venosus   Chamber at the inferior end of the primitive heart tube; site of confluence of the left and right common cardinal, vitelline, and umbilical veins prior to remodeling of the inflow region of the heart; left sinus horn forms the coronary sinus, and right horn forms the sinus venarum and thus the definitive right atrium.

Sinusal tubercle   Endodermal thickening at the posterior wall of the pelvic urethra in the region of contact of the paramesonephric ducts; expands to form the sinuvaginal bulbs, which later form the inferior segment of the vagina.

Soft palate   Most posterior region of the secondary palate; contains muscle that differentiates from its enclosed mesenchyme.

Somatic efferent   Characterizes cranial nerves III, IV, VI, and XII, which provide motor innervation to striated muscles that do not develop within the pharyngeal arches.

Somatic nervous system   Subdivision of the peripheral nervous system responsible for carrying conscious sensations and for innervating the voluntary (striated) muscles of the body.

Somites   Appear at about day 20 as blocks of segmental mesoderm developed from somitomeres; cervical, thoracic, lumbar, and sacral somites establish segmental organization of the body by giving rise to most of the axial skeleton (including vertebral column), part of the dermis, and the voluntary musculature.

Somitomeres   Segmental whorls produced prior to segmentation of paraxial mesoderm into somites; all but the first seven cranial pairs differentiate into somites.

Special somatic afferent   Neuronal function served by the olfactory (I: smell), optic (II: vision), and vestibulocochlear (VIII: hearing and balance) nerves.

Special visceral afferent   Characterizes sensory pathways that serve the sense of taste (gustatory function) provided by cranial nerves VII, IX, and X.

Spermatic duct (vas deferens)   Arises from the mesonephric ducts in the male (see **Vas deferens).**

Spermatic fascia   Processus vaginalis elongates and pushes this inguinal "sock," composed of internal (from transversalis fascia), cremasteric (from internal oblique muscle), and external (from the external oblique muscle) spermatic fascia, into the scrotal swelling.

Spermatogenesis   The nuclear and cytoplasmic changes that transform primordial germ cells of the male germ line into mature spermatocytes.

Spermiation   The release of the spermatozoon from the seminal epithelium into the lumen of the seminiferous tubule.

Spermiogenesis Process of cytoplasmic maturation that converts a spermatid to a spermatozoon.

Sphenoid bone Arises from the hypophyseal cartilages; greater and lesser wings have evolved from the optic capsule.

Sphenoid sinuses Extensions of the ethmoid sinuses into the sphenoid bone; first appear during the fifth fetal month and enlarge during infancy and childhood.

Sphenopalatine ganglion Parasympathetic ganglion of the facial nerve (VII); houses the peripheral neurons of the pathway that provides parasympathetic motor innervation to the lacrimal glands and mucous glands within the nasal cavity.

Spina bifida Spectrum of anomalies including spina bifida occulta, meningocele, meningomyelocele, rachischisis, and cranioschisis arising from failure of complete development and closure of the vertebral arches in one or more segments.

Spinal accessory nerve (XI) Classified as branchial efferent since it is located within the same plane of the brain stem as motor columns serving the trigeminal (V), facial (VII), glossopharyngeal (IX), and vagus (X) nerves.

Spinal nerves Originate at the point where dorsal and ventral roots join to form bundles of nerve fibers containing sensory, motor, and, in most cases, postganglionic sympathetic fibers.

Stapes bone Auditory ossicle arising from Reichert's cartilage of the second pharyngeal arch.

Stellate neuroblasts Final population of neuroblasts produced by the external germinal layer of the developing cerebellum; found in both the molecular and granular layers of the definitive cerebellar cortex.

Stem villus At 11 days, proliferation of syncytiotrophoblast and cytotrophoblast produce primary stem villi that evaginate into the trophoblastic lacunae; by day 16, an innermost core of extraembryonic somatopleuric mesoderm transforms these into secondary stem villi; by day 21, extraembryonic mesoderm differentiates into blood vessels and blood cells, converting these into tertiary stem villi.

Stratum corneum See **Horny layer.**

Stratum germinativum See **Germinative layer.**

Stratum granulosum Production of keratin and envelope proteins ceases as cells move from the stratum spinosum into this layer; produce filagrin, which helps to bundle keratin filaments within the cell.

Stratum spinosum Layer of keratinocytes overlying the stratum germinativum; as cells move into this layer they produce large amounts of keratin and envelope proteins that cover the inner surface of the plasma membranes.

Stylohyoid ligament Connects the tip of the styloid process to the lesser horn (cornua) of the hyoid; formed by Reichert's cartilage within the second pharyngeal arch.

Styloid process Inferior extension of the temporal bone; formed by Reichert's cartilage within the second pharyngeal arch.

Subarachnoid space Space between the arachnoid and pia layers of the brain and spinal cord; filled with cerebrospinal fluid.

Sublingual (salivary) glands Form from endodermal invaginations in the paralingual sulci of the oral cavity.

Submandibular ganglion Parasympathetic ganglion of the facial nerve (VII); houses peripheral neurons that provide parasympathetic postganglionic fibers to the submandibular and sublingual salivary glands.

Submandibular (salivary) glands Arise from endodermal invaginations in the floor of the oral cavity.

Subplate See **Cerebral cortex.**

Subventricular zone Layer of proliferating cells between the ventricular and intermediate layers of the cerebellum that supersedes the ventricular zone.

Sulcus dorsalis Shallow groove that appears in the sixth week to demarcate the epithalamus from the thalamus; obliterated by enlargement of the thalamus.

Sulcus limitans Narrow groove running longitudinally along the inner surface of the lateral wall of the neural tube that divides the dorsal (alar) columns from the ventral (basal) columns.

Superficial ring (of inguinal canal) Inferior medial boundary of the inguinal canal; deficiency of the external oblique muscle from which the external spermatic fascia evaginates into the scrotum.

Superior colliculi Paired swellings within the roof plate of the mesencephalon formed by proliferation of alar column neuroblasts; receive fibers from the retinas and mediate ocular reflexes.

Superior ganglion of cranial nerve IX (glossopharyngeal) Relays general sensory and special sensory (taste) impulses from the glossopharyngeal nerve to the visceral afferent nuclei; serves cranial nerve IX and the nucleus of the tractus solitarius, respectively.

Superior ganglion of the vagus (X) Relays general sensory, interoceptive, and special sensory (taste) impulses from the vagus nerve to the general afferent, visceral afferent nuclei, and nucleus of the tractus solitarius, respectively; serves cranial nerve X.

Superior laryngeal branch of the vagus nerve Innervates the musculature that develops in association with the fourth pharyngeal arch, including the cricothyroid, levator veli palatini, and pharyngeal constrictors; provides general and special (taste) sensory innervation to the very posterior region of the tongue and general sensory fibers to the epiglottis and mucous membrane of the larynx.

Superior parathyroid glands Named for their final position superior to the inferior parathyroids in the dorsal wall of the thyroid gland.

Superior vena cava Vessel arising from the proximal end of the right anterior cardinal vein.

Sweat glands First appear at about 20 weeks as buds of the stratum germinativum grow into the dermis to form unbranched highly coiled glands; secrete fluid by an eccrine mechanism; found in virtually all regions of the body except the nipples.

Sympathetic chain ganglion Paired ganglia formed at almost every segment from the cervical region to the first coccygeal level.

Sympathetic nervous system Two-neuron subdivision of the autonomic nervous system composed of central motor neurons within intermediolateral columns of the spinal cord (T1 to L2) and peripheral neurons within sympathetic chain ganglia or prevertebral ganglia; central neurons sprout preganglionic fibers that synapse with neurons in peripheral ganglia; neurons within peripheral ganglia produce postganglionic fibers that innervate target organs; termed a thoracolumbar system and is active during periods of "fight and flight."

Sympathetic trunk Composed of chain ganglia and the preganglionic fiber tract that interconnects them on either side of the vertebral column; paired sympathetic trunks run from the first cervical to the first coccygeal vertebral segment.

Synchondroidal joint Union of two bones comprised of hyaline cartilage or fibrocartilage.

Syncytiotrophoblast Expanding peripheral syncytial layer produced by mitoses within cells of the cytotrophoblast at the embryonic pole of the blastocyst beginning at day 6; secretes human chorionic gonadotropin maintaining thickened endometrium of uterus until placental membranes later usurp this function.

Syndactyly Insufficient cell death within the radial necrotic zones between digital rays results in fusion of the digits; may be manifested in webbing of the skin; bony elements of the digits may be fused.

Synovial (diarthroidal) joint Contains a cavity lined by a synovial membrane that in turn contains a slippery, lubricating fluid permitting unfettered movement between joined bones.

T

Tela choroidea   Thin membrane covering the roof of the fourth ventricle; formed by ependyma and a well-vascularized layer of pia matter.

Telencephalon (end-brain)   Secondary brain vesicle arising from the prosencephalon; forms the cerebral vesicles and the rhinencephalon (nose-brain).

Telopharyngeal (ultimobranchial) body   Formed from a controversial fifth pharyngeal pouch; migrates into the thyroid gland to form the calcitonin-secreting parafollicular (C) cells.

Temporal lobes   First appear as a forward growth of the caudal end of the lengthening cerebral hemisphere in the fourth month; involved in hearing, language, and perception.

Temporal squamosa   Dermal bone that forms in association with the maxillary process of the first pharyngeal arch.

Temporomandibular joint   Arose in evolution with the emergence of mammals; replaces the incus and malleus, which served as the jaw joint of vertebrates other than mammals.

Teratogen   Agent that acts on the developing embryo, causing abnormal development.

Terminal bronchial   Bronchial branches formed after about 17 generations of branchings of the lung bud by the 16th week; between weeks 16 and 28 they each subdivide into two or more respiratory bronchioles.

Terminal sac   See **Mature alveoli.**

Terminal sulcus   Transverse groove that demarcates the boundary between the anterior two-thirds and posterior one-third of the tongue.

Terminal villi   Lateral branches of the mature intermediate villi; contain folded, coiled capillaries.

Thalamus   Region of the diencephalon initially separated superiorly from the epithalamus by the sulcus dorsalis and from the inferior hypothalamus by the hypothalamic sulcus; relays information to the cerebral cortex and nuclei within the thalamus; functions in sight (lateral geniculate body) and hearing (medial geniculate body).

Third trimester   Seventh through the ninth month of gestation.

Third ventricle   Expansion of the neural canal enclosed within the diencephalon.

Thymus gland   Arises from endoderm within the third pharyngeal pouch; descends to a position just dorsal to the sternum, where it grows to a maximum size at puberty and then regresses.

Thyroglossal cyst (sinus)   Formed when the normally degenerating thyroglossal duct persists.

Thyroglossal duct   See **Thyroid gland** and **thyroglossal cyst.**

Thyroid gland   Forms at the apex of the thyroglossal duct as it elongates from the foramen cecum of the tongue; elongation of the thyroglossal duct places the thyroid just ventral and inferior to the developing larynx by the seventh week of development.

Tooth bud   Specialization of the dental lamina that may give rise to a primary or secondary tooth in collaboration with a dental papilla; derived from neural crest cells and an investing layer of dermal mesenchyme called the dental sac; forms the enamel organ of the growing tooth and the epithelial root sheath.

Transgenic animal   Produced by introducing foreign DNA into its genome by direct injection of the DNA into the male or the female pronucleus or by using DNA targeting techniques.

Tricuspid valve   See **Atrioventricular valves.**

Trigeminal nerve (V)   Innervates the maxillary process and mandibular process; contains branchial efferent and general sensory fibers; general sensory innervation provided by the mandibular division to the anterior two-thirds of the tongue and by the maxillary division to the nasal passages and primary and hard palates.

Trigeminal placode   Ectodermal placode that gives rise to the neurons within the distal part of the semilunar ganglion.

Trigone (of the bladder)   Smooth-walled region of the posterior bladder wall (between the orifices of the two ureters and the opening into the pelvic urethra); formed by the intussusception of the inferior ends of the mesonephric ducts.

Trilaminar germ disc   Three-layered (trilaminar) embryo consisting of ectoderm, mesoderm, and definitive endoderm.

Triploid   Nucleus contains three copies of all 23 chromosomes (69 chromosomes).

Trisomy   Results from the presence of two of the same kind of chromosome in one of the gametes forming a zygote containing three copies of the same kind of chromosome.

Trochlear nerve (IV)   Somatic efferent fibers within this cranial nerve innervate the superior oblique muscle of the eyeball.

Trophic substance   Supports the growth or viability of a cellular subpopulation such as brain-derived neural growth factor (BDNF)

Trophoblast   Arises from the outer cell mass during the morula stage and initially lines blastocyst cavity but then forms the syncytiotrophoblast and cytotrophoblast of the chorionic plate; development is largely under control of the male genome.

Trophoblastic lacunae   Cavities formed within the syncytiotrophoblast in the second week that then join with maternal sinusoids to establish uteroplacental circulation.

Tropic substance   Attracts cells or growth cones to the target structures that secrete them such as netrin.

True ribs   First seven ribs that articulate with the sternum via costal cartilages.

Truncoconal septa   Septa of the outflow tracts formed from neural crest cells migrating to the truncus arteriosus through the third, fourth, and sixth aortic arches; fusion simultaneously separates the right and left ventricular chambers along with their respective outflow tracts the pulmonary trunk and aorta.

Truncus arteriosus   Distal segment of the bulbus cordis, which is divided into the ascending aorta and pulmonary trunk by formation and fusion of the truncoconal septa between weeks 5 and 9.

Tuberculum impar   See **Median tongue bud.**

Tubotympanic recess   Develops from the first pharyngeal pouch; further differentiates into the eustachian (auditory) tube and the tympanic cavity.

Tubulobulbar complexes   Formed by Sertoli cells to siphon cytoplasm from spermatids, reducing the cytoplasmic-nuclear ratio during maturation of the spermatozoon.

Tunica vaginalis   Inferior remnant of the processus vaginalis in males; enwraps the testis but is also enclosed (like the spermatic cord) in three layers of spermatic fascia; potential lumen may become filled with serous fluid following injury or disease of the serosal membrane.

U

Ultimobranchial body   See **Telopharyngeal (ultimobranchial) body.**

Ultrasonography   Body is scanned with an ultrasound beam (3 to 10 MHz); computer analyzes returning echoes imaging internal structures.

Umbilical Cord   Formed by association of the connecting stalk and neck of the yolk sac (vitelline duct) as they become invested in amniotic membrane at the conclusion of embryonic folding in week 8.

Uncinate process   Hook-like region of the pancreas; derived from the ventral pancreatic bud; contains the main pancreatic duct.

Urachus (median umbilical ligament) Vestige arising from obliteration of the allantois; may rarely remain patent.

Ureter Duct that drains the kidneys into the bladder; derived from the ureteric bud.

Ureteric buds Sprout from the mesonephric ducts; lengthen to penetrate the metanephric blastema; undergo a prescribed series of bifurcations to form the renal pelvis, major and minor calyces, and collecting tubules of the metanephros; tips (ampullae) induce development of the metanephric excretory units.

Urethral (urogenital) folds Arise from the cloacal folds; give rise to the labia minora (females) and shaft (spongy urethra) of the penis (males).

Urogenital membrane Arises from the anterior end of the cloacal membrane in the seventh week as the urorectal septum fuses with the cloacal membrane.

Urorectal septum Mesenchymal septum that divides the cloaca composed of a Tourneaux fold, which grows inferiorly to the presumptive pelvic urethra, and left and right inferolateral Rathke folds that subdivide the inferior cloaca.

Uterovaginal (genital) canal Single cavity formed within the developing vagina and uterus by fusion of the paramesonephric ducts; produces the inferior end of the vaginal lumen.

Uterus Formed by fusion of the paramesonephric (müllerian) ducts.

V

Vagina Composite structure primarily arising from fusion of the paramesonephric ducts; smaller inferior segment is formed by growth of the sinusal tubercle.

Vaginal (sinuvaginal) bulbs Hollow expansions of the sinusal tubercle; give rise to the inferior segment of the vagina.

Vaginal plate Endodermal proliferation that occludes the inferior end of the genital canal; later canalized by desquamation to form the lower end of the vaginal canal.

Vagus nerve (X) Relays interoceptive information from the trachea, larynx, esophagus, and thoracic and abdominal viscera and stretch and chemoreceptors within the aortic arch and aortic bodies, respectively; transmits impulses from the skin behind the ear, external acoustic meatus, external surface of the tympanic membrane, and pharynx; innervates striated muscles of the fourth and sixth pharyngeal arches, glands, and smooth muscle of the pharynx, larynx, and thoracic and abdominal viscera.

Vas deferens (pl. vasa deferentia; also Spermatic duct) Male genital ducts that arise from the mesonephric ducts; differentiate in response to testosterone.

Vasculogenesis Blood vessels form throughout the entire embryo as endoderm induces overlying splanchnopleuric mesoderm to form networks of vasculature characteristic of each specific region; angioblasts form angiocysts that coalesce to form angioblastic cords and then angioblastic plexuses.

Ventral mesentery Fold of peritoneum derived from the inferior septum transversum; initially suspends the abdominal esophagus and stomach from the anterior abdominal wall; forms the falciform ligament, the visceral peritoneum of the liver and coronary ligament, and the lesser omentum.

Ventral pancreatic bud Endodermal diverticulum that sprouts just inferior to the cystic diverticulum on the ventral duodenal wall at the end of the fourth week; forms the uncinate process and main pancreatic duct.

Ventral primary ramus Ventral branch of any spinal nerve that innervates muscles of the lateral and anterior trunk and muscles of the upper and lower extremities; contains motor, sensory, and sympathetic fibers.

Ventral roots Paired bundles of nerve fibers emanating from the left and right ventrolateral wall of the spinal cord at every segmental level from the first cervical to first coccygeal level; contain motor axons of the ventral (basal) columns and preganglionic sympathetic fibers of the intermediolateral cell columns from T1 to L2.

Ventricular layer Layer of neuroepithelium located adjacent to the neural canal; gives rise to neurons, supporting cells, and ependyma of the central nervous system.

Vermis Median region of the cerebellum bounded laterally by the cerebellar hemispheres and caudally by the posterolateral fissure that separates it from the flocculonodular lobe.

Vernix caseosa See **Periderm.**

Vestibular ganglion of cranial nerve VIII Serves the special sensory function of balance; neurons arise from the otic placode (mainly) along with the neural crest.

Vestibule of the vagina Entrance to the vagina between the labia minora; derived directly from definitive urogenital sinus.

Vestibulocochlear nerve (VIII) Serves the special senses of hearing and balance.

Visceral afferent Part of the nervous system receiving interoceptive impulses via the glossopharyngeal (IX) and vagus (X) nerves from thoracic, abdominal, and pelvic viscera.

Visceral efferent Function served by cranial nerves III, VII, IX, and X; preganglionic fibers innervate parasympathetic ganglia that emit postganglionic fibers that innervate smooth muscles and glands of viscera from the head to the left colic flexure.

Vitelline arteries Initially vascularize the yolk sac; become the chief arteries of the gastrointestinal tract.

Vitelline duct Formed as growth of the embryo overtakes the stagnating yolk sac; connection between the yolk sac and midgut of the developing gastrointestinal tract narrows into this slim duct.

W

White matter Contains myelinated nerve fibers that arise from neuronal cell bodies within ventral gray column, nuclei, and specialized cortical layers of the higher centers.

White ramus communicans Connection between spinal nerves and chain ganglia at spinal cord levels T1 to L3 containing preganglionic sympathetic fibers originating from neurons within the intermediolateral column at each respective level.

Z

ZIFT (Zygote intrafallopian transfer) Male and female gametes are collected and combined in a culture dish for fertilization and subsequently introduced into the oviduct where they develop during transport to the uterus (see also **GIFT).**

Zona pellucida Protective shell around the oocyte initially formed during early stages of folliculogenesis.

Zygomatic bone Bone of the upper jaw that develops within the maxillary process; composed of dermal bone that has superseded the function of the palatopterygoquadrate bar in this location.

Index

Page numbers followed by f *indicate figures; those followed by* t *indicate tables.*

G